MANUAL OF SMALL ANIMAL EMERGENCY AND CRITICAL CARE MEDICINE

D1220088

DOUGLASS K. MACINTIRE, MS, DVM

Diplomate ACVIM and ACVECC
Director of Intensive Care
College of Veterinary Medicine
Department of Small Animal Surgery and Medicine
Auburn University
Auburn, Alabama

KENNETH J. DROBATZ, DVM, MSCE

Diplomate ACVIM and ACVECC
Director, Trauma Emergency Service
Veterinary Hospital, University of Pennsylvania
Philadelphia, Pennsylvania

STEVEN C. HASKINS, MS, DVM

Diplomate ACVA and ACVECC
Director, Small Animal Intensive Care Unit
Veterinary Medical Teaching Hospital
University of California
Davis, California

WILLIAM D. SAXON, DVM

Diplomate ACVIM and ACVECC
Telemedicine Consultant, IDEXX
Graton, California

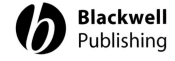

Blackwell Publishing

Blackwell Publishing Professional
2121 State Avenue, Ames, Iowa 50014, USA

Orders:	1-800-862-6657
Office:	1-515-292-0140
Fax:	1-515-292-3348
Web site:	www.blackwellprofessional.com

Blackwell Publishing Ltd
9600 Garsington Road, Oxford OX4 2DQ, UK
Tel.: +44 (0)1865 776868

Blackwell Publishing Asia
550 Swanston Street, Carlton, Victoria 3053, Australia
Tel.: +61 (0)3 8359 1011

Printed in Singapore

Library of Congress Cataloging-in-Publication Data
Macintire, Douglass K.
   Manual of small animal emergency and critical care medicine / Douglass K. Macintire,
Kenneth J. Drobatz, Steven C. Haskins.
     p. cm.
   ISBN-13: 978-0-397-58463-5
   ISBN-10: 0-397-58463-6
   I. Veterinary emergencies—Handbooks, manuals, etc. 2. Veterinary critical care—Handbooks, manuals, etc. I. Drobatz, Kenneth J. II. Haskins, Steve C. III. Title.

SF778.M33 2004
636.089'6025—dc22   2004048529

The last digit is the print number: 9 8 7 6 5 4

I dedicate this book to my parents who have always encouraged me and believed that I could succeed in any endeavor, and to my Savior, Jesus Christ, who gives me the strength to persevere and the hope to carry on.

Douglass K. Macintire

I dedicate this book to Lita, Alyssa, and Lianna. They give meaning to everything that I do.

Kenneth J. Drobatz

I dedicate this book to Soleil Clemons Yax. She is hope, love, and grace.

William D. Saxon

PREFACE

Writing a textbook on veterinary emergency medicine and critical care seemed like a great idea the first time Ken Drobatz and I talked about it a few years ago. Little did we know that we had committed ourselves to a monumental task. When it became apparent to us that we might have bitten off more than we could chew, we enlisted the capable help of two very good friends, Steve Haskins and Bill Saxon. The end result is a book that reflects the combined wisdom and experience of four people with different but very complimentary backgrounds.

Manual of Small Animal Emergency and Critical Care Medicine is designed to provide a textbook for veterinary students, new graduates, and veterinary practitioners that will offer guidance in the management of common emergencies. The book is divided into sections, first covering initial stabilization and life support of the whole animal and then providing a systems approach to common emergencies. Each section begins with an overview of the general approach to patients exhibiting emergent signs in each system and then provides protocols for specific conditions. This manual also provides information on monitoring and continuous care of critically ill patients.

The book is in outline format for quick reference and ease of implementation. It is extensively indexed and cross-referenced to provide thorough coverage of various emergency conditions, and useful formulas, tables, drug dosages, and illustrations are included throughout the text.

The authors have a wealth of experience in emergency medicine and critical care. Ken Drobatz directs the busy Emergency Service at The University of Pennsylvania, and I am the senior member of the staff of the Critical Care Service at Auburn University. Steve Haskin's background is in anesthesiology, and he brings with him a wealth of experience gained through establishing the Intensive Care Unit at the University of California at Davis. Bill Saxon is the practical member of our team. He has worked in the trenches in emergency practices in the Northeast and West Coast and currently works as a veterinary consultant for internal medicine and critical care cases. I am thrilled to be part of such a dedicated group.

This resource should be indispensable to any veterinarian treating emergencies—either new graduate or seasoned professional—because of the convenience of having the necessary information easily accessible and in a single volume. We worked hard to make this book convenient and user friendly for busy emergency clinicians. We hope you like it.

Douglass K. Macintire
Auburn, Alabama

ACKNOWLEDGMENTS

I am most grateful to my secretary, friend, and confidante, Billie Wood. Without her encouragement and expertise, this book never would have been completed.

Douglass K. Macintire

I thank all the residents, interns, and students with whom I have worked with over the years. I have learned more from them than they have from me.

In addition, I thank my good friend Paul, who has always been an inspiration for me throughout my veterinary career.

Kenneth J. Drobatz

My contribution to this book would not have been possible without the assistance of Norma Jean Saxon who is, quite simply, my hero.

William D. Saxon

CONTENTS

PART II: SPECIFIC PROTOCOLS AND PROCEDURES FOR EMERGENCY CONDITIONS

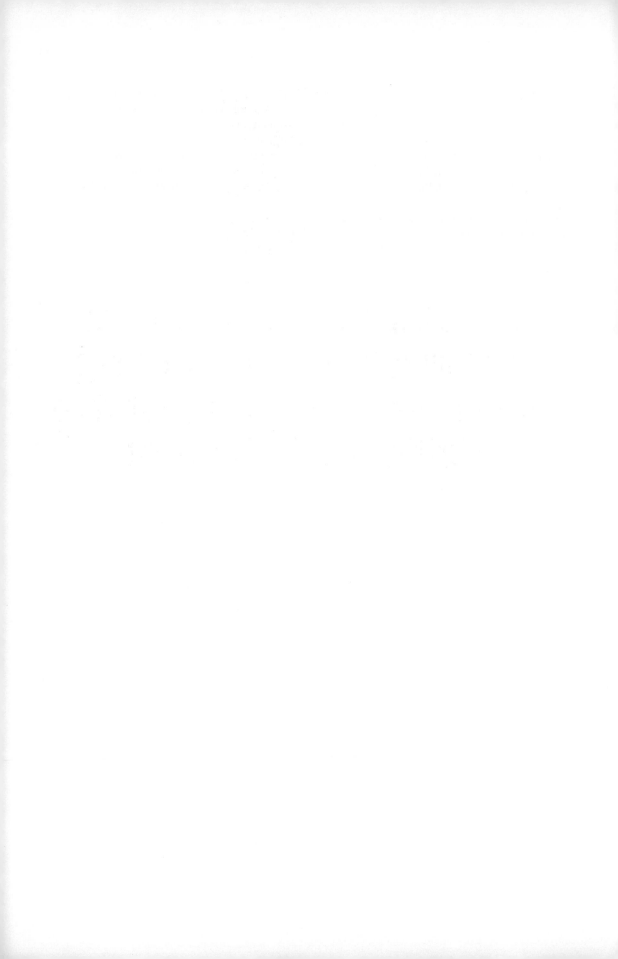

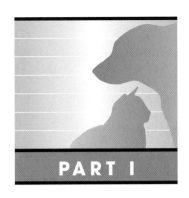

PART I

Life Support and Initial Stabilization, Monitoring and Intensive Care of the Critically Ill Patient

CHAPTER 1

APPROACH TO THE EMERGENCY PATIENT

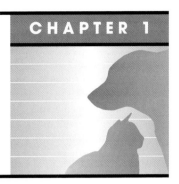

I. TRIAGE—DERIVED FROM FRENCH WORD MEANING "TO SORT"

A. Method used to classify patients according to urgency of need for emergency care

B. Allows rapid identification and treatment of life-threatening problems

C. Stable patients must wait to be treated; those with life-threatening problems are seen without delay.

D. All animals should be evaluated by either a veterinarian or a veterinary technician within 1 minute after arrival at the emergency hospital.

E. Patients with life-threatening problems (*Table 1-1*) can be taken directly to the emergency treatment area for immediate therapy; stable patients can wait with the owner.

II. IDENTIFICATION OF LIFE-THREATENING PROBLEMS: INITIAL EXAMINATION

A. Primary survey, assessment of breathing and vital signs

1. When the emergency or trauma patient is first presented, perform a rapid primary evaluation with special attention to the ABCs (Airway, Breathing, Circulation).
    a. This examination should concentrate on abnormalities that might be an immediate risk to the life of the patient (*Table 1-1*).
    b. Life-threatening abnormalities should be stabilized without delay.

    c. A secondary, more exhaustive physical and laboratory examination can be completed once the life-threatening problems have been stabilized (*see box, p. 7*)
    d. Semicomprehensive examinations should be repeated at regular intervals to keep pace with the changing condition of the patient. Just because something was not a problem at the time of the last examination does not mean that it is not a problem now.

2. Determine whether the animal is attempting to breathe.
    a. If not, clear the airway, intubate, and ventilate with 100% oxygen.
    b. If unable to intubate, perform emergency tracheostomy (p. 118).
    c. Apnea is a sign of a central nervous system (CNS) lesion or a peripheral problem with the neuromuscular axis.

3. If the animal is breathing, is it effective?
    a. Administer supplemental oxygen (p. 115) while completing physical examination.
    b. Classify the breathing pattern (*see box, p. 6*).
    c. Normal respiratory rate is 16–30 bpm. If respirations are labored, lung sounds are absent or increased, or animal is cyanotic or tachypneic, see "Respiratory Emergencies" (p. 115).
    d. Life-threatening respiratory insufficiency can exhibit any of the following signs:
        1) Orthopaedic stance—extended head and neck
        2) Apnea
        3) Restlessness or anxiety
        4) Open-mouth breathing; gasping

TABLE 1.1
PROBLEMS IDENTIFIED AT TRIAGE THAT REQUIRE IMMEDIATE ATTENTION

Cardiovascular
Cardiac arrest (no pulse, no auscultable heartbeat)
Pale mucous membranes
Slow capillary refill time (>2 seconds)
Weak, thready, or absent pulses
Active Hemorrhage
Brick-red membranes, capillary refill <1 second, bounding pulses
Tachycardia (dog >180; cat >250)
Bradycardia (dog <60, cat <150)
Pulse deficits, arrhythmias
Collapse

Respiratory
Rapid, shallow respirations
Upper airway obstruction
Labored breathing, gasping, open mouth breathing
Cyanosis
Pulmonary crackles and wheezes on auscultation
Chest trauma—rib fractures, penetrating chest wounds, flail chest

Neurologic
Seizures or history of seizures
Stupor
Coma

Head trauma
History of toxin ingestion
Acute paraparesis/paraplegia

Urinary
Inability to urinate
History of ethylene glycol ingestion
Large, painful bladder on palpation
No palpable bladder posttrauma

Other
Hyperthermia (T >105°F), heat stroke
Dystocia
Snake bite
Poisonings
Profuse vomiting or diarrhea
Burns
Fractures
Automobile-related injuries
Fall from height
Dehiscence of abdominal surgical wound
Frostbite
Drowning
Smoke inhalation
Electrocution
Organ prolapse
Gastric distension
Ocular emergencies—glaucoma, proptosis
Recent toxin ingestion

---

5) Cyanosis
6) Pa_{CO_2} above 80 mm Hg
7) Pa_{O_2} below 60 mm Hg (21% inspired oxygen at sea level)
    a) Sa o_2 below 90 (as measured with pulse oximetry)
    b) The ratio of Pa_{O_2} to percentage inspired oxygen is <3 while breathing enriched inspired oxygen

4. After stabilizing airway and breathing, evaluate other **vital signs.**
  a. Evaluate **mucous membrane color.**
    1) Pale membranes can occur with anemia, shock, pain, or poor perfusion.
    2) Blue membranes indicate cyanosis, which can occur with impaired respiration, methemoglobinemia (acetaminophen, nitrates), shunt, or congenital heart defect. (See "Cyanosis," p. 155.)
    3) "Muddy" or brown membranes can occur with sepsis or acetaminophen toxicity (cats).
    4) Hyperemic (brick red) membranes occur with hyperdynamic shock, cyanide or carbon monoxide toxicity, heatstroke, or other hypermetabolic states (pheochromocytoma, "thyroid storm")
  b. Assess **capillary refill time (CRT)**
    1) This should be performed by applying pressure to cause blanching of pink oral mucous membranes and counting the number of seconds for the pink color to return. It is better to perform this test on the gums rather than the lips, because tension on the lip may affect refill time. It is difficult or impossible to perform on animals with dark-pigmented gums.
    2) Assessment of CRT provides a crude indication of hydration status and peripheral perfusion.

TABLE 1.2
TREATMENT PRIORITIES IN EMERGENCY PATIENTS

A—Airway and arterial bleeding
Provide patent airway, 100% O_2
Apply pressure to areas of active hemorrhage

B—Breathing
Auscult chest, characterize breathing pattern
Perform thoracocentesis or emergency tracheostomy if indicated

---

C—Circulation
Place IV catheter, obtain samples for PCV/TS, BUN, glucose, Na, K, blood gases, ± coagulation tests and blood smear, urinalysis
Treat for shock if cardiac failure is ruled out as the cause of poor perfusion
Fluid guidelines for shock
    Crystalloid resuscitation—hypovolemic shock
        Dog, 90 mL/kg/h—Administer in 25% increments and assess patient response
        Cat, 60 mL/kg/h—Administer as above
    Acute blood loss, PCV <20%
        20 mL/kg fresh whole blood transfusion
    Shock with head trauma or pulmonary contusions
        Minimize crystalloid fluid, 10–20 mL/kg IV maximum
        7.5% hypertonic saline, 5 mL/kg IV
        Small-volume resuscitation with colloids
            Give 5 mL/kg hetastarch or dextran 70 q5–10 min until HR, color, pulses, and BP improve (generally up to 20 mL/kg)
Monitor PCV/TS q20–30 min in trauma patients
Place abdominal compression bandage if dropping PCV indicates internal hemorrhage.
Transfusion ± surgery for uncontrollable hemorrhage

D—Disability assessment
Neurologic examination
    Brain, spinal cord, peripheral nerves
    Rule out lesions with poor prognoses
    Treat head trauma or spinal cord injury
Musculoskeletal examination
    Antibiotics, cleaning, debridement for open fractures
    Splint, stabilize distal limb fractures
    Bandage, clean lacerations
    Radiograph when stable

E—Evaluate for abdominal injuries, urinary tract trauma, oliguria
Abdominocentesis, diagnostic peritoneal lavage, radiographs, ultrasound
Radiographic contrast studies
Monitor urine output

---

3) Normal CRT = 1.0–1.5 seconds
4) Rapid CRT (<1.0 second) is characteristic of hyperdynamic shock or hypermetabolic states (hyperthermia, sepsis, hyperthyroidism).
5) Slow CRT (>1.5 seconds) is associated with poor perfusion—dehydration, hypovolemia, cardiac disease, peripheral vasocon-striction, hypothermia, pain, exogenous catecholamines, hypoxia, or shock. CRT >3 seconds indicates serious peripheral vasoconstriction and poor perfusion.
c. Determine **pulse quality**
1) Palpable femoral pulse estimates mean blood pressure of at least 50 mm Hg. A

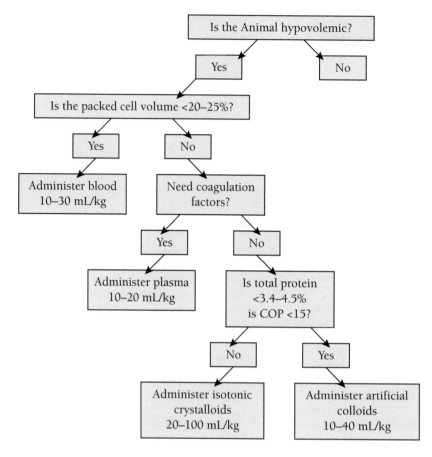

FIGURE 1.1 Deciding which fluids to administer.

palpable dorsal metatarsal pulse means that systolic blood pressure is at least 80 mm Hg.
2) Strong, bounding pulses—seen with hyperdynamic/early shock
3) Weak, thready pulses—seen with decompensating shock, pneumothorax, pericardial effusion

4) Pulse deficits—
Ausculted heartbeat does not match palpated pulses. Perform an electrocardiogram (ECG) to check for arrhythmias (p. 161).
   a) Premature ventricular contractions and ventricular tachycardia are common causes of pulse deficits in emergency

---

CHARACTERIZATION OF BREATHING PATTERNS

Upper airway obstruction: Noisy breathing, inspiratory dyspnea—
   Low-pitched snoring (large airway obstruction)
   High-pitched squeaking (very severe large airway obstruction)
Restrictive or pleural space disease: Rapid, shallow respirations, muffled heart sounds
Lower airway disease: Expiratory dyspnea, forced abdominal press—
   Mid-pitched wheezing
   History of coughing

Parenchymal disease: Crackles, wheezes, labored inspiration and expiration—
   Crepitation—fluid in alveoli
   Fluid rales—larger amount of fluid in lower airways
Secondary: Tachypnea: rapid rate, clear lung sounds—pain, anxiety, trauma, fever, anemia, acidosis

patients. *Causes include hypoxia, pain, trauma, myocardial contusion, shock, electrolyte imbalance, and gastric dilation–volvulus complex.*
  b) Atrial fibrillation is a common cause of pulse deficits in dogs with congestive heart failure.
  5) Absent pulses
    a) If no auscultable heartbeat, perform CPR (p. 26, Appendix C, p. 419).
    b) If heartbeat is auscultable but pulses are absent, consider thromboembolic disease (p. 179).
 d. Measure **heart rate** (If abnormal, see "Cardiac Emergencies," p. 160).
  1) Tachycardia: >160 (large-breed dog), >180 (small-breed dog), >200 (puppy), >220 (cat)
    a) Common causes of tachycardia include hypovolemia, pain, hypoxemia, hypercapnia, hyperthermia, sepsis, anemia, stress, hyperthyroidism, and heart failure.
  2) Bradycardia: <60 (dogs), <80 (cats)
    a) This is an unexpected finding in a stressed emergency patient.
    b) Rule out hyperkalemia, urethral obstruction, hypoadrenocorticism, organophosphate toxicity, severe hypothermia, and drug overdose (opioids).
    c) Other causes include head trauma, atrioventricular conduction disturbances, and excessive vagal tone.
 e. Determine **body temperature**
  1) Hyperthermia
    a) Temperatures up to 104°F could be an appropriate response to infection and should not be treated specifically.
    b) Active cooling is necessary to bring down body temperatures that exceed 106°F.
    c) Body temperatures >108°F can result in decompensation of enzyme systems and multiple organ failure.
  2) Hypothermia
    a) Active rewarming is necessary when temperatures drop below 94°F and cerebral obtundation occurs.
    b) Temperature <82°F can result in arrhythmias and coagulopathies.
    c) Hypothermia is common in cats with poor perfusion (severe dehydration, urethral obstruction, cardiomyopathy, ketoacidosis). Because external heating causes peripheral vasodilation, heat should not be

applied to hypovolemic patients until volume replacement therapy has been administered (preferably with warmed intravenous fluids).
    d) Hypothermia is common in pediatric patients and should be corrected before feeding is attempted.
    e) Delta T (ΔT), or the difference between core body temperature and toe web temperature, >8°F indicates serious peripheral vasoconstriction.

5. Use mnemonic **A CRASH PLAN** to carry out complete patient evaluation (*see box below*).

6. While performing the initial triage evaluation, the technician or veterinarian should obtain a **brief history** from the client that includes the following:
 a. What is the presenting complaint?
 b. When was the animal last normal? What is the duration of signs?
 c. Obtain a brief systems review (e.g., coughing, wheezing, polyuria, fecal consistency).
 d. Are any other animals showing similar clinical signs?
 e. Is the animal currently on medication or does it have a previously diagnosed medical condition?

7. External or internal hemorrhage must be controlled.
 a. Place a pressure bandage directly over the bleeding area.

MNEUMONIC TO AID IN PERFORMING COMPLETE PATIENT EVALUATION FOR SECONDARY SURVEY "A CRASH PLAN"

A	Airway
C	Cardiovascular/circulatory
R	Respiratory
A	Abdomen
S	Spine
H	Head (including eyes, ears, and neck)
P	Pelvis (including rectal examination)
L	Limbs (including tail)
A	Arteries
N	Nerves (including cranial nerves, reflexes, pain sensation)

b. Consider using a temporary tourniquet (<5 min) to stop arterial hemorrhage until artery can be clamped and ligated.

c. Apply a pressure wrap over fracture sites that appear to be enlarging because of ongoing hemorrhage.

d. Intrathoracic bleeding may be associated with respiratory distress—thoracocentesis may be required (p. 130).

e. Consider the possibility of ongoing abdominal hemorrhage in patients that fail to stabilize with intravenous fluids and have dropping hematocrits.

   1) Removal of the blood from the abdomen is generally not recommended.

      a) It will be reabsorbed (red cells intact)

      b) 40% in 24 h

   2) Three indications to remove blood from the abdomen

      a) When the accumulation is sufficient to impair respiration.

      b) When the patient requires a blood transfusion and the abdominal blood is the only available source

      c) When it is necessary during laparotomy to clear the field for visualization

   3) A snug "belly bandage" can be applied to limit ongoing abdominal hemorrhage as long as it does not compress the diaphragm and compromise respiration, but is contraindicated in patients with diaphragmatic hernia.

f. A coagulopathy should be suspected if there are petechial hemorrhages and/or bleeding from multiple sites (See p. 279).

B. Perform **emergency data base**—Fill four to five capillary tubes with blood while placing an intravenous catheter to obtain STAT blood work.

1. Packed cell volume, total solids (PCV/TS): Allows clinician to differentiate anemia from poor perfusion in animals with pale gums. Provides baseline values for monitoring trends (e.g., ongoing hemorrhage, correction of dehydration). Repeat every 20–30 minutes initially in shock/trauma patients receiving fluids, until values stabilize.

2. Blood urea nitrogen, blood glucose (BUN, BG): These values can be obtained from reagent strips or from in-house analyzers. These tests may help identify the cause of non-specific signs such as anorexia and vomiting by suggesting renal failure or diabetes mellitus, rather than primary gastrointestinal (GI) disease. Hypoglycemia can be a life-threatening cause of stupor or coma and may also indicate overwhelming sepsis. Early recognition allows immediate correction of hypoglycemia.

3. Serum electrolytes (Na^+, K^+, Cl^-, Ca^{2+}): These values can be used to detect life-threatening electrolyte abnormalities such as hyperkalemia, hypocalcemia, hypercalcemia, and sodium:potassium ratios in hypoadrenocorticism (see "Metabolic Emergencies"). Knowing these values helps the clinician choose appropriate fluid therapy.

4. Blood gases (see "Arterial Blood Gases".
   a. Recognition and correction of abnormalities may avert patient decompensation and possible cardiac arrest. (See "Metabolic Emergencies.")
   b. In general, 0.9% saline should be used for alkalosis, and a buffered solution (such as lactated Ringer's) should be used for acidosis.

5. A **blood smear** can be evaluated for leukocytosis, leukopenia, platelet estimate, presence of blood-borne parasites, and red blood cell (RBC) abnormalities.

6. In-house **coagulation tests** include activated clotting time (ACT), proteins induced by vitamin K antagonism (PIVKA; Thrombotest, Burroughs-Wellcome) and ACT, prothrombin time (PT), and activated partial thrombo-plastin time (APTT) (SCA 2000, Synbiotics Corp, San Diego, CA). These tests can be used to detect underlying coagulation defects such as disseminated intravascular coagulation (DIC) or anticoagulant rodenticide toxicity.

7. An **electrocardiogram** will help determine if arrhythmias or underlying cardiac disease are responsible for poor perfusion.

8. Urinalysis: A urine sample should be taken before fluids (if possible) to evaluate the animal's ability to concentrate urine. Urine sediment and dipstick results can be evaluated for casts, evidence of urinary tract infection, hematuria, glucosuria, ketonuria, and proteinuria.

III. A SECONDARY SURVEY OF THE PATIENT, INCLUDING A COMPLETE PHYSICAL EXAMINATION, SHOULD BE PERFORMED AS SOON AS THE RESPIRATORY AND CARDIOVASCULAR SYSTEMS HAVE BEEN ADDRESSED

A. Neurologic evaluation

1. Assess the patient for serious neurologic abnormalities of the brain.

a. Look for evidence of head trauma .
  1) Epistaxis, blood, or cerebrospinal fluid (CSF) in the ear canal
  2) Head tilt, nystagmus, strabismus
  3) Obtundation, decreasing mental activity
  4) Anisocoria
  5) Absent or slow pupillary light reflex
  6) Depressed or absent menace, palpebral, corneal, or nasal reflexes
b. Assess the level of consciousness—(AVPU)
  1) A: Alert
  2) V: Responds to voice or visual stimuli
  3) P: Responds to painful stimuli only
  4) U: Coma, unresponsive
c. For cases of head trauma, the following list is in order of increasing severity of lesion and decreasing prognosis (i.e., best to worst):
  1) Normal pupil size and PLR
  2) Slow PLR
  3) Bilateral miosis, responsive to light
  4) Pinpoint, unresponsive
  5) Bilateral mydriasis, unresponsive
d. Brainstem involvement warrants a very poor prognosis and is characterized by the following:
  1) Unconsciousness
  2) Bilaterally unresponsive miotic or mydriatic pupils
  3) Absent gag, swallow, and laryngeal reflexes
  4) Strabismus
  5) Absent physiologic nystagmus; spontaneous or positional nystagmus
  6) Irregular breathing rhythms/apnea
  7) Decerebrate rigidity
e. Computed tomography (CT) or magnetic resonance imaging (MRI), if available, will help characterize the nature and extent of the intracranial abnormalities and help identify the surgical candidates.
f. Brainstem auditory evoked potentials may be used to evaluate auditory and brainstem pathways. Electroencephalography has been used to evaluate cortical function but is difficult to interpret.

2. Assess the patient for serious neurologic abnormalities of the spinal cord and peripheral nerves
  a. Palpate spinal vertebrae checking for pain, misalignment
  b. Check spinal reflexes, panniculus response, voluntary motor movement, and pain perception in all limbs in any animal with a suspected back injury.
  c. Always stabilize the spine when doing radiography or transporting the patient.
  d. Perform a rectal examination, checking for pelvic fractures, anal tone, tail tone.
  e. Evaluate toe pinch for animal's recognition of deep pain sensation and assessment of crossed-extensor reflexes.
  f. Peripheral nerve function should always be assessed prior to bandaging patients with limb fractures (see "Neurologic monitoring" p. 87-88).

3. Serial neurologic examinations should be performed on animals that exhibit the following:
  a. Slow or absent pupillary light reflex
  b. Anisocoria
  c. Abnormal level of consciousness—depression, stupor, or coma
  d. Head trauma—hemorrhage on otic examination
  e. Depressed spinal reflexes—motor and sensation
  f. Acute spinal cord injuries

4. Notify owners at the earliest opportunity—before performing expensive diagnostics, therapeutics, and surgery—if the animal has neurologic lesions that warrant a poor-to-grave prognosis. The following lesions have a grave prognosis:
  a. Decerebrate rigidity is characterized by unconsciousness and extensor rigidity in all four legs. It is associated with severe cerebral trauma that is generally irreversible. This must be differentiated from cerebellar injury, in which the animal exhibits extensor rigidity of all four legs but is conscious. The prognosis is much better for cerebellar disease.
  b. Shiff-Sherrington syndrome is characterized by extensor rigidity of the forelimbs and flaccid paralysis of the rear limbs. This posture denotes a severe spinal cord lesion between T2 and L4.
  c. Fixed and dilated or midrange pupils that do not respond to light are associated with severe injury to the midbrain
  d. Lack of deep pain sensation and crossed extensor reflexes are seen with severe spinal cord damage.
  e. Hyperthermia or depressed respiration following severe neurologic injury may indicate hematomyelia (necrosis of cord).

f. Loss of anal or bladder tone, although not usually life threatening, can result in an unacceptable pet because of bowel and bladder incontinence. Owners may decide to consider euthanasia.

B. Emergency management of open wounds and fractures

1. Identify and treat open wounds and fractures. A cage muzzle is useful in preventing injury to the veterinarian during disability assessment. Cage muzzles are preferred because they do not compromise breathing by holding the mouth closed.

    a. Control bleeding

        1) Best method is direct pressure over wound with clean towels or gauze.

        2) Tourniquets should generally be avoided.

        3) Arterial bleeders may need to be clamped until animal is stable enough for ligation and definitive repair.

    b. Prevent further contamination

        1) Wounds should always be covered to prevent contamination with resistant hospital bacteria, even if the initial bandage is only temporary.

        2) Debris and contaminants are best removed by copious lavage with sterile saline. Sprayed tap water can be used in cases of massive wound contamination.

        a) Povodine iodine (1:9) or chlorhexidine (1:40) can be added to the lavage solution for severely contaminated wounds.

        b) Wound cleaning should be done with pressurized lavage using a 35-mL syringe and 18-gauge needle. Rapid filling can be accomplished by using a three-way stopcock and extension tubing leading to the saline reservoir.

        c) The importance of copious lavage cannot be overstated.

        d) Temporary wound management can be accomplished in the emergency room by packing the wound with gauze pads moistened with one of the above solutions, clipping the hair from the wound area, and covering with a sterile bandage. The wet dressing should be changed every 8 hours until definitive repair under general anesthesia can be accomplished.

        e) Dead or devitalized tissue should be removed from the wound as soon as possible

to prevent further bacterial growth and contamination.

        f) For contaminated wounds or open fractures, bacterial cultures can be obtained and empirical antibiotic therapy started with cephalothin sodium 20–40 mg/kg IV q8h pending culture results.

    c. Immobilize limb fractures

        1) Prevents further injury to nerves and tissue from bone fragments, controls bleeding, minimizes pain

        2) Temporary splints can be made with magazines, newspapers, cardboard, a stick, etc.

        3) A padded Robert Jones bandage is used to stabilize fractures below the elbow and stifle.

        4) Fractures of the proximal limbs or pelvis have more soft tissue "padding" and can often be managed with cage rest.

        5) A spica splint is a proximal extension of the Robert Jones bandage over the shoulder or hip and can be used to stabilize a femoral or humeral fracture.

C. Evaluation of the abdomen and urinary tract

1. Progressive abdominal distension may indicate gastric dilation–volvulus or abdominal hemorrhage. Bruising of the umbilicus is often noted with hemoabdomen.

2. A four-quadrant abdominocentesis is indicated in the following instances:

    a. Shock, painful abdomen: Cytology consistent with peritonitis will reveal abundant neutrophils, intracellular bacteria, and possibly vegetable fibers.

    b. Blunt abdominal trauma, dropping PCV: The hematocrit of the fluid is compared with that of the peripheral blood. Surgery can often be avoided by stabilizing the animal with blood transfusions and a belly bandage.

    c. Density of abdominal fluid: Fluid is evaluated to determine if it is a transudate, modified transudate, exudate, or hemorrhage. It should also be analyzed for creatinine and bilirubin.

    d. Azotemia or inability to visualize bladder posttrauma may indicate a ruptured bladder, especially in male dogs. Creatinine, potassium levels, and BUN will all be higher in the abdominal fluid than in blood.

3. Diagnostic peritoneal lavage (p. 191) or ultrasound-guided needle aspiration can be performed if abdominocentesis is negative.

4. Urinary tract trauma
a. Ruptured bladder should be suspected in patients with painful abdomen, abdominal bruising, and vomiting 24–48 hours posttrauma.
1) This is more common in males.
2) It is a possible complication of pelvic fractures.
3) A positive contrast cystogram (p. 227) confirms the diagnosis
b. Urethral tear usually results in extensive edema and bruising of the rear limbs and pelvis. Diagnosis is by positive-contrast urethrogram. Do **NOT** pass the catheter all the way to the bladder or the lesion may be missed.

c. Injury to the kidneys or ureters will cause lumbar pain, increased fluid density in the retroperitoneal area, and azotemia. Diagnosis is by intravenous urogram or abdominal ultrasound.

5. Palpate bladder, monitor urine output
a. Oliguria (<0.5 mL/kg/h of urine) may indicate dehydration, hypotension, inadequate resuscitation, acute renal failure, postrenal obstruction, or ruptured bladder.
b. Determine the underlying cause of oliguria by radiographs, contrast studies, ultrasound, blood work, urinalysis, and measurement of blood pressure.
c. Hyperkalemia, acidosis, dehydration, and uremia must be corrected.

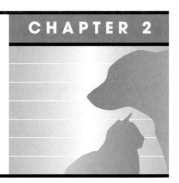

CHAPTER 2

EMERGENCY ROOM READINESS

I. THE IMPORTANCE OF READINESS

A. Resuscitation endeavors must be organized in advance

1. Necessary equipment, drugs, and supplies should be located in one place at all times.

2. Equipment must be in working order.

3. All available personnel should be trained to be a functional part of the resuscitation team.
    a. Periodic "fire drills" should be conducted.
    b. Typical "setup" for an emergency includes
        1) Oxygen
        2) Crash cart
        3) ECG
        4) IV catheter setup
        5) Fluids and administration set
        6) Heat source

B. The hospital should have a designated area for receiving emergency cases that includes a large sink and grate for wetting hyperthermic animals or removing topical poisons.

C. The hospital should also have a designated "arrest station" with crash cart, oxygen, and monitors at the ready.

II. EQUIPMENT RECOMMENDATIONS TO PROVIDE OPTIMAL CARE TO CRITICALLY ILL EMERGENCY PATIENTS

EQUIPMENT RECOMMENDATIONS FOR EMERGENCY HOSPITALS

Means of providing oxygen
    Flow meters
    Oxygen source
    Face masks
    Laryngoscope and assortment of blades
    Assortment of endotracheal tubes
    Tracheostomy tubes
    Nasal catheters
    Bubble humidifiers
    AmBU resuscitation bag
Anesthetic machine

Means of providing positive-pressure ventilation
Electrocardiograph
Stethoscope
Esophageal stethoscope
Penlight
Mouth speculum
Pressure bag for fluids
Clippers and blades
Vacuum for hair removal

(continued)

EQUIPMENT RECOMMENDATIONS FOR EMERGENCY HOSPITALS *(continued)*

Waste containers
Surgical gowns
Retractors—manual and self-retaining
Radiograph unit and automatic processor
Centrifuge
Ability to perform CBC and chemistries
Otoscope
Ophthalmoscope
Ability to take cultures
Gram stain, Diff-Quick stain
Fluid warmer
Endoscope/bronchoscope
Blood pressure measuring equipment: indirect and direct
Hemoglobinometer
Refractometer
Chemistry strips for blood glucose and urea nitrogen
Suction apparatus and catheters
Defibrillator with small and large external and internal paddles
Assortment of stomach tubes and stomach pumps

Circulating warm water blankets; forced-air warming blankets
Blood gas analyzer
Pulse oximeter
Electrolyte analyzer
Osmometer
Colloid oncotic pressure analyzer
Lactate analyzer
Coagulation testing method
Fluid infusion pumps
Syringe pump
Ventilator
Microscope
Ophthalmoscope
Nebulizer (ultrasonic)
Sterile surgical instruments and towels—major and minor packs
Surgical lights
Surgical table
Instrument stand
Neonatal incubator
Dextrometer
Thermometers

III. RECOMMENDED SUPPLIES

RECOMMENDED SUPPLIES FOR EMERGENCY HOSPITALS

Full assortment of syringes and needles, spinal needles with stylet, intraosseous needles
Full assortment of peripheral and jugular venous catheters
  Outside-the-needle catheters for peripheral veins: 2.5 inch, 18 and 20 gauge
  Outside-the-needle catheters for small peripheral veins: 1.75 inch, 22 and 24 gauge
  Outside-the-needle catheters for temporary chest or abdominal drains, tracheal catheters, jugular veins, femoral arteries or veins, peritoneal lavage, catheters, or pericardiocentesis (5.5 inch, 14 or 16 gauge)
  Inside-the-needle catheters for jugular veins or tracheal catheters, 8 and 12 inch; 17, 19, and 21 gauge
  Butterfly catheters: 19, 21, 23 gauge

Wide selection of fluids
  Extracellular replacement solution
    Lactated Ringer's
    Plasmalyte 148
    Normosol R
  0.9% Saline
  5% Dextrose in water
  Maintenance solution
    Plasmalyte 56
    Normosol M
    0.45% NaCl and 2.5% dextrose
  Wide selection of concentrates
    Potassium chloride
    Potassium phosphate
    Sodium chloride (7.5%)
    Sodium bicarbonate

(continued)

RECOMMENDED SUPPLIES FOR EMERGENCY HOSPITALS (*continued*)

50% dextrose in water	Casting material, Mason metasplints, aluminum rods
Mannitol	
Colloid solutions	Sandbags for positioning
Dextran 70®	Water-trap chest drain system
Hetastarch®	Assorted sutures
Oxyglobin®	Sterile gloves, latex examination gloves
Source of whole blood and plasma	Urinalysis strips
Administration sets—regular and pediatric	CVP manometers
Blood filter sets	Microscope slides
Calibrated burettes	Hematocrit tubes
Extension sets	ACT tubes
Three-way stopcocks	Buccal mucosal bleeding time lancet
Catheter caps	Blood-typing cards
T-ports	FeLV/FIV test kits
Chest drain cannulas	Ethylene glycol test kit
Urinary catheters: assorted red rubber tubes and	Glucose test strips
Foley catheters	Azostix
Closed urine collection bags	Superglue
Nasal and nasoesophageal catheters	Staple gun and staples
Tape, cotton, gauze, and other bandaging	Nebulizer
materials	Pediatric asthma inhalation chamber
Fleece pads for cage padding	

IV. RECOMMENDED DRUGS

RECOMMENDED DRUGS FOR EMERGENCY HOSPITALS

Epinephrine	Diltiazem
Atropine	Nifedipine
Sodium bicarbonate	Oxymorphone or Hydromorphone
Dopamine	Fentanyl
Dobutamine	Morphine
Phenylephrine	Butorphanol
Norepinephrine	Buprenorphine
Nitroprusside	Domitor
Nitroglycerine ointment	Antesedan
Hydralazine	Propofol
Calcium (gluconate or chloride)	Ketamine
Digitalis	Diazepam
Heparin	Acepromazine
Lidocaine	50% Dextrose
Procainamide	Eye lubricant
Amiodarone	Metoclopramide
Bretylium	Prochlorperazine
Propranolol	Pentobarbital
Esmolol	Phenobarbital
Verapamil	

(continued)

RECOMMENDED DRUGS FOR EMERGENCY HOSPITALS *(continued)*

Naloxone	Succimer
Nalbuphine	Methocarbamol
Doxapram	Vinegar (for neutralizing alkalis)
Dexamethasone phosphate	Kaolin pectate
Prednisolone sodium succinate	Vitamin K
Furosemide	Broad-spectrum, effective antibiotics
Mannitol	Diphenhydramine
Hydrogen peroxide	Aminophylline
Apomorphine	Fomepazole
Ipecac	Imidocarb
Cimetidine, ranitidine, or famotidine	Terbutaline
Activated charcoal	Albuterol
Pralidoxime (for organophosphates)	Acetylcysteine
Athamil calcium–disodium (CaEDTA)	B complex vitamins, Thiamine
(for lead)	Ethanol
Mercaprol (for arsenic)	Regular Insulin
Sodium nitrite and sodium thiosulfate	Euthanasia solution

CHAPTER 3

CARDIOPULMONARY–CEREBRAL RESUSCITATION (CPCR)

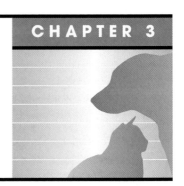

I. DEFINITION

A. Cardiopulmonary arrest (CPA) is the cessation of functional ventilation and effective circulation.

II. PREDISPOSING FACTORS

A. Cardiac arrest may be caused by any disease, carried to its extreme. Precipitating factors include:

1. Hypoxia

2. Acid–base, fluid, and electrolyte imbalance

3. Autonomic nervous system imbalance (e.g., vagal stimulation)

4. Drug reaction/overdose

5. Cardiac disease or arrhythmias

6. Trauma

III. CLINICAL SIGNS

A. Prevention of cardiac arrest is always more successful than treatment of it. Signs of impending arrest include

1. Agonal gasping

2. Cyanotic, gray, or pale white membranes

3. Nonresponsive dilated pupils

4. Weak, barely palpable pulses

5. Darkening of oozing blood

6. Lack of bleeding at surgical site

IV. PROGNOSIS/GENERAL RECOMMENDATIONS

A. Resuscitation reportedly generates a "return of spontaneous rhythm" rate of 30–60%. The number of human medical cardiac arrest patients that survive to discharge, however, only ranges from 2 to 14%. Numbers for dogs and cats are similar. Many of these patients, unfortunately, are discharged in a persistent vegetative state or with significant neurologic deficits.

B. Resuscitation is not recommended for all instances of cardiac arrest. The decision not to resuscitate should be made in advance on the merits of each individual case, and in consultation with the owner.

C. A cardiopulmonary resuscitation (CPR) flow sheet or checklist should be posted at the "CPR station" to ensure that essential components are not omitted from the resuscitation endeavor.

1. A CPR record should also be readily available and filled out with each resuscitation.

D. Resuscitation should continue for at least 20 minutes but not longer than 30 minutes.

V. TREATMENT

A. *Immediate basic life support* includes the ABCs (Airway, Breathing, Circulation)

1. **Airway:** Secure the airway by endotracheal intubation and give the animal two long breaths.

2. Breathing: Institute positive-pressure ventilation with 100% oxygen if spontaneous respiration does not begin. Sometimes breathing can be stimulated by placing a 25-gauge needle in the nasal philtrum and twisting it.

   a. One ventilation should be delivered for approximately every three to five chest compressions.

   b. Current human recommendations are to deliver breaths between chest compressions without pausing the compression procedure, but studies in animals show improved cardiac output when compressions are delivered simultaneously with ventilations.

   1) Simultaneous ventilation and chest compression is not recommended as first-order therapy because of its potential for inducing barotrauma and pneumothorax, especially in smaller patients.

   2) May be more effective in barrel-chested breeds or large-sized animals when it is difficult to generate an effective increase in intrathoracic pressure by conventional external compression methodologies.

   c. If the resuscitation is being conducted by one person, two ventilations should be delivered approximately every 15 chest compressions. Studies in pigs showed that compression alone (without ventilation) was also effective.

   d. The goal of artificial ventilation is to provide moderate hyperventilation.

   e. Recommended inspiratory pressure is 15 cm H_2O (cat) and 20 cm H_2O (dog). Higher pressures (20–30 cm H_2O) are required with simultaneous ventilation/compression, pleural fluid, or pulmonary edema.

   f. Inspiratory time should not exceed 1.5 seconds. Expiratory pressure should fall to 0 cm H_2O between compressions.

3. Circulation

   a. External chest compression

   1) External chest compression should be accomplished by applying pressure directly over the heart at a rate of 80–120 times per minute. The diameter of the chest is compressed by 25–30%.

   2) This may be done in lateral or dorsal recumbency.

   3) Compression should be held for a brief time to maximize the elimination of blood from the heart and the chest, and pressure must be fully released between compressions.

   4) Time must be allowed between compressions for adequate diastolic filling of the ventricles.

   5) The specific technique that will cause effective forward blood flow varies markedly from patient to patient.

   a) *If the initial technique does not generate palpable pulses or an improvement in mucous membrane color, Doppler blood flow, or pulse oximetry readings, an alternate technique should be used.*

   The compression force could be increased or decreased
   The rate could be increased or decreased
   The duration of systole could be increased
   The position of the animal could be changed
   The position of the hands could be changed
   The compressor could be changed
   Ventilations could be delivered simultaneously with every third to fifth compression.

   b. The heart pump mechanism of forward blood flow is the primary means of circulation in cats, exotic species, and small dogs (<10 kg) undergoing CPR.

   1) Compression of the ventricles causes blood to flow out of the ventricle and into the aorta.

   2) Backward flow is prevented by closure of the atrioventricular (AV) valves.

   c. The thoracic pump mechanism of forward blood flow is the primary means of blood flow in dogs >10–15 kg undergoing CPR.

   1) The generalized increase in thoracic pressure causes blood to move out of the heart and aorta.

   2) Backward flow is prevented by the pressure-induced collapse of the great veins in the chest and the presence of valves in the veins that prevent backflow of blood.

   3) Several of the artificial circulation techniques discussed below are based upon the thoracic mechanism of blood flow.

   d. Augmenting techniques

   1) Abdominal counterpressure helps splint the abdomen, preventing expansion when the chest is compressed and decreasing posterior displacement of the diaphragm when the chest is compressed.

   a) *This prevents the dissipation, through the abdomen, of the intrathoracic pressure induced by external chest compression by*

enhancing the generalized increase in intrathoracic pressure and improves cardiac output and cerebral blood flow.
b) *Abdominal counterpressure can increase diastolic arterial blood pressure during external chest compression by as much as 20 mm Hg.*
c) *Abdominal counterpressure can be applied by the hands of an assistant, a sandbag, or a large book.*
d) *Interposed abdominal compressions should alternate with chest compressions to increase diastolic filling of the heart. Simultaneous compression of the abdomen and heart could potentially result in hepatic trauma by pushing the liver into the chest during compressions, so interposed abdominal compressions are safer than continuous counterpressure of the abdomen.*

2) Antishock trousers have been reported to improve systemic blood pressure
 a) *By returning a small amount of blood from the peripheral pool to the central circulation*
 b) *By preventing the runoff of central blood volume into the periphery.*
 c) *Antishock trousers can be simulated by wrapping the hind legs and caudal abdomen with elastic bandaging material or towels.*
 d) *Do not wrap too far forward on the abdomen because it will cause anterior displacement of abdominal contents. Thoracic compression is then likely to fracture the liver, resulting in abdominal hemorrhage.*

3) A single abdominal tourniquet may be just as efficacious as shock trousers.
 a) *A rope, belt, or gauze can be placed tightly around the lower abdomen, just anterior to the pelvis.*
 b) *The wraps should be tight enough to compress the descending aorta.*
 c) *Wraps and tourniquets can be removed 10–20 minutes after restarting the heart; after hemodynamics have had a chance to stabilize.*

Wraps and tourniquets should be removed slowly.
Rapid exposure of a precariously balanced cardiovascular system to the hypoxic vasodilated tissues caudal to the tourniquet or

under the wrap may result in excessive hypotension.

e. Internal heart compression is associated with better cardiac output, arterial blood pressure, cerebral and coronary perfusion, myocardial perfusion, and peripheral tissue perfusion, higher mixed-venous Po_2, less arterial and mixed-venous metabolic acidosis, lower mixed-venous lactate concentrations, higher mixed-venous and end-tidal Pco_2, and higher survival rates with improved neurologic recovery than with external techniques.

1) Coronary blood flow is particularly difficult to achieve during closed chest compression. When aortic and right atrial pressure are increased equally, there is no pressure gradient across the heart, and therefore there is no coronary blood flow. Myocardial blood flow will only occur to the extent that right atrial pressure falls faster than aortic pressure between chest compressions.

2) Perform a thoracotomy if there is no evidence of effective artificial circulation and tissue perfusion within 5 minutes of cardiac arrest.
 a) *It should be performed after 10 minutes if there is no return of an effective spontaneous heart beat.*
 b) *A thoracotomy is also indicated when there is an open pneumothorax, a closed pneumothorax, chest trauma with broken ribs, diaphragmatic hernia, pleural effusion, or pericardial effusion or when the size or shape of the thorax precludes effective external chest compression techniques.*

3) There are additional advantages to a thoracotomy.
 a) *The adequacy of diastolic filling can be assessed between each compression. The heart should fill as rapidly as it is released. If this does not occur, it is objective evidence of the lack of venous return and the need for a fluid bolus or an α-receptor agonist.*
 b) *An accumulation of fluids or blood within the pericardial sac can be observed. The pericardial sac can be opened to prevent pericardial tamponade during or after resuscitation.*
 c) *The descending aorta can be depressed with the index finger of the opposite hand or clamped, directing essential blood flow*

to the brain and heart. This compression should remain for the duration of the resuscitation. It should be removed only after spontaneous activity has been determined to be stable and then should be removed gradually over 10–20 minutes.

***d)** Fibrillation can be diagnosed by direct observation, and internal defibrillation efforts may be more effective than external.*

***e)** Flaccidity can be assessed by direct visualization and palpation.*

4) A thoracotomy should only be done in a fully equipped central hospital with properly trained personnel.

5) Time is limited, yet the thoracotomy must be done safely so as not to generate additional life-threatening complications.

***a)** It measurably facilitates closure to clip a strip of hair along the line of the intended incision at the fifth intercostal space on the right side.*

***b)** Hair and loose dirt can be removed with a quick swab with an antiseptic solution (or water).*

***c)** The incision is made midway between the ribs down to, but not through, the pleura. Avoid the big intercostal vessels at the caudal edge of the rib.*

***d)** Pleural penetration should be accomplished with a finger or a hemostat (between positive-pressure ventilations). Incising with a scalpel endangers the lung.*

***e)** The incision is then extended dorsally and ventrally with scissors, taking care to avoid the internal thoracic artery, which runs longitudinally about 1 cm lateral to the sternum.*

***f)** Cardiac compression is facilitated by removing the heart from the pericardial sac. The sternopericardial ligament is snapped with digital pressure ventral to the heart, and the heart is gently lifted toward the operator. The pericardial sac is opened, carefully avoiding the phrenic and vagus nerves, and the heart is removed from the sac.*

***g)** The heart should be compressed between the flats of the fingers and the palm of the hand, taking care not to shift or rotate the natural position of the heart.*

Small hearts can be compressed between two fingers and the thumb.

Large hearts can be compressed between the palm and the opposite chest wall.

Do not use the fingertips, which can easily penetrate the wall of an atrium or ventricle.

The heart should be compressed from apex to base, allowing filling to occur between compressions.

B. *Advanced cardiac life support* includes drugs, defibrillation, and electrocardiography to enhance airway, breathing, and circulation.

1. Fluids

a. Cardiac arrest is a rapidly vasodilating disease process secondary to tissue anoxia. This increasing blood volume capacity must be filled with exogenous fluids to maintain an effective central circulating volume.

b. Notwithstanding preexisting anemia or hypoproteinemia, an isotonic extracellular replacement crystalloid fluid should be administered rapidly intravenously in aliquots of approximately 10–40 mL/kg for a dog and 10–20 mL/kg for a cat.

1) This bolus volume may need to be repeated periodically throughout the resuscitation endeavor in quantities sufficient to maintain an effective circulating volume.

2) Excessive fluid volumes predispose to pulmonary edema and should be avoided.

c. A hypertonic saline solution, such as 6 mL/kg of 7.5% saline or 5–10 mL/kg of 20–25% mannitol, might be more efficacious in this situation than isotonic solutions.

d. Colloidal solutions, such as 10 mL/kg of 6% dextran 70 or 6% hetastarch, might also be more efficacious because their retention within the vascular compartment is greater than that of crystalloid solutions.

2. Sympathomimetics

a. Epinephrine is the most efficacious catecholamine in cardiac arrest (*Table 3-1*).

1) The conventional dose of epinephrine is 0.01–0.02 mg/kg; 1 mL of 1:1000 epinephrine is mixed with 9 mL of saline to create a 1:10,000 dilution and is given at a dose of 1 mL per 10–20 pounds.

2) Higher doses of epinephrine (0.2 mg/kg) may be more efficacious with regard to maximizing cerebral blood flow, improving aortic diastolic to right atrial pressure gradient,

TABLE 3.1
AGONISTS USEFUL IN CARDIOPULMONARY RESUSCITATION

Drug	Receptor α	Activity β	Dosage
Epinephrine	+++	+++	0.02–0.2 mg/kg 1–10 μg/kg/min
Dopamine	++	+++	0.2–0.5 mg/kg 5–20 μg/kg/min
Norepinephrine	+++	+	0.1–0.2 mg/kg 1–10 μg/kg/min
Phenylephrine	+++	0	0.1–1.0 mg/kg

and resuscitation rates (1 mL/20 lb undiluted 1:1000 epinephrine).

　　a) Higher doses are also associated with a higher incidence of ventricular arrhythmias and ventricular fibrillation.
　　b) It is recommended to start with the conventional dose and, if ineffective, titrate upward with each successive dose to the high dose.

b. Catecholamines with only α-agonist activity (phenylephrine) or with α- and limited β-agonist activity (norepinephrine) or dopamine could also be used. Norepinephrine and phenylephrine might be considered in situations in which one needs peripheral vasoconstriction without the β-receptor effects on the heart.

c. Isoproterenol and dobutamine are not recommended because of their peripheral vasodilating properties.

d. Venoconstriction (α-agonism) redistributes blood from the venous capacitance vessels into the active arterial circulation.

e. Arterial constriction (α-agonism) increases arterial blood pressure and diminishes the loss of arterial blood volume into the periphery.

f. β-Agonist activity stimulates pacemaker activity and enhances contractility (when the heart is beating).

g. Vasopressin and angiotensin II might be effective in increasing myocardial blood flow and restoring spontaneous cardiovascular function. The CPR dose for vasopressin is 0.4–0.8 U/kg IV (0.1–0.2 mL/10 lb IV).

3. Route of administration for small volume drugs during CPCR

a. There are six routes by which small volume emergency drugs can be administered: peripheral venous, central venous, intraosseous, sublingual, intracardiac, and intratracheal.

b. Peripheral venous routes are those most commonly available during an unplanned resuscitation.

　　1) There is a time delay associated with their delivery to the heart.
　　2) The vein closest to the heart should be used.
　　3) Venous cutdown is often necessary to place the catheter.
　　4) If a catheter is not already in place, drugs should be administered by another route (sublingual, intraosseous, or intratracheal) while the cutdown is being performed.

c. The anterior vena cava, via a jugular catheter, is an ideal route for small-volume emergency drug administration because it is close to the heart and it avoids the problems inherent in the other routes.

d. The intracardiac route is associated with a number of potential problems.

　　1) Blind intracardiac injections may be associated with lung laceration, coronary artery laceration, and atrial or right ventricular laceration.
　　2) Intramyocardial deposition of epinephrine may cause refractory ventricular fibrillation.

3) Multiple myocardial injections cause trauma and may predispose to ventricular ectopic beats or ventricular fibrillation.
4) Intracardiac injection requires discontinuing the compressions during the injection.
5) It is technically difficult because there is no apex beat.
6) It is the method of choice during open-chest CPR as long as the myocardial vessels are avoided.
e. The intratracheal route has been recommended, but drug uptake is entirely dependent upon local blood flow and so is unpredictable and undependable. For intratracheal drug administration, the drug dosage should be doubled and diluted in saline to promote absorption. Drugs that can be given by this route include epinephrine, atropine, vasopressin and lidocaine.
f. Drugs and fluids can be delivered via the intraosseous route (see "Pediatric Emergencies") in animals when intravenous catheterization is difficult.
g. Emergency drugs can be administered by the sublingual route—injected into the meaty part of the tongue—where they will be absorbed rapidly because of preferential circulation to the head area.

4. Anticholinergics
   a. Excessive vagal tone and the lack of an idioventricular (escape) rhythm may cause and maintain asystole.

1) A low dose of atropine may cause a centrally mediated increase in vagal tone.
2) A high dose, particularly if given in the vicinity of epinephrine, may cause sinus tachycardia or ventricular fibrillation.
b. The dose of atropine is 0.04 mg/kg of body weight (0.5–1.0 mL/20 lb).
c. To avoid excessive tachycardia in animals with respiratory arrest and bradycardia, use a lower dose of atropine (0.1 mL/10 lb).

5. Sodium bicarbonate
   a. Alkalinization is recommended to combat the metabolic acidosis generated by the lack of tissue perfusion.
   b. Dogs develop a moderate-to-severe mixed-venous and cerebral metabolic acidosis within 15–20 minutes of cardiac arrest and resuscitation. Resuscitation is prompter and 24-hour neurologic recovery better when the metabolic acidosis is controlled.
   c. Several potential problems are associated with administration of sodium bicarbonate (*Table 3-2*). It is important to avoid them.
   d. There are alternative alkalinizing agents.
   1) Tromethamine (THAM) binds directly with hydrogen ion, which decreases rather than increases carbon dioxide levels.
   2) Carbicarb is an equimolar combination of sodium carbonate and sodium bicarbonate and therefore produces less CO_2.

TABLE 3.2 POTENTIAL PROBLEMS ASSOCIATED WITH SODIUM BICARBONATE	
The Problem	**What to Do about It**
Metabolic alkalosis	Don't give more than 0.5 mEq/kg per 5 min
Hypercapnia via carbonic acid equilibration	Can't prevent CO_2 generation; make sure that the animal is well ventilated to blow off CO_2
Intracellular/CSF acidosis due to rapid transcellular diffusion and reequilibration of the carbonic acid equation	Making sure that the animals are well ventilated will prevent hypercapnia in the first place
Hypokalemia due to intracellular redistribution secondary to the decrease in H^+	In hypokalemic patients, potassium must be simultaneously infused
Hypocalcemia (ionized) due to increased albumin binding	In hypocalcemic patients, calcium must be simultaneously infused
Hypernatremia; hyperosmolality	Not a problem; the animal will experience the alkalosis problem before it develops the hypernatremia problem

3) Dichloroacetate enhances activity of pyruvate dehydrogenase and the metabolism of lactic acid.

4) So far, sodium bicarbonate has not been shown to be bad enough nor the alternatives to be good enough to warrant replacing the former with the latter.

e. The administration of an alkalinizing agent may not be efficacious for short-duration cardiac arrests but may improve survival in long-duration cardiac arrests. Control of intracellular acidosis also improves myocardial function.

f. The current recommendation for sodium bicarbonate is none for the first 5 to 10 minutes and then 0.5 mEq/kg per 5 minutes of cardiac arrest thereafter. If it is known or suspected that metabolic acidosis predated the cardiac arrest, then the bicarbonate dosing should start right away.

6. Calcium
   a. Calcium should not be administered as a matter of routine during CPR. It does not improve the rate of return of spontaneous rhythms and is ineffective for ventricular fibrillation and asystole. Some subsets of electromechanical dissociation do benefit from calcium administration.

   b. Intracellular calcium concentrations increase rapidly during cardiac arrest. Calcium administration will augment this problem. This may be associated with
   1) Sustained muscular contraction of the heart (systolic arrest)
   2) Sustained coronary and cerebral artery vasoconstriction, which further diminishes blood flow to and oxygenation of these vital organs during the low-flow resuscitation period and following an otherwise successful resuscitation.
   3) Cytotoxicity appears to be increased following the use of calcium during CPR.
   a) *Calcium is an early player in the generation of toxic oxygen radicals.*
   b) *Large concentrations of cytosolic calcium interfere with mitochondrial function and ATP generation.*

   c. Calcium administration might be indicated in the following circumstances:
   1) Life-threatening hyperkalemia
   2) Severe hypocalcemia
   3) Electromechanical dissociation
   4) Overdose of calcium channel blockers

5) If the heart is observed to be flabby and atonic

6) At the end of the drug list, when all other pharmacologic endeavors have failed to achieve a spontaneously beating heart.

d. The recommended dose of calcium is 0.2 mL of 10% CaCl or 0.6 mL of 10% calcium gluconate per kilogram of body weight.

7. Magnesium
   a. Many conditions are known to be associated with intracellular hypomagnesemia, especially chronic anorexia and increased GI or renal losses.

   b. Empiric administration has been recommended in refractory arrhythmias, including ventricular flutter, ventricular fibrillation, and in nonresponsive cardiac arrest.

   c. The recommended dosage is 0.15–0.3 mEq/kg IV slowly, then 0.75–1.0 mEq/kg/day

8. Antiarrhythmics
   a. Lidocaine (1–3 mg/kg IV) may help reduce the heterogeneity of ventricular refractoriness and may occasionally be useful after CPR if the ventricular arrhythmias are severe.

   b. Bretylium (5–10 mg/kg IV) can be used to treat post-CPR arrhythmias but can also be used during CPR to treat ventricular fibrillation and to lower the threshold to defibrillation. Bretylium is also associated with a blockade of the release and reuptake of norepinephrine at the sympathetic nerve endings (vasodilation/hypotension). This effect appears about 20 minutes after bretylium administration and peaks at about 45–60 minutes.

9. Corticosteroids
   a. There is much laboratory evidence that high-dose corticosteroids "improve membrane stability" in models of tissue ischemia.

   b. There have been very few studies regarding the use of corticosteroids in cardiac arrest. Steroids might improve survival in patients with electromechanical dissociation or pulseless idioventricular rhythm.

10. Avoid glucose administration unless hypoglycemia is present. Modest hyperglycemia following resuscitation in both dogs and cats diminishes neurologic outcome. The mechanism is attributed to enhanced intracellular lactic acidosis.

TABLE 3.3
TYPES OF CARDIOPULMONARY ARREST

Type	Electrical Activity	Coordinated Mechanical Contraction?	Visual Appearance of Heart	Treatment
Ventricular asystole	None	No	Standstill	β Agonist
Ventricular fibrillation	Chaotic	No	Fine/coarse myocardial rippling	Defibrillation
Electromechanical dissociation	Normal	No	Standstill	?
Cardiovascular collapse	Normal	Yes	Normal	Fluids, positive inotrope

11. Electrical activity of the heart.
   a. There are several different kinds of cardiac arrest which must be identified so that therapy can be more directed (*Table 3-3*).
   b. A fibrillating heart consumes a great amount of oxygen during a time when myocardial blood flow is minimal to nonexistent. The longer the duration of ventricular fibrillation, the more difficult the heart is to defibrillate.

12. Defibrillation
   a. Early defibrillation of the fibrillating heart is so important that blind defibrillation has been recommended in humans if no ECG monitor is available,.
   b. In humans, defibrillation within 1 minute of CPA has a 98% chance of conversion; within 4 minutes, a 50% chance; and within 10 minutes, a 1% chance.
   c. Direct-current defibrillation is indicated as soon as ventricular fibrillation is identified.
      1) A critical quantity of energy is required to defibrillate a heart successfully, and this is not affected by the prior administration of epinephrine.
      2) Excessive energy and repeated defibrillations can cause myocardial damage. Start with lower settings and try to find the effective setting as soon as possible.
      3) The recommended dosages are a good place to start, but higher settings are commonly necessary.
         a) External dose: 5–10 joules/kg
         b) Internal dose: 0.5–2 joules/kg

      4) For refractory ventricular fibrillation
         a) Defibrillate 3 times in rapid succession, increasing the dose by 25–50% each time.
         b) If no response, give epinephrine (0.2 mg/kg IV) and repeat defibrillation at highest dose. Also consider magnesium chloride (0.15 mg/kg IV).
         c) If no response, give lidocaine 1–2 mg/kg IV, repeat epinephrine, and repeat defibrillation.
         d) If no response, give bretylium (5 mg/kg IV) and defibrillate.
   d. Pharmacologic defibrillation
      1) Unlikely to be effective. Use only as a "last ditch effort" when there is no defibrillator available.
      2) Potassium chloride (1 mEq/kg) followed by calcium (0.2 mL/kg 10% CaCl or 0.6 mL/kg 10% calcium gluconate), with or without preadministration of lidocaine (1 mg/kg) or bretylium (5 mg/kg)
      3) A sharp thump to the chest may, rarely, restore a normal rhythm in the case of ventricular tachycardia, A-V heart block, and ventricular fibrillation, but may also cause a beating heart to fibrillate.

C. *Recommendations for postresuscitative care*

1. The nature of cell injury during cardiac arrest
   a. Lack of perfusion injury. The lack of oxygen and other cellular metabolic substrates disables the cell's ability to maintain energy stores for essential cellular functions.

1) Such cells initially lose the ability to pump sodium out and, as a result, develop intracellular edema.

2) If the process continues unabated, such cells will die.

b. It has long been observed that certain organ systems (brain and heart, most notably) seem to function reasonably well immediately after resuscitation but then deteriorate in the ensuing hours.

1) The biphasic increases in blood–brain barrier permeability in a rat cardiac arrest model suggest an early ischemic insult followed by a delayed "reperfusion" insult.

2) Initially, in reperfusion failure, there are multifocal areas of "no-reflow," followed by a phase of global hyperemia; delayed nonhomogeneous global hypoperfusion follows and finally brain death. Miliary hemorrhages and diffuse brain edema are evident short term by high-field MRI; diffuse brain atrophy is evident long term.

3) There are several possible reasons for this:

a) Reperfusion injury secondary to the generation of reactive oxygen intermediate metabolites

b) Leukocyte activation and sequestration due to the liberation of cytokines and other inflammatory mediators

c) DIC

c. There is no clinically proven way to deal with toxic oxygen radicals.

1) Calcium channel blockers (such as lidoflazine) may reduce the conversion of xanthine dehydrogenase to xanthine oxidase.

2) Allopurinol and its long-acting metabolite oxypurinol, and folic acid and its photolytic metabolite pterin aldehyde are competitive inhibitors of xanthine oxidase.

3) Polyethylene glycol and superoxide dismutase hasten the metabolism of superoxide to hydrogen peroxide, and catalase and glutathione peroxidase speed the metabolism of hydrogen peroxide to water and molecular oxygen.

4) Deferoxamine is an iron chelator that limits the conversion of superoxide and hydrogen peroxide to the relatively more toxic hydroxyl radical.

5) Dimethyl sulfoxide, mannitol, dimethylthiourea (DMTU; a sulfhydryl com-

pound), N-acetylcysteine, captopril, and N-2-mercaptopropionylglycine (MPG) are hydroxyl radical scavengers.

6) α-Tocopherol, β-carotene, and the 21-amino steroids are potent inhibitors of membrane lipid peroxidation.

2. What can be done to minimize pulmonary consequences?

a. First evaluate the animal's ability to ventilate. Apnea or bradypnea is due to central neurologic dysfunction. The animal will require positive-pressure ventilation.

b. Next evaluate the lungs' ability to oxygenate.

1) Is there a pneumothorax?

2) Is there severe pulmonary edema from aggressive fluid therapy?

3) Are there pulmonary contusions from the external chest compression?

4) The extent of these complications should be assessed via chest radiography and arterial blood gas analysis.

c. Provide oxygen therapy as necessary to alleviate the hypoxemia.

d. Pneumonia has been reported to occur in about ⅓ of human patients within 7 days of resuscitation.

3. What can be done to maximize tissue perfusion?

a. The adequacy of tissue perfusion is assessed by the clinical signs of vasomotor tone, urine output, and metabolic monitors such as base deficit, blood lactate, and venous oxygen.

b. Adequate venous pressure is assessed by measuring central venous pressure (CVP) or

---

DRUGS USED TO TREAT REPERFUSION INJURY (EXPERIMENTAL DOSES)

Allopurinol (Burroughs Welcome, 30 mg/kg divided q8–12 h

Mannitol 20% (Baxter), 0.5–2 g/kg IV slowly

Dimethyl sulfoxide (Syntex Animal Health), 1 g/kg IV over 45 minutes

Deferoxamine mesylate (CIBA), 5–15 mg/kg IV during CPR, 50 mg/kg IV over 5 minutes to prevent reperfusion injury in dogs with gastric dilatation volvulus

ultrasonographic evaluation of end-diastolic filling volume.

c. Myocardial function is assessed by pulse quality, arterial blood pressure, cardiac output, and ultrasonographic evaluation of systolic performance. Administer catecholamines (dobutamine or dopamine) as necessary to support arterial blood pressure or forward blood flow.

4. What can be done to maximize myocardial recovery?

a. Myocardial cells rapidly develop a severe hypercarbic acidosis during cardiac arrest. The mechanism is thought to be via in situ bicarbonate buffering of metabolic acids.

b. Significant myocardial systolic and diastolic dysfunction occurs following global ischemia after resumption of a spontaneously beating heart. This myocardial stunning may either spontaneously resolve within 48 hours or cause progressive myocardial failure.

c. Norepinephrine-induced hypertension improved myocardial perfusion and oxygenation in a swine cardiac arrest model.

d. Providing supplemental nasal oxygen and antiarrhythmics as needed (most commonly lidocaine 50–75 μg/kg/min as a constant rate infusion (CRI) for ventricular arrhythmias) is often beneficial.

5. What can be done to maximize neurologic recovery?

a. Cardiac arrest produces cerebral hypoxia in 10 seconds, depletes glucose and glycogen stores in 2–4 minutes, and depletes ATP stores in 4–5 minutes. The energy-deficient cell accumulates sodium, calcium, and iron and eventually dies.

b. The most important aspect of cerebral resuscitation is to commence effective artificial circulation as early as possible and to restart effective spontaneous circulation as soon as possible.

c. Postresuscitation cerebral failure has been attributed to

  1) Global ischemia and ATP depletion (lack of perfusion injury)

  2) Reperfusion injury (reactive oxygen radicals, leukoactivation, coagulopathies)

  3) Extracerebral derangements (hypertension, hypotension, hypoxemia, acidemia, absorbed gut toxins, an overwhelmed retic-

uloendothelial (RE) system, coagulopathies, activated inflammatory cascades, and other organ failures).

d. Postarrest consciousness should begin to return within about 15–30 minutes (good prognostic indicator). If consciousness does not return, or if the resuscitation exceeded 15 minutes, the existence of cerebral damage should be assumed.

e. Following return of spontaneous circulation, the most important aspects of cerebral resuscitation involve the physiologic management and support of the patient.

  1) Avoid severe hypervolemia/hypertension, hypovolemia/hypotension, hypercapnia/hypocapnia, hypoxia, hyperthermia, and excessive activity.

  2) Avoid venous outflow obstruction and head-down positioning.

  3) Avoid the use of ketamine, inhalational anesthetics, and xylazine.

  4) Mannitol (0.5 g/kg; administered slowly IV) osmotically decreases cerebral edema and scavenges hydroxyl radicals.

  5) Furosemide (0.5–1 mg/kg) is a weak vasodilator and redistributes blood away from the brain. Both diuretics remove fluids from the body. Monitor for post-diuretic hypotension.

  6) Hyperventilation may be efficacious in some patients for a brief time (2 hours). It should not be used as a matter of routine. Monitor end-tidal CO_2 and keep above 20 mmHg.

  7) Moderate hypertension, mild hemodilution, normocapnia, and mild hypothermia (34°C) gave better neurologic recovery and less histopathologic brain damage than in the normotensive, hypocapnic, and normothermic group in one study.

  8) Hyperoxia, surprisingly, diminished neurologic recovery in one study.

  9) Corticosteroid administration did not improve neurologic recovery in several studies.

  10) The efficacy of reactive oxygen radical inhibitors, scavengers, or blockers has not been validated.

f. Trends of neurologic competence should be monitored closely in the hours and days following the arrest.

PROCEDURE FOR WITNESSED CARDIOPULMONARY ARREST

1. Call for help and move animal to arrest station

2. Establish airway; intubate and give two breaths

3. Feel for pulses; apply ECG leads; auscult chest

4. Continue breathing 20–30 breaths per minute

5. Asystole: Epinephrine (0.02 mg/kg), atropine (sublingual or intratracheal if no IV catheter), precordial thump, defibrillation

6. Ventricular fibrillation
   Defibrillate immediately—5 joules/kg
   Repeat at 7 J/kg if no response
   Repeat at 10 J/kg if no response

7. If no response, electromechanical dissociation (EMD), asystole, or pulseless idioventricular rhythm (PIVR), begin external chest compressions, 80–120/min

8. Establish venous or intraosseous access. Place pulse oximeter on tongue and end-tidal CO_2 monitor on endotracheal tube. Administer fluids (5–10 mL/kg colloids or 10–90 mL/kg crystalloids, depending on underlying cause of CPA). Repeat epinephrine (0.2 mg/kg IV), atropine (.02 mg/kg IV), sodium bicarbonate (0.5 mEq/kg IV), lidocaine (2–4 mg/kg IV).

9. Repeat defibrillation up to 3 times.

10. If no response, improve external compressions.
   Pulse oximeter should read >90 or be increasing.
   Add interposed abdominal compressions, simultaneous ventilation/compressions.

11. If no response, perform thoracotomy at 5th intercostal space. Grasp heart and manually compress until cardiac muscle tone and filling return.

12. Internal defibrillation, 1–2 J/kg using saline-soaked gauze to protect heart from paddles.

13. If no response, compress dorsal aorta and give epinephrine and atropine intracardiac; repeat 1 mEq/kg sodium bicarbonate IV.

14. Repeat internal defibrillation. If no response, discontinue efforts. If there is return of spontaneous circulation, proceed with postresuscitative care.

RECOMMENDATIONS FOR POSTRESUSCITATIVE CARE

Support cardiovascular system
Dopamine 5 µg/kg/min CRI OR
Epinephrine 1–10 µg/kg/min CRI (wean as soon as possible)
Supraventricular tachycardia: diltiazem 0.5–2.0 mg/kg IV, then 1–10 µg/kg/min CRI
Ventricular arrhythmias: lidocaine 2–4 mg/kg IV, then 25–75 µg/kg/min CRI
Continue IV fluids—Do not overhydrate (e.g. 3 mL/kg/h)

Minimize brain damage
Mannitol 0.5 g/kg IV slowly over 5–10 minutes q4h × 3
Corticosteroids (controversial)
   Dexamethesone sodium phosphate 2 mg/kg IV q8h × 3 OR
   Prednisolone sodium succinate 10–30 mg/kg IV q8h × 3
Furosemide 1 mg/kg IV following mannitol

Monitor urine output
Should be >1 mL/kg/h
Dopamine and mannitol should help prevent acute renal failure
Continue fluid diuresis
Taper off pressor agents ASAP

Protect the GI tract
If animal can swallow, give sucralfate slurry, 1 g/20 kg PO
If animal is unconscious, give injectable H_2 blockers (ranitidine 0.5 mg/kg IV q12h or famotidine 1 mg/kg IV or SC q12h)

If the animal has survived internal cardiac massage, the thoracotomy should be closed under sterile conditions following copious lavage and administration of broad-spectrum systemic antibiotics.

CHAPTER 4

SHOCK

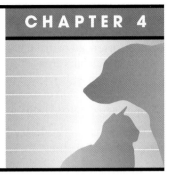

I. DEFINITION

Shock is defined as inadequate cellular energy production resulting from inadequate perfusion to meet the cellular metabolic requirements.

II. CATEGORIES OF SHOCK

A. General considerations

1. Poor tissue perfusion can be caused by many different mechanisms.

    a. Categorizing causes of shock helps organize your thoughts, but categories should not be considered to be distinct entities because they contain significant overlapping mechanisms.

        1) Published categorization schemes vary from author to author, and their somewhat arbitrary nature should not distract or concern the reader.

        2) A single patient may have more than one type of shock.

B. Hypovolemic shock is due to a low effective circulating volume of blood and poor venous return.

1. Hypovolemia may be due to

    a. External crystalloid losses (vomiting, diarrhea, diuresis)

    b. Internal crystalloid losses (abdomen, thorax)

    c. Albumin losses (external, internal)

    d. Whole blood losses (external, internal)

2. A relative or functional hypovolemia can be caused by

    a. Increased volume capacity or vasodilation

        1) Anaphylaxis

        2) Vasodilator drugs

        3) Neurogenic

    b. Maldistribution of the available blood volume (trauma)

    c. This is often referred to as distributive shock.

3. Absolute or relative hypovolemia should be treated with aggressive fluid therapy

    a. 0.5–1.0 blood volume equivalents of isotonic extracellular fluid-replacement crystalloids.

        1) Blood volume dog: 80–90 mL/kg

        2) Blood volume cat: 50–60 mL/kg

    b. 0.1–0.4 blood volume equivalents of a colloid solution.

C. Cardiogenic shock is low forward flow due to "periheart" related problems.

1. Cardiogenic shock may be due to

    a. Dilated cardiomyopathy (poor contractility)

    b. Hypertrophic cardiomyopathy (impaired relaxation)

    c. Backflow regurgitation (valvular insufficiency)

    d. Forward flow obstruction (stenosis)

    e. Pericardial tamponade or fibrosis (impaired filling)

    f. Severe bradycardia, tachycardia, or ventricular arrhythmias

    g. Myocardial depression (general anesthetics, sepsis)

    h. Myocardial damage (traumatic stunning, adriamycin)

D. Metabolic shock

1. Low blood oxygen
   a. Low arterial partial pressure of oxygen
   b. Hemoglobin carriage problems (methemoglobin, carboxyhemoglobin)
   c. Severe left shift of oxyhemoglobin dissociation curve (stored blood)

2. Hypoglycemia—inadequate energy substrate for cerebral metabolism

3. Anemia—inadequate oxygen-carrying capacity

4. Sepsis—interferes with intermediary metabolism

5. Heat stroke—the metabolic rate exceeds the animal's ability to deliver energy substrates

6. Cyanide poisoning interferes with mitochondrial cytochromic oxidative phosphorylation.

E. Septic shock is discussed separately and extensively because it is common, is challenging, and encompasses all of the above-mentioned categories of shock.

1. The signs of septicemia are due to the *systemic inflammatory response syndrome (SIRS)*.
   a. This systemic response occurs when the localized inflammatory response gets out of hand and affects tissues remote to the original site of inflammation.
   b. The mediators of the systemic reaction are the same as the mediators of the local inflammatory response.
      1) Leukocyte and endothelial activation
      2) Cytokines (tumor necrosis factor, platelet activating factor, interleukins 1 and 6)
      3) Arachidonic acid metabolites (prostaglandins, leukotrienes)
      4) Reactive oxygen metabolites
      5) Activated coagulation and platelet cascades
      6) Complement activation
   c. These cascades, once activated, exert positive feedback loops on one another that "autoperpetuate" the entire process, with subsequent deleterious systemic effects.
   d. Rather than being a cesspool of proinflammatory cascades flaming out of control, SIRS is more likely an imbalance between proinflammatory cascades and antiinflammatory cascades.

2. The *multiple organ dysfunction syndrome (MODS)* results when the systemic inflammatory response syndrome becomes severe and remote tissue injury causes deterioration of organ function.

3. Causes of SIRS and MODS
   a. Sepsis (bacterial, viral, fungal, rickettsial, spirochetal)
   b. Heat stroke
   c. Trauma
   d. Pancreatitis
   e. Uremia
   f. GI ischemic or inflammatory disease
   g. Disseminated cancer
   h. Hypovolemic shock
   i. Autoimmune diseases (AIHA, ITP, SLE)

4. Clinical manifestations of SIRS
   a. Mild-to-moderate depression
   b. Poor appetite
   c. Fever
   d. Hyperglycemia
   e. Leukocytosis with a left shift and mild toxicity
   f. Vasodilation (red mucous membranes, accelerated capillary refill time)
   g. "Bounding" pulse quality
   h. Normal-to-high cardiac output
   i. Normal-to-low arterial and central venous blood pressure
   j. Tachycardia, tachypnea, hyperventilation
   k. Nonhemorrhagic diarrhea
   l. Heart murmur
   m. Normal-to-hyperactive coagulation
   n. Normal-to-mildly impaired organ function
   o. Nonspecific increase of liver enzymes (particularly alkaline phosphatase)
   p. Hypoalbuminemia

5. Clinical manifestations of MODS
   a. Moderate-to-severe depression
   b. No appetite
   c. Subnormal core temperature
   d. Hypoglycemia
   e. Leukopenia or a large, rapid decrease in leukocyte count with a marked left shift and toxic neutrophils
   f. Vasoconstriction
   g. Low cardiac output
   h. Low arterial and central venous blood pressure
   i. Tachycardia, tachypnea, hyperventilation
   j. High venous oxygen, reduced arterial–venous oxygen difference

k. Hemorrhagic diarrhea

l. Heart murmur

m. Hypoactive coagulation with clinical petechiae or bleeding

n. Lactic/metabolic acidosis

o. Moderate-to-severe impairment of organ function (heart, kidneys, gut, lungs)

p. Moderate increases of liver enzymes, hypoalbuminemia

6. These descriptions of the clinical presentations of SIRS and MODS are idealized.

   a. Not every patient will have every sign

   b. Given the permutations of patient disease, and since these two "syndromes" are actually a continuum of the same mechanistic disorder, most patients exhibit overlapping signs.

III. TREATMENT OF SHOCK

A. Fluids: Restoration of an effective circulating blood volume is a first priority in hypovolemic, traumatic, and septic shock.

1. Combinations of crystalloids (0.5–1.0 blood volume equivalents) (to restore vascular and interstitial fluid deficits) and colloids (0.1–0.4 blood volume equivalents) to restore vascular volume and maintain packed cell volume, colloid oncotic pressure, and hemostasis are often indicated.

2. The endpoint of fluid administration for a specific patient is the alleviation of the peripheral vasoconstriction, the restoration of an acceptable pulse quality, and a return of urine output. An increase in the CVP to a high-normal level (8-10 cm H_2O) suggests that an adequate volume load is being presented to the heart.

3. *Aggressive fluid therapy is contraindicated in cardiogenic shock (e.g., cardiomyopathy and pericardial fibrosis).*

B. Sympathomimetics are seldom required in hypovolemic or traumatic shock but are occasionally required to support myocardial function, oxygen delivery, vasomotor tone, and tissue perfusion in septic shock and dilated cardiomyopathy or after cardiac arrest. They are contraindicated in hypertrophic cardiomyopathy.

1. First-choice drugs are dopamine or dobutamine. (See Appendix E, "Constant Rate Infusions," p. 422.)

   a. Dopamine (3+β-agonist, 2+α-agonist) works well in some patients. It is a modest vasoconstrictor in higher dosages.

      1) It is the better than dobutamine for arterial blood pressure support.

      2) It is not as effective as dobutamine for promoting forward blood flow.

      3) Dosage: 1–3 µg/kg/min for enhancing renal blood flow and urine output; 4–7 µg/kg/min for augmentation of blood pressure

   b. Dobutamine (3+β$_1$-agonist; 1+β$_2$-agonist) is a mild vasodilator and a better flow drug. It is the preferred drug for cardiogenic shock or myocardial depression secondary to sepsis.

      1) Arterial blood pressure does not usually change much

      2) Dosage: 5–15 µg/kg/min (dogs) 2.5–5 µg/kg/min (cats). Higher doses may cause seizures in cats.

C. Antibiotics

Antibiotics are indicated if the patient is known or suspected to have an infection or is significantly contaminated.

1. The range of organisms involved is usually unknown in the initial phases of treatment.

2. Antibiotics or antibiotic combinations should be broad spectrum and highly likely to be effective (*Table 4-1*).

D. Glucocorticosteroids have been shown to have beneficial effects in different forms of shock in animals, but their use remains highly controversial because of conflicting results in various scientific studies. The following discussion presents a brief overview for the interested reader.

1. The experimental evidence

   a. Antiinflammatory

      1) Diminish activation of the complement cascade

      2) Inhibit nitric oxide synthase

      3) Inhibit platelet aggregation

      4) Inhibit leukoactivation

      5) Decrease plasma levels of platelet activating factor and tumor necrosis factor

      6) Inhibit phospholipase A and prostaglandin/leukotriene generation

   b. Improved membrane stability

      1) Decreased absorption of endotoxin from the gut

TABLE 4.1
SPECTRUM OF ANTIBIOTIC ACTIVITY FOR USE IN SEPTIC SHOCK

| | Gram-negative | Gram-positive | | Anaerobic |
		Staph spp.	Strep spp.	
Penicillins				
Penicillin, ampicillin, amoxicillin	No	Yes	Often	Yes (except some *Bacteroides fragilis* and actinomyces)
Oxacillin, methicillin, nafcillin, cloxacillin	No	Yes	Yes	No
Carbenicillin ticarcillin, azlocillin, piperacillin, mezlocillin	Yes	Yes	Yes	Yes
Cephalosporins				
First generation	Some	Yes	Yes	No
Second generation	Yes (except *Pseudomonas* spp.)	Yes	Yes	No
Third generation	Yes	Yes	Yes	Yes
Imipenem/Cilastin	Yes	Yes	Yes	Yes
Aminoglycosides	Yes	Yes	No	No
Fluoroquinolones	Yes	Yes	No	No
Azteonam	Yes	No	No	No
Metronidazole	No	No	No	Yes
Clindamycin	No	Yes	Yes	Yes

2) Decreased leakage of lysosomal enzymes
3) Decreased platelet and red blood cell aggregation
4) Decreased loss of fluid from the vascular fluid space (reduces capillary permeability)
c. Improved microcirculation
1) Improved RBC, endothelial cell, platelet, and white cell membrane integrity decreases microcirculatory "sludging"
2) Modulates and normalizes vasomotor tone (lessens the vasoconstriction)
3) Improves cardiac output
d. Improved intermediary metabolism
1) Enhances gluconeogenesis
2) Enhances lactate metabolism and diminishes lactate production
3) Increases oxygen consumption

4) Increases ATP production
5) Normalizes a left-shifted oxygen-hemoglobin dissociation curve
e. Improved survival in numerous experimental studies

2. The clinical evidence
a. Wilson GL, White GS, Kosanke SD, et al. Therapeutic effects of prednisolone sodium succinate vs dexamethasone in dogs subjected to *E. coli* septic shock. J Am Anim Hosp Assoc 1982;18:639–648.

Compared saline, prednisolone sodium succinate (11 mg/kg at 15, 75, 255, and 435 min), and dexamethasone in propylene glycol (8 mg/kg at 15, 240, and 435 min) in a septic abdomen canine model ($n = 8$ per group).

TABLE 4.2
Sprung et al (1984): Effects of High-dose Corticosteroids in Patients with Septic Shock

	Shock Reversal (%)	Mortality (%) 5.5 days	Mortality (%) 25 days
Saline	0	69	69
MP	19	33	76
Dex	32	45	77

TABLE 4.3
Luce et al (1988): Ineffectiveness of High-dose Methylprednisolone in Preventing Parenchymal Lung Injury and Improving Mortality in Patients with Septic Shock

	Developed ARDS (%)	Mortality (%)
Saline	38	54
MP	34	58

Three-day mortality rates: saline, 75%; prednisolone, 0%; dexamethasone, 75%

b. Schumer W. Steroids in the treatment of clinical septic shock. Ann Surg 1976;184: 333–339.

Compared saline ($n = 86$), methylprednisolone (MP) sodium succinate (30 mg/kg) ($n = 43$), and dexamethasone (Dex) sodium phosphate (3 mg/kg) ($n = 43$) in clinical human septic shock; 40% of the patients received a second dose of steroid (½ dosage approximately 4 hours later).

Mortality rates: saline, 38%; MP, 12%; Dex 9%

c. Hoffman SL, Punjabi NH, Kumala S, et al. Reduction of mortality in chloramphenicol treated severe typhoid fever by high dose dexamethasone. N Engl J Med 1984;310:82–88.

Compared saline ($n = 18$) and dexamethasone (3 mg/kg; followed by 8 doses of 1 mg/kg every 6 hours) ($n = 20$) in typhoid fever.

Mortality rates: saline, 56%; Dex, 10%

d. Sprung CL, Caralis PV, Marcial EH, et al. The effects of high-dose corticosteroids in patients with septic shock. N Engl J Med 1984;311: 1137–1143 (*see Table 4-2*).

Compared saline ($n = 16$), methylprednisolone (30 mg/kg) ($n = 21$), and dexamethasone (6 mg/kg) ($n = 22$) in septic shock

e. Lucas CE, Ledgerwood AM. The cardiopulmonary response to massive doses of steroids in patients with septic shock. Arch Surg 1984;119:537–541.

Compared dexamethasone-treated patients (2 mg/kg loading dose plus 2 mg/kg/24 h × 2 as an infusion) ($n = 23$) with non-steroid-treated ($n = 25$) patients with septic shock.

Mortality rates: Dex, 22%; placebo, 20%.

f. Luce JM, Montgomery AB, Marks JD, et al. Ineffectiveness of high-dose methylprednisolone in preventing parenchymal lung injury and improving mortality in patients with septic shock. Am Rev Resp Dis 1988;138: 62–68 (*see Table 4-3*).

Compared placebo (mannitol) ($n = 37$) with MP (30 mg/kg q6h × 4) ($n = 38$) in septic shock.

g. Bone RC, Fisher CJ, Clemmer TP, et al. A controlled clinical trial of high-dose methylprednisolone in the treatment of severe sepsis and septic shock, N Engl J Med 1987;317: 653–658.

Compared saline ($n = 191$) and methylprednisolone (30 mg/kg q6h × 4) ($n = 191$) in severe sepsis and septic shock.

Incidence of secondary infection was the same; chance of dying from it was greater in the methylprednisolone group.

TABLE 4.4
Bone et al (1987): A Controlled Clinical Trial of High-dose Methylprednisolone in the Treatment of Severe Sepsis and Septic Shock

	Shock Development (%)	Shock Reversal (%)	14-Day Mortality (%) Overall	14-Day Mortality (%) Gram-neg	14-Day Mortality (%) Gram-pos
Saline	37	73	25	29	24
MP	45	65	34	33	33

TABLE 4.5
VA Study Group (1987): Effect of High-dose Glucocorticoid Therapy On Mortality in Patients with Systemic Sepsis

	14-Day Mortality (%)	Gram-neg	Gram-pos
Saline	22	27	18
MP	21	7	26

h. VA Study Group. Effect of high-dose glucocorticoid therapy on mortality in patients with clinical signs of systemic sepsis. N Engl J Med 1987;317:658–665.

Compared saline ($n = 111$) and methylprednisolone (30 mg/kg plus 5 mg/kg/h $\times$ 9) ($n = 112$) in septic shock.

Incidence of secondary infection was the same; chance of dying from it was greater with methylprednisolone (*see Table 4-5*).

i. Bollaert PE, Charpentier C, Levy B, et al. Reversal of late septic shock with supraphysiologic doses of hydrocortisone. Crit Care Med 1998;26:645–650.

Compared saline ($n = 19$) and hydrocortisone (HC) (100 mg q8h $\times$ 5 days) ($n = 22$)

No difference in incidence of GI bleeding or secondary infections (*see Table 4-6*).

j. Bennett IL, Finland M, Hamburger M, et al. The effectiveness of hydrocortisone in the management of severe infections. JAMA 1963;183: 462–465.

Compared saline ($n = 89$) and hydrocortisone (300 mg day 1; 250 mg day 2; 200 mg day 3; 150 mg day 4; 100 mg day 5; and 50 mg on day 6) ($n = 80$).

Mortality rates: saline, 37%; HC, 40%

TABLE 4.6
Bollaert et al (1998): Reversal of Late Septic Shock with Supraphysiologic Doses of Hydrocortisone

	7-Day Shock Reveral (%)	28-Day Mortality (%)
Saline	21	63
HC	68	32

3. The meta-analyses

a. Lefering R, Neugebauer EAM. Steroid controversy in sepsis and septic shock; a meta-analysis. Crit Care Med 1995;23:1294–1303.

b. Cronin L, Cook DJ, Carlet J, et al. Corticosteroid treatment for sepsis: a critical appraisal and meta-analysis of the literature. Crit Care Med 1995;23:1430–1439.

Corticosteroids appear to increase mortality in overwhelming infection.

They have no overall beneficial effect in septic shock.

They may improve survival somewhat in gram-positive sepsis.

There was no difference between "low-dose" and "high-dose" steroid therapy.

There was no difference between hydrocortisone, methylprednisolone, and dexamethasone.

There was no increased incidence of
Gastrointestinal bleeding
Secondary infections
Hyperglycemia

There was a trend toward increased mortality due to the secondary infection in the steroid-treated group.

Mortality rates ranged from 7.1% to 78.1% in the analyzed studies.

4. Why is there such a difference between the results of experimental and clinical studies?

a. Early experimental studies established that steroids were most effective if given before the shock event. Delayed therapy was proportionately less efficacious. All clinical trials represent delayed therapy.

1) Timing is important.

2) Most immunomodulator therapy (antiendotoxin antisera; antitumor necrosis antibodies; etc.) were very promising in the laboratory but did not improve survival in clinical trials.

b. Experimental studies are well defined and of singular insult. Clinical sepsis comes with permutations of additional underlying disorders—many of them lethal. It is not fair to expect corticosteroids to cure heart failure, liver failure, or cancer.

c. The inclusion criteria (the definition of "sepsis" and "septic shock") vary considerably from study to study, which makes it difficult to compare studies and helps explain differences in results.

1) Steroids would not be demonstrated to be efficacious if none or all of the patients in both control and treatment groups survived; there would be no difference.

2) If the magnitudes and permutations of disease(s) in each group studied were not the same, maybe the results cannot be trusted.

d. Mortality may not be the best endpoint of therapeutic efficacy in clinical septic shock.

1) Particularly when death is counted 2 to 4 weeks after the shocking event

2) As an analogy, if a patient was hypo-glycemic and was given glucose to restore blood glucose to normal but died anyway, is it appropriate to conclude that glucose therapy was not efficacious? It didn't improve survival!

3) The problem with corticosteroid therapy is that there is no interim marker of thera-peutic efficacy.

e. The view that shock (multiple organ failure) is solely a consequence of a hyperactive inflam-matory process (SIRS) is probably wrong. It is probably a consequence of the imbalance be-tween proinflammatory processes and anti-inflammatory processes.

1) "Out-of-control" antiinflammatory processes are probably as damaging to the body as out-of-control inflammatory processes.

2) The administration of antiinflammatory drugs may be beneficial in some instances and detrimental in others. The problem is that we do not know which animals might benefit.

f. That corticosteroids might not be effective overall in septic shock does not preclude possi-ble effectiveness in certain subgroups. Their ef-fectiveness seems to have been established in

1) Typhoid fever
2) Bacterial meningitis
3) *Pneumocystis carinii* infection in AIDS patients

5. Shock is a complex disease and, consequently, the efficacy of treatments such as corticosteroids is a complex question whose answer is not yet known.

E. Antiprostaglandins

1. Prostaglandins that are released into the sys-temic circulation during shock cause marked he-modynamic changes, including decreased cardiac output, systemic hypotension, pulmonary hyper-tension, and increased vascular permeability.

2. Treatment with antiprostaglandins ameliorates these cardiovascular changes and improves sur-vival but generally does not affect the leukopenia, thrombocytopenia, acidosis, or coagulopathies that develop during septic shock.

3. The adverse effects of antiprostaglandins include

a. GI tract hemorrhage and ulceration, which are augmented by coadministration of corticosteroids.

b. Renal afferent vasoconstriction also has been reported when ibuprofen was adminis-tered during septic shock in dogs.

4. It would seem that the narrow spectrum of beneficial effects in the face of real and serious dis-advantageous effects would limit the efficacy of this group of drugs in the treatment of shock.

F. Glucose

1. A bolus of glucose (0.25–0.5 g/kg IV) should be given to increase the ECF glucose concentra-tion to approximately 100 mg/dL.

2. Blood glucose concentration can then be main-tained by an infusion of a 2.5–10% glucose solution.

G. Bicarbonate

1. Administer sodium bicarbonate if metabolic acidosis becomes severe.

2. If the base or bicarbonate deficit is known, the dose of bicarbonate to administer can be calcu-lated by the formula

$$\text{mEq bicarbonate} = \text{Base deficit} \times 0.3 \times \text{Body weight (kg)}.$$

3. If the magnitude of the metabolic acidosis can-not be measured but is estimated on the basis of the severity of the clinical signs to be moderate or severe, 1–2 mEq of bicarbonate per kg of body weight, respectively, could be administered.

4. Administer bicarbonate slowly (over 20 min).

5. There are several potential problems associated with the administration of sodium bicarbonate. It is important to avoid them (see *Table 3-2*)

H. Positive inotropes

1. Myocardial depression can occur secondary to systemic consequences of disease (sepsis, general anesthesia, "toxemia" secondary to severe visceral organ disease).

2. Treatment involves correcting the underlying disease process in so far as possible.

3. If blood pressure remains low despite adequate fluid loading, sympathomimetics are indicated (first choice: dopamine or dobutamine).

I. Acute vasogenic **renal failure prevention**

1. Urine output is an indirect indicator of renal blood flow. Place a urinary catheter aseptically to verify and quantitate urine output.

2. Adequate fluid administration is the mainstay of renal perfusion, maintaining urine output, and minimizing the incidence of renal failure.

3. If restoring effective circulating volume does not generate an acceptable urine flow, administer diuretics.
  a. Mannitol (0.5 g/kg, IV, over 10–20 min) os-motically increases blood volume and renal perfusion and subsequently acts as an osmotic diuretic. If urine flow is not detected within 10

minutes following the end of the mannitol in-fusion, another diuretic agent should be administered.
  b. Furosemide (1–2 mg/kg, IV) promotes mild renal (and visceral) vasodilation and is a potent loop diuretic. If urine flow is not detected within 10 minutes, a different diuretic should be administered.
  c. Dopamine (5 µg/kg/min, IV) causes renal (and visceral) vasodilation via dopaminergic-receptor stimulation.
  d. If each diuretic individually fails to induce an acceptable urine output, perhaps simultane-ous administration of all three diuretics may be effective.

J. **Gastrointestinal tract protection**

1. GI tract (GIT) mucosal ulceration and slough-ing are common consequences of septic shock. Mechanisms of damage include
  a. Tissue hypoxia and diminished organ perfusion

TREATMENT GUIDELINES FOR SEPTIC ANIMALS

Maximize oxygen delivery to tissues
Provide supplemental oxygen
Maintain hematocrit ≥30%
Optimize pH (check blood gases)
Restore tissue perfusion
    Volume replacement
        Lactated Ringer's, 90 mL/kg to resuscitate, then 10–20 mL/kg/h to maintain BP and CO.
        Colloids—plasma, hetastarch, or dextran 70: 7 mL/kg initial bolus with 15 mL/kg LRS; then 20 mL/kg/day CRI
    Positive inotropes (see Appendix)
        Dobutamine, 5–20 µg/kg/min IV CRI (cat 2.5–5.0 µg/kg/min)
        Dopamine, 5–10 µg/kg/min IV CRI
    Vasopressor agents
        Dopamine, 10–30 µg/kg/min CRI
        Norepinephrine, 1–10 µg/kg/min IV CRI
        Vasopressin, .001–.004 U/kg/min CRI

Remove septic focus
Identify septic focus: radiographs; ultrasound; diagnostic peritoneal lavage, bronchoalveolar lavage; culture urine, blood, catheter tips; aspiration/cytology/culture of abscesses/masses

Bacteriocidal intravenous antibiotic combinations
    Effective vs. gram-negative organisms
        Enrofloxacin, 5 mg/kg q12h IV (diluted, given slow)
        Gentamicin, 6 mg/kg q24h IV
        Amikacin, 10 mg/kg q8h IV
        Tobramycin, 2–4 mg/kg q8h IV
    Effective vs. gram-positive organisms
        Ampicillin, 20–40 mg/kg q8h IV
        Cefazolin, 20 mg/kg q8h IV
        Imipenem, 2–5 mg/kg q8h IV
        Cefoxitin, 30 mg/kg q5h IV
    Effective vs. anaerobes
        Clindamycin, 11 mg/kg q8h IV
        Metronidazole, 10 mg/kg q8h IV

Prevent complications
Altered clotting function
    Heparin, 150–250 U/kg SC q8h
    Fresh frozen plasma incubated with 10 U/kg heparin for 30 minutes (if AT III or clot-ting factors decreased)
GI bleeding
    Cimetidine, 5–10 mg/kg IV q6–8h
    Ranitidine, 2 mg/kg IV q8–12h
    Sucralfate, 0.25–1 gr q8h PO

(continued)

b. Oxygen radical–induced lipid peroxidation

c. Diffusion of luminal hydrogen ions into mucosal cells

d. Deterioration of the effectiveness of the mucous barrier

e. Destructive action of bile acids and pancreatic proteases

2. The mainstay of GIT protection is the restoration of an effective circulating blood volume and the reestablishment of adequate perfusion and oxygenation of the viscera.

3. Sucralfate react\s with hydrochloric acid to form a complex that binds to proteinaceous exudates at ulcers and protects the site from further damage by pepsin, acid, or bile.

    a. It may also stimulate prostaglandin E_2 and I_2 activity and therefore has a cytoprotective effect similar to misoprostol.

    b. It does not alter acid, trypsin, or amylase secretion.

    c. Sucralfate decreases the bioavailability and absorption of other drugs and may also cause constipation.

    d. The recommended dosage is 0.25–1 g q8–12h.

4. Cimetidine, ranitidine, and famotidine block the H_2 receptor on the basolateral membrane of the parietal cells of the stomach.

    a. These agents, by virtue of increasing gastric fluid pH, may allow repopulation of the stomach and mouth with potentially pathogenic organisms, which in turn predisposes to nosocomial pneumonia.

    b. Dosages

Cimetidine: 5–10 mg/kg PO, IV, or IM q6–8h
Ranitidine: 0.5–2 mg/kg PO, IV, or IM q8–12h
Famotidine: 0.5–1 mg/kg PO, SC q12–24h

5. Omeprazole is a gastric proton pump inhibitor. In an acid environment, it is activated to a sulfonamide that binds irreversibly to the H^+/K^+ ex-

---

TREATMENT GUIDELINES FOR SEPTIC ANIMALS (*continued*)

Oliguria despite adequate volume replacement
  Low-dose dopamine (1–3 μg/kg/min CRI)
  Mannitol, 0.5–2 g/kg IV
If desired, administer either glucocorticoids OR NSAIDS (controversial—see text for discussion)
Correct hypoglycemia
  0.25–0.5 g/kg 50% dextrose as needed or 5–10% drip
  Consider glucose–insulin–potassium infusion (3 g glucose + 1 U insulin + 0.5 mEq KCI per kg given over 4–6 h)
Correct acid–base and electrolyte imbalance
  Do not exceed 0.5 mEq/kg/h of KCI infusion
  Base deficit × 0.3 × BW (kg) = mEq NaHCO₃ to correct deficit. Give ¼ by slow IV bolus and remainder over 6–12 h.
For hypotension despite adequate fluid loading, consider pressor agents, narcotic antagonist
  Dopamine, 5–10 μg/kg/min
  Norepinephrine, 1–10 μg/kg/min
  Naloxone, 2 mg/kg IV bolus followed by 2 mg/kg/h infusion
  Vasopressin, begin at .001 U/kg/min CRI. Decrease to .0003 U/kg/min or increase to .004 U/kg/min to effect

For peripheral edema
  7% NaCl in 6% dextran 70, 5 mL/kg IV slowly
  Plasma, hetastarch, dextran 70, 10–20 mL/kg IV
For reperfusion injury (experimental doses)
  Allopurinol, 15–25 mg/kg IV
  Mannitol, 0.5–2 g/kg (20% solution) IV slowly
  Deferoxamine, 25–50 mg/kg IV over 5 minutes
  Dimethyl sulfoxide (DMSO), 1 g/kg IV over 45 minutes
  Superoxide dismutase, 5 mg/kg IV
For respiratory decompensation (ARDS)
  Positive-pressure ventilation
  Avoid fluid overload

Provide nutrition
Consider placing gastrostomy or jejunostomy tube in animals undergoing abdominal surgery
Caloric requirement = 30 × BW (kg) + 70

Monitor trends closely
PCV, TS, BUN, glucose, electrolytes, blood gases
Mm color, CRT, heart rate, respirations, pulse quality
Blood pressure, CVP, pulse oximetry
Urine output

change ATPase enzyme on the secretory surfaces of the parietal cells. Dosage: 0.5–1 mg/kg PO q24h

6. Misoprostol directly inhibits gastric parietal cell acid secretion and is cytoprotective by increasing secretion of gastric mucous and bicarbonate. Dosage: 1–5 μg/kg PO q8h

K. Diffuse infiltrative pulmonary parenchymal disease, often referred to as **acute respiratory distress syndrome (ARDS)**, is a common sequela to several of the shock processes.

1. Pulmonary complications may be associated with
   a. Contusions secondary to trauma
   b. Hemorrhage secondary to coagulopathies
   c. Increased pulmonary capillary permeability as a consequence of the systemic inflammatory reaction
   d. Elevated pulmonary capillary hydrostatic pressure due to backward failure of the left heart or aggressive crystalloid fluid therapy
   e. Low colloid oncotic pressure

2. This diffuse infiltrative process decreases lung compliance and increases the work of ventilation.

3. As the process worsens, it causes small airway and alveolar collapse and increases venous admixture and hypoxemia. Oxygen therapy, initially, is palliative, but as the parenchymal involvement worsens, positive-pressure ventilation becomes necessary to reexpand small airways and alveoli.

L. Disseminated intravascular coagulation is caused by endothelial damage that exposes basement membrane collagen or by tissue damage that causes the release of tissue thromboplastin into the systemic circulation.

1. This activates the coagulation and platelet aggregation cascades.

2. DIC is an activated, hypercoagulative, thrombotic state associated with miliary microthombosis.
   a. This is seldom severe enough to cause measurable organ dysfunction, but it is associated with microangiopathic RBC fragmentation (schistocytes) and intravascular and extravascular hemolysis.
   b. Endogenous fibrinolysis leads to a rise in plasma fibrin degradation products, which tend to inhibit thrombin activity.
   c. Postmortem fibrinolysis may negate histologic demonstration of these microinfarctions.

3. A later hypocoagulative state (hemorrhagic diathesis) is induced by the depletion of platelets and coagulation precursors and the accumulation of thrombin-inhibiting fibrin degradation products.

MANAGEMENT OF ANAPHYLACTIC SHOCK

Clinical signs occur within minutes after exposure to offending antigen
   Restlessness, vomiting, diarrhea, shock
   Urticaria, facial edema

Possible causes: antibiotics (especially penicillin, sulfas, cephalosporins), vaccines, foreign proteins (antitoxins), exogenous ACTH or TSH, procaine, benzocaine, lidocaine, salicylates, antihistamines, tranquilizers, insect or snake venom, vitamins, heparin, iodinated contrast material, blood transfusions

If possible, remove offending agent (e.g., stop blood transfusion)

Peracute shock: add 1 mL 1:1000 epinephrine to 9 mL saline (1:10,000 dilution) and give 0.1 mL/kg IV

Severe hypotension: add 0.1 mL 1:1000 epinephrine to 9.9 mL saline (1:100,000 dilution) and give 0.1 mL/kg IV

IV fluids
Dog: 90 mL/kg/h to effect
Cat: 50 mL/kg/h to effect

Diphenhydramine: 1 mg/kg IM

Prednisolone sodium succinate 5–10 mg/kg IV

If hypotension continues, consider colloid infusion (5–10 mL/kg), epinephrine drip (1–10 μg/kg/min) or dopamine infusion (5–10 μg/kg/min)

Wean from pressor agent as soon as possible

a. This phase is associated with multifocal hemorrhage, prolonged coagulation times, and impaired clot formation.

4. Treatment
   a. Treatment of the underlying disease. Generous administration of crystalloid fluids to maximize microcirculation and to induce modest hemodilution is important.
   b. Heparin is used to treat the hypercoagulative phase: 200–250 units/kg SC q6–8h
   c. Fresh plasma is used to treat the hypocoagulative phase: 10 mL/kg

M. Nutrition should be started within 24–48 hours of onset of a critical illness.

1. Enteral feeding may be preferable to intravenous feeding because it preserves gut mucosal mass, gut impermeability, and mucosal immunity; reduces infectious complications and release of cytokine inflammatory mediators associated with a critical illness; and improves survival over that with intravenous feeding. Many critically ill patients develop a gastric stasis that limits the efficacy of feeding by this route.

2. Intravenous feeding is preferable to acute malnutrition, infection, organ failure, and death.

N. Adjunctive Therapies

1. Antisera to endotoxin, tumor necrosis factor, and platelet activating factor are protective when tested in the laboratory, but they were not demonstrated to be efficacious in the management of clinical sepsis.

2. Reactive oxygen-radical blockers, scavengers, and inhibitors have not yet been validated.

CHAPTER 5

ANESTHETIC PROTOCOLS FOR SHORT PROCEDURES

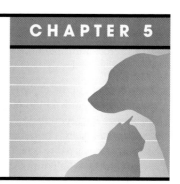

I. OVERVIEW OF ANESTHETIC DRUGS USED IN CRITICAL PATIENTS

A. There are six groups of anesthetic drugs—opioids, ketamine, barbiturates, etomidate, propofol, and the inhalationals—and three groups of adjunctive agents—benzodiazepines (diazepam), phenothiazines (acepromazine), and α_2-agonists (xylazine, detomidine, metdetomidine) from which to choose.

1. Drug selection is usually based on familiarity, patient needs, drug characteristics, convenience, and cost.

2. The choice of induction agent is the best match of pharmacologic drug-induced effects versus the preexisting physiologic disease-induced derangements.

3. As there is always a steep learning curve associated with any new anesthetic or technique, there is reduced efficiency and safety associated with them. New agents/techniques should not be learned on critically ill patients, which exhibit reduced tolerance for mistakes.

B. All anesthetic agents are dangerous and may be associated with adverse effects (including death) in precariously balanced critically ill patients.

1. It is most important to know the mechanisms behind the harmful effects of the drugs that you use.
    a. Most-common mechanisms include myocardial depression, excessive vasodilation (hypotension) or vasoconstriction (impaired tissue perfusion), hypotension, hypoventilation or hypoxemia

    b. Drug selection is most commonly based on avoiding additive or synergistic harmful drug and disease effects.

2. More important than the choice of agent is the manner in which it is administered. Give less and give it more slowly than you would to a normal patient.

3. Patient response to an anesthetic agent is unpredictable. Monitor patient response very closely.

C. The approximate order (least to most) in which the various choices are likely to induce excessive hypotension or impaired tissue perfusion

1. Anesthetic agents: opioids < ketamine, etomidate < barbiturates, mask induction with a gaseous agent < propofol

2. Sedative agents: opioids < benzodiazepines < phenothiazines, α_2-agonists

All anesthetics should be considered respiratory depressants with opioids > propofol > inhalational anesthetics in the lead. Respiratory depression is easy to manage as long as it is recognized.

II. GUIDELINES FOR ANESTHESIA IN CRITICAL PATIENTS

A. The generic anesthetic induction technique: Rules that apply regardless of the agent(s) chosen

1. Stabilize the underlying disease process as much as possible in the time available prior to induction.

a. Preoxygenate animals with respiratory compromise.

b. Correct severe anemia with transfusion or hemoglobin solution.

c. Volume replace hypovolemic animals.

d. Correct acid–base and electrolyte abnormalities in animals with impaired renal function.

e. Monitor ECG, pulse oximetry, end-tidal CO_2, and blood pressure during anesthesia.

2. Premedication may or may not be helpful or necessary.

    a. The animal should be outwardly and inwardly tranquil. Excited animals require higher induction dosages, predisposing them to overdosage or sympathetic-induced arrhythmias.

    b. Often this is accomplished by the underlying disease process, but if the animal is relatively awake and alert, a sedative should be administered.

        1) Opioids are a common choice.

        2) Benzodiazepines are unpredictable tranquilizers in dogs and cats without preexisting CNS depression when given alone but are often effective when given in combination with other agents.

        3) α_2-Agonists should probably be avoided in this group of patients because of their arrhythmogenic, early vasoconstriction (hypertension, reduced visceral perfusion), and late hypotensive effects.

        4) Phenothiazines and butyrophenones (e.g., droperidol) should probably be avoided in this group of patients because of their unpredictable α-blocking/hypotensive effects.

    c. Anticholinergics are controversial.

        1) They should be administered when an opioid anesthetic technique is used or when there is preanesthetic bradycardia.

        2) They should not be administered when a patient has hypertrophic cardiomyopathy, aortic stenosis, preanesthetic tachycardia, or tachyarrhythmias.

3. Draw the calculated dose of the primary anesthetic into a syringe, and into another syringe, draw a benzodiazepine (diazepam 0.2 mg/kg).

4. Administer about one-fifth of the calculated dose of the primary anesthetic. Thirty seconds later, administer the whole dose of benzodiazepine.

5. Redose the primary anesthetic at 30-second intervals until the desired effect is achieved (usually "intubatability" but not necessarily profound muscle relaxation [ketamine; opioids]). Monitor, monitor, monitor!

6. The animal can now be maintained by any of the above six anesthetic choices.

III. SPECIFIC DRUGS USED IN CRITICAL PATIENTS

A. Opioids used in "anesthetic" dosages are notable for their centrally mediated bradycardia and respiratory depression; but cardiac output, arterial blood pressure, and tissue perfusion are fairly well maintained.

1. Agonist opioids produce a state of deep narcosis but are not complete anesthetics like barbiturates and inhalationals.

    a. Animals that are well narcotized will move spontaneously and in response to noise.

    b. Immobility and total unresponsiveness are thus not suitable endpoints for the titration of induction doses of an opioid, as they are for the more traditional anesthetics.

    c. Opioid "anesthesia" commonly necessitates administration of an adjunctive sedative such as diazepam.

2. Oxymorphone and fentanyl are common choices for induction of anesthesia.

    a. Meperidine exhibits potent hypotensive qualities (myocardial depression and histamine release) and is not used to induce anesthesia.

    b. Morphine has been used but is also a potent liberator of histamine in the dog and may, therefore, cause hypotension when used to induce anesthesia.

3. *The large dosages of opioid necessary to induce an animal under general anesthesia precludes the use of this induction procedure in cats.*

4. Opioids are generally associated with a decrease in heart rate due to a centrally mediated increase in vagal tone, and an anticholinergic should be administered prior to the opioid.

5. Opioids are generally associated with minimal changes in cardiac output, systemic blood pressure, and oxygen delivery.

    a. Except for those that release histamine, opioids cause minimal changes in vasomotor tone.

    b. Opioids are considered agents of choice for induction of critically ill patients.

6. Agonist opioids are potent respiratory depressants, and animals should be oxygenated before and after their administration. Some patients may require positive-pressure ventilation.

7. Opioid inductions are slower than barbiturate or ketamine inductions. **Opioid inductions are not recommended for use in patients with upper airway obstructions or pulmonary disease or in patients with megaesophagus or full stomachs, when rapid access and control of the airway are necessary.**

8. Oxymorphone (0.2 mg/kg) or fentanyl (0.02 mg/kg) is administered IV in approximately ¼ of the calculated dosages until the desired endpoint is attained; diazepam (0.2 mg/kg) is administered after the first dose of oxymorphone. Remember, these patients may still respond to environmental noise and stimuli by jumping, raising their heads, or even sitting up, even though they may be quite intubatable (with finesse).

9. For maintenance, oxymorphone (0.1 mg/kg IV) or fentanyl (0.01 mg/kg IV) could be administered at about 20-minute intervals. Diazepam (0.2 mg/kg IV) must also be administered at periodic intervals.

10. To reverse or not at the end of the procedure:
   a. If there is excessive CNS and respiratory depression, the opioid should be partially reversed.
      1) Titrated doses of naloxone (0.01–0.04 mg/kg IM) or nalbuphine (0.25–0.75 mg/kg)
      2) Naloxone can also be diluted in 9 mL of saline and administered slowly IV to effect.
   b. If the animal can maintain its ventilatory and oxygenation requirements, it is best to allow it to sleep off the effects of the opioid and enjoy the residual effects of the analgesia.

B. Ketamine is notable for its centrally mediated stimulation of most cardiovascular parameters, with little change in systemic vascular resistance and only transient respiratory depression.

1. When used alone, muscle tone is always high and spontaneous movement is common; *always use an adjunctive sedative (usually diazepam) for muscle relaxation.*

2. Ketamine has a direct myocardial depressant effect and an indirect, centrally mediated, sympathomimetic effect that usually (but not always) more than compensates for the direct depressant effect.
   a. Ketamine increases heart rate and has a variable effect on contractility; this usually results in an increase in cardiac output. It is an induction agent of choice for patients with dilative cardiomyopathy.
   b. Ketamine should not be used in cats with hypertrophic cardiomyopathy or hyperthyroidism because of its sympathomimetic activity.

3. Ketamine causes minimal changes in peripheral vascular resistance and usually increases blood pressure and tissue perfusion.

4. **Ketamine is a transient respiratory depressant but may cause prolonged apnea in some patients. In critical patients, always be prepared to intubate and ventilate if respiratory arrest occurs.**

5. Ketamine is a rapid inducer and an agent of choice in patients with pulmonary parenchymal disease or upper airway obstruction.

6. It minimizes the laryngospasm, bronchospasm, and coughing reflexes. Animals under the influence of ketamine will swallow, and thus the incidence of aspiration may be lower than that with other anesthetics.

7. In most mammals, ketamine is metabolized in the liver to a metabolite I, which has 10% of the anesthetic activity of ketamine, and then to a metabolite II, which has 1% of the anesthetic activity of ketamine; the metabolites are mostly excreted in the bile.
   a. In the cat, ketamine is only metabolized to the level of metabolite I, which is mostly excreted in the bile. Very little ketamine or metabolite I is excreted in the urine in the cat.
   b. Intravenous ketamine is not contraindicated in a cat with a urethral obstruction but rather is indicated because of the critical condition of these cats.
   c. High doses of ketamine (IM or repeated IV boluses) should not be given to cats with renal disease, as prolonged recovery can result.

8. Ketamine is probably a good analgesic and an antiarrhythmic.

9. It is seizurogenic and should not be used in patients with seizure activity or patients undergoing myelography.

10. Ketamine should not be used in patients with head trauma or increased intracranial pressure because it increases arterial blood pressure and cerebral blood flow.

11. For induction of anesthesia, ketamine (10 mg/kg) is administered intravenously in 2-mg/kg increments at 30-second intervals until the desired effect is achieved; diazepam (0.2 mg/kg IV) is administered after the first dose of ketamine.

12. For maintenance, ketamine (2 mg/kg IV) may be required occasionally to smooth out the anesthetic. Recovery will be somewhat prolonged if repeated injections have been administered, since ketamine is cumulative.

C. Telazol is a combination of tiletamine (50 mg/mL) (a dissociative agent) and zolazepam (50 mg/mL) (a benzodiazepine).

1. The recommended doses are 2.5 mg/kg SC or IM for premedication, 2.5–5 mg/kg IV for induction, and 10–15 mg/kg SC or IM for induction; it may be repeated (1 mg/kg IV) for maintenance.

2. Telazol has all of the relative advantages and disadvantages of ketamine (see above).

D. Etomidate has minimal cardiopulmonary effects when administered in recommended dosages.

1. Etomidate is a carboxylated imidazole formulated in 35% propylene glycol (osmolality 4640 mOsm/L). Its **hypertonicity may cause pain** when administered via small peripheral veins and therefore *it should be administered by central vein or along with fluids in a peripheral vein.*

2. When administered intravenously in doses of 1–3 mg/kg, it causes a rapid, smooth induction of general anesthesia.

3. It undergoes rapid hepatic hydrolysis, resulting in rapid recovery and minimal cumulative effects following repeated dosages.

4. Etomidate is not a myocardial depressant or vasodilator; thus **it is a drug of choice in patients who are candidates for induction hypotension.**

5. Etomidate causes minimal respiratory depression. It does not cause histamine release.

6. Etomidate suppresses corticosteroid production for several hours following its use; however,

no detrimental effects have been attributed to this characteristic. If an animal "crashes" after receiving etomidate, corticosteroids should be administered during resuscitation.

7. Etomidate decreases cerebral blood flow and cerebral oxygen consumption as much or more than do the barbiturates; it is therefore **recommended in patients with head trauma or cerebral edema.** It also has anticonvulsant properties.

8. Muscle relaxation is generally good; however, myoclonic muscle twitching is not uncommon.

9. It does not have analgesic properties.

E. Barbiturates can cause acute myocardial and respiratory depression when administered as a bolus, but the stable, compensated anesthetic state exhibits mild hypertension and peripheral vasoconstriction; cardiac output and respiratory parameters are well maintained.

1. Barbiturates cause mild sedation to anesthesia, depending upon the dose.

2. Barbiturates can be potent myocardial depressants and peripheral vasodilators when given in intravenous boluses and therefore are not a favorite induction drug for patients prone to induction hypotension.
    a. Barbiturates should be titrated to effect with small (1/5 of the calculated dose) incremental dosages when administered to hypotension-prone patients.
    b. The barbiturate dosage can be decreased by adjunctive administration of diazepam (0.2 mg/kg) after the first small dose of barbiturate.

3. Barbiturates are also profound respiratory depressants, as are most anesthetics.

4. Barbiturates are arrhythmogenic and probably should not be used in patients with preexisting arrhythmias.

5. Barbiturates will cause a decrease in the packed cell volume due to the redistribution of interstitial fluids and splenic vasodilation and *should probably not be used in patients with borderline anemia and/or hypoproteinemia.*

6. Barbiturates are not analgesic.

7. Barbiturates enhance laryngeal reflexes, making endotracheal intubation more difficult, and bronchial reflexes, making *bronchospasm more likely in animals with preexisting asthma.*

8. Barbiturates will be more potent if there is an increase in the un-ionized portion (acidosis), if there is a decrease in the protein-bound portion (hypoproteinemia, antiprostaglandin or sulfonamide administration, in patients with hepatic or renal failure), or in situations in which the proportion of cardiac output distributed to the brain is increased (peripheral vasoconstriction).

9. Barbiturates might be preferred in upper airway obstructive or pulmonary diseases in which rapid access and control of the airway is important.

10. Barbiturates neither increase intracranial pressure nor alter vasomotor reactivity and do decrease cerebral metabolic oxygen consumption. **Barbiturates are indicated in patients with increased intracranial pressure or cerebral edema.**

F. The **inhalants** are also potent myocardial depressants, peripheral vasodilators, hypotensive agents, and respiratory depressants as a class of drugs, compared with the injectables. There are some differences within the ranks in that isoflurane is associated with the least myocardial depression but the most peripheral vasodilation.

1. Mask induction should be avoided in patients for which induction excitement would constitute a problem and in patients with airway obstruction or pulmonary disease.

2. Chamber induction can be used for very excitable or dangerous animals, but it increases environmental pollution considerably.

3. The rumor that the inhalational anesthetics might be safer induction choices than injectables is derived not from the inherent pharmacodynamics of these agents (they are more hypotensive than most injectable agents), but from the fact that mask induction takes time (homeostatic mechanisms have longer to compensate for the depressant effects of the anesthetic), and the inhalational agents are retrievable should the patient experience an adverse response to them.

4. As a class of drugs, the inhalant anesthetics are potent, dose-related myocardial depressants, hypotensive agents, and respiratory depressants.
  a. Apneic and cardiac arrest therapeutic thresholds: isoflurane > methoxyflurane ≥ halothane > enflurane
  b. Myocardial depression: enflurane > halothane ≥ methoxyflurane > isoflurane
  c. Reductions in cardiac output: enflurane > halothane ≥ methoxyflurane > isoflurane
  d. Reductions in systemic vascular resistance: isoflurane > enflurane > methoxyflurane ≥ halothane
  e. Hypotension: enflurane > isoflurane > halothane ≥ methoxyflurane
  f. Impaired tissue oxygenation: enflurane> isoflurane = halothane = methoxyflurane
  g. Respiratory depression (by steady-state Pa_{CO_2} measurements): enflurane > isoflurane > methoxyflurane > halothane
  h. Respiratory depression (by apneic thresholds, carbon dioxide–ventilatory response curves, and/or hypoxia–ventilatory response curves): All inhalational anesthetic agents are quantitatively similar.

5. Isoflurane is the least soluble of the commonly used inhalational anesthetics.
  a. Induction, changes in level of anesthesia, and recovery occur more rapidly. This may be disadvantageous, since deep levels of anesthesia can be achieved very rapidly and rapid recoveries can sometimes be excessively rough and hyperreflexive.
  b. Isoflurane and halothane have the same vapor pressure; thus it can be used in a halothane vaporizer, since dial settings accurately reflect vaporizer output.
  c. The MAC value for isoflurane is higher than halothane (1.5% versus 0.9%) and so higher vaporizer settings are required to maintain general anesthesia (1.6 to 2.0%) in the normal animal.
  d. Isoflurane is a good analgesic, like methoxyflurane, but unlike halothane.
  e. Isoflurane does not sensitize the heart to catecholamine-induced arrhythmias as does halothane.
  f. Isoflurane is approximately as hypotensive as halothane and methoxyflurane, but it has the least myocardial depressant activity of the three and is the most potent peripheral vasodilator.
  g. Isoflurane is the least metabolized of the three (methoxyflurane, 45%; halothane, 20%; isoflurane, 0.2%); it is least likely to be associated with "inhalational–anesthetic-agent" hepatotoxicity or nephrotoxicity.

6. All inhalant anesthetic agents are considered harmful to your health with exposure to very low concentrations for prolonged periods. Hospital exposure to trace amounts of these anesthetics must be minimized.

7. Inhalant anesthetic agents may be toxic to some organs.

a. Excessive myocardial depression and hypotension may impair organ perfusion, causing ischemia and hypoxia.

b. Reactive metabolites of several anesthetic agents have been associated with renal (methoxyflurane and to a much lesser extent enflurane) and hepatic (methoxyflurane, halothane, and enflurane) toxicity. These toxicities are rare and, for the most part, unpredictable.

G. Propofol is a potent myocardial depressant and peripheral vasodilator and, therefore, hypotensive agent.

1. Propofol is a substituted isopropyl phenol in an lipid emulsion.

2. Propofol is associated with very short (5–10 minutes), smooth recoveries, even after repeated doses (*propofol is not cumulative in the dog, but it is in the cat*). Rapid recovery is attributed to rapid redistribution and extensive metabolism.

3. Propofol causes some myocardial depression and is a potent peripheral vasodilator and hypotensive agent. **Although this hypotension is transient in the normal patient, propofol should not be used in patients predisposed to induction hypotension.**

4. **Propofol is a potent respiratory depressant, and apnea is not uncommon in critically ill patients. Be prepared!**

5. Propofol decreases cerebral blood flow and cerebral oxygen consumption and increases cerebral vascular resistance; like barbiturates and etomidate, it is indicated in patients with head trauma and cerebral edema. Propofol has anticonvulsant properties and is indicated in patients with uncontrolled seizures.

6. Propofol may cause myoclonic muscle twitching.

7. It does not have analgesic properties.

8. Induction may be associated with transient lipemia.

9. The dose of propofol for induction is 4.0 mg/kg with premedication and 6.0 mg/kg without. For maintenance, it can be redosed intermittently (1 mg/kg) or can be infused continuously (0.1–0.4 mg/kg/min).

H. Diazepam has minimal cardiopulmonary effects.

1. Benzodiazepines are not very good sedatives in dogs and cats that do not have preexisting CNS depression (disease or drug induced). They seldom tranquilize and frequently cause CNS excitation when used as a sole agent.

2. Benzodiazepines are most commonly used in critical patients concurrently with a more potent sedative, thus allowing decreased dosage of the primary drug.

I. Acepromazine is an unpredictable vasodilator/hypotensive agent. Phenothiazine tranquilizers should be avoided in hypotension-prone patients.

J. α_2-Agonists (medetomidine, xylazine) cause myocardial depression, lower the threshold to ventricular arrhythmias, and initially cause peripheral vasoconstriction and then centrally mediated vasodilation.

1. **α_2-Agonists should be avoided in visceral organ disease, dilative cardiomyopathy, head trauma, and ventricular arrhythmias.**

2. Depressed cardiac function limits the use of xylazine and medetomidine to young healthy animals. In this group fully reversible profound chemical restraint can be achieved.

3. Xylazine causes emesis in 85% of cats.

4. Reversal agents
a. Yohimbine: use the same volume as xylazine slowly IV
b. Antipamezole: 0.75–1 mg/m^2 (see chart on bottle)

IV. ANESTHESIA CONCERNS AND PROTOCOLS FOR COMMON CONDITIONS

A. Appendix K lists problems by system that are commonly encountered in critically ill patients and the precautions and recommendations for choosing appropriate anesthetic drugs for these patients (p. 485).

B. Dosages of recommended drugs can be found in the next section, "Anesthetic Dosages for Healthy Patients" (p. 44).

C. The clinician is encouraged to read about precautions listed for individual drugs in the preceding section, "Specific Drugs Used in Critical Patients" (p. 39).

V. ANESTHETIC DOSAGES FOR HEALTHY PATIENTS

(*Note:* Dosage reduction may be needed in critical patients.)

A. Premedications. (Table 5.1)

1. Used to minimize stress, ease restraint, provide smoother induction and recovery, allow dosage reduction of induction drugs, and minimize side effects

2. Premedication combinations

Acepromazine 0.02–0.05 mg/kg + butorphanol 0.1 mg/kg IM; dog

TABLE 5.1
PRE-ANESTHETIC DRUG DOSAGES FOR HEALTHY PATIENTS

Drug	Dosage	Onset/Duration	Comments
Anticholinergics:			
Glycopyrrolate (0.2 mg/mL)	0.01 mg/kg SC, IM, IV—dog, cat	20–40 min IM/ 2–4 h	Does not cross blood-brain barrier; preferred in C-sections
Atropine sulfate (0.4 mg/mL)	0.02–0.04 mg/kg SC, IM 0.02 mg/kg IV—dog, cat MAX DOSE: 3 mL	Route dependent/ 60–90 min	Reduces secretions; prevents bradycardia; use with narcotics, xylazine, ketamine and in brachycephalic dogs (excess vagal tone)
Sedatives/tranquilizers/dissociatives			
Acepromazine	0.05–0.1 mg/kg SC, IM 0.02–0.05 mg/kg IV—dog, cat MAX DOSE: 3 mg	Route dependent/ 2–3 h	Use lower doses in geriatric and large dogs; can cause hypotension; lowers seizure threshold
Diazepam	0.1–0.2 mg/kg SC, IM—dog, cat	minutes/1–2 h	Caution with severe liver disease. May form precipitate if mixed with other drugs. Use separate syringe
Midazolam	0.1–0.2 mg/kg SC, IM—dog, cat	minutes/30 min	Commonly used as combination agent with Ketamine or Opioids
Droperidol	0.03–0.02 mg/kg SC, IM—dog		
Ketamine	3–8 mg/kg SC, IM—cat	5–10 min	Poor muscle relaxation; contraindicated in head trauma, epilepsy, myelography
Telazol	2.5–5.0 mg/kg SC, IM—dog, cat	Minutes/40 min	Similar to Ketamine/Valium combinations
Oxymorphone (1.5 mg/mL)	0.04–0.06 mg/kg SC, IM—dog, cat	Route dependent/ 2–6 h	Often causes panting respiration; do not exceed 4 mg/dog
Fentanyl (0.05 mg/mL)	5–10 μg/kg SC, IM—dog		Expensive but very safe

Acepromazine 0.02–0.05 mg/kg + oxymorphone 0.04 mg/kg SC IM; dog
Acepromazine 0.02–0.05 mg/kg + fentanyl 5–10 μg/kg SC, IM; dog, cat
Acepromazine 0.02–0.05 mg/kg + meperidine 4.0–5.0 mg/kg SC, IM; dog, cat

Acepromazine 0.02–0.05 mg/kg + ketamine 3.0–5.0 mg/kg IM; cat

B. Induction agents: Rapid induction is preferred in dyspneic patients when airway must be secured quickly. Titrate to effect (Table 5-2).

TABLE 5.1
(continued)

Morphine (15 mg/mL)	0.5–1.0 mg/kg SC, IM—dog	15 min/2–4 h	May cause vomiting and diarrhea, then constipation
Butorphanol (10 mg/mL)	0.2–0.4 mg/kg SC, IM—dog, cat	15–30 min/ 2–4 h	Ceiling effect at 0.4 mg/kg (do not exceed)
Buprenorphine (0.3 mg/mL)	5–20 μg/kg SC, IM—dog, cat	15–30 min/ 6–8 h	Long lasting; least respiratory depression of opioids
Innovar-vet	0.02–0.04 mg/kg SC, IM—dog	15–30 min/ 1–2 h	
Meperidine	2.0–5.0 mg/kg SC, IM—dog		

TABLE 5.2
INDUCTION AGENT DOSAGES FOR HEALTHY PATIENTS

Drug	Dosage	Onset/Duration	Comments
Thiamylal	10 mg/kg IV	Seconds/minutes	Use 2% dog, 1% cat
Thiopental	10–15 mg/kg IV with premeds; 20 mg/kg IV without—dog, cat	Seconds/minutes	Give ½ rapidly, then titrate; redistributed to fat; avoid redosing sighthounds, lean animals; apnea and arrhythmias; extravasation causes tissue damage
Methohexital	6.0 mg/kg IV—dog (2%)	Seconds/minutes	Ultrashort acting; requires premeds for smooth induction and recovery
Propofol	4.0 mg/kg IV with premeds; 6.0 mg/kg IV without—dog, cat	Seconds/minutes	Discard unused portion; no excitement phase; give 25% q30s until intubation; can maintain with 100–400 μg/kg CRI or intermittent boluses of 0.5–2 mg/kg IV
Ketamine	2.2–10.0 mg/kg IV— dog, cat	Seconds/dose dependent–30 min	Never sole agent in dog; mix 50:50 with diazepam and give 1 mL/10 kg IV

(continued)

TABLE 5.2
INDUCTION AGENT DOSAGES FOR HEALTHY PATIENTS (continued)

Drug	Dosage	Onset/Duration	Comments
Telazol	8 mg/kg IV	Seconds/30–40 min	Similar to Ketamine/Valium
Etomidate	1 mg/kg IV + diazepam 0.2–0.5 mg/kg IV— dog, cat	Seconds/30–60 min	Expensive, painful (give with fluids); safe drug for critical patients but cannot reverse
Innovar-Vet	0.04 mL/kg IV—dog	Minutes/1–2 h	
Oxymorphone or Hydromorphone	0.2 mg/kg IV + diazepam 0.2 mg/kg IV—dog	Minutes/30–60 min	Can repeat 0.05–0.1 mg/kg IV q20 min prn
Fentanyl (0.05 mg/mL)	10 μg/kg IV + diazepam; 0.2–0.5 mg/kg IV—dog	Seconds/30–60 min	Can maintain with 0.5–1.0 μg/kg/min CRI or give 5–10 μg/kg IV bolus q20 min
Halothane box	3.0–5.0% plus oxygen 6.0–8.0 L/min—dog, cat	Minutes/hours	Good for fractious cats; can place IV catheter for sedation when cat is manageable; contaminates environment
Isoflurane box	4.0–5.0% + oxygen 6.0–8.0 L/min—dog cat	Minutes/hours	Good for fractious cats; preferred over halothane in older animals with cardio-vascular or liver disease
Isoflurane mask	0% increasing to 4% + oxygen ± nitrous oxide—dog, cat	Minutes/hours	Slow induction; use with premeds in old or debilitated animals
Halothane mask	0% increasing to 3% + oxygen ± nitrous oxide—dog, cat	Minutes/hours	Catecholemine-induced arrhythmias; use acepromazine as premed

C. Maintenance anesthesia

Inhalation Anesthetic	Loading Dose	Maintenance Dose
Methoxyflurane	1.5–3.0% Circle 1.0–2.0% Nonrebreathing	0.5–1.0% Circle 0.2–1.0% Nonrebreathing
Halothane	2.0–3.0% Circle 1.5–2.0% Nonrebreathing	1.5–2.5% Circle 1.0–1.75 Nonrebreathing
Isoflurane	2.0–3.0% Circle 1.5–2.0% Nonrebreathing	1.5–2.5% Circle 1.0–2.0% Nonrebreathing
Oxygen		20–30 mL/kg/min (min. 1 L/min) Circle
		200 mL/kg/min (min. 1 L/min) Nonrebreathing
Nitrous oxide		50–67%

D. Neuromuscular blocking agents (Table 5.3)

TABLE 5.3
NEUROMUSCULAR BLOCKING AGENTS

Drug	Dosage	Onset/Duration	Comments
Atacurium	0.25 mg/kg IV loading dose, then 3.0–8.0 μg/kg/min or 0.1 mg/kg redose	Seconds/15–20 min	Used for ventilator patients; must be ready with respiratory support
Pancuronium	0.06 mg/kg IV loading dose; 0.03 mg/kg IV redose	Seconds/30 min	
Vercuronium	50–100 μg/kg IV loading dose; 33 μg/kg redose or 1–1.7 μg/kg/min CRI	Seconds/	

E. Reversal of neuromuscular blocking agents (Table 5.4)

TABLE 5.4
REVERSAL AGENTS FOR NEUROMUSCULAR BLOCKING AGENTS

Drug	Dosage	Onset/Duration	Comments
Atropine Edrophonium	0.01–0.02 mg/kg IV 0.5 mg/kg IV	IV 20 sec	Administer atropine 5 min before edrophonium
Atropine Neostigmine	0.04 mg/kg IV 0.06 mg/kg IV	5 min	More muscarinic effects than edrophonium

F. Reversal of opioid anesthetics (Table 5.5)

TABLE 5.5
REVERSAL AGENTS FOR OPIOD ANESTHETICS

Drug	Dosage	Onset/Duration	Comments
Naloxone (0.4 mg/mL)	0.01 mg/kg; give ½ IV and ½ IM or SC 0.02–0.04 mg/kg IM—dog, cat	Minutes	Can dilute 1 mL in 9 mL saline and give slowly IV to effect, remainder SC
Buprenorphine	10–20 μg/kg IV given 15–20 min before reversal		Can retain analgesic effects and reverse CNS depression

G. α_2 Blocking agents (Not for use in critical, debilitated or geriatric patients)

TABLE 5.6 ALPHA-2 BLOCKING AGENTS			
Drug	Dosage	Onset/Duration	Comments
Medetomidine (1 mg/mL) (Domitor)	0.75 mg/m^2 IV, 1.0 mg/m^2 IM—dog (as per label dose)	Minutes/30–40 min	Severe bradycardia
Atipamezole (5 mg/mL) (Antisedan)	0.75–1 mg/m^2 IM	Minutes	Use chart on label to reverse medetomidine
Xylazine (20 mg/mL)	0.22–0.44 mg/kg IV, IM, SC	Route dependent/ minutes	Bradycardia, cardiac + respiratory depression
Yohimbine	Equal volume to xylazine IV	Minutes	Reversal agent

VI. INJECTABLE DRUG COMBINATIONS FOR SHORT PROCEDURES

A. Ketamine 6 mg/kg IV and diazepam 0.3 mg/kg IV; mix 50:50 volume, and administer 1 mL/20 lb, IV (cats and dogs)

B. Acepromazine 0.05 mg/kg IV or IM mixed with oxymorphone (0.05 mg/kg IV or IM) OR butorphanol (0.2 mg/kg IV or IM). Reverse with naloxone. Hydromorphone can be used in place of oxymorphone.

C. Atropine 0.04 mg/kg IM mixed with acepromazine 0.05 mg/kg IM. Wait 10–15 minutes, then give xylazine 0.22 mg/kg IV with butorphanol 0.22 mg/kg IV

1. Use for bandage change, radiographs, etc. in cardiovascularly stable patients

2. Reverse with yohimbine.

D. BAG: butorphanol 4 mL (40 mg), acepromazine 0.5 mL (5 mg), glycopyrrolate 5 mL (or atropine 8 mL). Fill to 20 mL with sterile water. Administer 1 mL/20 lb (0.1 mL/kg) IV or IM for sedation/ restraint. Can be given orally (1 mL/10 lb) to unruly patients.

E. Glycopyrrolate 0.02 mg/kg IM, then medetomidine 10–20 μg/kg IM and butorphanol 0.2–0.4 mg/kg IM; use only in young healthy animals.

F. Ketamine 3 mg/kg IM and medetomidine 30 μg/kg IM (dog). Anticholinergic is not needed, as ketamine keeps the heart rate up.

G. "Cat cocktail"—equal volume of medetomidine 25 μg/kg IM, ketamine 2.5 mg/kg IM, and butorphanol 0.25 mg/kg IM. You can reduce dose of medetomidine for less sedation.

H. For older patients: butorphanol 0.2–0.4 mg/kg IM or oxymorphone 0.11–0.22 mg/kg IV or IM AND diazepam or midazolam 0.2–0.4 mg/kg IV or IM. General anesthesia can be induced with 2–3 mg/kg of thiopental or ketamine IV following the initial examination or diagnostic procedure.

VII. PAIN MANAGEMENT IN CRITICAL PATIENTS

A. Overview, recognition of need for analgesia

1. Discomfort encompasses a broad range of adverse sensory and emotional experiences, of which pain is only one form. When discomfort is great enough or prolonged enough to alter normal behavior or activity, the recipient is said to be suffering.

2. Nocioception is the neural response to a noxious stimulus that causes tissue damage.

3. Pain is the perceived unpleasantness of a physical noxious stimulus that would evoke a protective avoidance response.

   a. The pain perception threshold is approximately the same for most mammalian species.

   b. The pain tolerance threshold varies widely, even within a species; environment and personality have a great deal to do with it.

4. The presence of pain in an animal and the need for analgesic therapy depends upon the observation of behavioral changes or abnormalities in the animal that can be reasonably attributed to pain.

   a. Since pain is a perceptual thing (it is in the eyes of the beholder), it cannot be defined precisely in another being or animal.

   b. Client-owned dogs and cats are untrained in the ways to pain, as laboratory animals can be.

5. Mild pain is subclinical and unidentifiable because it is not associated with any behavioral changes.

   a. It might be equated with the amount that is a nuisance, for which persons wouldn't go out of their way to seek an analgesic.

   b. Animals will go about their daily activity.

6. Severe pain is intolerable.

   a. The animal may throw itself about its cage in an apparent mindless frenzy simply because it cannot deal with it in any other way.

   b. Unprovoked vocalizing (crying, whimpering) in an animal that does not have CNS disease and is not recovering from anesthesia, and does have a disease that might be painful, is also taken as evidence of severe pain.

7. Moderate pain is the area in which caregivers need to be the most vigilant.

   a. The pain signs may be very subtle.

   b. Pain signs are not specific to pain.

   c. History of surgery or disease that is reported to be painful in humans is reason to suspect that an animal might be in pain, but it is not the *definition* of pain in that animal.

   d. Pain signs (in no particular order):

      1) Increased activity—animal assumes abnormal postures or positions in an attempt to relieve the pain.

      2) Decreased activity—animal may move, but infrequently and stiffly, as if to guard and protect the painful area.

      3) Decreased appetite

      4) An anxious, "worried" expression

      5) A disinterested expression ("staring off into space")

      6) Doesn't rest comfortably or sleep

      7) Less tolerant of caregiver manipulation

      8) Responds inappropriately when area is touched

        a) Splints body against "the assault"

        b) Moves away from stimulus

        c) Cries out

        d) Bites

      9) Responds inappropriately when area is approached (before it is touched) (as above)

      10) Tachycardia, tachypnea, hypertension, arrhythmias, dilated pupils, salivation, and/or hyperglycemia

      11) A positive response (a normalization of one or several of the above signs) to the administration of an analgesic.

8. None of the "pain signs" are specific to pain, and there are many nonpainful situations in which they might appear.

   a. When it is not clear whether an animal is experiencing pain and thus not clear whether analgesics should be administered, it is appropriate to administer a test dose of an analgesic and monitor the response closely.

   b. A favorable response supports the diagnosis.

   c. A favorable response necessitates continued therapy.

9. Analgesics should be administered on a regular schedule and based on their duration of action rather than allowing them to wear off so that the animal exhibits clinical signs of discomfort.

   a. Stimulation of nociceptive pathways can result in hyperalgesia and reduce the efficacy of analgesic drugs.

   b. Sustained pain can delay recovery and should be addressed as soon as critical patients are stabilized.

B. Specific drugs used for analgesia

1. Agonist opioids, including oxymorphone, morphine, meperidine, methadone, and codeine, have been the drugs primarily used for analgesia therapy over the years.

   a. These agents, while very effective analgesics, cause dose-dependent CNS depression (dogs, primates, rats, and rabbits) or CNS excitation (cats, horses, ruminants, and swine).

      1) This difference in effect may be due to differences in the distributions of the various opioid receptors within the CNSs of the various species.

2) Very little of either CNS effect is seen with recommended doses of these analgesic drugs.

b. Opioids are associated with euphoria and psychologic as well as physical dependency in species that exhibit CNS depression. For this reason, these drugs are regulated by the Federal Bureau of Narcotics and Dangerous Drugs, and very careful records of their use must be kept.

c. Opioid agonists cause a dose-dependent respiratory depression, except when they cause CNS excitation.

1) Panting is often seen in the dog after administration of some opioids; this response is attributed to an effect on the thermoregulatory center, rather than a lack of respiratory depression. These animals generally are neither hypoventilating nor hyperventilating.

2) Very little of either CNS effect is seen with recommended doses of these analgesic drugs.

d. Opioid agonists generally have little adverse cardiovascular effect, although larger doses can induce a centrally mediated, atropine-responsive, increase in vagal tone and bradycardia. Hypotension may (rarely) occur due to bradycardia, venous pooling (morphine), histamine release (morphine, meperidine), myocardial depression (meperidine, fentanyl), and/or a central sympatholytic effect.

e. Emesis and/or defecation commonly occurs following opioid administration to a dog and occasionally a cat, because of stimulation of the chemoreceptor trigger zone. Vomiting is much more commonly seen in awake, healthy patients than in animals that are immobile.

f. Opioids (morphine) increase resting smooth muscle tone (peristalsis is decreased; bladder, biliary, pancreatic sphincter tone is increased). Constipation, tolerance, and physical dependence may be a problem with prolonged small-dose administration.

g. Dosages (see Table 5-7, Appendix E, p. 422)

h. Fentanyl patches (Duragesic, Janssen Pharmaceuticals)

1) Four transdermal absorption rates: 25, 50, 75, 100 μg/h (see Table 5-8 for dosages)

2) Onset of action: dog, 12–24 hours; cat, 6 hours

3) Duration of action: 3 days

4) Offset of action: 12 hours

5) Wear gloves when applying patches

6) If the animal is going home, warn owners about dangers of removal and accidental ingestion.

7) This is still a schedule II drug, and accurate record keeping is essential.

8) Uptake is probably variable, but the effectiveness is just like that of any other analgesic; it is a balance between the amount of pain and the amount of analgesic "on board." Ineffective dosing schedules should be supplemented with another patch or parenteral agonist analgesics.

TABLE 5.7
DOSAGES FOR AGONIST OPIODS FOR ANALGESIA

Agonist Opioid	Intermittent Dosing	Continuous Infusion
Oxymorphone	0.02–0.05 mg/kg IM, SC q4h	5–10 μg/kg/h
Hydromorphone	0.05–0.2 mg/kg IM, SC q4h	5–10 μg/kg/h
Morphine	0.2–0.5 mg/kg IM, SC q4h	50–100 μg/kg/h
Fentanyl	0.002–0.005 mg/kg IM, SC q2h	0.5–1.0 μg/kg/h
Methadone	0.2–0.5 mg/kg IM, SC q4h	50–100 μg/kg/h
Meperidine	2–5 mg/kg IM, SC q4h	0.5–1.0 mg/kg/h
Codeine	0.5–2 mg/kg PO q6h	NA

μg/h	Recommended Animal Size

TABLE 5.8
FETANYL PATCH DOSAGES

μg/h	Recommended Animal Size
25	Cat
50	Small dog
75	Medium-sized dog
100	Large dog

i. Oxymorphone has been our choice of the agonist opioids for analgesia, although it is more expensive than meperidine or morphine. Hydromorphone has recently become the opioid of choice replacing oxymorphone because it is less expensive and more readily available.

1) Morphine and methadone are reasonable alternatives.

a) *They are cheaper.*

b) *They may or may not be associated with more vomiting.*

2) Meperidine is not a very impressive analgesic.

2. *Agonist-antagonist opioids*

a. At least six classes of opioid receptors have been identified (Table 5-9):

TABLE 5.9
OPIOID RECEPTORS

Opioid Receptor	What It Mediates
μ_1	Supraspinal analgesia
μ_2	CNS depression, supraspinal analgesia, bradycardia, miosis, respiratory depression, hypothermia, constipation, indifference, euphoria and physical dependency
κ	Spinal analgesia, some CNS and respiratory depression, and miosis
σ	CNS excitation, anxiety, tachypnea, tachycardia, delirium, dysphoria, and mydriasis
δ	Spinal analgesia
ε	Unknown

b. Different opioids with different receptor affinities (weak, strong) and effects (stimulate, inhibit) in different species induce different clinical effects.

c. The commercially available agonist–antagonist opioids are σ-receptor antagonists and κ-receptor agonists, with variable μ-receptor effects (from weak agonism to weak antagonism). In general, they should be viewed as weak opioids.

1) They are not very good for severe pain.

2) They exhibit a ceiling effect within the dose range commonly recommended for clinical use.

a) *Higher doses are not associated with greater CNS or respiratory depression.*

b) *Higher doses are also not associated with any greater degree of analgesia.*

3) When mixed with an agonist opioid, the result is an analgesic state that is somewhere between the two.

a) Adding an agonist to an agonist–antagonist will enhance the analgesia.

b) Adding an agonist–antagonist to an agonist will diminish the analgesia.

4) Butorphenol has antiemetic properties and may be preferred in vomiting animals.

5) Buprenorphine is the longest-acting opioid and may be difficult to reverse, sometimes requiring up to 10 times the naloxone dose.

d. Dosages (see Table 5-10)

3. Antiprostaglandin drugs are effective analgesics for mild-to-moderate, but not severe, chronic somatic pain of an inflammatory nature in most species and for acute colic pain in horses.

TABLE 5.10
AGONIST/ANTAGONIST OPIOID DRUG DOSAGES

Agonist–Antagonist Opioid	Dosage
Butorphanol	0.2–0.6 mg/kg IM q4h
Buprenorphine	0.01–0.02 mg/kg IM q8–12h
Nalbuphine	0.2–0.8 mg/kg IM q4h
Pentazocine	2–5 mg/kg IM q4h

a. They are associated with GI ulceration, hemorrhage, and perforation due to the inhibition of mucous secretion.

   1) There is considerable interspecies difference with regard to this effect. Naproxen, tolmetin, indomethacin, and flurbiprofen are so prone to do this in the dog and cat that their use is not recommended.

   2) Antiprostaglandins may also be associated with afferent arteriolar vasoconstriction, especially when angiotensin II and norepinephrine levels are high (shock). This may result in a prerenal or vasogenic renal failure.

   3) Antiprostaglandins also impair platelet adhesion because of impaired production of thromboxane.

b. Recent interest has focused on different isoenzymes of cyclooxygenase.

   1) COX-1 (a constitutive enzyme) is responsible for maintaining healthy GI mucosa, functional platelets, and blood flow to certain tissues.

   2) COX-2 (an inducible enzyme) is synthesized by inflammatory cells.

   3) Nonsteroidal antiinflammatory drugs (NSAIDs) that selectively inhibit COX-2 (carprofen, etodolac) are safer antiinflammatory analgesics.

c. Dosages of clinically recommended antiprostaglandins (see Table 5-11)

d. Acetaminophen is an antiprostaglandin-like analgesic.

   1) It does not inhibit platelet aggregation nor cause GI ulceration or acute renal failure.

   2) Metabolism is associated with the production of a reactive metabolite that is normally scavenged by glutathione.

     a) Cats are deficient in glucuronyl transferase (for glucuronide conjugation). Toxic effects can occur after a single dose of acetaminophen.

     b) There is a limited supply of glutathione in all species.

     c) When glucuronyl transferase is depleted, the reactive metabolite oxidizes cellular protein, causing hepatotoxicosis; sulfur groups, causing further glutathione depletion; and hemoglobin iron, causing methemoglobinemia.

     d) Acetaminophen intoxication can be treated with activated charcoal, N-acetylcysteine, cimetidine, and urine alkalinization.

4. **Regional analgesic techniques** (Table 5-12)

a. Local anesthetics may be injected locally as a field or regional block for analgesia purposes.

b. Local anesthetics may be deposited into the epidural space, either in a single administration or repeatedly via a preplaced catheter. Lidocaine (1-hour duration) and bupivacaine (4-hour duration) have been used. The duration of action can be prolonged by admixing epinephrine (1:100,000 or 1:200,000 dilution).

TABLE 5.11 DOSAGES OF CLINICALLY RECOMMENDED ANTIPROSTAGLANDINS	
Antiprostaglandin	**Dosage**
Aspirin	10 mg/kg PO (dog: q12h; cat q48h)
Etodolac	5–15 mg/kg q24h (dog)
Carprofen	1–2 mg/kg PO q12h (dog); limit to 2 days in cat. For surgical pain: 4 mg/kg IV initially once, then 2.2 mg/kg PO, IV, SC, IM q12h if needed.
Ketoprofen	1–2 mg/kg PO, IM, SC IV q24h for ≤ 5 days
Ketoralac	0.3–0.5 mg/kg IV, IM q8–12h for 1–2 doses (dogs <30 kg); 5–10 mg/dog PO (dogs >30 kg) 0.25 mg/kg q8–12h IM for 1–2 doses (cats)
Acetaminophen	10 mg/kg (dogs only; do not use in cats)
Meloxicam	0.2 mg/kg PO, IM, SC, IV (first dose), then 0.1 mg/kg—Limit use to 2–3 days.
Deracoxib	3–4 mg/kg q24h for up to 7 days (dog)

TABLE 5.12
REGIONAL ANALGESIC TECHNIQUES

Techniques	Drug/Dose	Indication
Epidural opioid administration	Morphine 0.1 mg/kg in 1 mL saline/4.5 kg	Rear limb fracture and pelvic orthopaedic repair
Interpleural block	Bupivacaine (0.5%) 1.5 mg/kg and 2 mL saline injected	High abdominal surgery and postthoracotomy
Intercostal nerve block (two intercostal nerves, cranial and caudal)	Bupivacaine (0.5%), 0.25–1.0 mL per site (not to exceed 3 mg/kg)	Postthoracotomy
Brachial plexus block	Bupivacaine (0.5%; 2–3 mL) or lidocaine (2.0%; 2–3 mL)	Forelimb fracture repair
Intraarticular injection	Bupivacaine (0.5%; 1–2 mL) or morphine (0.1 mg/kg) in 1 mL saline/4.5 kg	Cruciate ligament surgery or postarthroscopy examination

c. Needle or catheter insertion into the epidural space is easy to learn and is well tolerated by the animal, although recognized problems include:

1) Sympathetic paralysis causes peripheral vasodilation and hypotension.

2) Motor paralysis to the hind limbs. Paresthesias while the block is wearing off may incite the animal to chew at the appendage.

3) If the block gravitates too far anteriorly in the epidural space, intercostal paralysis and ventilatory impairment may occur.

d. Other agents can also be used to provide epidural analgesia: agonist opioids, agonist–antagonist opioids, and α-2 agonists. The proposed advantage is analgesia without the adverse effects noted above for the local anesthetics.

5. Go-home analgesics (see Table 5-13)

a. Many of the familiar analgesic options are available only for parenteral administration, which limits their use after the patient leaves the hospital.

b. However, many oral analgesics can be prescribed for at-home use:

1) Butorphanol, morphine, hydromorphone, codeine, oxycodeine, propoxyphene, pentazocine, fentanyl patches, tramadol.

2) Aspirin, aspirin/codeine, acetaminophen, acetaminophen/codeine, ketoprofen, ketorolac, carprofen.

TABLE 5.13
USEFUL ORAL, TRANSDERMAL OPIOID AND NSAID/OPIOID COMBINATIONS

Drug	Dose (mg/kg)	Dose Interval (h)	Formulations
Opioid Agonists			
Morphine	Dog: 0.3–1.0	4–8	Tablets (various manufacturers): 15, 30 mg
	Cat: 0.1–1.0	4–8	Solution (Roxane Laboratories): 4, 20 mg/mL; suppositories (Roxane Laboratories): 5, 10, 20, 30 mg

(continued)

TABLE 5.13
(continued)

Drug	Dose (mg/kg)	Dose Interval (h)	Formulations
Morphine (oral) sustained release	Dog: 1.5–3.0	8–12	MS Contin (Purdue Frederick): 15, 30, 60, 100 mg: Oramorph SR (Roxane Laboratories): 30, 60, 100 mg
Codeine	Dog: 1.0–4.0	4–8	Tablets (various manufacturers): 15, 30, 60 mg
Codeine with acetaminophen	Dog: 1.0–2.0	6–8	Tablets (various manufacturers): 60 mg codeine and 300 mg acetaminophen; dose is mg/kg of codeine; toxic to cats!
Fentanyl transdermal patch	Cat: 25 mg Dog (<10 kg) 25 µg Dog (10–20 kg): 50 µg Dog (20–30 kg): 75 µg Dog (>30 kg): 100 µg	72–120	Duragesic (Jansen Pharmaceutica): 25, 50, 75, 100 µg patches; variation in transdermal uptake may be quite large; many factors influence rate and efficacy of absorption
Opioid Agonist-Antagonists			
Butorphanol	Dog/Cat: 0.2–1.0	4–6	Tablets (Torbutrol), Fort Dodge Laboratories): 1, 5, 10 mg
Pentazocine	Dog: 2.0–10	4–6	Tablets (Talwin Nx, Sanofi Winthrop): 50 mg pentazocine and 0.5 mg naloxone

6. Anxiolytics do not provide any analgesia, per se, but decrease the animal's concern about its environment.

   a. The clinical signs of anxiety are indistinguishable from those of pain.

b. When the "pain" signs persist after the administration of a suitable dose (or two) of an analgesic, it would be appropriate to administer an anxiolytic.

c. Dosages (see Table 5-14)

TABLE 5.14
DOSAGES OF ANXIOLYTIC AGENTS

Anxiolytic	Dose	Comment
Diazepam	0.2 mg/kg IM, IV	May be anxiogenic in animals without preexisting CNS depression
Midazolam	0.1–0.2 mg/kg IM, IV	Similar to diazepam
Acepromazine	0.01–0.03 mg/kg IM	May unpredictably cause hypotension
Pentobarbital	1–2 mg/kg IV	Higher doses may cause excess CNS depression
Xylazine	0.05–0.1 mg/kg IM	May have untoward cardiovascular effects

CHAPTER 6

FLUID THERAPY

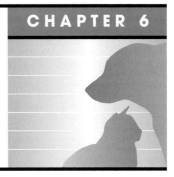

I. CRYSTALLOID SOLUTIONS

A. Crystalloids are fluids containing electrolytes or glucose molecules that are capable of entering all body fluid compartments.

1. Electrolytes are small: sodium has a molecular weight (MW) of 23 and that of glucose is 180.

2. Colloids are much larger, with molecular masses starting at about 10,000 kilodaltons (kDa). These molecular size differences have huge physiologic implications (described below).

B. They may be isotonic, hypertonic, or hypotonic.

1. These terms relate the sodium concentration (usually) of the fluid or the osmolality (for fluids that contain no sodium) to that of normal plasma.

2. Isotonic solutions have a sodium concentration or osmolality about equal to that of normal plasma. Because the electrolyte composition is similar to that of plasma, these fluids are considered replacement fluids and can be administered rapidly to treat shock or dehydration.

3. Hypertonic solutions have a sodium concentration/osmolality that exceeds that of normal plasma. This hypertonicity causes a temporary and immediate fluid shift from the interstitium to the vascular space.

4. Hypotonic solutions have a sodium concentration/osmolality that is less than that of normal plasma. These fluids should not be administered rapidly as replacement fluids, as red blood cell lysis may occur. Indications include hypernatremia, hyperkalemia, hyperosmolality, congestive heart failure, and liver disease.

5. Dextrose-in-water solutions are considered separately

a. They have no sodium (or any other electrolytes)

b. Their osmolality in the bottle depends upon the glucose concentration.

    1) Each 1% increment contributes 50 mOsm/kg.

    2) A 2.5% solution would be hypotonic (125 mOsm/kg).

    3) A 6% solution would be isotonic (300 mOsm/kg).

    4) A 10% solution would be hypertonic (500 mOsm/kg).

    5) A 50% solution would be very hypertonic (2500 mOsm/kg)

c. In the body, however, the glucose is metabolized fairly rapidly leaving just the water.

    1) In the body, all dextrose-in-water solutions behave as if they are hypotonic.

    2) Therefore, irrespective of their concentration or osmolality in the bottle, all dextrose solutions are considered hypotonic solutions with regard to generic fluid therapy recommendations.

    3) None of these fluids are used for blood volume restoration because the hypotonicity can cause hemolysis.

d. 5% dextrose in water is primarily used for drug admixtures and as a free water source.

e. 50% dextrose in water is used primarily to supplement existing fluids to a desired glucose concentration.

    1) Add 50 mL of 50% dextrose to 1L of fluids to make a 2.5% dextrose solution.

    2) Add 100 mL of 50% dextrose to 1L of fluids to make a 5% dextrose solution.

TABLE 6.1
SODIUM CONCENTRATION AND OSMOLALITY OF COMMON CRYSTALLOID REPLACEMENT FLUIDS

Product (Company)	Sodium Concentration (mEq/L) (osmolality [mOsm/L])
Lactated Ringer's solution (many)	130 (280)
0.9% Saline (many)	155 (310)
Ringer's solution (many)	147 (314)
Plasmalyte 148 (Baxter)	140 (296)
Normosol R (Abbott)	140 (299)

TABLE 6.3
SODIUM CONCENTRATION AND OSMOLALITY OF COMMON MAINTENANCE SOLUTIONS

Product (Company)	Sodium Concentration (mEq/L) (Osmolality [mOsm/kg])
0.45% strength saine (Many)	77 (154)
Plasmalyte 56 (Baxter)	40 (110)
Normosol M in 5% Dextrose (Abbott)	40 (364)

C. The vascular endothelium provides virtually no barrier to the diffusion of sodium, other crystalloids, or water.

1. When isotonic crystalloids are infused into the intravascular fluid compartment, they rapidly equilibrate with the interstitial fluid compartment within 30 minutes.

2. The volume remaining in the intravascular fluid compartment is only 20–30% of the infused volume. The rest is in the interstitial fluid space.

3. This is why such large volumes need to be administered to achieve important and sustained augmentation of circulating blood volume.

TABLE 6.2
SODIUM CONCENTRATION AND OSMOLALITY OF HYPERTONIC SOLUTIONS

Product (Company)	Sodium Concentration (mEq/L) (Osmolality [mOsm/kg])
23.4% saline (Baxter)	2800 (5600)
7.5% saline	1200 (2400)
3% saline	513 (1026)
25% mannitol	0 (1250)

4. It is not that these fluids are ineffective blood volume expanders, it is that they are not very efficient, compared with other fluid choices.

5. They are, however, the only fluids that can be used to restore an interstitial fluid deficit.

D. The idea behind polyionic, isotonic ECF **replacement fluids** is that large volumes can be administered to a patient without adverse effects on normal electrolyte concentrations. Blood loss should be replaced by at least 3 times as much crystalloid. Not all ECF replacement solutions are created equal (Table 6-1).

1. To the extent that individual electrolyte concentrations of the various fluids vary from normal, the infusion of these fluids, especially in large volumes, will cause proportional changes in the patient's electrolyte concentrations.

2. Saline contains a high normal concentration (compared with normal plasma) of sodium and a very much higher than normal concentration of chloride, and nothing else.
   a. Large-volume infusion of saline should cause the patient's sodium to increase a little, the chloride to increase a lot, and the bicarbonate and potassium to decrease a moderate amount.
   b. Given some time or slower infusions, the kidneys will compensate for this fluid insult.
   c. Saline might be the fluid of choice if the preexisting status of the patient involves hypochloremia, hyponatremia, or hypernatremia metabolic alkalosis.

3. Lactated Ringer's solution contains calcium (3 mEq/L). To avoid formation of calcium precipitates, do not administer sodium bicarbonate solution or blood transfusions containing citrate anticoagulant through the same intravenous line.

4. Normosol-R and Plasmalyte 148 contain magnesium (3 mEq/L) instead of calcium and may help prevent magnesium deficiency in critical anorexic patients receiving prolonged fluid therapy.

E. The usual crystalloid fluids of choice for acute blood volume restoration are those whose electrolyte concentrations are close to those of plasma with regard to sodium, potassium, chloride, and a "bicarbonate-like" anion (bicarbonate, lactate, gluconate, or acetate).

1. Lactated Ringer's, Plasmalyte 148, Normosol R.

2. These solutions are economical and readily available and can be safely administered in large volumes to normal animals.

3. Other electrolyte concerns such as calcium, magnesium, and phosphorus are rarely an important consideration in the choice of fluids to administer to patients needing acute volume restoration.

F. Polyionic, isotonic, crystalloid fluids often need to be administered in large volumes to achieve blood volume restoration goals.

1. It may be necessary to administer 0.5–1 blood volume equivalent or more, titrated to the individual needs of the patient.
   a. Canine blood volume: 80–90 mL/kg
   b. Feline blood volume: 50–55 mL/kg

2. The endpoint of fluid administration for a specific patient is determined by the alleviation of the peripheral vasoconstriction, the restoration of an acceptable pulse quality, return of urine output to at least 1–2 mL/kg/h, and an elevation of CVP) to a high normal level (8–10 cm H_2O).

3. The restoration of preload does not, in and of itself, guarantee acceptable forward flow parameters (cardiac output, arterial blood pressure, and tissue perfusion). These parameters should be evaluated once preload to the heart has been reestablished, and further therapy implemented as necessary (a β_1-agonist if contractility is considered too low; a vasodilator/constrictor if systemic vasomotor tone is thought to be too high/low).

G. Isotonic crystalloid fluids can cause harm.

1. They are substantially redistributed to the interstitial fluid compartment.
   a. Interstitial edema, pulmonary edema, and cerebral edema are potential complications of large volume administration.
   b. Patients with low plasma colloid oncotic pressure, pulmonary contusions, cerebral trauma, fluid-nonresponsive renal disease, or backward heart failure are particularly susceptible.

2. Hemodilution of blood constituents that are not in the crystalloid fluid occurs.
   a. Anemia
   b. Hypoproteinemia (low colloid oncotic pressure)
   c. Hypocoagulopathy
   d. If any of these abnormalities occur, red cells, colloids, or coagulation factors, respectively, must be added to the fluid therapy regimen.

3. Heart failure patients are susceptible to fluid overload with any fluid, including crystalloids. High-sodium fluids should be avoided.

4. Renal failure patients are susceptible to crystalloid fluid overload if they cannot respond to the fluid load with diuresis.

5. Freshly lacerated/ruptured blood vessels (within the last hour) may exhibit rebleeding if subjected to an aggressive fluid therapy plan with any fluid.
   a. An increase in vascular hydrostatic pressure causes the rebleeding.
   b. Pulmonary and cerebral contusions, lacerated livers and spleens, etc. are very susceptible to this problem.
   c. Fluid therapy in these patients should be "conservatively aggressive."
      1) The goal is to be aggressive enough to pull cardiovascular function away from the "death line" and yet conservative enough to avoid rebleeding.
         a) Enough to make one complication non–life threatening without making the other one life threatening
         b) As in "partial resuscitation"
      2) The mean blood pressure should be maintained between 80 and 100 mm Hg. Hypertension should be avoided to prevent rebleeding.

H. Hypertonic saline is indicated when it is difficult to administer a sufficient volume of fluid rapidly enough to resuscitate the patient or when it is desirable to obtain the greatest cardiovascular benefit with the least volume of infused fluids (Table 6-2).

1. Large animals; ambulatory practices;

2. Hypertonic saline (volume for volume compared with isotonic replacement solutions) provides better volume expansion, higher cardiac output and blood pressure, and better tissue perfusion.

3. Hypertonic saline also causes prominent vasodilation.

4. As with isotonic crystalloids, the effects are short lived, but plateau effects are superior to those of normal saline.

5. Indications include head trauma and pulmonary contusions, when it is important to minimize interstitial edema from large volumes of crystalloid fluids.

6. The commonly recommended dose of 7.5% hypertonic saline is 4–6 mL/kg.

7. 23.4% saline can be diluted with two parts of hetastarch or dextran to create an effective solution for immediate resuscitation (4–6 mL/kg IV). This bolus is followed with 6–20 mL/kg/h of crystalloid fluids initially and decreased to 2–4 mL/kg/h after the patient stabilizes.

8. Hypertonic saline can cause harm.
   a. An increase in sodium and chloride concentration and osmolality, and a decrease in potassium and bicarbonate concentration
      1) Changes are moderate and of minimal clinical importance unless the patient has preexisting electrolyte abnormalities or repeated doses are administered.
      2) Hypertonic saline is contraindicated in dehydrated patients who have depleted interstitial reserves.
   b. Arrhythmias might be a problem if hypertonic solutions are administered close to the heart.
   c. Hemolysis might occur if hypertonic solutions are administered in small peripheral veins.

I. Maintenance fluids are rarely indicated in emergency situations but can be used for daily fluid therapy needs following replacement efforts (Table 6-3).

1. Electrolyte solutions are high in K^+ and low in Na^+ and CL^-

2. These fluids must be administered slowly (usually 2.2 mL/kg/h)

3. Normosol-M, Plasmalyte 56, 0.45% NaCl and 2.5% dextrose with 20 mEq of KCl added

II. COLLOID SOLUTIONS

Colloid therapy is indicated when the total protein is below about 3.5–4.5 g/dL or the colloid oncotic pressure is below 15 mm Hg or is likely to be reduced below this level with crystalloid therapy.

A. The colloids are also more effective blood volume expanders than are the crystalloid fluids and should be considered when the patient does not appear to be responding appropriately to crystalloid fluid infusion or if edema develops prior to adequate blood volume restoration.

B. A plasma substitute (dextran 70 or hetastarch) should be administered as a part of the fluid therapy.

C. Colloids, although more expensive per bottle than crystalloids, provide a better blood volume expansion effect and less interstitial expansion than crystalloids and maintain a higher colloid oncotic pressure. Their "cost:effect" ratio is not bad; they are cost effective.

D. Commercial colloidal solutions are isoosmotic (they are suspended in saline) and hyperoncotic in the bottle (Table 6-4).

The progressively higher colloid oncotic pressure of hetastarch and dextran 70 is due to greater quantities of smaller–molecular weight molecules.

TABLE 6.4 COLLOID ONCOTIC PRESSURE OF COMMON COLLOIDAL SOLUTIONS	
Colloids	**Colloid Oncotic Pressure (mm Hg)**
Plasma	Low 20s
6% Hetastarch	Low 30s
6% Dextran 70	Low 60s

TABLE 6.5
MOLECULAR SIZES OF COMMON COLLOIDAL SOLUTIONS

Colloid	kDa Range (thousands)	Average MW	Number-averaged MW
Albumin	69	69	69
Hetastarch	10–1000	450	69
Dextran 70	15–160	70	41
Oxypolygelatin	5.6–100	30	—
Oxyglobin	64–500	250	—

E. The artificial colloid solutions contain a wide range of molecular sizes (Table 6-5).

1. The number-averaged molecular weight represents the clinically relevant number.

2. Colloids below MW 50,000 are rapidly excreted in the urine and exhibit a short duration of action (2–4 hours).

   a. Left behind are the larger molecules of each fluid type.
   b. The sustained volume expansion effect of each colloid is remarkably similar, suggesting that the number of fewer, larger molecules remaining for each fluid type is approximately the same.
   c. Dextran 40 (MW 40,000) is readily filtered through the glomerulus and may cause tubular obstruction or acute renal failure in dehydrated patients. Its use is not recommended.

3. The initially greater increase in blood volume with dextran 70, as predicted from the much higher in-the-bottle colloid oncotic pressure is short lived and not clinically important except in patients susceptible to the harmful effects of acute volume overload.

4. The greater sustained blood volume expansion with hetastarch, as predicted from its larger molecular size is marginal and unlikely to be clinically significant, unless hetastarch is administered repeatedly on a daily basis, resulting in a large population of high–molecular weight polymers in circulation.

F. Cost is, of course, an issue when selecting a colloid. Costs vary with vendor, and veterinarians should determine their own specific costs. As an example, our "to-the-client" costs are shown in Table 6-6.

G. The artificial colloids produce a dose-related defect of primary hemostasis that is somewhat greater than that due to simple dilution when administered in large volumes.

1. They induce a von Willebrand's–like syndrome. Prolongation of APTT is attributed to a reduction in factor VIII:C activity. Prolonged bleeding time and decreased platelet adhesiveness is attributed to inhibition of the vWf:antigen activity.

2. While it is not expected that even large doses would induce bleeding in normal patients, these products should be used conservatively, if at all, in patients with von Willebrand's disease.

3. They may be viewed as therapeutic for the hypercoagulable phase of DIC.

4. The evidence would support only a small difference between the two colloids in this regard (dextran 70 having slightly more effect than hetastarch).

TABLE 6.6
COST TO CLIENT OF COMMONLY USED COLLOIDAL SOLUTIONS

Colloids	Cost per 500 mL
Dextran 70	$37
Hetastarch	$54
Plasma	$400

H. Dextrans are mixtures of straight-chain polysaccharides produced by the bacteria *Leuconostoc mesenteroides* or lactobacilli grown on sucrose media. Products with different molecular weights can be produced by acid hydrolysis of macromolecules.

1. Recommended dosage: not exceeding 22 mL/kg/day (dog) or 15 mL/kg/day (cat)

2. Can be given as a slow IV bolus for patients in shock (7–10 mL/kg) or as a constant infusion

3. Half-life of Dextran 70 is 12–24 hours

4. It is generally the least expensive colloid.

I. Hetastarch is a modified branched glucose polymer.

1. Starches are metabolized by plasma and interstitial α-amylase.

2. The half-life is 24–36 hours, but larger polymers may remain in circulation for weeks. Serum amylase levels rise to two to three times normal during infusion and may persist for 5 days.

3. Not associated with clinical bleeding but will prolong coagulation tests

4. Dosage
  a. 10–40 mL/kg/day IV bolus to effect (dogs)
  b. 5 mL/kg increments given over 5–10 minutes, repeated to effect, up to 40 mL/kg total dose
    1) Used for cats, animals with pulmonary contusions, head trauma, or hypovolemic cardiogenic shock
    2) Use the smallest dose possible to maintain mean arterial blood pressure at 80 mm Hg.
  c. Following the initial bolus, animals with SIRS can receive 10–20 mL/kg/day CRI.
  d. Usually administered with twice the colloid volume in crystalloids.

J. Gelatins

1. Oxypolygelatin is a bovine bone gelatin–based colloid in balanced electrolyte solution.

2. It does not interfere with platelet function.

3. Dosage: 5 mL/kg over 15 minutes to effect, combined with crystalloid fluids and continued at a slower rate to a total dose of 10–20 mL/kg/24 h

4. Volume effect lasts 4 hours

K. Albumin constitutes 50% of the total plasma protein and 80% of the plasma colloid oncotic pressure.

1. There are approximately 5 g of albumin per kilogram of body weight in the ECF; 40% in the intravascular space and 60% in the interstitial space.

2. The plasma albumin concentration is about 2.5–3.5 g/dL; that of interstitial albumin is about 1–1.5 g/dL.

3. Albumin synthesis is regulated by osmoreceptors in the hepatic interstitial space. Other intravascular colloids (hypergammaglobulinemia and artificial colloid administration) will decrease albumin synthesis.

4. Albumin has a strong negative charge and is an important carrier of certain drugs, hormones, metals, and enzymes and certain chemicals and toxins such as cations, anions, toxic oxygen radicals, and toxic inflammatory substances.

5. Human serum albumin is available in a 5% or 25% solution.
  a. The 5% solution is similar to the synthetic colloids in dosage and indications.
  b. The 25% solution increases vascular volume by five times the volume administered. The maximum dose is 2 mL/kg
  c. Although these solutions have been used in dogs, they are expensive and may result in anaphylaxis if given repeatedly.

L. Oxyglobin (Biopure, Cambridge, MA; 212-614-4673) is a synthetic colloid that also carries oxygen. It is:

1. Sterile and ultrapurified; there is no potential for the transmission of infectious disease.

2. Stroma-free
  a. It is nonantigenic and does not require blood typing or cross-matching prior to administration.
  b. Adverse reactions that have been associated with its administration include discoloration of sclera and urine, and vomition.

3. Polymerized
  a. It extends half-life in the body; once administered, it has a half life of approximately 24 hours at a dosage of 20–30 mL/kg.
  b. No renal toxicity

4. Bovine hemoglobin solution

5. Oxyglobin is supplied in packages of two 125 mL single-dose bags.
  a. It is deep purple.
  b. It can be stored at room temperature for up to 3 years. This is a real advantage for individuals who do not use much blood.

6. It is a plasma-phase, oxygen-carrying solution.
  a. The plasma or serum will appear red when the blood is centrifuged.
  b. Because it is carried in the plasma, it will not increase packed cell volume measurements, but will directly and proportionately effect hemoglobin concentration measurements.
  c. Because it is carried in the plasma, it may improve oxygenation of tissues in which vessel pathology does not permit passage of whole red blood cells. This may constitute a real advantage of this product compared with whole blood. More research needs to be done.

7. Useful for resuscitation from acute blood loss or severe anemia.

8. Plasma color change can affect blood chemistries that depend on colorimetry. Collect blood before administration or consult the company for interpretation of blood values.

9. It is expensive.

10. A dose is 10–30 mL/kg; repeated in 24 hours if needed.

11. PCV will decrease with dilution, but plasma hemoglobin can be monitored with a hemoglobinometer. (Should be ≥ 7.0 g/dL). A blood hemoglobin concentration of 7.0 correlates to a hemocrit of 21% (3X[Hb] = effective PCV).

M. Plasma also contains coagulation factors.

1. While all plasma is created equal, it does not remain so, depending upon how it is stored (Table 6-7).

2. In addition to albumin and clotting factors, plasma contains fibronectin, α-macroglobulins, antithrombin III, and antitrypsin.

3. Indications for plasma include sepsis, pancreatitis, other causes of SIRS, coagulation defects, DIC, hypoalbuminemia, and increased third-space losses.

4. The recommended dosage is 20–30 mL/kg/day, which can be administered over 2–4 hours if needed rapidly.

5. It takes approximately 22 mL/kg to raise serum albumin by 0.5 g/dL.

N. RBCs should be administered if the packed cell volume is below 20–25% (hemoglobin below 7–8 g/dL) or is likely to be reduced below this level with crystalloid fluid therapy. (See "Transfusion Medicine," pp. 284–286.)

III. SPECIFIC CONDITIONS REQUIRING FLUID THERAPY

A. Shock fluid therapy (blood volume restoration)

1. Recognition of hypovolemic shock
  a. History of blood, protein, or crystalloid loss
    1) Evidence of dehydration if it was a crystalloid loss

TABLE 6.7 EFFECT OF STORAGE ON PLASMA PROPERTIES		
Plasma Product	**What It Has Lost**	**Which Coagulopathies It Could Be Used For**
Refrigerator stored	Platelets and labile factors (V, VIII and vonWillebrands)	Pancreatitis, Hypoproteinemia
Fresh frozen (up to 1 year)	Platelets	Above plus hemophilia A, DIC, vonWillebrand's disease, and Vitamin K antagonism
Fresh (within about 6 hours of collection)	Nothing lost—it has everything	Above plus DIC and thrombocytopenia

2) Hemoconcentration (polycythemia, hyperproteinemia) if it was a pure crystalloid loss

b. Evidence of vasoconstriction
   1) Pale color
   2) Prolonged capillary refill time
   3) Cool appendages
      a) To the touch
      b) Toe web temperature/core temperature gradient
   4) Oliguria/anuria
c. Poor pulse quality
d. Low measured central venous pressure
e. Low measured arterial blood pressure
f. Low measured cardiac output
g. Small anterior and posterior vena cava and heart on imaging techniques such as radiography and ultrasound
h. Low venous oxygen
i. High blood lactate
j. Metabolic acidosis

2. Treatment: combinations of adequate volumes of fluids
   a. Fluids should be titrated to the needs of the individual patient, to achieve the desired goal.
   b. Treatment goal is to restore an effective circulating volume while maintaining concentrations of the various blood constituents.

B. Dehydration

1. Recognition of dehydration (Table 6-10)
   a. Decrease in skin turgor
      1) Tendency for the skin to stand in a fold after it is released
         a) Animals are, on average, 5% dehydrated when the skin returns to its resting position just barely detectably slow.
         b) Animals are, on average, 12% dehydrated when the skin stands in a fold after it is released.
      2) Be sure to check the same area (thorax) with the animal in the same position (recumbent) each time.
      3) There is very large individual variation in this sign.
         a) Variance can be as much as ± 10% points.
         b) We don't use this monitor because it is accurate, but because often it is the only even remotely quantitative parameter available.
         c) Emaciation also manifests as decreased skin turgor (you cannot differentiate).
         d) Obesity obscures the decreased skin turgor due to dehydration.
   b. Dry mucous membranes: Digitally evaluate the moistness of the gums and mouth inside the cheeks, compared with normal.
      1) Dry, tacky mucous membranes in the absence of panting or anticholinergics indicate dehydration.
      2) Excess saliva does not indicate overhydration; it may indicate nausea
   c. Oliguria in the absence of renal disease suggests dehydration. A normal response to dehydration is to reabsorb as much of the glomerular filtrate as possible to conserve water.
   d. High urine specific gravity is an expected finding with dehydration.
      1) Obtain a urine sample before fluids are administered if possible.
      2) Normal urine specific gravity for a dehydrated animal is >1.030.
         a) If urine is not concentrated, renal disease should be suspected and

---

TABLE 6.8
FLUID RESUSCITATION OPTIONS FOR SHOCK/TRAUMA

Crystalloids
   Dogs: 80–90 mL/kg
   Cats: 50–55 mL/kg
7.5% hypertonic saline: 4–6 mL/kg
Synthetic colloids
   Dogs: 10–40 mL/kg
   Cats: 5 mL/kg over 15 minutes; up to 4 doses
Plasma: 10–40 mL/kg
Whole blood: 10–30 mL/kg
Red blood cells: 5–15 mL/kg
Oxyglobin: 10–30 mL/kg, not to exceed 10 mL/kg/h

TABLE 6.9
TREATMENT GOALS FOR FLUID RESUSCITATION OF CRITICAL PATIENTS

Parameter	Optimal	Minimum/maximum
Loss of skin turgor due to dehydration	Normal skin turgor	Barely noticeable decrease
Packed cell volume (%)	30–40	20/60
Total protein (g/dL)	6–7	3.5/9
Albumin (g/dL)	2.5–3.5	1.5/5.5
Colloid oncotic pressure (mm Hg)	18–24	14/30
Vasomotor tone	Normal	Barely noticeable vasoconstriction
Urine output (mL/kg/h)	1–2	0.5/6
Central venous pressure (cm H_2O)	5–10	0/12
Arterial blood pressure (mm Hg, mean)	80–120	60/140
Cardiac output (L/min/M^2)	4.5	3.5/NA
Venous oxygen (mm Hg)	40–50	30/60
Blood lactate (mM/L)	<2.5	NA/3–5 mild; 5–10 moderate; >10 severe
Base deficit (mEq/L)	0 to –5	NA/–10

further workup of the kidneys performed.

b) Other reasons for inability to concentrate urine effectively include diuretic administration, hypoadrenocorticism, hyperadrenocorticism, diabetes mellitus, diabetes insipidus, and medullary washout.

e. Evidence of coexisting hypovolemia (but not necessarily shock): see "Recognition of hypovolemic shock" above

f. An acute change in body weight

1) Lean body (muscle) mass can be neither gained nor lost fast enough to effect important changes in body weight on a daily basis.

a) Day-to-day changes in body weight are mostly attributed to shifts in water balance.

b) The term "water" here does not refer to free water without electrolytes (which will always herein be referred to as "free water") but to water with electrolytes (mostly sodium and associated ions—variable concentrations of chloride and bicarbonate).

c) To distinguish them from loss of "free water," electrolyte-rich water losses such as those from vomiting, diarrhea, and diuresis will herein be referred to as "sodium and water" losses (or gains, as they relate to crystalloid fluid therapy).

2) The problem with day 1 assessments of dehydration is that we seldom know yesterday's body weight.

3) It is, however, an ideal way to track fluid therapy over the course of a hospital stay.

4) Third-space fluid losses can substantially reduce functional extracellular fluid volume but not be associated with a decrease in body weight (and may even be associated with increased body weight, depending upon circumstances).

5) If weight loss can be accurately assessed, dehydration can be accurately replaced by administering 1L per kilogram of short-term loss in body weight.

g. Electrolyte concentrations may change, depending on the nature of the fluid loss.

1) They are variable (hypernatremia and hypokalemia are common but not universal).

TABLE 6.10 PHYSICAL ASSESSMENT OF DEHYDRATION	
Estimated % Dehydration	**Clinical Signs**
<4	Not detectable
4–5	Earliest detectable signs: Subtle loss of skin elasticity; mucous membranes may be "tacky"
6–8	Decreased skin turgor, slight delay in return to normal position; dry mucous membranes; slight prolongation of capillary refill time; eyes may appear dull
10–12	Prolonged capillary refill time (>2 sec); dry mucous membranes; sunken eyes; tented skin stands in place; possible tachycardia and weak pulses
12–15	Pale mucous membranes, capillary refill time >3 seconds; signs of shock, dementia; death imminent

2) They are not good indices upon which to base the determination that the animal is dehydrated.

h. Measurement of packed cell volume and total protein usually reveals hemoconcentration and hyperproteinemia in dehydrated patients. Obtain serial measurements to assess the effectiveness of fluid therapy. Assessment of dehydration with this parameter can be masked by anemia and hypoproteinemia.

2. Quantifying the magnitude of the dehydration (deciding how much fluid to administer to correct it)

a. If an accurate, recent body weight is known, the deficit can be calculated from the difference between the current and the previous body weight.

b. If an estimate of the percentage dehydration based on skin turgor has been made, this number, multiplied by the current body weight in kg, is the volume of fluid that should be administered to correct the dehydration. Remember that volumes based on changes in skin turgor may well be inaccurate.

c. If there is reason to believe that the skin turgor sign is inaccurate because of obesity, emaciation, etc, then, based on other findings including history, make a best-guess estimate of the deficit—pick a number between 5 and 12%.

d. The accuracy or inaccuracy of deficit assessments will be based on the animal's response to therapy in the coming hours.

3. Sample calculations for correction of dehydration

a. Dehydration replacement:

% dehydration × body weight (kg) = liters needed

or

% dehydration × body weight (lb) × 500 = mL needed

b. Maintenance—various formulas are used; choose ONE

1) 1 mL/lb/h or 2.2 mL/kg/h

2) 30 mL/lb/day or 66 mL/kg/24 h for small dogs

3) 20 mL/lb/day or 44 mL/kg/24 h for large dogs and cats

4) Use chart (Table 6-11, p. 68).

c. Continuing losses: Estimate the amount lost through vomiting, diarrhea, polyuria, excessive drooling, etc., and add to maintenance needs and dehydration replacement fluid requirements.

4. Use a balanced electrolyte, isotonic, replacement fluid. Animals with acute dehydration should have their deficits replaced fairly rapidly (over 2–6 hours), while animals with chronic dehydration, hypernatremia, or hyperosmolality should have slower replacement (over 10–12 hours).

SAMPLE FLUID THERAPY CASES

Example 1: A 10-kg, puppy with acute onset of vomiting and diarrhea, 7% dehydrated (mm tacky, CRT—2 sec). Estimated losses of 50 mL q2h from vomiting and diarrhea. PCV, 48; TS, 8.0; Na, 150; K, 3.5; BUN, 40; glucose, 120

Solution: Use balanced electrolyte solution and replace the deficit over 4 hours
  Dehydration: % dehydration x BW (kg) = liters needed

0.07×10 kg = 0.7 L	= 700 mL
Maintenance (2.2 mg/kg/h): 2.2 mL/kg $\times$ 10 kg $\times$ 4 h	= 88 mL
Losses over 4 h = 50 mL/2 h $\times$ 2	= 100 mL
	888 mL ÷ 4 = 222 mL/h

The puppy is given 222 mL/h for 4 hours and reevaluated
  PCV, 39 TS, 6.5; Na, 150; K, 3.1
  mm pink, CRT - 1 sec, urine in cage

At this time, the puppy is considered rehydrated, and fluid therapy should be adjusted to cover maintenance needs plus continuing losses.

Maintenance: 66 mL/kg/24 h	= 660 mL
Losses:	= 600 mL
	1260 mL ÷ 24 h = 53 mL/h

Potassium is added to the fluids, since the dog has excessive losses and decreased intake. We add 28 mEq/L according to the KCl replacement chart. Effectiveness of therapy will be monitored by PCV, TS, Na$^+$, K$^+$, BUN, glucose, urine output, mm color, CRT, pulses, heart rate, and continuing losses.

Dextrose will be added to fluids to prevent hypoglycemia, or PPN solution will be given in place of maintenance fluids.

Example 2: A 10-year-old male castrated ketoacidotic, diabetic cat weighing 6 lb. The cat is 12% dehydrated (mm dry and tacky, CRT—3 sec) PCV, 42; TS, 9.5; BUN, >80; glucose, 450; Na, 160; K, 3.8; osmolality, 360 mOSm/L

Solution: Use balanced electrolyte solution and replace deficit over 12 hours

Dehydration: % $\times$ BW (lb) $\times$ 500 = 0.12 $\times$ 6 $\times$ 500	= 360 mL
Maintenance: 1 mL/lb/h = 1 $\times$ 6 $\times$ 12 h	= 72 mL
Continuing losses (polyuria) = 1.5 mL/lb/h $\times$ 6 lb $\times$ 12 h	= 108 mL
	540 mL ÷ 12 h

This cat will receive 45 mL/h over the first 12 hours to correct dehydration. At that point, the rate can be decreased to supply maintenance and losses (72 mL + 108 mL = 180 mL) over the next 12 hours, for a rate of 15 mL/h. Potassium will be added as needed, because insulin therapy, polyuria, and anorexia will make this cat prone to hypokalemia.

C. Potassium supplementation

1. Hypokalemia is the most common electrolyte abnormality in critical patients.

2. Common causes of hypokalemia in critical patients include
  a. Translocation of K$^+$ into the cell—alkalosis, insulin treatment, glucose infusions, diabetes mellitus.
  b. Decreased K$^+$ intake—anorexia, K$^+$-deficient fluids
  c. GI losses—vomiting and diarrhea
  d. Urinary losses—renal disease, osmotic diuresis, hypomagnesemia

3. Clinical signs of hypokalemia include
  a. Skeletal muscle weakness—cramps, rear limb weakness, ventroflexion of head and neck (cats)

b. Smooth muscle weakness—ileus, anorexia, vomiting, constipation
c. Mental depression, lethargy, confusion
d. Polyuria, decreased renal concentrating ability.
e. Death from respiratory muscle paralysis can occur with extreme hypokalemia.
f. Arrhythmias, myocardial necrosis

4. Potassium replacement can be administered orally, subcutaneously, or intravenously
   a. Oral K$^+$ supplementation: Elixer should be mixed 1:1 with water to prevent vomiting (solution is very irritating). Flavored potassium gel (Tumil-k) is more palatable.
   b. Subcutaneous K$^+$ supplementation: Solutions containing up to 30 mEq/L of KCl can be administered safely
   c. Intravenous K$^+$ replacement
     1) Rate of supplementation must not exceed 0.5 mEq/kg/h, or arrhythmias, cardiac arrest, or sudden death may result.
     2) See Table "Guidelines for Potassium Supplementation"
     3) Mix concentrate thoroughly when adding to fluids, to prevent iatrogenic hyperkalemia from high concentrations at the bottom of solution

D. Bicarbonate supplementation

1. Causes of metabolic acidosis
   a. Bicarbonate anion loss (diarrhea) or hydrogen ion retention (renal tubular acidosis). An inorganic acidosis such as this is not associated with an anion gap (hyperchloremic metabolic acidosis)
   b. Addition acidoses (organic acidoses) such as lactic acidosis, ketoacidosis, or renal failure acidosis are associated with an anionic, as well as an osmotic, gap, because of the accumulation of unmeasured anions/osmols (normochloremic acidosis).

2. The treatment of metabolic acidosis is primarily aimed at correcting the underlying disease process.
   a. If the metabolic acidosis and the pH disturbance are severe (base deficit > 10 mEq/L; bicarbonate < 14 mEq/L; pH < 7.2), the animal may benefit from alkalinization therapy.
     1) The decision to administer an alkalinizing agent depends heavily on the underlying disease process.

GUIDELINES FOR POTASSIUM SUPPLEMENTATION

(Use either scale to determine required amount)

Sliding Scale of Cornelius
The total daily dose of potassium is based on the prevailing K$^+$ concentration as follows:
   Mild K$^+$ depletion (K$^+$ = 3.0–3.7 mEq/L)
      Add 1–3 mEq/kg/day of K$^+$
   Moderate K$^+$ depletion (K$^+$ = 2.5–3.0 mEq/L)
      Add 4–6 mEq/kg/day of K$^+$
   Severe K$^+$ depletion (K$^+$ <2.5 mEq/L)
      Add 7–9 mEq/kg/day of K$^+$

Modified Sliding Scale of Scott

Serum K$^+$ (mEq/L)	mEq K$^+$ to add to 250 mL of fluid	mEq K$^+$ to add to 1 L of fluid	Maximum infusion rate (0.5 mEq/kg/h)
<2.0	20	80	6 mL/kg/h
2.1–2.5	15	60	8 mL/kg/h
2.6–3.0	10	40	12 mL/kg/h
3.1–3.5	7	28	18 mL/kg/h
>3.5 to <5.0	5	20	25 mL/kg/h

a) In diseases that are relatively easy to treat (diabetic ketoacidosis or moderate hypovolemic shock), alkalinizing therapy should be conservative.

b) In diseases that are relatively difficult to treat (severe hypovolemic shock or septic shock), alkalinizing therapy should be relatively aggressive.

2) The mEq of bicarbonate to administer can be calculated by multiplying the base or bicarbonate deficit that you want to restore by 0.3 × body weight (kg) or by 1–3 mEq/kg of body weight for mild-to-severe metabolic acidosis, respectively.

3) This dose must not be administered faster than it can be redistributed from the vascular fluid compartment to the interstitial fluid compartment (20–30 minutes), lest it cause alkalosis in the vascular fluid compartment. If administered as an intravenous bolus, severe hypotension and even death can result, presumably due to the rapid change in hydrogen ion concentration, hypokalemia, or hypo(ionized)calcemia.

b. There are several potential problems associated with the administration of sodium bicarbonate, including hypernatremia, hyperosmolality, shifting of oxygen-hemoglobin disociation curve to the left, drop in ionized calcium, transcellular shift of serum potassium, and paradoxical CSF acidosis.

E. Maintenance fluid therapy

1. The nature of normal ongoing losses

a. The net sodium concentration of the fluids normally lost over the course of the day (mostly urine and insensible losses) is 40–50 mEq/L.

b. The net potassium concentration is 15–20 mEq/L.

c. Replacement of normal daily losses should ideally mimic these electrolyte concentrations. Administering an ECF replacement solution with an electrolyte concentration close to that of normal plasma represents too much sodium and too little potassium.

1) Hypernatremia is rarely a problem, however, since a well-hydrated patient with reasonable renal function can readily eliminate the excess sodium.

2) Hypokalemia, however, is almost always a problem if the animal is not eating, because the kidney is not very good at conserving potassium.

2. Estimating the volume of the normal ongoing losses:

a. The volume of fluids required to replace the normal ongoing losses can be determined from predictive charts.

b. If a chart is not available, formulas used to construct those charts are

1) Dog: mL/day = $132 \times BW_{kg}^{0.75}$
2) Cat: mL/day = $80 \times BW_{kg}^{0.75}$
3) The range of daily fluid requirements is 50–75 mL/kg/day.

a) The chart will deliver higher values for smaller dogs and lower values for larger dogs and cats.

b) Fluid maintenance needs can be approximated by giving 2–3 mL/kg/h.

3. The kind of fluid for replacement
a. A commercial maintenance solution
b. An ECF replacement solution supplemented with 20 mEq of potassium per liter.
c. A homemade maintenance solution: 1 part ECF replacement solution and 1–2 parts 5% dextrose in water.

4. NEVER administer a potassium-supplemented maintenance solution rapidly for blood volume or deficit volume replacement.

F. Abnormal-ongoing-loss therapy

1. The nature of normal ongoing losses
a. Most vomiting, diarrhea, and diuresis exhibit similar concentrations for sodium and potassium. Bicarbonate is variable.

1) A "duodenal vomiter" regurgitates duodenal fluids into the stomach and then vomits a combination of duodenal and gastric fluids.

a) The net fluid is very alkaline.
b) Most vomiting animals are in this category.
c) Check for color in the vomitus.
d) Check the pH of the vomitus.

2) A "gastric vomiter" vomits only gastric fluids, which are acidic.

b. Third-space fluid accumulations have electrolyte concentrations which are the same as those for the ECF.

2. The volume of the abnormal ongoing losses can be estimated visually or measured volumetrically or by weight.

3. Abnormal crystalloid fluid losses should be replaced with an ECF replacement solution (lactated

TABLE 6.11				
MAINTENANCE FLUID REQUIREMENTS FOR DOGS				
Body Weight (kg)	mL/day	mL/kg/day	mL/h	mL/kg/h
1	132	132	6	6
2	222	111	9	4.5
3	301	100	13	4.3
4	373	93	16	4
5	441	88	18	3.6
6	506	84	21	3.5
8	628	78	26	3.3
10	742	74	31	3.1
12	851	71	35	2.9
14	955	68	40	2.9
16	1056	66	44	2.8
18	1153	64	48	2.7
20	1248	62	52	2.6
25	1476	59	61	2.4
30	1692	56	71	2.4
35	1899	54	79	2.3
40	2100	52	87	2.2
50	2481	50	103	2.1
60	2846	47	119	2.0
80	3531	44	147	1.8
100	4174	42	174	1.7

Ringer's solution is best because it has the lowest sodium concentration) with supplemental potassium (10–14 mEq/L).

G. Fluid therapy diuresis

1. Goal is to maximize renal perfusion and assist in excretory function.

2. An increased glomerular filtration rate (GFR) will result in decreases in BUN and serum creatinine and phosphorus.

3. First, rehydrate the patient.
  a. Oliguria is a normal response to dehydration.
  b. Oliguria is defined as <1 mL/kg/h.

4. If the animal is not clinically dehydrated but is not producing urine, administer a fluid challenge

$$5\% \times BW \text{ (kg)} = \text{liters to administer}$$

5. Once the animal is rehydrated, "Ins and Outs" can be used to determine continued fluid therapy needs.

  a. Place a urinary catheter with a closed system drainage bag.
  b. Measure output every 2–4 hours.
  c. The volume of urine measured is replaced with IV fluids plus 1 mL/kg/h added for insensible losses.
  d. Expected urine output is 2–6 mL/kg/h during fluid diuresis.

6. Fluid choice
  a. Initial fluid should be replacement fluid.
  b. Consider using maintenance fluids, half-strength saline, or alternating with 5% dextrose in water if hypernatremia develops.
  c. Following rehydration, 14–20 mEq of KCl are usually added to the fluids to maintain serum potassium in the normal range.
  d. Serum potassium should be checked initially and during fluid diuresis.
    1) Hyperkalemia is common in oliguric patients with acute renal failure.

TABLE 6.12
MAINTENANCE FLUID REQUIREMENTS FOR CATS

Body Weight (kg)	mL/day	mL/kg/day	mL/h	mL/kg/h
1	80	80	3	3
2	135	67	6	3
3	182	61	8	2.7
4	226	57	9	2.3
5	267	53	11	2.2
6	306	51	13	2.1
7	344	49	14	2
8	381	48	16	2
9	416	46	17	1.9

TABLE 6.13
ELECTROLYTE CONCENTRATIONS OF SOME COMMON ABNORMAL CRYSTALLOID FLUID LOSSES

Type of loss	Sodium	Potassium	Bicarbonate
Diarrhea	60–120	10–20	30–50
"Duodenal" vomitus	60–120	10–20	30–50
"Gastric" vomitus	60–120	10–20	0
Diuresis	60–120	10–40	0–24

2) Hypokalemia is common in anorexic polyuric patients with chronic renal failure.
e. During fluid diuresis, the patient must be monitored closely to avoid overhydration (see box "Signs Associated with Overhydration").

H. Partial parenteral nutrition (PPN)

1. Goal is to minimize ongoing destruction of body tissue in critical animals until recovery occurs or enteral food intake is possible.
    a. Recommended for short term use (<7 days).
    b. Not recommended for debilitated animals. These fluids will not provide enough calories to reverse ongoing weight loss.

2. Indications
    a. Malnourished patients, unlikely to eat for >3 days
    b. Patients that cannot tolerate enteral nutrition (vomiting, malabsorption, GI obstruction, pancreatitis, high risk of aspiration)

SIGNS ASSOCIATED WITH OVERHYDRATION

- Shivering, restlessness
- Serous nasal discharge
- Labored breathing, tachypnea, moist cough
- Chemosis, exophthalmos
- Nausea, vomiting
- Ascites
- Tachycardia—followed by bradycardia and cardiac arrest with severe overload
- Subcutaneous edema—especially hock joint and intermandibular space
- Pulmonary crackles and edema
- Pleural effusion (especially cats)
- Polyuria—dilute urine specific gravity
- Depressed mentation
- Weight gain
- Central venous pressure >13 cm H_2O or increase of >3 cm in 1 hour

c. These solutions can be used to supplement enteral feeding in patients that cannot tolerate full caloric intake enterally.

3. Definition

a. Provides partial energy needs (usually 50% of caloric requirement) and can be administered through a peripheral vein.

b. TPN solutions (total parenteral nutrition) provide 100% of caloric requirements and must be administered through a central vein because the solution is very hyperosmolar.

4. Available commercial products

a. Clinimix (Clintec Nutrition Co.; Deerfield, IL) contains 2.75% amino acids and 5% dextrose.

b. Quickmix (Clintec Nutrition Co.; Deerfield, IL) contains 2.75% amino acids and 5% dextrose.

c. Procalamine (Mcgaw Inc.; Irvine, CA) contains 3% amino acids and 3% glycerol.

d. Administer at maintenance fluid rates (e.g., 50 mL/kg/day, cats; 66 mL/kg/day, dogs).

5. "Homemade" PPN solutions

a. Formula 1: (Makes 1L of non-lipid-based PPN)

- Remove 352 mL from LRS with 5% dextrose

- Add 352 mL of 8.5% amino acid with electrolytes (Travesol, Baxter Healthcare, 1-800-544-6108 or Abbott 1-888-299-7416).
- May add 1–2 mL of vitamin B complex
- Solution is good for 48 hours if refrigerated, 24 hours at room temperature.

b. Formula 2: (Makes 1L of lipid-based PPN)

- 400 mL of 10% dextrose
- 300 mL of lactated Ringer's solution
- 200 mL of 8.5% amino acids with electrolytes
- 100 mL of 20% lipid emulsion
- May add 10–20 mEq of KCl
- Final solution is 546 mOsm/L and provides 337 nonprotein calories and 17 g of protein per liter.

6. Sterile technique is mandatory when preparing solutions.

7. Special attention must be directed to catheter care and maintenance in animals receiving PPN solutions, as complications of therapy include thrombophlebitis and catheter occlusion. If redness, heat, or swelling is detected at the catheter site, a new line should be placed and the old one removed.

CHAPTER 7

MONITORING CRITICAL PATIENTS

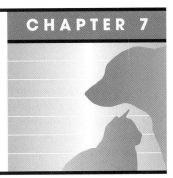

I. CARDIOVASCULAR MONITORING

A. Physical parameters

1. Mucous membrane color
  a. Red (injected)
    1) Suggests vasodilation (sepsis, drugs, heat stroke) and well-oxygenated hemoglobin
    2) Cyanide poisoning, carbon monoxide toxicity
    3) Hypermetabolic state (hyperthermia, pheochromocytoma, hyperthyroidism, hypertension, drugs)
  b. Pale to very pale—suggests that there is not much hemoglobin in the capillary beds of these tissues; anemia or vasoconstriction
  c. White—suggests that there is no hemoglobin in these tissues (SEVERE anemia or vasoconstriction)
  d. Blue
    1) Suggests that the hemoglobin in the capillary beds is not well oxygenated
    2) This may be attributed to hypoxemia or methemoglobinemia.
    3) Cyanosis may be peripheral (local ischemia) or central (global hypoxia).
  e. Grey ("blue + white")—suggests sluggish local blood flow and unoxygenated hemoglobin
  f. Purple ("red + blue")—suggests vasodilation and unoxygenated hemoglobin (sepsis)
  g. Brown—methemoglobinemia (acetaminophen toxicity)
  h. Yellow or orange
    1) Hepatic disease, bile duct obstruction, or hemolysis
    2) Hemoglobin-based oxygen-carrying solution

2. Capillary refill time (CRT)
  a. CRT is the time it takes for a capillary bed to refill with blood after the blood has been pushed out of the capillary bed with digital pressure.
  b. The dominant determining factor is precapillary arteriolar vasomotor tone. A prolonged CRT equates to peripheral vasoconstriction and vice versa.
  c. Vasoconstriction has many causes: hypovolemia, hypothermia, poor cardiac output, pain, and vasoconstrictor drugs.
  d. Normal CRT is 1.5–2 seconds.
  e. Dry, tacky membranes are consistent with dehydration.

3. Heart rate
  a. If the heart rate is too slow, cardiac output will diminish and hypotension may ensue.
    1) Bradycardia may be a problem in this regard when the heart rate is less than 40–60 beats/min.
    2) Bradycardia may be caused by excessive vagal tone (opioids, pain, vagovagal reflexes, oculovagal reflexes), atrioventricular conduction disturbances, hyperkalemia, severe hypothermia, terminal hypoxia, drugs (opioids, α_2-agonists, cholinergics, β-blockers), organophosphate or carbamate poisoning, or increased cerebrospinal fluid pressure (head trauma, neoplasia).
  b. If the heart rate is too fast, the heart will not have time to fill adequately and cardiac output will diminish.
    1) In addition, the short diastolic filling time leads to poor coronary artery perfusion at a time when myocardial oxygen and nu-

trient demands are increased. Failure to address this problem can lead to progressive cardiac dysfunction.

2) Tachycardia may be a problem in this regard when the heart rate exceeds about 180 in a large-breed dog, about 200 in a small-breed dog, or about 240 in a cat.

3) Tachycardia may be caused by hypovolemia, pain, hypoxemia, hypercapnia, hyperthermia, sepsis, drugs (ketamine, anticholinergics, sympathomimetics), hyperthyroidism, pheochromocytoma, shock, or heart disease.

4. Pulse quality reflects stroke volume.
   a. The "quality" or "fullness" of the pulse assesses both the height (the difference between diastolic and systolic blood pressure) and the width of the pressure waveform.
   b. Small stroke volumes can be attributed to poor contractility, hypovolemia, tachycardia, poor ventricular diastolic performance, ventricular arrhythmias, and aortic stenosis.
   c. A weak, thready pulse is consistent with poor cardiac output.
   d. The pulse should be palpated while the heart is being ausculted. Pulse deficits (heart rate and pulse rate are different) indicate an arrhythmia.

5. Toe web temperature
   a. Cool appendages suggest vasoconstriction.
   b. Appendage temperature can be assessed subjectively by palpation.
   c. Appendage temperature can be measured subjectively by comparing toe-web temperature to core temperature. The normal difference is 4° C (8° F).

B. Electrocardiogram (ECG)

1. An ECG records electrical activity in the heart and serves to identify arrhythmias. It does not measure mechanical performance of the heart: myocardial performance, cardiac output, or blood pressure.

2. Precise placement of the ECG leads is not necessary for monitoring purposes.
   a. The right arm lead may be placed on the right arm or anywhere on the right, cranial quadrant of the body; the left leg lead may be placed on the left leg or anywhere on the left, caudal quadrant of the body; etc.

b. Alligator clips provide satisfactory short-term patient attachments if the teeth have been filed and the jaws bent or padded to prevent pain and tissue ischemia.
   1) Disposable adhesive electrodes are better for long-term monitoring.
   2) Loose sutures of stainless steel with long ends can be used to attach the alligator clips when continuous monitoring is required.
   c. In an emergency, leads can be placed rapidly by remembering that Christmas (red and green) is in the back (comes at the end of the year) and black and white in the front, with grass (green) and snow (white) on the down side. The animal should be in right lateral recumbency.

3. Evaluation of the EGC
   a. Is the rhythm regular or regularly irregular (normal), or is it irregularly irregular (abnormal)? Atrial or ventricular ectopic pacemakers are often premature (follow the preceding complex too closely) and are followed by a longer-than-normal pause.
   b. Is the PQRST waveform consistently present and/or approximately normal in size and shape?
   1) Wide, bizarre QRS waveforms are due to ventricular ectopic pacemaker activity or conduction disturbances. Premature ventricular contractions may be caused by: endogenous release of catecholamines secondary to any stress, exogenous catecholamine therapy, hypoxia or hypercapnia, hypovolemia or hypotension, digitalis toxicity (potentiated by hypokalemia and hypercalcemia), hypokalemia (potentiated by respiratory or metabolic alkalosis, glucose or insulin therapy), hyperkalemia (potentiated by acidosis, hypocalcemia, or succinylcholine or iatrogenic), certain anesthetics lower the threshold to endogenous or exogenous catecholamines (halothane, xylazine, thiamylal, thiopental), myocardial inflammation, disease or stimulation (intracardiac catheters, pleural tubes), thoracic and nonthoracic trauma, dilative or hypertrophic heart failure, visceral organ disease (gastric volvulus/torsion), intracranial disorders (increased pressure, hypoxia), pheochromocytoma, or heart failure.
   2) Tall T waves may be due to hyperkalemia, myocardial hypoxia, or concentric or eccentric hypertrophy.

c. Is there a P wave prior to each QRS; does the P-R interval appear normal? Absent P waves may indicate a supraventricular pacemaker or hyperkalemia.

d. S-T segment depression is often attributed to myocardial hypoxia or potassium or calcium abnormalities but commonly occurs in dogs with no other demonstrable problems.

e. Is there synchrony between the ECG and the palpated pulse? Pulse deficits may be caused by premature atrial contractions, premature ventricular contractions, or variable diastolic ventricular filling suggesting a relative hypovolemia or electromechanical dissociation.

C. Arterial blood pressure (ABP)

1. ABP is the luminal pressure of the blood in a large artery.

2. ABP is the product of cardiac output, vascular capacity, and blood volume. Impairment of one of these is usually compensated for by the other two to maintain adequate blood pressure.

3. ABP is important for cerebral and coronary perfusion. Precapillary arteriolar vasomotor tone, not ABP, is the main determinant of peripheral organ perfusion.

4. ABP can be measured by indirect sphygmomanometry.
   a. This involves applying an occlusion cuff over an artery in a cylindrical appendage.
      1) The width of the occlusion cuff should be about 40% of the circumference of the leg.
      2) The occlusion cuff should be placed "snugly" around the leg. If it is applied too tightly, the pressure measurements will be erroneously low. If too loose, the pressure measurements will be erroneously high.
   b. Inflation of the cuff applies pressure to the underlying tissues and will totally occlude blood flow when the pressure exceeds the systolic blood pressure. The cuff is placed on one of the following locations: midforeleg, just distal to the hock, base of tail, or below the stifle (cats).
   c. As the cuff pressure is gradually decreased, blood will begin to flow intermittently when the cuff pressure falls below the luminal systolic pressure.

   d. Detection of flow distal to the cuff is evidenced by
      1) Needle oscillations on the manometer
      2) Digital palpation of a pulse distal to the cuff
      3) Doppler instrumentation involving the application of two small ultrasound crystals over an artery. The energy frequency reflected from moving tissues is shifted slightly from that which was transmitted, and this frequency difference is converted electronically to an audible signal.
      4) Oscillometric technology involves the interpretation of changes in intracuff pressure associated with changes in appendage volume as the cuff is slowly deflated.
      5) Using a Doppler flow meter, the first sound auscated when the pressure is decreased is the systolic blood pressure. Further reduction of cuff pressure results in a change in sound quality that correlates with the diastolic pressure.
   e. All external techniques are least accurate when vessels are small, when blood pressure is low, and when vessels are constricted.

5. Direct measurement of ABP is more accurate and continuous than indirect methods.
   a. Requires introducing a catheter into an artery
      1) The dorsal metatarsal artery is most commonly used.
      2) The catheter site must be clipped and prepared aseptically.
      3) Lidocaine should be infiltrated to minimize pain and reduce reflex vasospasm.
   b. Indwelling catheters must be flushed with heparinized saline continuously or at frequent intervals (hourly).
   c. The measuring device could be
      1) A long fluid-administration set suspended from the ceiling
      2) An aneroid manometer attached to the catheter by a couple of lengths of sterile extension tubing and a stopcock at each junction
      3) A commercial transducer and recording system
   d. The zero level of the transducer must be set at heart level.

6. Systolic, diastolic, and mean ABP in normal animals are approximately 100–160, 60–100, and 80–120 mm Hg, respectively.

7. Hypotension can be caused by hypovolemia, poor cardiac output, or systemic vasodilation.

   a. Systolic pressures below 80 mm Hg and mean pressures below 60 mm Hg warrant therapy.

     1) Primary therapy should be directed at the underlying disease process.

     2) Sympathomimetic drugs can be used if the underlying disease cannot be stabilized in a timely manner.

   b. Hypovolemia could be caused by extracellular fluid deficits or vascular volume deficits.

   c. Decreased cardiac output may be due to myocardial failure, valvular disease, pericardial tamponade, severe bradycardia or tachycardia, or arrhythmias.

   d. Peripheral vasodilation may be caused by sepsis, anaphylaxis, or vasodilatory drugs.

8. Hypertension may cause retinal detachment, hemorrhage, increased intracranial pressure, and excessive afterload. Mean blood pressures above about 140 mm Hg should be treated.

   a. Hydralazine, nifedipine, and esmolol are commonly used.

   b. Nitroprusside is sometimes used and is a potent vasodilator.

   c. All vasodilators are hypotensive agents and ABP should be monitored to ensure adequate therapy without excessive hypotension.

D. Central venous pressure (CVP)

1. CVP depends on intravascular volume, venous tone and compliance, intrathoracic pressure, and cardiac function.

2. The primary indication for measuring CVP is assessment of fluid therapy, particularly in conditions of renal disease, pulmonary disease, heart disease, and septic shock.

3. Normal CVP is from 0 to 5 cm H_2O. Trends are more important than single measurements, but a measurement of 7–10 generally indicates adequate fluid loading.

4. Elevated CVP is caused by volume overload, pleural or pericardial effusion, pulmonary edema, pulmonary thromboembolism, pneumothorax, and pulmonary hypertension.

5. Peripheral venous pressure bears no correlation to CVP and should not be used for this purpose.

6. Verification of a well-placed, unobstructed catheter can be obtained by observing small fluc-

tuations in the fluid meniscus within the manometer synchronously with the heartbeat and larger excursions associated with ventilation. Large fluctuations synchronous with each heartbeat may indicate that the end of the catheter is positioned within the right ventricle, and will record erroneously high CVP measurements.

7. CVP measurements should be made between ventilatory excursions, since changes in pleural pressure during spontaneous or positive-pressure ventilation affect the luminal pressure within the anterior vena cava.

8. CVP measurement requires a jugular catheter with the tip at the level of the right atrium. This is connected to a three-way stopcock with extension tubing. A manometer is attached to the stopcock perpendicular to the catheter line, and the intravenous fluids are attached to the third portal of the stopcock.

9. The zero point should be level with the right atrium.

   a. Sternum in lateral recumbency

   b. Point of shoulder in sternal recumbency

10. The CVP is measured when the manometer is filled from the fluid bag, and the stopcock is turned "off" to the fluid bag, allowing the fluid in the manometer to equilibrate with the patient. The CVP reading is the point at which the meniscus stops descending.

11. If the CVP is below zero, the manometer should be lowered so that the zero point is now at the 5-cm mark, allowing readings between 0 and 5 to be negative values.

12. CVP readings should always be taken with the animal in the same position.

13. The normal CVP in small animals is 0–10 cm H_2O.

   a. Values in hypovolemic patients may range from −5 to + 3 cm H_2O.

   b. Measurements must be evaluated with respect to other cardiovascular evaluations.

   c. Trends are very important. Increases exceeding 3–5 cm per hour warrant slowing the fluid rate.

   d. Values of 12–15 indicate overhydration or volume overload. A CVP of 20 is consistent with heart failure. Values >20 are seen with cardiac tamponade.

E. Cardiac output, pulmonary artery pressure, and pulmonary capillary wedge pressure.

1. Cardiac output is usually measured by thermodilution.

    a. Thermodilution catheters are expensive and not commonly used in veterinary practice. These are balloon-tipped, flow-directed catheters (Swan-Ganz, Edwards Labs, Santa Ana, CA).

        1) The catheter is inserted via the jugular vein, usually through a preplaced sheathed introducer catheter, through the right ventricle into the pulmonary artery.

        2) When the balloon is deflated, pulmonary artery pressure is measured.

        3) When the balloon is inflated and the branch of the pulmonary artery is occluded (pulmonary artery occlusion pressure) pulmonary venous pressure (close to left atrial pressure) is measured. Pulmonary artery occlusion pressure represents the filling pressure to the left side of the heart (as CVP represents the filling pressure to the right heart). Normal range is 6–12 mm Hg.

    b. Cardiac output is measured by rapidly injecting a small volume (3, 5, or 10 mL, depending upon the size of the patient) of room-temperature saline into the proximal port (located in the right atrium).

        1) The saline mixes with the blood and flows past the thermistor located in the pulmonary artery.

        2) The computer calculates the average change in temperature and then calculates the cardiac output.

2. Cardiac output may be reduced by

    a. Insufficient venous return and end-diastolic ventricular filling volume (hypovolemia, positive airway and pleural pressure, or disease-induced or surgical inflow occlusion)

    b. Ventricular restrictive disease (hypertrophic restrictive cardiomyopathy, pericardial tamponade, or pericardial fibrosis)

    c. Decreased contractility

    d. Excessive bradycardia, tachycardia, or arrhythmias

    e. Regurgitation (retrograde flow) of part of the end-diastolic blood volume due to insufficient atrioventricular valves

    f. Outflow tract obstruction (stenosis)

F. Oxygen delivery and oxygen consumption

1. Oxygen delivery is the product of cardiac output and oxygen content. Oxygen content is usually calculated: ([hemoglobin in g/dL $\times$ 1.34 mL/g] $\times$ % saturation) + (0.003 $\times$ Pao_2).

2. Although oxygen delivery is a most important parameter, it is seldom calculated in veterinary medicine because cardiac output is seldom measured.

3. Adequate oxygen delivery is the goal of coordinated cardiovascular and pulmonary function (*Fig. 7-1*).

    a. Single abnormalities such as hypovolemia, bradycardia, heart failure, or hypoxemia are normally compensated for by the other determinants of oxygen delivery.

    b. Multiple abnormalities have a compounding effect on oxygen delivery.

4. Adequate oxygen delivery is that which meets the oxygen requirements of the tissues.

5. One of the compensatory mechanisms for reduced oxygen delivery is an increased extraction percentage.

    a. Venous oxygen is reduced when oxygen delivery is reduced. Causes include anemia, hypoxemia, hypovolemia, poor contractility, bradycardia, ventricular arrhythmias, and poor cardiac output.

    b. Venous oxygen is also reduced when oxygen consumption is increased: increased muscular activity, elevated body temperature, and hyperthyroidism.

    c. Venous oxygen is increased when oxygen delivery is increased, when oxygen consumption is reduced, or with arteriovenous shunting.

    d. Venous Po_2 reflects tissue Po_2 and bears no correlation to arterial Po_2. Mixed or central venous Po_2 normally ranges between 40 and 50 mm Hg (*Table 7-1*).

    e. Peripheral venous Po_2 cannot be interpreted, but low values should be investigated to determine cause and appropriate therapy (Table 7-1).

G. Lactic acid

1. Pyruvate is produced in the cytosol by anaerobic glycolysis and is then normally taken up by the mitochondria, converted to acetyl-CoA, and incorporated into the tricarboxylic acid cycle.

2. Under anaerobic conditions, when oxidative pathways are obstructed, pyruvate is converted to

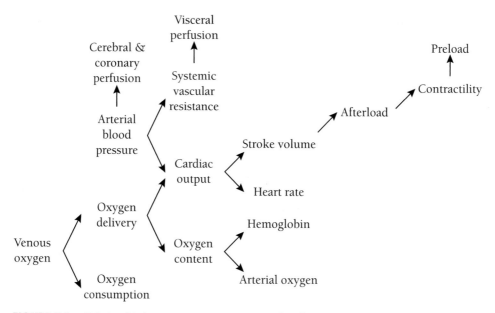

FIGURE 7-1.   Relationship between various parameters of perfusion and oxygenation.

lactate to regenerate oxidized nicotinamide adenine dinucleotide (NAD^+).

3. Lactic acidosis is most commonly associated with inadequate tissue oxygenation, and both skeletal muscle and the gastrointestinal (GI) system are major sources of it.

4. Blood lactate is normally <1.0 mmol/L
   a. It is considered to be high when it measures above 2.5 mmol/L.
   b. The magnitude of the elevation, in general, corresponds with the severity of the underlying problem.
      1) Since severe disease, in general, is associated with a poor prognosis, high blood lactate concentrations may be statistically associated with a poor prognosis.

2) Blood lactate does not, however, define the poor outcome, the disease does. If the disease is severe but easily treatable, so is the high lactate level, and the prognosis is good.
3) Lactate measurements should be viewed as a position statement rather than a prognostic indicator.
4) High lactate levels warrant aggressive therapy to correct the underlying cause. A decreasing trend toward normal is a good sign, whereas rising lactate levels in the face of aggressive treatment warrant a poor-to-guarded prognosis.
5) There may also be a poor correlation between blood lactate concentration and the magnitude of the metabolic acidosis. Lactate production and H^+ production are not linked processes; many other causes of metabolic acidosis exist.

H. Gastric P_{CO_2}

1. The partial pressure of carbon dioxide can be measured on a fluid sample that has been equilibrated with the gas composition of the lumen of the stomach.

2. Since carbon dioxide is a very soluble gas, it is presumed that the gastric mucosal P_{CO_2} is the same as the P_{CO_2} measured in the fluid.

3. Gastric mucosal and arterial bicarbonate concentrations are presumed to be equal.

TABLE 7.1
SIGNIFICANCE OF VENOUS P_{O_2} MEASUREMENTS

Venous P_{O_2} (mm Hg)	Importance
>60	High
40–50	Normal
30–40	Low
25–30	Low, probably warrants treatment
20–25	Very low, definitely warrants treatment
<20	Extremely low, do something!

4. The pH is calculated from the measured P_{CO_2} and the assumed bicarbonate by the Henderson-Hasselbalch equation: $6.1 \times \log [HCO_3]/ P_{CO_2}$.

5. Many studies have reported that gastric P_{CO_2} increases and mucosal pH decreases with intestinal ischemia. Some studies have reported a statistical correlation between a mucosal pH <7.23 and mortality.

6. Gastric tonometry requires specialized equipment. A tonometer is a nasogastric tube with a CO_2-permeable silicon balloon at the end.

7. The balloon must be in contact with the gastric mucosa for at least 30 minutes. After CO_2 equilibration, a sample of saline is removed to measure P_{CO_2}. This value is used to approximate gastric intramucosal P_{CO_2}. Normal gastric intramucosal pH is 7.35–7.41.

8. This technique appears to give a reasonably accurate assessment of regional blood flow.
   a. Like lactate determination, it is a "position measurement" rather than a prognostic indicator, per se.
   b. The technique requires specialized equipment and is time consuming.

I. Packed cell volume/total protein (PCV/TP)

1. Baseline PCV/TP should be determined for all emergency patients on admission to the critical care ward, and trends should be monitored.

2. Elevations in both hematocrit and total protein are seen with dehydration. Serial measurements should show a decrease to normal range with appropriate hydration.

3. Pale mucous membranes can be seen with either poor perfusion or anemia. A low hematocrit documents anemia.
   a. Blood loss anemia exhibits a decrease in both hematocrit and total solids.
   b. Hemolytic anemia has a decreased hematocrit, but total solids are usually in the normal range. Serum may be hemolyzed or icteric.
   c. With acute severe blood loss, the drop in total solids precedes the drop in red blood cells because of splenic contraction. Serial hematocrits should be monitored if ongoing hemorrhage is suspected.
   d. In acute blood loss, a transfusion is usually warranted when the hematocrit drops below 20% in dogs or 15% in cats.
   e. When the total protein is <3.5%, plasma or synthetic colloid administration is usually indicated. Administration of crystalloid solutions alone in this situation usually results in tissue edema.
   f. Severe hyperproteinemia may indicate hyperglobulinemia from chronic disease (feline infectious peritonitis, ehrlichiosis) or neoplastic disease (plasma cell myeloma). Neurologic signs from hyperviscosity syndrome can result from extreme hyperproteinemia.
   g. Polycythemia can be seen secondary to cardiac disease or pulmonary disease resulting in chronic hypoxemia. Other causes include renal neoplasia, chronic pyelonephritis, or hyperadrenocorticism. If dehydration is ruled out as the cause, other rule-outs include hypoxemia, renal disease, and myeloproliferative disease.
      1) Extreme polycythemia may cause neurologic disturbances or retinal hemorrhage.
      2) Phlebotomy may be necessary to reduce the hematocrit below 60%.
      3) Removal of 20 mL/kg of blood reduces the hematocrit approximately 15%.

J. Hemoglobin

1. Hemoglobin concentration is quantitatively the most important component of blood oxygen content.

2. "Minimal" hemoglobin concentration depends upon the status of cardiac output.
   a. In a singular disease like immune-mediated anemia, a low hemoglobin concentration (5 g/dL) can be allowed because cardiac output can increase to compensate for the anemia.
   b. If the ability to increase cardiac output is compromised for any reason, the hemoglobin concentration cannot be allowed to drop so low.
      1) In sepsis, for instance, it is recommended to maintain the hemoglobin concentration above 8 g/dL (equivalent to a packed cell volume of about 25%).
      2) In sepsis, it is recommended to maintain the oxygen delivery above 600 L/min/m2 (*Table 7-2*).

3. Hemoglobin products (whole blood, packed red blood cells, Oxyglobin) improve both volume (venous return and cardiac output) and oxygen content.

TABLE 7.2
EFFECT OF REDUCED HEMOGLOBIN ON OXYGEN DELIVERY AT VARIABLE CARDIAC OUTPUTS

Cardiac Output Hb (PCV)	High (6.5 L/min/m^2)	High Normal (5.5 L/min/m^2)	Normal (4.5 L/min/m^2)	Low normal (3.5 L/min/m^2)	Low (2.5 L/min/m^2)
13 (40)	1161	982	804	625	447
10 (30)	871	737	603	469	335
8 (25)	726	614	503	391	279
7 (20)	580	491	401	312	223
5 (15)	436	369	302	235	168
3 (10)	276	233	191	148	106

4. Hemoglobin measurement provides a more accurate assessment of tissue oxygen delivery than hematocrit when Oxyglobin is used.

K. Colloid osmotic pressure (oncotic pressure)

1. Colloids are responsible for the osmotic "holding power" of fluids within the vascular fluid compartment.

    a. Large colloidal molecules, principally albumin, are not freely permeable across the vascular membrane and therefore are maintained in higher concentration in the vascular fluid compartment than in the interstitium.

    b. Several diseases increase capillary permeability to albumin and other colloids in the systemic or pulmonary vasculature.

    c. As the permeability increases, the transvascular albumin concentrations equilibrate, and plasma albumin concentration or oncotic pressure becomes less important.

2. Hypoproteinemia may be associated with hypovolemia, subcutaneous edema, and ascites. This is not a straight-line relationship, since decreased plasma albumin concentration is initially offset by a dilutional decrease in perivascular albumin concentration.

3. Measurement of total plasma solids using a refractometer allows a general estimate of colloid oncotic pressure. Values below 3.5 g/dL indicate the need for colloid fluids or edema may result.

4. If systemic colloids are used (e.g., hetastarch, dextrans), refractometer readings no longer provide a valid estimate of colloid oncotic pressure.

5. A colloid osmometer uses a semipermeable membrane and measures the change in pressure in the reference chamber when an unknown solution is placed in the test chamber. The membrane pore size in these instruments is 20 or 30 kilodaltons (kDa).

    a. These membranes are freely permeable to the small electrolytes, and this analyzer is "blind" to changes in osmolality.

    b. The colloid osmometer (Wescor 4400 colloid Osmometer, Wescor, Inc., Logan, UT) is the only way to monitor the effect of synthetic colloids.

6. Normal colloid osmotic pressure is 20–25 mm Hg.

    a. Values in the high "teens" are common in critically ill patients but are not considered worthy of treatment, per se.

    b. Values in the low "teens," or single digits are considered too low and warrant treatment with an artificial colloid or plasma.

L. Osmolality

1. Osmolality is determined by the total number (concentration) of solutes in a solvent.

2. Osmolality is measured in an osmometer that uses the principle of freezing point depression caused by concentrated solute solutions.

    a. Colloids do not contribute measurably to osmolality because they are not present in high enough concentrations to affect freezing point depression. An osmometer is "blind" to the amount of colloid in the solution.

    b. Normal range is 290–310 mOsm/kg.

3. Osmolality is also calculated: $2 \times [Na^+] +$ glucose (mg/dL)/18 + BUN (mg/dL)/2.8.

a. The predominant contributor to the osmolality is sodium and its related anions (predominantly chloride and bicarbonate).

　1) Hyperglycemia and uremia can contribute considerably to the osmolality.

　2) Because urea equilibrates across semipermeable membranes, it is considered an ineffective osmole and exerts no osmotic "pull" on free water.

b. The calculated osmolality is subtracted from the measured osmolality to determine if there is an accumulation of other unmeasured osmoles (an osmolar gap).

　1) The osmolar gap is normally less than 10–15 mOsm/kg

　2) Hypermannitolemia, ketoacidosis, lactic acidosis, phosphate and sulfate acidosis (oliguric renal failure), radiocontrast solutions, ethylene glycol intoxication, ethanol/methanol intoxication, and salicylate intoxication can cause an increase in the osmolar gap because of the presence of unmeasured osmolar substances.

4. Hyponatremia is the only cause of hypoosmolality.

5. Hyperosmolality may be caused by an increase in any of the above-mentioned measured or unmeasured solutes.

6. Extracellular osmolality (or its predominant determinant, sodium concentration) is primarily responsible for the osmotic attraction to, and retention of, water within the extracellular fluid compartment. Extracellular sodium is maintained by the cell membrane sodium-potassium-ATPase pump. If this pump fails secondary to ATP depletion, sodium will accumulate within the cell, causing intracellular edema, lysis, and cell death.

7. Acute changes in extracellular osmolality result in transcellular fluid fluxes (hypoosmolality causes cellular edema; hyperosmolality causes cellular dehydration). The endothelial membrane is freely permeable to crystalloids; thus osmolality has no impact upon the transvascular fluid flux.

8. Brain cells are protected from shrinkage in hyperosmolar states through the generation of osmotically active substances called idiogenic osmoles. To prevent cerebral edema, hyperosmolar states must be corrected slowly over 48 hours (see Hypernatremia p. 423, Hyperosmolar diabetes p. 304).

II. RESPIRATORY MONITORING

A. Physical signs

1. Auscultation at the larynx, thoracic inlet (trachea), anteroventral quadrant of the thorax (bronchial), and all lung fields (small airways) is important to localize abnormal sounds.

a. Tracheal sounds are loud, high-pitched, harsh sounds of air passing through the trachea; the expiratory phase is slightly longer than the inspiratory phase.

b. Bronchial sounds are loud, high-pitched sounds. The exhalation phase is longer than the inspiratory phase, and there is a distinct pause between inspiration and exhalation.

c. Small airway sounds are subtle. Air flowing through the lobar and segmental bronchi is heard as soft, low-pitched, gentle rustling sounds. The inspiratory phase is longer than the expiratory phase, and there is no pause between inspiration and exhalation.

d. Bronchial and vesicular sounds are usually heard simultaneously.

TABLE 7.3 OSMOLALITY VERSUS COLLOID ONCOTIC PRESSURE		
Terminology	**Osmolality**	**Colloid Oncotic Pressure**
Units of measure	mOsm/L	mm Hg
Method of measurement	Freezing point depression	Pressure change associated with a fluid flux across a semipermeable membrane
Solute	Crystalloids	Colloids
Importance	Transcellular fluid flux	Transvascular fluid flux

2. Abnormal sounds
   a. Crackles are caused by the sudden opening and closing of small airways.
   b. Pleural friction rubs, caused by inflammation of the serosal surfaces, can be confused with crackles but are generally lower pitched and longer in duration. Pleural friction rubs occur in reverse order during exhalation.
   c. Wheezes are caused by vibration of the airway walls and result from airway narrowing. Wheezes have a musical quality. They may be high-pitched or low-pitched, and they may be loud and polyphonic or subtle and monophonic.

3. Breathing rate
   a. Normal breathing rate is considered 15–30 breaths per minute for a dog or cat at rest.
   b. Breathing rate, per se, is of limited value without some reference to tidal volume and previous trends.
   c. A change in breathing rate is, however, a sensitive indicator of a change in the underlying patient status.

4. Arrhythmic breathing patterns indicate a disorder of the medullary central pattern generator.
   a. Cyclic hyperventilation and hypoventilation (Cheyne-Stokes breathing)
   b. An inspiratory hold (apneustic breathing) may be seen during ketamine anesthesia.
   c. Tachypnea interspersed with apnea
   d. Cyclic hypoventilation and apnea
   e. Central neurogenic tachypnea
   f. Agonal gasping, characterized by a gaping of the mouth and, sometimes, spasmodic contraction of the diaphragm, is not considered a real breathing effort even if there is movement of some air.
   g. Medullary dysfunction is often associated with other signs of intracranial disease.
   h. Phrenic nerve "irritability" is associated with hiccoughs—the diaphragm contracts with each heartbeat.

5. Breathing is normally free, easy, and subtle.
   a. Inspiration is normally less than 1 second.
   b. Inspiration is usually associated with simultaneous expansion of both the chest and the abdomen (diaphragm).
      1) The volume of the chest and abdominal expansion is usually minimal.
      2) Upper thoracic spinal cord disease may cause an abdominal (or diaphragmatic) breathing pattern due to intercostal motor paralysis.

   3) Cervical cord disease or peripheral neuropathy may interfere with both intercostal and diaphragmatic function resulting in weak or absent ventilatory efforts.
   c. Prolonged inspirations may indicate upper airway disease.
   d. Prolonged exhalations may indicate lower airway disease.
   e. Exaggerated breathing effort may indicate hyperventilation or difficult ventilation.

6. Cyanotic mucous membrane color
   a. Cyanosis may be due to hypoxemia (central) or to stagnant tissue blood flow (peripheral—congestive heart failure, end-stage of hypovolemic or septic shock; cardiac arrest).
   b. Cyanosis is always a late sign.
   c. Anemic animals may not exhibit cyanosis even with severe hypoxemia because the bluish tint of mucous membranes generally occurs when the reduced hemoglobin concentration exceeds 5 g/dL.
   d. Any animal may appear cyanotic with poor or fluorescent lighting; you must use a good, consistent light source.

B. Blood gas evaluation

1. Partial pressure of carbon dioxide in arterial blood (Pa_{CO_2}) is a measure of ventilatory status.
   a. Reference range: 35–45 mm Hg
      1) $Pa_{CO_2} < 35$ mm Hg indicates hyperventilation. Pa_{CO_2} values below 20 mm Hg are associated with severe respiratory alkalosis and decreased cerebral blood flow, which may impair cerebral oxygenation.
      2) $Pa_{CO_2} > 45$ mm Hg indicates hypoventilation. Pa_{CO_2} values above 60 mm Hg may be associated with excessive respiratory acidosis and hypoxemia (when breathing room air) and are usually considered to represent sufficient hypoventilation to warrant ventilation therapy.
   b. Venous P_{CO_2} is usually 3–6 mm Hg higher than arterial P_{CO_2}.
      1) It is variably higher in transition states, during anemia, and with carbonic anhydrase inhibitor therapy.
      2) It reflects tissue P_{CO_2}, which represents a combination of arterial P_{CO_2} and tissue metabolism.
   c. End-tidal P_{CO_2} is an estimate of Pa_{CO_2} and is often somewhat lower than Pa_{CO_2} (2–5 mm Hg).
   d. Hypercapnia may be caused by
      1) Dead space rebreathing

2) Hypoventilation
   a) *Neuromuscular disease*
   b) *Airway obstruction*
   c) *Thoracic or abdominal restrictive disease*
   d) *Pleural space filling disorder*
   e) *End-stage pulmonary parenchymal disease*

2. The arterial P_{O_2} (Pa_{O_2}) is a measure of the oxygenating ability of the lungs.
   a. It is the partial pressure (vapor pressure) of oxygen dissolved in the plasma, irrespective of the hemoglobin concentration.
   b. Economical, portable, reliable, battery-operated blood gas analyzers are available.
   c. The normal Pa_{O_2} ranges between 80 and 110 mm Hg for an animal breathing room air. Hypoxemia is defined as Pa_{O_2} < 80 mm Hg, and may be attributed to
      1) Decreased inspired oxygen concentration
      2) Hypoventilation (while inspiring 21% oxygen)
      3) Decreased pulmonary oxygenating ability
   d. A Pa_{O_2} of 60 mm Hg is a commonly selected minimum value below which support procedures such as oxygen therapy or ventilation therapy should be instituted.

3. Blood sampling technique
   a. The dead space of a 3-mL plastic syringe is filled with heparin, and the excess is eliminated.
      1) The dead space of a 3-mL syringe is 0.08 mL (80 units of heparin; enough to anticoagulate 80 mL of blood). If the syringe is filled, there will be a 3% dilution (0.08/3) of the blood sample; 0.08/1 mL is an 8% dilution.
      2) Dilution of the blood sample changes the measured blood gas values and should be minimized.
   b. An artery is located and percutaneously punctured using a 22- to 25-gauge needle.
   c. A consistent volume of blood is collected, using minimal negative pressure to avoid P_{O_2} reduction and red cell lysis.
   d. The sample is either analyzed immediately or placed in ice water.

4. *Venous admixture* is the collective term for all of the ways in which blood can pass from the right to the left side of the circulation without being properly oxygenated.
   a. Venous admixture can be estimated from the difference between the calculated alveolar P_{O_2} and the measured arterial P_{O_2} (A-a P_{O_2}). This is the alveolar-arterial oxygen gradient (A-a gradient).
      1) PA_{O_2} is calculated via the alveolar air equation: Alveolar P_{O_2} = Inspired P_{O_2} – Pa_{CO_2} (1.1), where inspired P_{O_2} = barometric pressure – water vapor at 39°C (50 mm Hg) $\times$ 21%, and 1.1 = 1/RQ, assuming RQ = 0.9.
      2) The A-a P_{O_2} is normally 10 mm Hg when the animal is breathing 21% oxygen and about 100 mm Hg when the animal is breathing 100% oxygen.
      3) A higher A-a P_{O_2} indicates reduced ability of the lung to oxygenate blood.
      4) A table for determining PA_{O_2} (alveolar oxygen concentration) based on the measured Pa_{CO_2} value for animals breathing room air at sea level is presented in *Table 7-4*.
   b. If an animal is breathing 21% oxygen at sea level, a simplified version of the alveolar air equation is to add the measured Pa_{O_2} and Pa_{CO_2} values.
      1) If the added value is less than 120 mm Hg, there is venous admixture.
      2) The lower the added value, the greater the venous admixture.
   c. Patients breathing an enriched oxygen mixture should have an elevated Pa_{O_2}.
      1) The Pa_{O_2} should be at least five times the inspired oxygen concentration when it is expressed as a pecentage (ie, an animal breathing 20% oxygen should have a Pa_{O_2} of approximately 100 mm Hg.
      2) A Pa_{O_2} measurement below this value indicates venous admixture.
      3) The Pa_{O_2}/Fi_{O_2} ratio is useful when animals are receiving supplemental oxygen. It is expressed as a ratio of arterial oxygen over fractional inspired oxygen concentration.
      4) Values < 300 are consistent with acute lung injury and < 200 ARDS.
      5) As an example, an animal receiving nasal oxygen has a Fi_{O_2} of 0.4 and a Pa_{O_2} of 200. This yields a ratio of 200/0.4 = 500 (normal ratio).
   d. If central venous oxygen is measured, venous admixture (%) can be calculated by the formula: $(Cc_{O_2} - Ca_{O_2})/ (Cc_{O_2} - Cv_{O_2})$; where C = content of oxygen in capillary (c), arterial (a), and pulmonary artery (mixed venous) (v) blood. Capillary P_{O_2} is assumed to equal alveolar P_{O_2} for the purposes of this calculation.

TABLE 7.4
ALVEOLAR OXYGEN (PAO_2) CALCULATIONS

To measure Alveolar-arterial oxygen gradient, take PAO_2 and subtract Pao_2; Normal: 0–10

PCO_2	PAO_2	PCO_2	PAO_2	PCO_2	PAO_2	PCO_2	PAO_2
10	137.5	33	108.75	56	80	79	51.25
11	136.25	34	107.5	57	78.75	80	50
12	135	35	106.25	58	77.5	81	48.75
13	133.75	36	105	59	76.25	82	47.5
14	132.5	37	103.75	60	75	83	46.25
15	131.25	38	102.5	61	73.75	84	45
16	130	39	101.25	62	72.5	85	43.75
17	128.75	40	100	63	71.25	86	42.5
18	126.25	41	98.75	64	70	87	41.25
19	125	42	97.5	65	68.75	88	40
20	123.75	43	96.25	66	67.5	89	38.75
21	122.5	44	95	67	66.25	90	37.5
22	121.25	45	93.75	68	65	91	36.25
23	120	46	92.5	69	63.75	92	35
24	118.75	47	91.25	70	62.5	93	33.75
25	117.5	48	90	71	61.25	94	32.5
26	117.5	49	88.75	72	60	95	31.25
27	116.25	50	87.5	73	58.75	96	30
28	115	51	86.25	74	57.5	97	28.75
29	113.75	52	85	75	56.25	98	27.5
30	112.5	53	83.75	76	55	99	26.25
31	111.25	54	82.5	77	53.75	100	25
32	110	55	81.25	78	52.5		

1) Oxygen content is calculated by the formula: [(Hb g/dL × 1.34) % hemoglobin saturation] + (0.003 × Po_2).

2) Venous admixture calculated in this way is normally less than 10%.

C. Pulse oximetry

1. The percent saturation of the hemoglobin with oxygen (Sao_2), like Pao_2, is a measure of the ability of the lung to deliver oxygen to the blood.

a. The relationship between the two is defined by the sigmoid oxyhemoglobin dissociation curve.

b. An Sao_2 of 95% is equivalent to a Pao_2 of 80 mm Hg; an Sao_2 of 90% is equivalent to a Pao_2 of 60 mm Hg.

c. *In vitro* oxygen–hemoglobin saturation analyzers are commercially available, economical, and easy to operate.

d. Pulse oximeters, like all external monitoring devices, accurately measure hemoglobin saturation under ideal circumstances. The accuracy of a pulse oximeter is greatest within the range of 80–95% and is determined by the empirical formula programed into the instrument.

1) One common reason for poor instrument performance is peripheral vasoconstriction; the instrument is not able to pick up a pulse.

2) Differences in tissue absorption or light scatter, different thicknesses of tissue, smaller pulsatile flow patterns, small signal/noise ratios, incompletely compensated light-emitting diodes, baseline read errors (motion), differences in sensor location, and electrical or optical interference may also account for inaccuracies.

3) If the pulse rate indicated by the instrument is not the same as that of the patient, the indicated saturation is probably not accurate either.

4) If the indicated pulse rate is the same as that of the patient, but the indicated saturation is low, move the probe to a new location. When pulse oximeters are in error, they are almost always erroneously low. The highest reading is most likely to be the most accurate.

D. Thoracic radiographs are often very illustrative in chest disease and should be procured if the patient is stable enough to tolerate the stress and the time delay.

1. Some patients are presented in such a severe life-threatening condition that it is not appropriate to obtain a chest radiograph prior to stabilizing the patient. The appropriate stabilization therapeutics are based on the physical examination findings and other rapid, simple diagnostic tests that can be accomplished on the examination table.

2. The chest radiograph should reveal the problem if it involves the pleural space, lung parenchyma, or lower airways. The chest radiograph often looks relatively normal in neuromuscular disease, upper airway obstruction, and pulmonary thromboembolism.

3. An abnormal chest radiograph detects an abnormality but does not necessarily define the physiologic performance of the lung. The lung, like most other organs in the body, can compensate for a great deal of disease and still function normally (oxygenate the blood normally).

III. UROLOGIC MONITORING

A. Urine output

1. Urine production is an excellent indicator of tissue perfusion.

2. Urine production of 1–2 mL/kg/h indicates good renal perfusion.

3. Acute renal failure is characterized by anuria or oliguria (<0.5 mL/kg/h). If there is no response to a fluid challenge, aggressive attempts to initiate urine flow are warranted.

4. Animals with polyuria, such as male cats with postobstructive diuresis, require higher rates of fluid administration to maintain hydration. Urine output should be monitored q2–4h so that fluid input can be adjusted to match losses.

5. Urine output can be monitored by placing an indwelling urinary catheter and attaching it to sterile tubing and a collection bag. Another way to estimate urine output is by weighing a urine-soaked disposable diaper and subtracting the weight of a dry diaper: 1 g = 1 mL of urine.

6. Urine output should be monitored closely in animals with a history of abdominal trauma, exposure to nephrotoxins, heatstroke, shock, or snakebite.

B. Urine specific gravity

1. In dehydrated animals, urine specific gravity will be very concentrated (dogs >1.035, cats >1.060).

2. The ability to concentrate urine is lost when > 66% of the functional nephrons are impaired. Inability to concentrate occurs before azotemia develops.

3. Classically, "fixed" or isosthenuric urine specific gravity (equal to that of plasma) is considered to be 1.008–1.012. This may increase slightly with dehydration or proteinuria but will not exceed 1.020 when there is renal insufficiency.

4. Before renal insufficiency can be diagnosed, other causes of inability to concentrate urine must be excluded, including diuretic administration, pyometritis, hypoadrenocorticism, diabetes mellitus, diabetes insipidus and hyperadrenocorticism.

5. The primary differential diagnoses for dilute urine (specific gravity <1.008) include hyperadrenocorticism, psychogenic polydipsia, diabetes insipidus and *Escherichia coli* urinary tract infection.

C. Urine sediment

1. An acute renal insult results in active urine sediment with tubular casts and degenerate epithelial cells. Granular casts can be seen with pyelonephritis and hyaline casts can be seen with nephrotoxicity.

2. Animals receiving nephrotoxic drugs such as aminoglycosides or amphotericin B should have the urine sediment checked daily for casts.

3. Animals with chronic renal failure usually have clear urine containing no cells or casts.

4. Animals with a urinary tract infection have increased numbers of white blood cells in the urine sediment, unless immunosuppression or hyperadrenocorticism is present.

5. Animals with portosystemic shunt or severe liver disease may have ammonium biurate crystals (golden brown, "flame"-shaped crystals).

6. Animals with ethylene glycol toxicity may have calcium oxalate crystals (coffin-shaped crystals).

7. Centrifugation of red urine will differentiate hematuria from hemoglobinuria. Higher numbers of red blood cells will be seen in the sediment of animals with hematuria.

D. Urine protein/creatinine ratio (U P/C)

1. This test should be performed in animals with proteinuria detected by urine dipstick.

2. The severity of proteinuria can be estimated with this test because protein and creatinine are excreted in relatively constant amounts through the glomerulus.

3. Normally, the U P/C ratio should be <1.0.

4. Urinary tract inflammation can cause proteinuria with a mild increase in U P/C (1–10).

5. The highest U P/C ratios (>25) are generally seen in cases of amyloidosis. Intermediate values (10–40) are seen with glomerulonephritis, although there is much overlap. There is a rough correlation between the severity of the glomerular lesion and the magnitude of proteinuria.

E. BUN, creatinine, potassium, phosphorus

1. BUN (blood urea nitrogen) is a crude estimate of glomerular filtration but is influenced by nonrenal factors.
  a. Increased BUN is associated with a high-protein diet, GI hemorrhage, catabolic states, dehydration, hypotension, and decreased cardiac output.
  b. Renal azotemia occurs when > 75% of the nephrons are nonfunctional.
  c. Postrenal azotemia occurs with urethral obstruction or ruptured bladder.
  d. Animals with prerenal azotemia should have concentrated urine unless extrarenal factors are influencing their ability to concentrate.
  e. Conditions associated with a low BUN include low-protein diet, hepatic dysfunction, medullary washout, and diuresis.

2. Serum creatinine
  a. Creatinine is an end product of muscle metabolism that is excreted through glomerular filtration.
  b. Creatinine level is less influenced by extrarenal factors than BUN.
  c. Prerenal causes of increased creatinine level include decreased cardiac output, hypotension, and dehydration. Renal and postrenal causes are the same as for BUN.

3. Potassium
  a. Hyperkalemia is common with postrenal obstruction and acute renal failure.
  b. Hypokalemia can result from anorexia, vomiting, and polyuria secondary to renal failure.

4. Phosphorus
  a. Hyperphosphatemia develops when the glomerular filtration rate decreases.
  b. Animals with renal failure should eat low-phosphorus diets.
  c. Phosphate binders, such as aluminum or calcium hydroxide, should be given with meals to effect (30–180 mg/kg/day).

IV. METABOLIC MONITORING

A. Glucose

1. Hyperglycemia can be seen in diabetic animals, stressed cats, head trauma patients, or hypermetabolic states such as seizures, early sepsis, or fever.

2. Hyperglycemia should be avoided in animals with head trauma because it is associated with a worse prognosis for neurologic recovery.

3. Hypoglycemia may be a cause of weakness, coma, seizures, or ataxia.

4. Juvenile hypoglycemia can be seen in young puppies, especially toy-breed dogs, or puppies with portosystemic shunt or glycogen storage disease.

5. In older animals, severe hypoglycemia may result from insulinoma, hepatic disease, or paraneoplastic syndromes.

6. Hypoglycemia may indicate sepsis or hypoadrenocorticism.

7. Baseline serum glucose should be checked in all patients presenting as emergencies.

8. Falsely low values will be obtained using whole blood from animals with hemoconcentration and elevated hematocrits in machines that require a drop of whole blood on a glucose strip. More accurate readings can be obtained by separating the serum and placing a drop of serum on the strip.

B. Albumin

1. Albumin is produced in the liver and is the determinant of colloid oncotic pressure in plasma.

2. When serum albumin <1.5 g/dL, there is a tendency toward edema formation and effusions.

3. Causes of hypoalbuminemia include chronic liver disease, protein-losing enteropathy, protein-losing nephropathy, generalized vasculitis, peritonitis, hemorrhage, severe burns or exudative skin disease, malnutrition, or starvation.

4. Animals with hypoalbuminemia may also have low antithrombin III, leading to a hypercoagulable state.

5. Treatment is with colloids: plasma, hetastarch, dextran 70 or 5% human serum albumin (20 mL/kg IV over 4–6 h or as CRI q24h).

C. Calcium

1. Serum calcium levels should be checked in animals with unexplained weakness, stiffness, polyuria, enlarged lymph nodes, seizures, or periparturient illness.

2. Hypercalcemia can be caused by neoplasia—(especially lymphosarcoma), anal sac adenocarcinoma, multiple myeloma, metastatic bone tumors—blastomycosis, primary hyperparathyroidism, acute or chronic renal failure, hypoadrenocorticism, or vitamin D rodenticide toxicity.

   a. Keeshonden and Siamese cats are at risk for primary hyperparathyroidism.

   b. Hemolysis and hyperlipemia falsely raise calcium concentration.

   c. In dogs, serum calcium should be corrected by the following formula: Corrected calcium = Ca (mg/dL) − albumin (g/dL) + 3.5.

   d. Serum phosphorus is usually normal to low in animals with hypercalcemia of malignancy or primary hyperparathyroidism.

   e. Serum parathormone (PTH) concentration is high with primary hyperparathyroidism and low with malignancy.

   f. Hypercalcemia can cause irreversible renal failure. Aggressive treatment with 0.9% sodium chloride, furosemide, and glucocorticoids is indicated. Glurocorticoids may mask diagnosis of neoplasia and their use should be avoided in undiagnosed cases. Calcitonin or bisphophates can also be used in acute cases (see Hypercalcemia p. 313).

3. Hypocalcemia

   a. Causes of hypocalcemia include hypoalbuminemia, vitamin D deficiency (GI malabsorption), hypoparathyroidism, eclampsia, acute pancreatitis, ethylene glycol toxicity, phosphate enemas, citrate toxicity, low-calcium/high-phosphorus diet, and renal failure.

   b. Clinical signs include seizures, tetany, weakness, ataxia, anorexia, vomiting, arrhythmias, panting, and muscle tremors.

   c. Eclampsia usually occurs in small-breed bitches within 21 days of whelping.

   d. Hypocalcemia may occur postthyroidectomy in cats if the parathyroids are inadvertently removed or damaged.

   e. Calcium gluconate 10% contains 9.2 mg/mL elemental calcium. Initial control of signs is usually achieved with 1.0–1.5 mL/kg administered slowly IV. The same amount can be diluted 1:1 with saline and given subcutaneously q8h until oral supplementation is begun (50–100 mg/kg/day).

   f. Calcium chloride 10% contains 27.2 mg/mL elemental calcium. Because it is more potent, a lower dose (0.4–0.6 mL/kg) is used to control signs. It should never be given subcutaneously because it is very irritating and causes tissue necrosis and skin sloughs.

   g. Calcium must be given very slowly (over 10 minutes) while monitoring the ECG. The infusion must be temporarily discontinued if bradycardia develops. Response to therapy (decreasing tremors, muscle relaxation, improved mentation) is fairly rapid and dramatic.

D. Electrolytes

1. Serum electrolytes should be measured in animals with vomiting and diarrhea, altered mentation, weakness, abnormal ventilation, renal disease, urethral obstruction, ruptured urinary bladder, or dehydration.

2. Measurement of serum electrolytes aids in fluid choice and diagnostic rule-outs.

3. Hypernatremia can be caused by dehydration, diabetes insipidus, or salt toxicity from ingestion.

   a. Rapid correction of hypernatremia can result in cerebral edema.

   b. Hypovolemia should be corrected first with isotonic fluids to replace dehydration deficits. Then, a hypotonic fluid (5% dextrose in water or 0.45% NaCl in 2.5% dextrose) can be used to replace free water deficits.

c. Severe hypernatremia should be corrected over 2–3 days at a rate of 0.5 mEq/h or 10–12 mEq/day.

d. Sodium concentration should be monitored frequently during correction.

4. Hyponatremia

a. Causes of hyponatremia include hypoadrenocorticism, diuretics, burns, third-space losses with repeated drainage, GI losses, psychogenic polydipsia, congestive heart failure, and severe liver disease.

b. An ACTH stimulation test can be done to check for hypoadrenocorticism.

c. The sodium concentration should be gradually raised at a rate of 0.5 mEq/L/h. Normal saline usually suffices, but hypertonic saline can be given to patients with severe hyponatremia (<110 mEq/L).

5. Hypokalemia

a. Hypokalemia is common in critically ill patients. It can result from excessive loss (renal disease, polyuria, diuretics, dialysis, vomiting, or diarrhea), decreased intake (anorexia, potassium-deficient fluids), or translocation from extracellular to intracellular fluid (insulin and glucose, bicarbonate, alkalosis, catecholamines).

b. Clinical signs associated with hypokalemia include weakness, lethargy, anorexia, and vomiting (from GI ileus), polydipsia, polyuria, and ventroflexion of the neck in cats. Respiratory paralysis can occur with severe potassium depletion.

c. Potassium should be added to the fluids of anorexic animals at a dose of 14–20 mEq/L.

d. More severe potassium deficits can be treated by following the chart for potassium supplementation (*Table 7-5*).

TABLE 7.5 POTASSIUM SUPPLEMENTATION CHART	
Serum K⁺ (mEq/L)	**Amount to add per Liter (mEq)**
3.5–4.0	20
3.0–3.5	30
2.5–3.0	40
2.0–2.5	60
<2.0	80

e. When giving potassium IV, do not exceed the rate of 0.5 mEq/kg/h or cardiac arrest may occur.

f. Oral potassium supplementation can be given initially at a dose of 1 mEq/kg q8h, then 0.5 mEq/kg q12h for maintenance.

g. Potassium can also be added to subcutaneous fluids, but concentrations >30 mEq/L are irritating to tissues.

6. Hyperkalemia

a. Causes of hyperkalemia include oliguric renal failure, ruptured bladder, urethral obstruction, administration of potassium-sparing diuretics, acidosis, crushing injuries, saddle thrombus, and hypoadrenocorticism.

b. Clinical signs include weakness, paralysis, collapse and death. The primary organ affected is the heart because of conduction disturbances.

c. Treatment

1) Sodium bicarbonate (1–2 mEq/kg slowly IV) will translocate potassium into the cells. Avoid this treatment in animals with a potential for hypocalcemia (cats with urethral obstruction).

2) Regular insulin (0.5 U/kg IV) with 50% dextrose (1 g/kg IV) also induces translocation into cells. Follow with 2.5% glucose in IV fluids.

3) Calcium gluconate 10% (0.5–1.0 mL/kg IV slowly) directly antagonizes the effect of potassium on the heart without lowering serum concentrations. It is used to treat life-threatening arrhythmias.

7. Hypochloremia

a. Severe hypochloremia can result from gastric vomiting. Consider pyloric outflow obstruction, duodenal foreign body, or severe pancreatitis. Another common cause of hypochloremia is administration of diuretics, such as furosemide.

b. Hypochloremia is associated with metabolic alkalosis because chloride concentration varies inversely with bicarbonate concentration.

c. Lipemia and hyperproteinemia can falsely lower laboratory values for chloride.

d. Treatment involves intravenous infusion of 0.9% NaCl to correct volume deficits.

8. Hyperchloremia

a. The most common cause of hyperchloremia is metabolic acidosis that occurs with bicarbonate loss through diarrhea and renal retention of chloride to maintain electrical neutrality.

b. Hyperchloremia can also occur when 0.9% saline is administered for several days as a maintenance fluid.

V. NEUROLOGIC MONITORING

A. Spinal cord

1. Animals with spinal trauma or acute disk herniation should have repeated neurologic evaluations to check for progression of disease.

2. Animals with limb or pelvic fractures or those in deep shock may not respond appropriately to the initial assessment, so the neurologic examination should be repeated following stabilization.

3. Check for peripheral nerve injuries (brachial plexus avulsion, radial nerve paralysis, loss of anal and bladder tone from pelvic trauma) before spending time and money to repair expensive fractures.

4. A complete neurologic examination cannot be performed on animals with extensive trauma. However, you should always check each of the limbs for deep pain sensation and check the anal sphincter reflex.

a. When checking for deep pain, remember that there must be recognition of pain sensation by the animal's brain to prove that spinal tracts are intact. The withdrawal reflex is segmental and may be intact despite severe cord damage above or below the reflex arc.

b. Progressive loss of deep pain sensation following spinal cord injury may indicate hematoma or worsening of spinal cord edema and is an indication for immediate surgery to decompress the spinal cord at the site of the lesion.

5. When checking for deep pain sensation, start with a toe pinch using your fingernails. If this does not elicit a response, use a hemostat at the base of the nail. Sometimes, the only cranial response exhibited by very depressed or moribund

	TABLE 7.6 SMALL ANIMAL COMA SCALE		
Variable	**Criteria**		**Score**
Motor activity	Normal gait, normal reflexes		6
	Hemiparesis, tetraparesis, or decorticate rigidity		5
	Recumbent with intermittent extensor rigidity		4
	Recumbent with constant extensor rigidity		3
	Recumbent with intermittent extensor rigidity/opisthotonus		2
	Recumbent, hypotonic with depressed/absent spinal reflexes		1
Brainstem reflexes	Normal pupillary light reflex and oculocephalic reflexes		6
	Slow pupillary light reflex and normal-to-reduced oculocephalic reflexes		5
	Bilateral/unresponsive miosis and normal-to-reduced oculocephalic reflexes		4
	Pinpoint pupils and reduced-to-absent oculocephalic reflexes		3
	Unilateral/unresponsive mydriasis and reduced-to-absent oculocephalic reflexes		2
	Bilateral/unresponsive mydriasis and reduced-to-absent oculocephalic reflexes		1
Level of consciousness	Occasionally alert and responsive		6
	Depressed/delirious, but capable of response to stimulus		5
	Obtunded/stupor, but responds to visual stimuli		4
	Obtunded/stupor, but responds to auditory stimuli		3
	Obtunded/stupor, but responds to noxious stimuli		2
	Comatose and unresponsive to noxious stimuli		1
Total score	3–8	9–14	15–18
Prognosis	Grave	Poor to guarded	Good

From Shores A. Small Animal Coma Scale Revisited. Tenth Annual ACVIM Forum 1992:748-749.

patients is pupillary dilation. An assistant should observe the animal's face to detect any sign of pain recognition. Lack of deep pain sensation carries a very poor prognosis.

6. Different areas of the limb should be evaluated to assess peripheral nerve function:
    a. Medial toe of forelimb—median nerve
    b. Lateral toe of forelimb—ulnar nerve
    c. Dorsum of paw—radial nerve
    d. Inner brachium of forelimb—musculoskeletal nerve
    e. Upper inner brachium—axillary nerve
    f. Lateral toe rear leg—tibial nerve
    g. Medial toe rear leg—peroneal nerve

B. Cranial nerves

1. Animals with head trauma may have loss of consciousness, palpable skull fractures, asymmetric pupils, altered pupillary light reflexes, hemorrhage from the nose or ears, bradycardia, or hypotension.

2. Cranial nerves should be serially evaluated to monitor for worsening of the brain injury.

3. Midrange or mydriatic pupils with no pupillary light reflex and no physiologic nystagmus (fixed and dilated) indicate a midbrain or brainstem lesion that carries a grave prognosis.

4. Miotic pupils that respond to light and exhibit physiologic nystagmus indicate a lesion above or below the midbrain. This finding carries a good-to-fair prognosis, as long as the signs are static or improving.

C. Serial neurologic evaluations should be assessed according to the Small Animal Coma Scale (*Table 7-6*).

CHAPTER 8

NUTRITIONAL SUPPORT OF CRITICAL PATIENTS

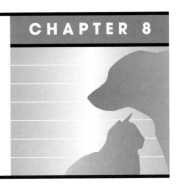

I. ACUTE MALNUTRITION

A. Acute protein–energy malnutrition predisposes to impaired immune competence; poor wound healing and an increased incidence of dehiscence; an increased incidence of wound infection and systemic sepsis; cardiac, skeletal, and smooth muscle weakness; and major organ failure and death. Hepatic lipidosis is a common consequence of acute malnutrition in the cat.

1. These occur without any of the overt signs of chronic malnutrition such as muscle wasting.

2. Critically ill animals are in a state of accelerated starvation because stress causes a hypermetabolic state.

B. When is nutrition therapy indicated?

1. No clinical or laboratory tests provide pathognomonic evidence of acute malnutrition.

2. It is assumed that nutritional supplementation is necessary whenever a critically ill patient has gone without nutrition for several (3) days (adults) or 1 day (neonates).

3. Clinical evidence of a "poor doer" in the absence of other more likely causes is also an indication for nutritional support.

4. Sepsis and wound dehiscence are common consequences of acute malnutrition and should be considered indications for improving nutrition.

5. The bottom line: When in doubt, feed!

C. Energy expenditure of the critically ill patient

1. Resting energy expenditure (REE) in the dog and cat is calculated as 70 kcal × body weight in $kg^{0.75}$ (*Table 8-1*). Normal maintenance energy requirement for dogs is about 132 kcal × $kg^{0.75}$ and for cats is about 80 kcal/$kg^{0.75}$. Minimum energy requirements for critically ill dogs and cats would be equal to REE. Maximum expected energy requirements may be as high as 1.5 × REE.

2. A second formula used for animals >2 kg to estimate resting energy requirement is

$$RER = 30 \, BW \, (kg) + 70$$

3. These formulas may overestimate RER for cats. In cats, a simple formula can be used to estimate energy needs:

$$REE = 40 \, BW \, (kg)$$

4. Because of the potential consequences of overfeeding, the REE is the amount fed. It is not necessary to multiply this value by an "illness factor" as previously recommended, although if the animal is losing weight, the amount fed can be increased toward the maximum energy expenditure from Table 8-1).

5. Consequences of overfeeding include vomiting, diarrhea, cramping, nausea, electrolyte disturbances, hyperglycemia, hepatic dysfunction, and respiratory distress.

TABLE 8.1
ENERGY REQUIREMENTS FOR DOGS AND CATS.

Body Weight (kg)	Minimum Energy (kcal/day)	Estimated Expenditure[a] (kcal/h)	Maximum Energy (kcal/day)	Estimated Expenditure[b] (kcal/h)
1	70	3	105	4
1.5	95	4	142	6
2	118	5	177	7
2.5	139	6	209	9
3	160	7	239	10
3.5	179	8	269	11
4	198	8	297	12
4.5	216	9	324	14
5	234	10	351	15
6	268	11	403	17
7	301	13	452	19
8	333	14	499	21
9	364	15	546	23
10	394	16	590	25
11	423	18	634	26
12	451	19	677	28
13	479	20	719	30
14	507	21	760	32
15	534	22	800	33
16	560	23	840	35
17	586	24	879	37
18	612	26	918	38
19	637	27	956	40

(*continued*)

II. METHODS AND PROCEDURES OF PROVIDING ENTERAL NUTRITION

A. Enteral feeding should be used any time the intestinal tract (motility, digestion, and absorption) is functional.

1. This approach is easier and cheaper and is associated with less infection risk than parenteral routes.

2. Enteral nutrition preserves gut epithelial structure and function better than does parenteral nutrition.

B. Voluntary food consumption is always preferable.

1. Small quantities of a commercial dog or cat food, respectively
   a. Commercial moist, semimoist, or dry food is preferable because they are nutritionally balanced.

   b. Human food (including beef, poultry) or baby food could be offered.
      1) These are single-source foods but are satisfactory for short-term feeding.
      2) Baby foods containing onion should be avoided because of the potential for Heinz body anemia.
      3) Dogs can do very well with a human diet, but cats have a higher protein (especially arginine and taurine) requirement and will develop nutritional deficiency.
   c. Many different kinds should be offered since one cannot predict which the patient will find appetizing.

2. It may help to warm the food or to provide a topping of chicken/beef broth to make it more appetizing.

3. Coaxing and hand-feeding are sometimes effective in encouraging the animal to eat.

4. Some conditions predispose to anorexia and should be minimized as much as possible

TABLE 8.1
(continued)

Body Weight (kg)	Minimum Energy (kcal/day)	Estimated Expenditure[a] (kcal/h)	Maximum Energy (kcal/day)	Estimated Expenditure[b] (kcal/h)
20	662	28	993	41
21	687	29	1030	43
22	711	30	1067	44
23	735	31	1103	46
24	759	31	1139	47
25	783	33	1174	49
26	806	34	1209	50
27	829	35	1244	52
28	852	36	1278	53
29	875	36	1312	55
30	897	37	1346	56
35	1007	42	1511	63
40	1113	46	1670	70
45	1216	51	1824	76
50	1316	55	1974	82
60	1509	63	2264	94
70	1694	71	2541	106
80	1872	78	2809	117
90	2045	85	3068	128
100	2214	92	3320	138

[a] $70 \times BW\ (kg^{0.75})$
[b] Maximum energy requirements for a critically ill patient; calculated as $1.5 \times REE$.

(hypokalemia, vitamin B and zinc deficiencies, uremia, pain, opioids, and drug-induced central nervous system (CNS) depression).

5. If a cat feels well enough to groom itself, the food material could be applied to the lips or feet and be consumed during grooming.

C. Appetite stimulants (*Table 8-2*)

1. Diazepam (0.05–0.15 mg/kg IV; 0.1–0.4 mg/kg IM, PO q12h) or oxazepam (2 mg PO q12h) have an immediate but short-lived appetite-stimulating effect.
2. Cyproheptadine (2–4 mg/cat PO q12–24h) is an antiserotonin agent with appetite-stimulating effects but has a slow onset (24 hours).
3. Prednisolone (0.2–0.4 mg/kg PO q24h) can be used for temporary appetite stimulation but can have potentially significant adverse effects.
4. Stanozolol (1–2 mg q12h PO, cats; 1–4 mg q12h PO, dogs) may be effective.

D. Force feeding

1. If the animal will not eat voluntarily, perhaps it will eat or swallow if the food is placed into the cheek pouch.
   a. The food should not be forced into the back of the mouth since the animal may not swallow it; the food may then cause airway obstruction or be aspirated into the trachea.
   b. Force feeding is usually not a satisfactory method of providing nutrition during prolonged illness.
   c. Force feeding may promote anorexia by causing food aversion.

2. For animals that cannot eat voluntarily, intermittent feeding can be accomplished with orogastric intubation. This is the primary method of feeding for neonates (*Figs. 8-1 and 8-2*).

E. A **nasogastric tube** or **nasoesophageal tube** can be inserted without general anesthesia and is normally well tolerated by dogs and cats.

TABLE 8.2
APPETITE STIMULANTS

Drug	Dosage	Potential Side Effects
Diazepam	0.1–0.2 mg/kg PO q12–24h (dog) 0.05–0.10 mg/kg IV 18–24h (cat, dog)	Nonpurposeful eating, sedation, hepatic encephalopathy, idiosyncratic hepatic necrosis
Oxazepam	1.25–2.5g PO q12–24h (cat) 0.3–0.4 mg/g PO q12–24h (dog)	As for diazepam
Flurazepam	0.1–0.2 mg/kg PO q12–24h (cat)	As for diazepam
Cyproheptadine	2–4 mg PO q12–24h (cat) 5–20 mg PO q12–24h (dog)	Excitability, aggression, vomiting
Cyanocobalamin	1000 μg SQ or in IV	Not reported
Boldenone	5 mg SQ or IM q24 h (cat, dog)	Delayed onset of activity, muscle pain at injection site
Stanozolol	1–2 mg PO q12–24 h (cat, dog)	Delayed onset of activity
Nandrolone	5 mg/kg IM weekly; dogs	Uncommon
Prednisolone	0.5–1 mg/kg q12–24 h	PU/PD, decreased wound healing

1. A soft, flexible tube of appropriate size (about 8 Fr for most dogs and 5 Fr for most cats) and length is selected.
   a. We use pediatric polyurethane infant feeding tubes (NCC Div., Mallinckrodt, Argyle, NY).
   b. Silicone tubes with weighted tips are also available (Biosearch Medical Prod., Somerville, NJ).

2. The tube can be placed into the stomach or the terminal esophagus.
   a. Gastric tubes allow assessment of residuals from the previous feeding.
      1) One of the common problems in critically ill patients is gastric stasis.
      2) Filling the stomach with food results in regurgitation or vomition, which inevitably leads to aspiration and pneumonia.
      3) Knowing whether the stomach has emptied itself of the last feeding is critical to whether the next feeding should be administered or not.

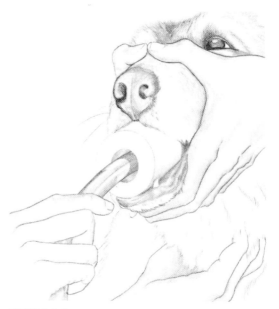

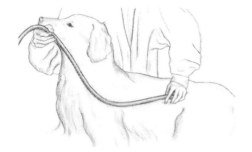

FIGURE 8-1. Prior to orogastric intubation, the tube should be measured from the mouth to the last rib and marked. (From Crow SE, Walshaw SO. Manual of Clinical Procedures in the Dog, Cat, and Rabbit. 2nd ed. Philadelphia: Lippincott Williams & Wilkins, 1997:169.)

FIGURE 8-2. A roll of 2-inch tape makes an excellent speculum for passing an orogastric tube. (From Crow SE, Walshaw SO. Manual of Clinical Procedures in the Dog, Cat, and Rabbit. 2nd ed. Philadelphia: Lippincott Williams & Wilkins, 1997:169.)

b. Terminal esophageal tubes diminish the risk of regurgitation of stomach acids into the terminal esophagus but do not allow checking of residuals and mandate that instillation be very slow.

3. Insertion technique (*Figs. 8-3, 8-4, and 8-5*)

a. A mark is made on the tube (measured from its tip) equivalent to the distance from the nasal meatus to the midcervical esophagus.

b. A second mark is made equivalent to the distance from the nasal meatus to the last rib (the stomach).

c. A small quantity of a 0.5–1% local anesthetic solution is dripped into the nostril; the nose should be elevated so that the solution will gravitate deep into the nasal cavity.

d. The tube is generously lubricated with lidocaine gel and introduced along the ventromedial aspect of the nasal cavity.

1) The introducing hand should be braced against the animal's snout or head so that when the animal moves or sneezes, the hand moves with the head.

2) The tube is released when the animal moves its head so that the tube will not be pulled out of the nose.

3) The catheter is introduced in short, well-controlled insertions, releasing the catheter between each insertion and allowing the animal to move and then settle down.

4) The tip of the tube is initially directed ventromedially. When the tip reaches the median septum at the floor of the nasal cavity, the external nares are pushed dorsally with the thumb, opening the ventral meatus for tube passage ("pig nose" technique, Fig. 8-5).

e. There will be some increased resistance when the catheter reaches the midnasal region.

1) This is the narrowest portion of the nasal cavity and it may require a little firm pressure to pass.

2) The tube may have passed into the dorsal nasal cavity, where it cannot be passed; it should be withdrawn and reinserted in a more ventral direction.

3) The tube may be too large for the nasal cavity of the patient; it should be removed and replaced with a smaller tube.

f. The head and neck should be in a neutral position, not flexed (impedes passage of the catheter through the pharynx) or extended (predisposed to passage of the catheter into the trachea).

g. When the catheter has been introduced to the first mark, the catheter tip should be positioned in the midcervical esophagus; aspiration of air through the catheter with a syringe

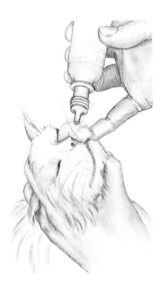

FIGURE 8-3. Topical anesthetic must be instilled into the nares before attempting to pass a nasogastric or nasoesophageal tube. Always elevate the head to allow the anesthetic to disperse by gravity flow. (From Crow SE, Walshaw SO. Manual of Clinical Procedures in the Dog, Cat, and Rabbit. 2nd ed. Philadelphia: Lippincott Williams & Wilkins, 1997:171.)

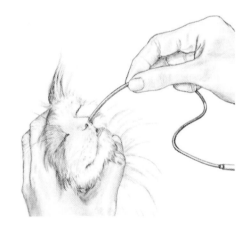

FIGURE 8-4. The animal's head is held with one hand while the other hand is used to insert the well-lubricated tube into the ventromedial aspect of the nostril. (From Crow SE, Walshaw SO. Manual of Clinical Procedures in the Dog, Cat, and Rabbit. 2nd ed. Philadelphia: Lippincott Williams & Wilkins, 1997:172.)

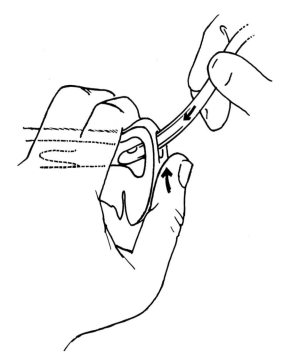

FIGURE 8-5.   In dogs, passage of a nasal tube is facilitated by using the "pig nose technique." (From Bojrab MJ, Ellison GW, Slocum BS, eds. Current Techniques in Small Animal Surgery. 4th ed. Baltimore: Williams & Wilkins, 1998:153.)

should not be possible (the esophagus should collapse around the end of the catheter and occlude it).

    1) If air is aspirated, the catheter tip is either in the trachea or coiled in the pharynx; it should be withdrawn and reinserted.

    2) Occasionally there is air in the esophagus, especially if the animal is having trouble breathing, and this could be confusing.

    3) If the catheter is kinked and occluded, aspiration of air will also not be possible, but there is no way that this can be established at this time.

h. Continue to advance the catheter. If the patient begins to cough or if the tube exits the mouth or the other nostril, it is clearly in the wrong place and should be withdrawn and reinserted.

i. When the catheter has been introduced to the second mark, the catheter tip should be positioned in the stomach.

    1) The position of the catheter tip is verified if gastric fluid can be aspirated.

    2) Aspiration of air does not preclude having the tube is in the stomach.

    3) Clearly audible gurgling sounds, auscultated over the left dorsal abdominal region, when air (3 mL in the cat; 5–10 mL in the dog) is rapidly injected into the tube verifies the position of the tube.

    4) The lack of coughing in response to insertion of the catheter or injection of a small volume of saline does not prove that the tube is not in the trachea; critically ill patients commonly do not cough with such stimuli.

    5) A radiograph will verify the location of the tube when its position cannot be absolutely verified by the above techniques.

j. Once the proper position of the nasogastric (NG) tube has been verified, its position should be fixed by suturing or stapling it first to the lateral aspect of the nasal cavity at the alar notch. The catheter is then sutured or stapled to the skin as it courses along the side of the face, or up between the eyes, over the top of the head.

    1) The tube should be out of the visual range of the animal.

    2) Tags of tape may be used for suturing the tube if desired, but they are most often not necessary.

    3) Super glue can be used but hair is removed when the catheter is removed and it may grow back a different color.

    4) Lengths of intravenous fluid extension tubing should be added if the catheter is too short to reach the neck of the patient.

    5) It is helpful to bandage a loop of catheter to the animal's neck to avoid tension and traction on the suture sites.

    6) An Elizabethan collar may be necessary to keep the patient from removing the catheter.

k. Because of the small tube diameter, only liquid diets such as Clinicare can be administered through NG tubes.

F. An **esophagostomy tube** is a better "go-home" tube but requires general anesthesia for placement.

1. A soft, flexible polyurethane or red rubber tube of appropriate length is selected (10–12 Fr, cats and small dogs; up to 22 Fr for large dogs).

2. The tube may be placed into the stomach or caudal esophagus (see related discussion under nasogastric tube).

3. Insertion technique (*Figs. 8-6 and 8-7*)

a. The skin on the left side of the dog's neck is clipped and surgically prepped.

b. A mark is made on the tube (measured from its tip) equivalent to the distance from the mid-cervical esophagus (insertion point) to the last rib (the stomach).

c. A curved Carmalt forceps (or similar instrument) is placed through the mouth down to a midpoint in the cervical esophagus on the left side of the neck and pushed outward to tent the skin over the esophagus.

d. The skin is incised over the tip of the forceps; the incision is extended through the subcuta-

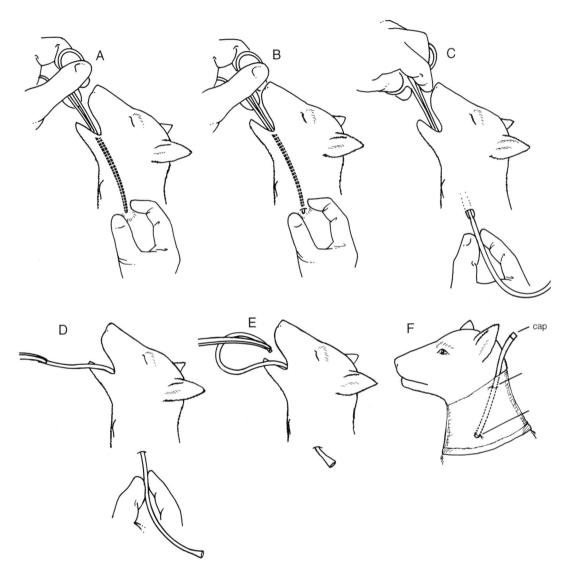

FIGURE 8-6. Drawing illustrating placement of a large-bore esophagostomy tube using curved hemostats. **A.** The hemostats are inserted into the oral cavity, oropharynx, and proximal esophagus, then the tips are pushed laterally. **B.** A skin incision is made, and the tips of the hemostats are pushed through the wall of the esophagus and the subcutaneous tissues. **C.** The flexible feeding tube is grasped with the tips of the hemostats. **D.** The tube is pulled out through the mouth with the hemostats. **E.** The tube's tip is regrasped with the hemostats and is guided down the pharynx and esophagus. **F.** The tube is pulled gently to straighten the curve in it, and after it is advanced so the tip is in the midthoracic esophagus, it is anchored with a suture that enters the fascia and periosteum around the wing of the atlas. (From Bojrab MJ, Ellison GW, Slocum BS, eds. Current Techniques in Small Animal Surgery. 4th ed. Baltimore: Williams & Wilkins, 1998:164.)

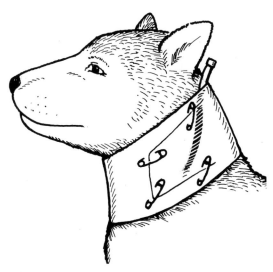

FIGURE 8-7.   Drawing illustrating the cervical dressing covering the esophagostomy tube. A trap door is made over the tube's exit site at the skin and is held closed with four safety pins when it is not needed. (From Bojrab MJ, Ellison GW, Slocum BS, eds. Current Techniques in Small Animal Surgery. 4th ed. Baltimore: Williams & Wilkins, 1998:165.)

neous connective tissues and through the wall of the esophagus. The esophageal incision should be as small as possible; just large enough to allow the tip of the forceps to be pushed through.
e. The forceps is pushed through the esophagus/skin incision.
f. The tip of the esophagostomy tube is grasped with the forceps and pulled up through the mouth.
g. The tip of the tube is then redirected down the esophagus to the predetermined length using the Carmalt forceps to direct the tube. As it is directed caudally into the esophagus, the end of the tube exiting the neck will "flip" from caudal to cranial.
h. Proper placement is judged in the same manner as for a NG tube.
i. The tube is sutured in place by an overlapping, interlocking suture pattern and bandaged to the neck.
j. Gruel diets can be administered through esophagostomy tubes.

4.   Specialized equipment for placing esophagostomy tubes is available from Cook Veterinary Products, Bloomington, IN.

G. Gastrostomy tubes may be placed surgically or percutaneously. Percutaneous gastrostomy tubes can be placed with or without an endoscope.

1.   Gastrostomy tubes are well tolerated by dogs and cats.

2.   Gastrostomy tubes can be large enough to allow instillation of gruels and blenderized commercial dog and cat foods.

3.   Gastrostomy tubes do not cause pharyngitis or esophagitis nor do they interfere with gastroesophageal sphincter or glottis function as NG and esophagostomy tubes might.

4.   A gastrostomy tube allows a patient to eat normally, which will facilitate weaning the animal onto normal nutrition prior to removing the tube.

5.   The usual protocol is to start with the instillation of small volumes (2 mL/kg) of water into the tube 12–24 hours after tube placement. In the absence of patient discomfort, regurgitation, vomiting, or residuals, feeding can start 24–48 hours after tube placement (see feeding protocol below).

6.   Percutaneously inserted tubes should be left in place for at least 5 days prior to removal.
   a. A firm adhesion should develop between the stomach serosa and the peritoneum.
   b. This should prevent leakage and peritonitis when the tube is used and when it is removed.
   c. The gastric fistula heals very rapidly after the tube is removed. If the tube is accidentally removed, it must be replaced within a few hours or else the hole will become too small.

7.   Potential problems with gastrostomy tubes include vomiting, infection, pressure necrosis at stoma site, and leakage of gastric contents into the abdominal cavity secondary to an incomplete seal.

8.   Insertion technique (*Figs. 8-8 through 8-15*)
   a. The patient is anesthetized and placed in right lateral recumbency.
   b. The left flank, caudal to the last rib, is clipped and surgically prepared.
   c. If a gastroscope is to be used, it is now introduced into the stomach, which is moderately inflated so that the stomach wall apposes the abdominal wall.
      1) Insert an outside-the-needle catheter into the lumen of the stomach.
      2) Pass a length of 2-0 or 1-0 nylon suture material through the catheter; grasp the end of the suture with endoscopic forceps and withdraw the endoscope and suture out through the mouth so that the suture now extends from outside the abdominal body

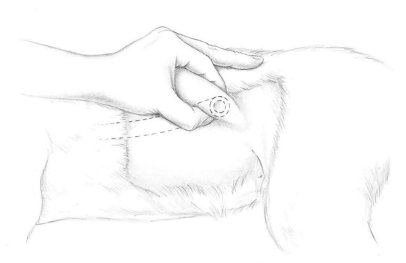

FIGURE 8-8. For blind placement of a gastrostomy tube, a rigid tube is passed into the stomach and the end of the tube is located behind the last rib on the left lateral abdominal wall, making certain that the spleen or other abdominal organs are out of the way. (From Crow SE, Walshaw SO. Manual of Clinical Procedures in the Dog, Cat, and Rabbit. 2nd ed. Philadelphia: Lippincott Williams & Wilkins, 1997:183.)

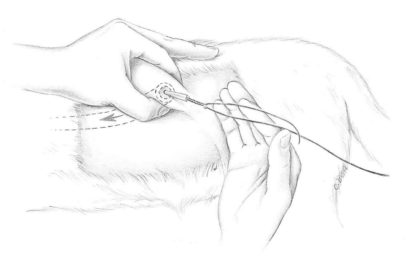

FIGURE 8-9. A needle or catheter is placed through the abdominal wall, stomach wall, and into the lumen of the tube. Stiff suture material is advanced through the needle into the tube until it comes out of the mouth. The needle and stomach tube are removed, leaving suture extending from the left lateral abdominal wall to the mouth. (From Crow SE, Walshaw SO. Manual of Clinical Procedures in the Dog, Cat, and Rabbit. 2nd ed. Philadelphia: Lippincott Williams & Wilkins, 1997:185.

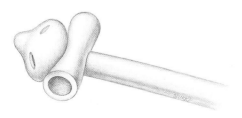

FIGURE 8-10. An extra flange can be added to the mushroom-tipped catheter to provide extra security against dislodgement. A segment of tubing is cut from the distal end of the stomach tube to make the flange as shown. (From Crow SE, Walshaw SO. Manual of Clinical Procedures in the Dog, Cat, and Rabbit. 2nd ed. Philadelphia: Lippincott Williams & Wilkins, 1997:181.)

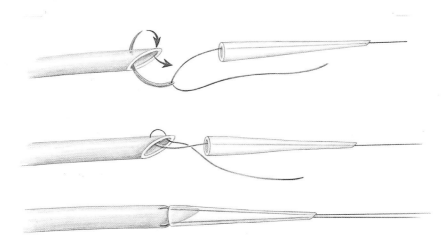

FIGURE 8-11. The suture that exits the animal's mouth is passed through a Sovereign catheter and then through the stomach tube. The beveled end of the stomach tube is pushed into the catheter, and the suture is tied together to form a firm knot. (From Crow SE, Walshaw SO. Manual of Clinical Procedures in the Dog, Cat, and Rabbit. 2nd ed. Philadelphia: Lippincott Williams & Wilkins, 1997:186.)

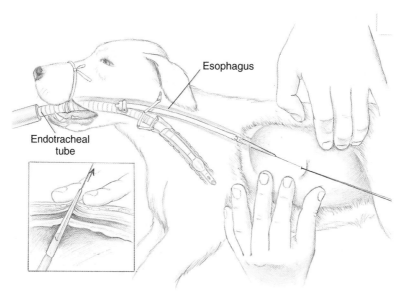

FIGURE 8-12. The lubricated catheter/tube assembly is pulled through the mouth and esophagus until it exits the abdominal wall. (From Crow SE, Walshaw SO. Manual of Clinical Procedures in the Dog, Cat, and Rabbit. 2nd ed. Philadelphia: Lippincott Williams & Wilkins, 1997:186.)

wall, up through the esophagus, and out the mouth.

d. If a nonendoscopic tube placement device is to be used (Cook Instruments, Bloomington, IN), it is now inserted into the stomach and then pushed outward so that it tents the skin.

  1) A length of a stiff plastic stomach tube could also be used for this purpose.

2) A long needle or trocar with an end hole (Jorgensen Laboratories, Loveland, CO) is passed through the placement device and is pushed through the abdominal wall.

3) Nylon suture material is passed through the trocar and into the stomach tube or insertion device, which is then removed so that the suture now extends from outside

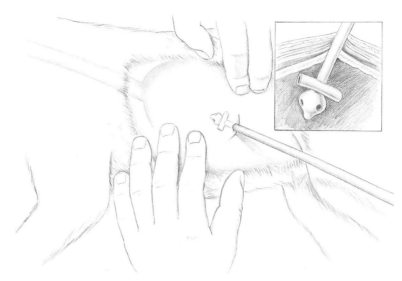

FIGURE 8-13. Steady pressure is applied to pull the inner flange snug with the abdominal wall. (From Crow SE, Walshaw SO. Manual of Clinical Procedures in the Dog, Cat, and Rabbit. 2nd ed. Philadelphia: Lippincott Williams & Wilkins, 1997:186.)

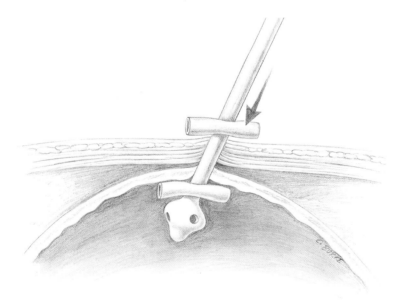

FIGURE 8-14. An outer flange is added to hold the tube in place. (From Crow SE, Walshaw SO. Manual of Clinical Procedures in the Dog, Cat, and Rabbit. 2nd ed. Philadelphia: Lippincott Williams & Wilkins, 1997:187.)

the abdominal body wall, up through the esophagus, and out the mouth.

e. Both techniques require care to ensure that the spleen is displaced behind the stomach before pushing needles and stylets through the abdominal wall. The gastroscope is used to highlight an area behind the last rib and below the lumbar muscles.

f. Tie the mouth end of the suture to the back end of the gastrostomy tube (the end that will be pulled through the abdominal wall; the end opposite the flanged end that will remain in the stomach).

g. Pull the abdominal suture and the gastrostomy tube out through the abdominal wall. You will have to enlarge the incision in the abdomi-

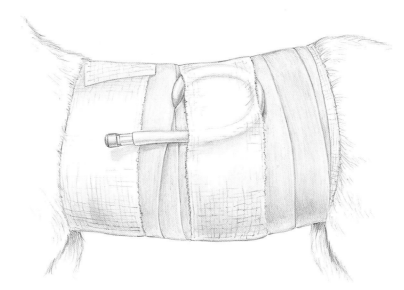

FIGURE 8-15.   An abdominal bandage is applied, and the end of the tube is capped. (From Crow SE, Walshaw SO. Manual of Clinical Procedures in the Dog, Cat, and Rabbit. 2nd ed. Philadelphia: Lippincott Williams & Wilkins, 1997:188.)

nal wall, taking care to make only a minimal incision in the stomach wall.

h. Gently pull the inner flange of the gastric cannula snugly up against the mucosa of the stomach and the stomach serosa up against the abdominal wall.

i. Place the external flange snugly so that the stomach is held in apposition to the abdominal wall.

j. The tube is sutured/bandaged to the abdominal wall and the wound site is cleaned once daily.

k. The tube should be left in place for at least 7 days to ensure that a good seal has formed between the stomach and the body wall. It can be removed once the animal is eating well on its own (*Fig. 8-16*).

l. For long-term feeding, a low-profile gastrostomy tube can be used (*Figs. 8-17* and *8-18*).

9. Supplies

a. 18–24 Fr Pezzer catheters (Mill-Rose Laboratories, Mentor, OH)

b. 18–24 Fr Bard Urologic Catheter, mushroom tipped (Bard Urologic Division, CR Bard, Inc., Covington, GA 30209).

c. Gastrostomy Tube Introduction Set (Cook Veterinary Products, Bloomington, IN 47402).

d. Eld Percutaneous Gastrostomy Device, Veterinary Medical and Surgical Supplies, 67 McMichael St., Maryville, NSW 2293, Australia. Fax: 011-61-49-622-292.

H. Enterostomy tubes

1. General anesthesia is required for tube placement.

2. May be placed at the time of abdominal surgery

3. Indicated if the stomach or small bowel must be avoided (pancreatitis, gastric neoplasia)

4. Cannot use blended diets—only liquid because of small tube lumen

5. Jejunal placement may require monomeric (elemental) diet instead of polymeric diet to avoid diarrhea.

6. Feeding must be by constant infusion. Bolus feeding can cause cramping and diarrhea.

7. Insertion technique (*Figs. 8-19* and *8-20*)

a. The tube is placed at the time of abdominal surgery.

b. A purse-string suture is placed through the antimesenteric border of the proximal jejunum, and a 12- gauge needle is directed aborally and tunneled subserosally for several centimeters before entering the bowel lumen. A 5 Fr red rubber or polyvinyl chloride catheter is advanced for 20–30 cm through the needle.

c. The purse string is tightened, and the needle removed from the bowel lumen.

d. The needle is placed through the right lateral abdominal wall from the prepared skin

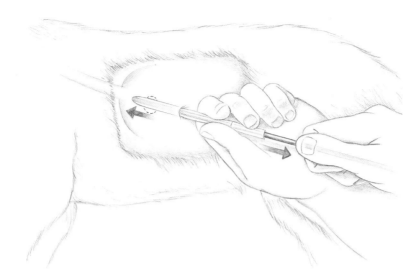

FIGURE 8-16. The gastrostomy tube can be removed by cutting off the excess tube and inserting a blunt metal rod (such as a Steinman pin) to stretch the mushroom tip and extract the tube. The inner flange will usually be passed in the feces in a few days. (In cats, endoscopic retrieval of the flange is preferred.) (From Crow SE, Walshaw SO. Manual of Clinical Procedures in the Dog, Cat, and Rabbit. 2nd ed. Philadelphia: Lippincott Williams & Wilkins, 1997:189.)

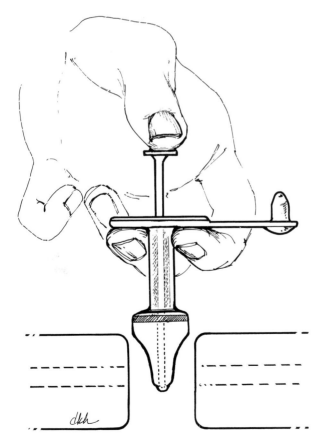

FIGURE 8-17. When long-term enteral feeding is necessary, it may be desirable to place a low-profile gastrostomy device (Bard Button Bard Interventional Products, CR Bard, Jewksbury, MA; Surgitek Button, Surgitek Cabot Medical Company, Racine, WI; Low Profile Button, Cook Instruments, Bloomington, IN). The gastrostomy tube is removed, and the low profile gastrostomy device is placed in the same stoma. (From Bojrab MJ, Ellison GW, Slocum BS, eds. Current Techniques in Small Animal Surgery. 4th ed. Baltimore: Williams & Wilkins, 1998:176.)

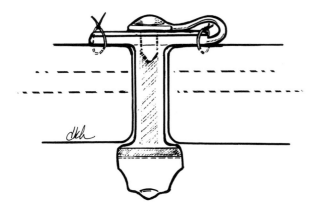

FIGURE 8-18.   The device is sutured to the skin and capped between feedings. (From Bojrab MJ, Ellison GW, Slocum BS, eds. Current Techniques in Small Animal Surgery. 4th ed. Baltimore: Williams & Wilkins, 1998:176.)

surface to the peritoneal cavity, and the catheter is threaded through the needle from the inside out and the needle removed. Simple interrupted or continuous sutures are used to fix the enterotomy site to the abdominal wall.

8. Begin feeding 24 hours after tube placement. Common tube-feeding complications are listed in *Table 8-3.*

I. Enteral feeding procedure (*Table 8-4*)

1. Determine how many kilocalories you want your patient to receive for the day.
a. Normally start with the column labeled "minimum energy requirements".
b. The kilocalorie estimate may be adjusted if there is reason to believe that the animal's metabolic expenditure is above or below this value.

2. Determine the kilocalorie density of the food product to calculate how much to feed (*Table 8-5*).

3. The calculated amount to feed divided by the number of feedings per day is the goal value for each feeding. The typical protocol is to start with a 4-hour feeding schedule to keep the volume per feeding minimal.

4. The nutritional materials can be introduced either as intermittent boluses or as a continuous infusion. Continuous infusion techniques may be associated with less adverse gastrointestinal (GI) consequences (vomiting, diarrhea).

5. Initial feeding volumes should be conservative (less than the goal value per feeding): 2 to 4 mL/kg/feeding or 1 mL/kg/h. Feed 1/3 of the calculated caloric amount on the first day.

6. If abdominal discomfort or restlessness develop or if the animal salivates, retches, or vomits, the volume of the nutrient solution or its concentration may be too high.

7. After 4 hours, or prior to the next feeding, the tube should be aspirated to ensure that the nutrient solutions are not accumulating at the site of deposition (stomach or esophagus).
a. Ideally, no residual solution should be aspirated.
b. If more than 50% of what has been administered is retrievable, the gut is not working properly. The material should be reinstilled, no additional solution should be administered, and residuals should be rechecked in 4 hours.

8. If, however, the GI tract appears to be moving the nutrient solutions forward, subsequent feedings can be increased in volume, toward the goal value per feeding calculated above. Once the goal value per 4-hour feeding has been reached, the volume per feeding can be further increased as the feeding frequency is decreased toward three to four times per day.

9. If diarrhea develops, it may be necessary to reduce the volume of intermittent feedings, to feed more frequently, or to switch to continuous infusions. It may be necessary to decrease the concentration (osmolality) of the fed solution, to correct hypoproteinemia, to change to a different carbohydrate (lactose-free) or protein source, or to change to an entirely different food product.

10. Tubes should be flushed with water between feedings; food retained within the tube may become stale or rancid. Tubes should be capped between feedings to prevent the aspiration of air or

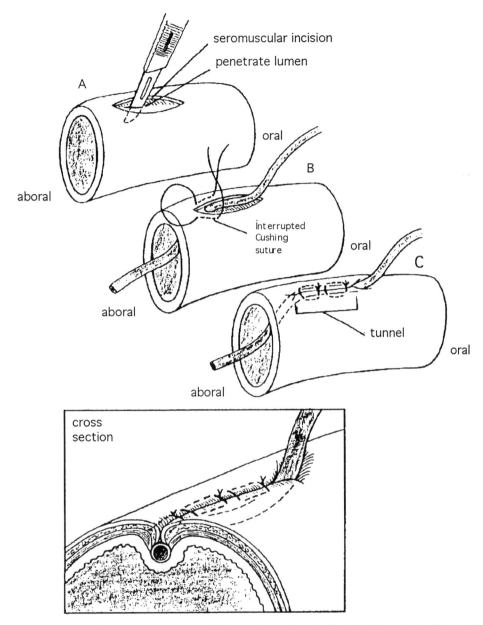

seromuscular incision

penetrate lumen

A

oral

B

aboral

interrupted
Cushing
suture

oral

C

aboral

tunnel

oral

aboral

cross
section

FIGURE 8-19. Steps in placing a jejunostomy tube (incision/tunnel method). **A.** A 2–3 cm longitudinal incision is made in the seromuscular layer of the antimesenteric border of an isolated segment of jejunum. **B.** A stab incision is made at the aboral end of the incision and a feeding tube is directed aborally into the gut lumen. **C.** A Cushing pattern with 3-0 to 4-0 monofilament suture is used to close the seromuscular incision. (From Bojrab MJ, Ellison GW, Slocum BS, eds. Current Techniques in Small Animal Surgery. 4th ed. Baltimore: Williams & Wilkins, 1998:178.)

the regurgitation of the nutrient material. For continuous feeding, open, unrefrigerated solutions should not hang for more than about 4 hours.

J. What to do if there is gastric/intestinal stasis

1. One common problem in critically ill patients is gastric stasis.

a. Gastric stasis is when residuals exceed 50% of what was previously introduced.

b. This cannot be assessed if the tube is in the terminal esophagus.

2. Motility inducers

a. Metoclopramide stimulates GI motility without stimulating gastric, pancreatic, and bil-

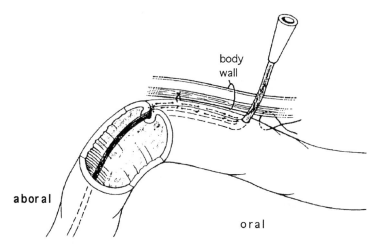

FIGURE 8-20.   Steps in placing a jejunostomy tube (continued). A submucosal tunnel is created for the feeding tube. A stab incision is made through the body wall and the catheter is exteriorized. The enterostomy site is sutured to the peritoneal surface of the adjacent body wall. The catheter is secured to the skin with a Chinese finger trap friction suture. The abdomen is closed, and a protective bandage is placed over the feeding tube exit site. (From Bojrab MJ, Ellison GW, Slocum BS, eds. Current Techniques in Small Animal Surgery. 4th ed. Baltimore: Williams & Wilkins, 1998:179.)

iary secretions by sensitizing the upper GI smooth muscle to the effects of acetylcholine.

    1) Gastric, duodenal, and jejunal tone and motility is increased; lower esophageal sphincter tone is increased; pyloric sphincter tone is decreased.

    2) Metoclopramide (0.05–0.1 mg/kg/h IV CRI) antagonizes dopamine at receptor sites in the CNS and can have sedative, central antiemetic, and extrapyramidal effects.

  b. Cisapride (0.1–0.5 mg/kg PO q8h) enhances the release of acetylcholine at the myenteric

TABLE 8.3
TUBE FEEDING COMPLICATIONS

Complication	Remedy
(1) Vomiting	Aspirate stomach contents before feeding; do not feed if full
	Stop feeding and restart more slowly
	Consider metoclopramide, sucralfate
	Correct hypokalemia, uremia
(2) Diarrhea	Check osmolality of diet; dilute to 200–400 mOsm/kg
	Consider adding fiber (Metamucil)
	Use CRI if animal cannot tolerate bolus feedings
(3) Tube ejection	Prevent vomiting—antiemetics
	Consider E-collar
(4) Aspiration pneumonia	Confirm tube placement and alveolar lung disease with radiographs
	Treat with antibiotics
(5) Clogged tube	Always flush with warm water before and after feeding
	Avoid giving pills in tube
	Instill carbonated beverage or cranberry juice
	Can try pancreatic enzymes
(6) Cellulitis	Change bandage regularly
	Monitor site for redness, swelling, and discharge
	Keep site clean and dry
	Antibiotics may be necessary

TABLE 8.4
GENERAL GUIDELINES FOR ENTERAL NUTRITION

1. Do not use tube for 24 hours
2. Begin by flushing tube with 5 mL/kg of water
3. On the first day, feed 1/3 of daily caloric requirement divided into 6 feedings (q4h)
4. Warm food and inject it slowly
5. Aspirate tube prior to each feeding; if > half of previous meal is aspirated, the feeding should be skipped—consider metoclopramide
6. Always flush tube before and after feeding with 5–10 mL of water
7. Increase feeding to 2/3 of requirement on day 2, and full feeding by day 3
8. Keep the skin wound clean and change the bandage as needed

---

plexus, increasing lower esophageal peristalsis and sphincter pressure, and gastric motility without increasing gastric secretions but is usually not available.

c. Erythromycin (0.5–1.0 mg/kg PO, IV q8h) is a bacteriostatic antibiotic that also enhances GI motility.

d. Bethanecol (0.1–3 mg/kg SQ q4h; 0.5–1.0 mg/kg PO q8h) is a synthetic cholinergic ester that directly stimulates cholinergic receptors.

1) It increases esophageal peristalsis and lower esophageal sphincter tone; increases tone and peristalsis of the stomach and intestinal tract; increases gastric and pancreatic secretions; and increases bladder detrusor muscle tone.

2) Bethanecol should not be used if there are GI ulcers, recent GI surgery, GI obstruction, urinary outflow obstructions, bradycardia, asthma, epilepsy, or hyperthyroidism.

e. Neostigmine (0.005–0.02 mg/kg SQ, IM q6h) is an acetylcholinesterase blocking agent that prolongs the longevity and effect of acetylcholine at all cholinergic and neuromuscular junctions. It is used most commonly to reverse the effects of neuromuscular blocking agents and in the treatment of myasthenia gravis.

1) Low doses of the drug can be used to obtain desirable enhancement of GI motility without inducing a muscarinic (vomiting, diarrhea, salivation, increased bronchial secretions, bronchospasm, bradycardia, increased gastric and pancreatic secretions) or a nicotinic (muscle cramps, twitching, tetany, paralysis) crisis.

2) Muscarinic effects can be blocked by prior administration of an anticholinergic such as atropine.

III. PARENTERAL NUTRITION

A. Parenteral nutrition is indicated whenever the gut is not working well enough to digest and absorb enough nutrients to meet the animal's daily requirements.

1. Parenteral nutrition is indicated if the animal is vomiting or regurgitating, if there is gastric stasis, or if the animal has pancreatitis or another reason to enforce bowel rest.

2. Parenteral nutrition may also be indicated in animals with coma or other neurologic deficits that increase the risk of aspiration.

B. Parenteral nutrition is more complicated and more expensive than enteral nutrition, is associated with a high risk of infection, and is associated with disuse villous atrophy of the small intestine.

C. There are two general approaches to intravenous nutrition:

1. To supply all of the calorie/amino acid requirements of the patient: total parenteral nutrition (TPN).

2. To supply only a portion of the calorie/amino acid requirements of the patient: partial parenteral nutrition (PPN).

3. TPN solutions are very hypertonic (1500–2000 mOsm/L) and must be given into a large central vein so that they can be rapidly diluted to minimize the incidence of phlebitis and thrombosis.

4. PPN solutions are designed for administration through peripheral veins and so must have much lower osmolality to minimize vessel damage, and thus they are not so calorie dense.

TABLE 8.5
COMPOSITION OF COMMERCIAL ENTERAL DIETS

Product	Caloric Content (kcal/mL or g)	Protein Content (g/100 kcal)	Protein Content (% prot/cal)	Fat Content (% fat /cal)	Carbo-hydrate Content (% CHO/cal)	Cost (¢/kcal)
Veterinary polymeric						
CliniCare Canine powder[a]	0.9	6.0	24	64	12	2.5
CliniCare Canine liquid	0.9	5.5	25	59	16	3.5
Renal Care Canine	0.8	2.8	14	66	20	3.7
CliniCare Feline powder[a]	0.8	9.1	36	53	11	2.6
CliniCare Feline liquid	0.8	8.6	36	48	16	4.2
Renal Care Feline	0.8	5.6	25	60	15	4.0
Eukanuba Nutritional Recovery Diet	2.1	7.4	29	41	30	
Prescription Diet a/d	1.3	8.8	36	51	13	0.5
Prescription Diet Feline p/d[a]	0.9	9.3	37	56	7	0.2
Prescription Diet Feline k/d[c]	0.9	4.4	21	67	13	0.2
Prescription Diet Feline c/d[c]	0.6	8.9	33	52	15	0.2
Prescription Diet Canine k/d[c]	0.6	3.1	13	49	39	0.2
Prescription Diet Canine u/d[c]	0.7	1.9	8	48	45	0.2
Prescription Diet Canine i/d[c]	0.6	5.9	24	31	45	0.2
Waltham Instant Concentration Diet [a]	1.5	9.3	37	37	25	
Nutri-Cal	4.6	0.3	1	62	37	1.2
Human polymeric						
Jevity	1.1	4.2	18	30	52	2.5
Pulmocare	1.5	4.3	17	55	28	2.5
Osmolite HN	1.1	4.4	17	30	53	2.5
Sustacal	1.0	6.8	24	21	55	2.5
Ensure HN	1.1	6.0	23	40	38	2.5
Baby food, turkey	1.0	14.6	58	42	0	1.0
Human monomeric						
Peptamen	1.0	4.4	16	33	51	5.0

[a]Diluted with water according to manufacturer's directions.
[b]Blenderized ½ can (224 g) + ¾ cup (170 mL) water.
[c]Blenderized ½ can (224 g) + ¾ cup (284 mL) water.

D. TPN formulas

1. For most critically ill dogs: 500 mL 50% dextrose; 500 mL 8.5% amino acid solution (Baxter; Abbott) with electrolytes; 250 mL 20% Intralipid; 1 mL multi-Vitamin B; 20 mEq potassium phosphate. Provides 1.2 kcal/mL; 19.7% glucose; 40 mEq K+/L; 2.8 g protein/100 kcal; kcal as 56% glucose and 33% fat.

2. For most critically ill cats: 250 mL 50% dextrose; 500 mL 8.5% amino acid solution with electrolytes; 250 mL 20% Intralipid; 1 mL multi-Vitamin B; 10 mEq potassium phosphate. Provides 1.08 kcal/mL; 12.4% glucose; 40 mEq K+/L; 3.9 g protein/100 kcal; kcal as 39% glucose and 46% fat.

3. For liver and renal failure dogs: 1000 mL 50% dextrose in water; 250 mL 8.5% amino acid solution; 250 mL 20% Intralipid; 500 mL lactated Ringer's; 1 mL multi-Vitamin B. For patients with renal failure with hyperkalemia, add no potassium; for patients with renal failure without hyperkalemia, add 66 mEq/L potassium chloride; for patients with liver failure, add 66 mEq/L of potassium phosphate. Provides 1.14 kcal/mL; 25% glucose; 0 or 40 mEq K$^+$/L; 0.93 g protein/100 kcal; kcal as 74% glucose and 22% fat.

4. For liver and renal failure cats: 500 mL 50% dextrose in water; 250 mL 8.5% amino acid solution; 250 mL 20% Intralipid; 500 mL lactated Ringer's; 1 mL multi-Vitamin B. For patients with renal failure with hyperkalemia, add no potassium; for patients with renal failure without hyperkalemia, add 46 mEq/L potassium chloride; for patients with liver failure, add 46 mEq/L of potassium phosphate. Provides 1.06 kcal/mL; 16.6% glucose; 0 or 40 mEq K$^+$/L; 1.34 g protein/100 kcal; kcal as 63% glucose and 32% fat.

5. An alternate method for calculating caloric needs for TPN is shown in the worksheet in *Table 8-6.*

E. PPN formula: Mix 500 or 1000 mL of ProcalAmine (McGaw) (3% glycerol; 3% amino acids) with 250 or 500 mL, respectively, of 20% lipid emulsion (Baxter, Abbott), plus 30 or 60 mEq potassium chloride, respectively.

1. Osmolality 580 mOsm/kg; 0.75 kcal/mL; 40 mEq K$^+$/L; 2.7 g protein/100 kcal; kcal as 10% carbohydrate and 80% fat.

2. This solution should be safe to administer through a peripheral venous catheter.

3. Fat-soluble vitamins and trace elements need not be added if parenteral nutrition is conducted for less than 1 week; if longer, vitamins A, D, and E, and a multi-trace element concentrate should be added to the parenteral nutrient solution. Vitamin K should not be added to the parenteral nutrient solution but should be administered subcutaneously once weekly.

F. Parenteral nutrient solutions must be mixed aseptically. The "All-in-One" mixing bags greatly facilitate the mixing of these solutions.

    a. Three separate ports are provided for admixing each of the three nutrient solutions (dextrose, amino acid, and lipid—always add the amino acid solution between the dextrose and lipid solutions). The order of mixing should be dextrose, amino acids, lipids, water and electrolyte solutions, and additives (KCl, vitamins, insulin, etc.).

    b. Assuming that it was mixed aseptically, the solution can be refrigerated for up to 7 days and administered at room temperature for as long as 2 days before discarding it.

    c. It has been recommended to cover the solution with a bag to protect the amino acids and lipids from light degradation.

G. An intravenous nutrition catheter is a dedicated catheter; it should not be used for any other purpose such as blood sampling or drug administration. Nutrition fluids are good growth media for accidental contaminants.

H. Parenteral nutrition procedures

1. Determine how many kilocalories your patient needs for the day. Normally use the column labeled "minimum energy requirements" (REE).

2. Choose a solution that seems most appropriate for your patient.

3. Divide the volume of solution to be administered for the day by 24 to obtain the hourly infusion rate (mL/h).

    a. Start the infusion at 50% of this value for the first 4 hours.

    b. Check the blood glucose level at the end of the 4 hours.

        1) If the blood glucose level is satisfactory (<250 mg/dL), increase the infusion rate to 75% of the calculated infusion rate and remeasure the blood glucose level in 4 hours.

        2) If the blood glucose level is satisfactory, increase the infusion rate to 100% of the calculated hourly infusion rate and remeasure the blood glucose level in 4 hours.

        3) If the blood glucose level is between 250 and 300 mg/dL during the weaning-on process, do not further increase the infusion rate; if the blood glucose level exceeds 300 mg/dL, decrease the glucose infusion rate.

    c. If the blood glucose level is consistently between 250 and 300 mg/dL during the maintenance phase, consider decreasing the glucose infusion rate; if the blood glucose level is consistently over 300 mg/dL, decrease the glucose infusion rate.

    d. If the animal is glucose intolerant (the predicted 100% infusion rate cannot be achieved without unacceptable hyperglycemia)

        1) Accept the highest infusion rate that the animal will tolerate—partial nutrition is better than no nutrition.

TABLE 8.6
PARENTERAL FEEDING WORKSHEET (ALTERNATE METHOD)

1. Calculate resting energy requirement (RER)(kcal/day): $70 \times BWkg^{0.75}$
   (For animals between 2 kg and 45 kg, can use abbreviated formula: $(30 \times BWkg) + 70$)

2. May add an illness/infection/injury factor to account for stress-induced increases in metabolism but the need for this is not well established.

Mild illness, infection, or injury:	no augmentation of RER
Moderate illness, infection, or injury:	$(1.1 \times RER) \times RER$
Severe illness, infection, or injury:	$(1.25 \times RER) \times RER$

3. Mix solution (can double the formula for large dogs)
   150 mL 50% dextrose
   250 mL 20% Intralipid
   500 mL 8.5% Travasol with electrolytes
   18 mEq Potassium phosphate
   5 mL Vitamin B complex

   This solution provides 1 kcal/mL. It has an osmolality of 1129 mOsm/L and should not be administered through a peripheral vein. It is 17% protein, 54% lipid, and 29% carbohydrate. It contains 20 mEq/L of potassium.

4. Calculate hourly infusion rate: (RER ± stress factor)/24

5. Begin infusion at 50% of this goal infusion rate and check blood glucose after 4 hours.

6. If blood glucose <200 mg/dL, increase infusion rate to 75% of goal and recheck blood glucose after 4 hours. If blood glucose is 200–250 mg/dL, do not increase the infusion rate; if blood glucose is >250 mg/dl decrease the infusion rate or treat with insulin.

7. After 4 hours, if blood glucose is <200 mg/dL, increase infusion rate to 100% of goal and recheck blood glucose after 4 hours.

8. If blood glucose <200 mg/dL, you have successfully weaned the patient on to the parenteral feeding solution. If blood glucose is >200 mg/dL decrease the infusion rate or treat with insulin.

9. If the patient is glucose intolerant as evidenced by hyperglycemia, the infusion rate should be slowed or insulin therapy should be instituted and the amount of glucose in the next preparation could be decreased.

10. If the patient is lipid intolerant as evidenced by lipemia, the infusion rate should be slowed and the amount of lipid in the next preparation should be decreased.

11. If the patient is protein intolerant (renal or hepatic insufficiency) as evidenced by either an unacceptable increase in blood urea nitrogen or ammonia, the infusion rate should be slowed and the amount of protein in the next preparation should be decreased.

2) Decrease the glucose concentration in the solution and replace its energy equivalents with lipid (1.7 mL 50% dextrose = 2 mL 20% Intralipid); or

3) Add exogenous insulin to the nutrient solution or the patient to supplement the animal's endogenous insulin output (1–2 U/kg/24 h regular insulin).

4. Amino acids are provided as a proportion of the diet; designated either as a percentage of the total diet or as a ratio of grams of protein or nitrogen to nonprotein kilocalories. Amino acids should be provided in a ratio of about 1.5–3 g of metabolizable protein per 100 kcal of energy in the dog and about 3–5 g of metabolizable protein per 100 kcal of energy in the cat. Animals with hepatic or renal failure may be amino acid intolerant (hyperammonemia and uremia, respectively) and it may be necessary to decrease the amino acid concentration of the nutrient solution.

5. Patients should be weaned off high-glucose infusions so that the high endogenous insulin levels do not precipitate a rebound hypoglycemia. Decrease the infusion rate by 50%, check a blood glucose level in 2 hours. If the blood glucose is OK, stop the glucose infusion and recheck the blood glucose level in 2 hours.

HOMEMADE LIQUID AND BLENDERIZED DIETS

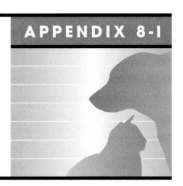

Recipe 1—Blenderized commercial pet food
½ can (224 g) Feline p/d
¾ c (170 mL) warm water
Blenderize for 1 minute at high speed
Strain one to two times through a kitchen strainer (1-mm mesh)
Provides 0.9 kcal/mL
Protein (% of total kcal)—36.9%
Fat (% of total kcal)—56.3%

Recipe 2—Blenderized commercial renal failure diet
½ can (224 g) Prescription Diet Feline k/d
1¼ c (284 mL) water
Blenderize at high speed for 60 seconds. Strain twice through a kitchen strainer (1-mm mesh)
Caloric density—0.9 kcal/mL
Protein (% of total kcal)—20.8%
Fat (% of total kcal)—66.6%
Carbohydrate (% of total kcal)—12.6%

Recipe 3—AMC feline diet
240 mL Pulmocare
240 mL Sustacal
5 T Casec powder
250 mg taurine
12 mL Pet- Tinic
Blenderize and feed 8 oz daily in divided feedings
8 oz provide 325 kcal and 24g protein

Recipe 4—AMC feline diet
240 mL Pulmocare
240 mL Sustacal
10 scoops ProBalance Maximum Feline
Blenderize and feed 8 oz daily in divided feedings
8 oz provide 325 kcal and 24g protein

Recipe 5—University of Florida feline diet
8 oz of a human enteral product (30–60 kcal/oz)
1000 mg arginine
500 mg taurine
140–500 mg carnitine
2000 mg fish oil
100–200 mg thiamine
7–8 mg zinc

Recipe 6—University of Florida feline diet
4.5 oz of a meat-based baby food (15–25 kcal/oz)
250 mg taurine
1000 mg fish oil
50–100 mg thiamine
3–4 mg zinc

Recipe 7—University of Pennsylvania tube feeding diet
8 oz Pulmocare
2 T dehydrated cottage cheese (ProMagic)
Blenderize
Provides 1.7 kcal/mL
31% protein, 46% fat DMB

Recipe 8 - University of California-Davis (Biourge)
8 oz Pulmocare
240 mL warm water
30 g micropulverized casein (Casec, Mead-Johnson)
5 g KCl
2 mL B vitamins
1 g citrulline
500 mg choline
250 mg taurine
Blend all ingredients with water, then *mix* with Pulmocare. DO NOT blend, to avoid foaming. Mix before each feeding. Keep refrigerated up to 72 hours. Warm the volume needed at each meal prior to feeding.
Provides 0.9 kcal/mL
42% protein, 22% fat DMB

CRITICAL CARE NUTRITION / ENTERAL FEEDING TUBES A/D TUBE FEEDING

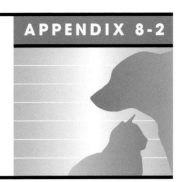

Product Description	Caloric Density (kcal/mL; as is)	Tube Size (French)						
		5	8	10	12	14	16	18
Undiluted a/d	1.2	−	−	−	±	±	+	+
2 cans a/d + 50 mL water	1.0	−	−	±	+	++	+++	+++
2 cans a/d + 100 mL water	0.9	−	±	+	++	++	+++	+++
2 cans a/d + 150 mL water[a]	0.8	−	+	++	+++	+++	+++	+++
1 can a/d + 150 mL water[b]	0.6	+	+	++	+++	+++	+++	+++
Strained meat	0.95	−	−	−	±	±	+	+
2 jars of baby food + 45 mL water	0.7	−	±	+	+	++	+++	+++

[a]Method of Dr. Karol Matthews, Ontario Veterinary College, University of Guelph; a/d is blended 60 seconds, not strained.
[b]Pediatric Feeding Tube Model K-32; (5 french × 38 cm), Baxter Health Care Laboratories, Deerfield, IL.
Legend: − flow, excessive pressure, really hard push; + flow, high pressure, hard push; ++ good flow, acceptable pressure, medium push; +++ good flow, low pressure, easy push.

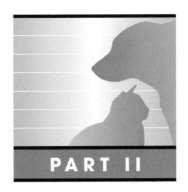

PART II

Specific Protocols and Procedures for Emergency Conditions

CHAPTER 9

RESPIRATORY EMERGENCIES

I. GENERAL APPROACH/METHODS OF OXYGEN DELIVERY

A. Clinical signs of respiratory distress

1. Tachypnea
2. Open-mouth breathing
3. Cyanotic mucous membranes
4. Loud breathing
5. Restlessness, anxiety
6. Glazed look
7. Extended head and neck
8. Paradoxical respiration (abdominal wall and chest wall move opposite one another during respiration)

Tachypnea is the most consistent sign. The severity of respiratory compromise is not always manifested clinically, although patients that are exhibiting any of the signs 1–8 are most likely in severe distress. Cats are more subtle in showing clinical signs of respiratory distress than dogs, unless they are stressed.

B. Oxygen supplementation

1. Supplemental oxygen should be provided for any animal with signs of respiratory distress. **When in doubt, supplement!** (See side effects below)
2. Precaution: When supplementing oxygen, make every effort to avoid prolonged exposure (>24 hours) at high concentrations (>60% FiO_2). The FiO_2 is the fractional inspired oxygen concentration. It is approximately 20% on room air, 100% on pure oxygen, and 40% on nasal insufflation. Oxygen toxicity can cause irreversible pulmonary fibrosis through the generation of oxygen free radicals and subsequent lipid peroxidation. The following recommendations should help to prevent oxygen toxicity:

a. After initial stabilization with 100% oxygen, reduce the level of fractional inspired O_2 in small increments to maintain the lowest FiO_2 compatible with adequate systemic and tissue oxygenation. Inspired concentrations less than 50% are generally considered safe.
b. If PO_2 cannot be maintained above 60 mm Hg without high concentrations of supplemental oxygen, consider mechanical ventilation with positive end-expiratory pressure (PEEP) or continuous positive airway pressure (CPAP). When more alveoli are open for gas exchange, the FiO_2 can usually be reduced to safer levels.
c. To optimize oxygen delivery to tissues, anemia should be corrected, cardiac output optimized, and alterations in acid–base balance, electrolytes, and body temperature normalized.
d. Current recommendations in small animals are to avoid giving 100% O_2 for more than 24 hours or 60% O_2 for more than 48 hours.

3. Methods of oxygen supplementation
   a. Oxygen mask
      1) Advantages: Inexpensive, easy to administer, can achieve high inspired oxygen concentrations with a tight-fitting mask
      2) Disadvantages: Requires restraint in awake patients, not well tolerated by some patients, cannot control inspired oxygen concentration
      3) Oxygen flow rate: 100–200 mL/kg/min
      4) Useful for providing short-term O_2 supplementation during initial assessment of an

emergency patient or as a means of preoxygenation before performing stressful procedures (such as radiographs or catheter placement).

b. Enriched oxygen environments

1) Oxygen cage

   a) Advantages: Nonstressful, high inspired oxygen concentrations can be achieved, humidity and temperature control, can control inspired oxygen concentration

   b) Disadvantages: Wasteful of oxygen, cages are expensive, the patient is isolated and cannot be monitored, oxygen supplementation is interrupted whenever the cage door is opened, most cages tend to overheat when large dogs are in them

   c) Intermittent oxygen supplementation can be helpful for some patients prior to diagnostic and therapeutic procedures. Stabilization in an oxygen cage, followed by a procedure with immediate placement back into the oxygen cage is particularly efficacious in cats.

2) Neonatal incubator

   a) Advantages: Inexpensive, nonstressful

   b) Disadvantages: Difficult to achieve high inspired oxygen concentration, cannot control inspired oxygen concentration, cannot control humidity, limited temperature control, patient is isolated

3) Oxygen blanket

   a) Most oxygen blankets used in veterinary medicine are plastic sheets or bags. The patient's head is placed in the bag, and oxygen is piped in to form an "oxygen tent."

   b) Advantages: Inexpensive, high inspired oxygen concentrations can be achieved, some patients tolerate this method well

   c) Disadvantages: Cannot control inspired oxygen concentration, patient can overheat, carbon dioxide and moisture can build up

4) Crowe collar (Fig. 9-1)

   a) Elizabethan collar with plastic wrap over the top. Leaving an opening at the top will allow heated gases and carbon dioxide to escape.

   b) Advantages: Inexpensive, well tolerated, high inspired oxygen concentrations, patient can be monitored and procedures performed without interrupting oxygen supply

   c) Disadvantages: Cannot control inspired oxygen concentration, patient can overheat, moisture and carbon dioxide can accumulate, some patients do not tolerate

5) Nasal oxygen insufflation

   a) Advantages: Inexpensive, moderately well tolerated, relatively high inspired oxygen concentrations can be achieved, patient can be monitored and procedures performed without interruption of oxygen supply

   b) Disadvantages: Some animals do not tolerate it, cannot control or measure inspired oxygen concentration, can cause nasal mucosal irritation, application of the catheter can sometimes be stressful to the patient

   c) Procedure

   1. Equipment: Oxygen source, in-line bubble humidifier, red rubber or other commercial pediatric feeding tube (largest bore possible for patient's naris), catheter adapter, 5- or 10-mL syringe barrel without plunger, sterile suction tubing, lidocaine (2%) or proparacaine, lubricant, medical adhesive tape and suture material, or cyanoacrylate adhesive

   2. Technique

   a. Infuse lidocaine into naris and elevate muzzle; wait 2–3 minutes.

   b. Premeasure and mark the catheter (with tape as a butterfly for securing the catheter) for the distance between the medial canthus of the eye and the naris.

   c. Lubricate the tip of the catheter.

   d. Insert the catheter into the ventromedial aspect of the naris. The first few centimeters are the most sensitive, and the catheter should advance quickly at first. An assistant should stabilize the animal's head. The catheter should be advanced to the predetermined distance.

   e. The catheter should be secured with skin staples or suture through the "butterfly" tape or tissue glue as close as possible to where it exits the naris. (Fig. 9-1)

   f. Secure a more proximal portion of the catheter in a similar manner to the skin, either ventral to the ear or on the forehead. The forehead avoids catheter

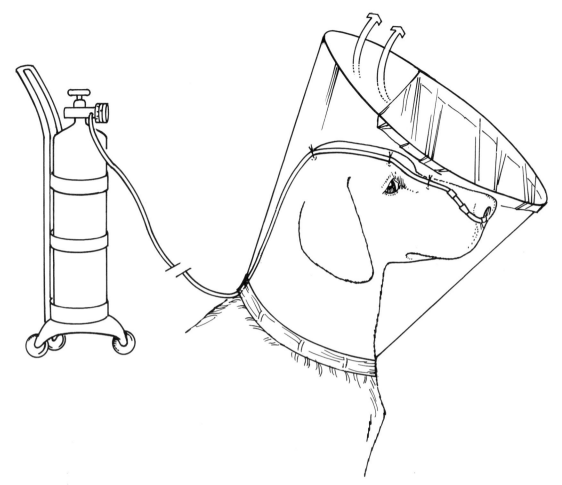

FIGURE 9.1 The "Crowe Collar" and Nasal Oxygen. Note the location of suture placement for the nasal oxygen tube. The "Crowe Collar" can also be used without nasal oxygen by piping oxygen directly into the closed-in area of the collar. (From Crowe DT, Devey JJ. Nasal, nasopharyngeal, nasotracheal, nasoesophageal, nasogastric, and nasoenteric tubes: insertion and use. In Bojrab MJ, Ellison GW, Slocum B, eds. Current techniques in small animal surgery. Baltimore: Williams & Wilkins, 1998:151-161.)

contact with the whiskers, which can be irritating, particularly to cats.

g. *Attach the syringe barrel to the proximal end of the catheter by use of the adapter.*

h. *Connect the syringe to the humidified oxygen source via the suction tubing.*

i. *Select the highest oxygen flow rate that the patient will tolerate to treat the hypoxemia (generally 0.5 to >5 L/min, or 100–200 mL/kg/min).*

j. *A second nasal line can be placed in animals that remain dyspneic. A "Y"-type connector can be used to attach the nasal lines to the flow tubing.*

6) **Positive-pressure ventilation**

a) *See Mechanical Ventilation*

b) *Advantages: Complete control of ventilation, inspired oxygen concentration can be controlled (in some ventilators PEEP may be used)*

c) *Disadvantages: Expensive, requires constant nursing care, invasive, generally requires complete anesthesia or sedation, may induce barotrauma*

C. Intravenous catheterization

1. Obtain intravenous catheterization in patients with respiratory distress. This allows administration of emergency drugs to these critically ill patients.

2. This procedure may be stressful and should be attempted only in patients that will tolerate the procedure after preoxygenation. Clinical judgment is required.

II. UPPER AIRWAY OBSTRUCTION (PHARYNX, LARYNX, TRACHEA)

A. Clinical signs

1. Loud breath sounds heard without the stethoscope.
2. Extrathoracic upper airway obstruction
   a. Breath sounds tend to be the loudest and distress the worst on **inspiration** with extrathoracic upper airway obstruction. Severe obstructions can cause distress and noise on **inspiration** and **expiration** (particularly fixed airway obstructions).
   b. Rarely, severe upper airway obstruction can result in minimal breath sounds because very little air is being moved. This can occur in some patients with severe laryngeal paralysis in which a minimal amount of air is moved on inspiration
   c. Duration of inspiration is much greater than that of expiration, and the animal appears to work harder to inspire than to expire.

3. Intrathoracic upper airway obstruction
   a. Breath sounds tend to be louder and distress worse on expiration with intrathoracic upper airway obstruction. Severe intrathoracic upper airway obstruction can cause distress and noise on expiration and inspiration (particularly fixed airway obstructions).
   b. Duration of expiration is much greater than that of inspiration.
4. Upper airway foreign bodies, inflammation, or infection can often cause coughing, retching, or hypersalivation.
5. A history of coughing/retching and voice change often accompanies laryngeal paralysis.

B. Diagnosis

1. Clinical signs, history, and physical examination are the most important clues for the diagnosis of upper airway obstruction.
2. Definitive diagnosis requires direct visualization of the obstruction or imaging techniques such as radiography and fluoroscopy.

3. Fluoroscopy allows visualization of dynamic airway problems. It is one of the standard ways to definitively diagnose a collapsing trachea. It may also be used to detect mainstem bronchus compression and diaphragm paralysis. This procedure is generally performed at referral hospitals only.
4. Bronchoscopy can aid in the diagnosis of collapsing trachea, tracheal stenosis, foreign body aspiration/granuloma, parasitic disease, or neoplasia either by direct visualization or through procurement of diagnostic samples.
5. Laryngoscopic examination under heavy sedation or light anesthesia is generally necessary to evaluate upper airway problems. (For technique, see "Laryngeal Paralysis," p. 121.)

C. Procedures

1. Emergency tracheostomy
   a. Emergency tracheostomy is defined as a tracheostomy performed without prior control of the airway. Most tracheostomies may be performed under more controlled circumstances in which orotracheal intubation has been achieved and airway control exists.
   b. Technique
     1) Under emergency conditions, a tracheostomy could be performed under mild tranquilization/sedation and a local block.
     2) If the animal is cyanotic, immediate oxygenation can be achieved by placing a needle between two tracheal rings and attaching it to a humidified oxygen source. As soon as the animal's color improves, anesthesia or sedation can be administered to allow placement of the tracheostomy tube.
     3) The patient should be positioned in dorsal recumbency, with a towel or sandbag placed under the neck to dorsiflex it to optimize the surgical site exposure.
     4) Ideally, clipping and surgical preparation of the site is preferred, but with true emergency tracheostomy, this time is not always available.
     5) Make a ventral, midline cervical skin incision from the cricoid cartilage to about the sixth tracheal ring. If in doubt, make the incision too long rather than too short.
     6) The muscles overlying the trachea are bluntly separated along the midline to visualize the tracheal rings.

7) Make an incision with a scalpel blade through the annular ligament between cartilage rings. Generally, the incision is made between the third and fourth tracheal cartilages or further down the trachea beyond the obstruction if indicated. The incision should extend approximately 65% of the circumference of the trachea. The tracheostomy tube is then placed through the incision and into the trachea. Tube placement is aided by placing stay suture loops around the tracheal rings above and below the tracheostomy site.

8) Administer ventilation with 100% inspired oxygen immediately.

9) Secure the tracheostomy tube to the neck with umbilical tape or gauze tied around the neck.

10) Once the animal is stabilized the surgical site can be more properly clipped and cleaned and the skin incision closed above and below the tracheostomy site. The skin closure should not make a complete seal around the tracheostomy tube. A tight seal will allow any air leaking around the tracheostomy tube to dissect subcutaneously as well as into the mediastinum, creating a pneumomediastinum.

11) A cuffed endotracheal tube with inner cannula is available (Shiley Pediatric tracheostomy tube with obturator, Mallinckrodt Medical TPI, 1595 Deere Ave, PO Box 19614, Irvine, CA 92713-9614). The cuff is only inflated if mechanical ventilation is required or during the first 24 hours after placement to prevent aspiration of tracheal secretions. High-pressure inflation of the cuff should be avoided, as tracheal necrosis may result.

2. **Tracheostomy tube care**

   a. Once a tracheostomy tube has been placed, the animal should be monitored continuously. The presence of the tube causes mucoid secretions that can dry and obstruct the tube. Airway obstruction, premature tube dislodgement, and aspiration of mucous plugs can be life-threatening consequences of tracheostomy tube placement.

   b. If possible, double-lumen tubes should be used so that the inner cannula can be cleared while the outer sleeve remains in place to keep the airway patent.

   c. If a double-lumen tube is not available, the single-lumen tube must be changed and cleaned up to two to four times daily, or even more often if tube blockage occurs. A second tube should be placed immediately when the first one is removed for cleaning.

   d. Traction sutures placed in the rings above and below the tracheostomy site are used to aid in tube placement.

   e. When a tracheostomy tube is removed, it can be soaked in disinfectant, but it must be thoroughly rinsed with sterile saline before being replaced in the patient.

   f. Postoperative care also includes humidification and suction. A heated humidifier system can be obtained from a human respiratory therapist, or 3–10 mL of sterile saline can be placed in the tube q3–4h to keep the epithelium moist, or nebulization with saline or diluted acetylcysteine can be performed every 4–8 hours. Hydration should be maintained with adequate fluid therapy to prevent drying of secretions.

   g. Suctioning is not a benign procedure, and it may result in cardiopulmonary arrest or severe hypoxemia. It should initially be done three to four times daily and then as needed.

   h. Before suctioning, the animal should be preoxygenated with 100% oxygen for 2–3 minutes, and saline placed into the tube to loosen secretions.

   i. The suction tubing should be long enough to extend to the bronchus. The operator should gently twirl the catheter while withdrawing it. Each suctioning episode should last 10 seconds.

   j. When the tracheostomy tube is finally removed, the animal must be watched closely for signs of dyspnea. Another technique involves placing a small-lumen tube and occluding it to make sure the animal is able to breathe before tube removal. The tracheostomy site is allowed to heal by granulation.

D. Specific conditions

1. **Elongated soft palate**

   a. Approximately 80% of elongated soft palates are found in brachycephalic dogs. It is often associated with other respiratory tract abnormalities such as stenotic nares, laryngeal saccule eversion, laryngeal collapse, tracheal stenosis, and tracheal collapse. Pharyngeal

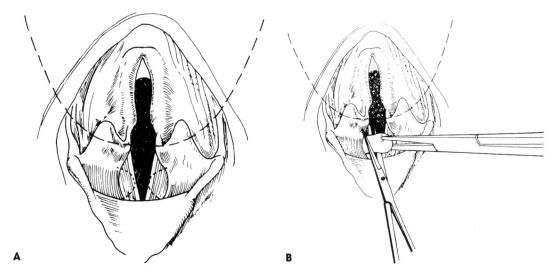

FIGURE 9.2 **A.** Elongated soft palate. The *dorsal dashed line* represents the position of an elongated soft palate obstructing the dorsal aspect of the larynx. Everted saccules (*ventral dashed line*) protrude from their crypts and partially obscure the vocal folds. **B.** Everted laryngeal saccules. The laryngeal saccule is grasped with tissue forceps and amputated at its base. (From Hedlund CS. Brachycephalic syndrome. In Bojrab MJ, Ellison GW, Slocum B, eds. Current techniques in small animal surgery. Baltimore: Williams & Wilkins, 1998:357-362.)

mucosal edema and protruding tonsils are also common. (*Fig. 9-2A*)

b. Pathophysiology

1) The elongated soft palate extends beyond the tip of the epiglottis and may be sucked into the glottis during inspiration, causing airway obstruction and interference with laryngeal function. Injury to the palate and larynx can result in edema and swelling.

2) Some patients may have increased body temperature because of inability to cool themselves through the respiratory system and the extra work of respiration.

c. Clinical signs

1) Severity depends upon length of the soft palate and degree of obstruction.

2) Gagging, coughing, snoring during breathing (particularly inspiration). Cyanosis is present in severely affected animals.

d. Treatment

1) Definitive treatment requires resection of the portion of the palate that is causing the obstruction. Surgical texts should be consulted, as excessive shortening of the soft palate will leave the patient prone to aspiration pneumonia.

2) Emergency stabilization may require anesthesia and intubation with severely affected patients.

3) Emergency stabilization in moderately to severely affected patients may include mild sedation with acepromazine (30–50 μg/kg IV or IM), oxygen supplementation, and whole-body cooling if the patient is overheated. Patients should be cooled to 39.5°C (103°F) to avoid rebound hypothermia.

4) Antiinflammatory doses of corticosteroids will help decrease pharyngeal and mucosal inflammation and edema.

2. Everted laryngeal saccules

a. Most frequently seen in brachycephalic dogs alone or in association with other upper respiratory tract abnormalities such as elongated soft palate or stenotic nares. Rarely seen in other breeds with laryngeal paralysis

b. Pathophysiology

1) Eversion of the saccules occurs in response to the increased negative pressure in the larynx during inspiration. The everted tissue becomes inflamed and edematous, causing airway obstruction.

2) The upper airway obstruction may cause increase in body temperature due to the inability to cool through the respiratory tract.

c. Treatment

1) Emergency stabilization in moderately to severely affected patients may include mild sedation with acepromazine (30–50 μg/kg IV or IM), oxygen supplementation, and whole-body cooling if the patient is overheated. Patients should be cooled to 39.5°C (103°F) to avoid rebound hypothermia.

2) Antiinflammatory doses of corticosteroids will help decrease pharyngeal and mucosal inflammation and edema.

3) Definitive therapy requires surgical removal of the saccules (*Fig. 9-2B*). The patient is positioned in sternal recumbency with the mouth open. The everted saccules can be visualized just behind the arytenoid cartilages of the larynx. Each saccule is grasped with long hemostats, retracted rostrally, and amputated at its base with scissors or a scalpel. Hemorrhage is minor and controlled by pressure. The electroscalpel causes more edema and inflammation and should be avoided.

3. Laryngeal paralysis

a. Laryngeal paralysis is failure of the laryngeal folds to abduct during inspiration. It is due to loss of innervation (from the recurrent laryngeal nerves) of the intrinsic musculature of the larynx. Laryngeal paralysis occurs in both dogs and cats. Unilateral paralysis occurs but rarely results in clinical signs.

b. Etiology

1) General causes of laryngeal paralysis include congenital, systemic neuromuscular, metabolic, traumatic, inflammatory, and idiopathic conditions. Idiopathic is by far the most common.

2) Congenital laryngeal paralysis occurs before 18 months of age and appears to be inherited in Bouvier des Flandres, Siberian Huskies, English Bulldogs, and possibly Bullterriers.

3) Laryngeal paralysis may occur in association with a generalized polyneuropathy and has been recognized with myasthenia gravis.

4) Hypothyroidism has been associated with laryngeal paralysis. Idiopathic laryn-

geal paralysis tends to occur in older, large-breed dogs such as Labrador Retrievers, Golden Retrievers, Irish Setters and Saint Bernards.

c. Diagnosis

1) History

Exercise intolerance, increased effort and noise on inspiration, coughing/gagging when eating or drinking, change in voice characterized by deeper and weaker bark sounds, and occasional syncope.

2) Cervical and thoracic radiography

a) *Seldom useful in the definitive diagnosis of laryngeal paralysis, but secondary changes can occur.*

b) *Secondary radiographic changes*

1. Air in the laryngeal saccules

2. Caudodorsal interstitial/alveolar pattern may result from neurogenic pulmonary edema secondary to the upper airway obstruction

3. Generalized increase of pulmonary radiodensity because of atelectasis

4. Aspiration pneumonia

5. Esophageal dilation with air

6. Rarely, hiatal hernia

3) Laryngeal muscle electromyography

a) *Used rarely to diagnose laryngeal paralysis*

b) *Correlation between electromyography and clinically apparent laryngeal paralysis is not always consistent*

4) Laryngoscopic examination

a) *The gold standard for the clinical diagnosis of laryngeal paralysis*

b) *Examination should be performed under light sedation with a short-acting barbiturate (thiamylal sodium, 2 mg/kg boluses or propofol 4–6 mg/kg IV). The sedation should be performed slowly using the lightest sedation necessary to visualize the larynx adequately. This allows the animal to breath spontaneously while the larynx is visualized. Laryngeal function cannot be assessed if the animal is not breathing spontaneously.*

c) *The larynx should be visualized through several respiratory cycles. It is helpful for an assistant to observe the animal's respiration while the clinician visualizes the larynx. The assistant notifies the clinician when an inspiration occurs.*

d) The arytenoid cartilages and vocal folds normally abduct in a coordinated fashion at the beginning of inspiration.

e) The arytenoid cartilages and vocal folds neither abduct nor adduct during inspiration in patients with laryngeal paralysis. Sometimes, in severe cases, they are sucked together during inspiration, narrowing the upper airway and obstructing inspiration.

f) Fluttering of the vocal folds or complete adduction of the folds during inspiration may be observed in the presence of laryngeal paralysis.

d. Treatment

  1) Emergency stabilization

    a) Immediate oxygen supplementation

    b) Sedation with acepromazine (30–50 μg/kg IV or IM).

    c) Cool patient if temperature exceeds 40.5°C (105°F). Cool only to 39.5°C (103°F) to avoid rebound hypothermia.

    d) Antiinflammatory doses of corticosteroids sometimes help decrease laryngeal swelling and edema.

    e) Rarely, anesthesia and intubation are necessary to stabilize the patient initially. Complete anesthesia should be avoided because animals with dynamic upper airway obstruction often reobstruct during the excitement phase of anesthetic recovery.

    f) Intubation should immediately relieve the respiratory problem. If it does not, then other causes of respiratory distress should be investigated.

    g) Submit blood for thyroid testing and for presence of antibodies against acetylcholine receptors (myasthenia gravis).

  2) Surgery

    a) Surgical options for laryngeal paralysis include vocal fold removal, castellated laryngofissure, and arytenoid lateralization. (Consult surgical texts.)

    b) Complications include scar tissue formation resulting in upper airway obstruction, swelling causing upper airway obstruction immediately postsurgery, and aspiration pneumonia.

4. **Nasopharyngeal polyp**

  a. Nasopharyngeal polyps are granulation tissue covered by variable types of epithelium arising from the eustachian tube. They may be accompanied by otitis media or sometimes even otitis externa. These primarily occur in cats.

  b. Clinical signs

    1) Chronic upper respiratory signs such as coughing, sneezing, nasal discharge, and stertorous breathing are often present. Clinical signs may develop at any age but tend to be more common in kittens or young cats. Nasopharyngeal polyps have been reported in kittens as young as 4 weeks.

    2) Episodes of respiratory distress may be severe in some cats, manifested with cyanosis and even syncope.

    3) Nasopharyngeal polyps may cause sudden death in some kittens.

    4) The severity of clinical signs may change with the position of the polyp. A cat with transient obstruction of the glottis will exhibit waxing and waning signs as the polyp moves over the airway.

  c. Diagnosis

    1) Diagnosis is based on history, clinical signs, and visual examination of the pharynx.

    2) Visual examination of the pharynx should be performed under general anesthesia to facilitate a thorough examination.

    3) The polyp may be seen protruding beyond the soft palate.

    4) Most often, ventral displacement of the soft palate is noticed. Gentle, forward retraction of the soft palate with a spay hook will reveal the polyp located dorsal to the soft palate. A dental mirror can help facilitate visualization of the dorsal aspect of the soft palate.

    5) Skull radiographs may reveal otitis media on the affected side (increased opacity of the ventral bulla) as well as a soft tissue mass in the area of the nasopharynx.

  d. Treatment

    1) Surgical treatment is the only option.

    2) An oral approach with forward retraction of the soft palate will often expose the polyp.

    3) A curved mosquito forceps is used to clamp the stalk of the polyp. Removal is achieved by gentle, steady pulling and twisting of the stalk.

    4) Postsurgical complications include transient (resolves after 3–6 weeks) or permanent

Horner's syndrome and persistent otitis media related to rupture of the tympanic membrane.

5) Otitis media may require surgical drainage (bulla ostectomy), culture and sensitivity testing, and antibiotic therapy.

5. Foreign body

a. Pharyngeal foreign bodies include needles, fish hooks, bones, toothpicks, wooden sticks, grass awns (foxtails), and grass blades. Conditions that can mimic upper airway foreign body include sublingual and oropharyngeal hematoma resulting from rodenticide coagulopathy or ranula from a zygomatic sialocele.

b. A common pharyngeal foreign body in dogs is a ball, particularly balls with a smooth surface.

c. Clinical signs

1) Usually, acute onset of gagging, repeated movements of the tongue, hypersalivation, repeated swallowing, shaking of the head, and pawing at the mouth

2) Pharyngeal foreign bodies can cause severe respiratory distress because of occlusion of the airway by the foreign body or because of inflammation and swelling in reaction to the foreign body.

d. Diagnosis

1) Diagnosis is based on history, clinical signs and direct visualization of the foreign body.

2) Pharyngeal and thoracic radiographs will help evaluate the rest of the respiratory tree.

3) Fiberoptic bronchoscopy will visualize the lower airways beyond the larynx.

e. Treatment

1) Removal of the foreign body generally requires immediate induction of general anesthesia and provision of a patent airway.

2) Expulsion of the foreign body may be aided by suspending the animal upside down and applying the Heimlich maneuver (quick forceful pressure) just behind the diaphragm.

3) Emergency tracheostomy may be needed if the patient is in severe respiratory distress and orotracheal intubation cannot be achieved to relieve the obstruction.

4) Manipulation of large foreign bodies, such as balls, can cause occlusion of the airway. Pay stringent attention to maintaining a patent airway at all times during foreign body retrieval. If airway occlusion does occur, dorsal displacement of the foreign body can sometimes open up the airway. If this does not help, perform emergency tracheostomy if orotracheal intubation is not possible.

5) A thorough, well lit examination of the pharyngeal area should be performed. Small grass blades can often be hidden in the pharyngeal mucosal folds. Grass awns (foxtails) can also lodge in the tonsillar crypts.

6) If significant trauma and inflammation are present, consider antiinflammatory doses of corticosteroids.

7) If severe penetration and mucosal damage have occurred, administer broad-spectrum antibiotics.

8) Monitor the patient closely during anesthetic recovery, for any respiratory compromise.

6. Neoplasia

a. Most tumors of the pharyngeal area are malignant. Common tumors are squamous cell carcinoma and lymphoma. Other pharyngeal tumors include fibrosarcoma, tonsillar carcinoma, and oral melanoma.

b. Primary laryngeal tumors in dogs include leiomyomas, rhabdomyosarcomas, squamous cell carcinomas, and melanomas. Lymphosarcoma and squamous cell carcinoma are the most common laryngeal tumors in cats.

c. Clinical signs

1) Dysphagia ± nasal discharge, sonorous respiration, respiratory distress

2) Other nonspecific clinical signs depend upon the extent of tumor involvement and include anorexia, lethargy, and weight loss.

d. Diagnosis

Visual examination of the pharynx and larynx, cytology, impression smears, and histopathologic examination of biopsies of the abnormal tissue

e. Treatment

1) Patients in extreme respiratory distress may require immediate intubation or emergency tracheostomy if intubation is not possible.

2) Definitive treatment depends upon the type of tumor and extent of involvement.

The three major modalities of therapy are local excision, radiation, and/or chemotherapy/immunotherapy.

3) Prognosis

Most tumors of the pharynx and larynx are malignant and carry a poor long-term prognosis. Take thoracic radiographs to check for pulmonary metastasis and aid in prognosis.

7. Laryngeal spasm

a. Laryngeal spasm is primarily a problem only in cats.

b. It is a spasmodic closure of the larynx.

c. The most common cause is manipulations of the pharynx and larynx during attempts to pass an endotracheal tube.

d. Certain anesthetics such as barbiturates may precipitate laryngospasm in cats.

e. Spontaneous laryngospasm has been reported in cats.

f. Clinical signs

1) Coughing and retching are the most common clinical signs noticed after manipulation of the larynx.

2) Clinical signs of spontaneous laryngospasm include sudden-onset respiratory distress lasting from several seconds to minutes. Wheezing, stridor, cough, and cyanosis occur during the episode. Frequency of the spontaneous episodes may range from very infrequent to several times per day.

g. Diagnosis

1) Unless directly witnessed by the clinician, diagnosis of spontaneous laryngospasm depends upon historic information.

2) Iatrogenic laryngospasm (intubation) can be directly witnessed by the spasmodic closure of the larynx after attempts at intubation.

h. Treatment

1) Reported treatment for spontaneous laryngospasm is to invoke a swallowing reflex by injection of 1–2 mL of tap water into the oral cavity of the cat. The response should be immediate.

2) Look for an underlying cause such as pharyngeal or laryngeal irritation and treat the cause of the irritation.

3) Iatrogenic laryngospasm can be prevented by administration of 1–2 drops of 2% lidocaine onto the laryngeal folds prior to intubation. Avoid excessive amounts of local anesthetics, as they can cause severe Heinz body hemolytic anemia in the cat.

8. Tracheal laceration

a. Common causes of tracheal laceration include neck bite wounds, transtracheal wash procedure, and traumatic intubation. Blunt trauma to the chest may cause tracheal rupture, most commonly just cranial to the carina.

b. Clinical signs

1) Air leakage from the tracheal tear often results in subcutaneous emphysema. Pneumomediastinum and pneumothorax are other sequelae to the leakage of air from the trachea. Pneumomediastinum is usually not associated with clinical signs, and the air is generally reabsorbed over time. However, rupture of the mediastinum can result in pneumothorax and severe dyspnea requiring thoracocentesis.

2) Subcutaneous emphysema in any patient without obvious skin wounds should alert the clinician that tracheal laceration has occurred.

3) The severity of respiratory distress depends upon the severity of the tracheal tear.

4) Head position may affect the degree of respiratory distress when there is complete disruption of the trachea.

c. Diagnosis

1) Tracheal rupture should be considered in any patient with subcutaneous emphysema and no evidence of skin wounds to explain the emphysema. Progressive subcutaneous emphysema should also alert the clinician to the possibility of tracheal tear.

2) Thoracic and cervical radiography

a) Peritracheal, intermuscular, and subcutaneous emphysema may be present.

b) Pneumomediastinum and pneumothorax may be present. With pneumomediastinum, intrathoracic structures such as the esophagus and descending aorta are clearly visualized because of the surrounding air. Pneumothorax classically results in loss of sternal contact of the heart on the lateral view and presence of air compressing the lungs.

c) Positive contrast studies using water-soluble organic iodide solutions may be helpful if the diagnosis is not obvious with plain radiography.

d) *Bronchoscopy may be used to diagnose and locate the tracheal lesion.*

e) *Tracheal tears from intubation are most commonly found on the dorsal aspect of the trachea.*

d. Treatment

1) Conservative therapy with cage rest and close observation is indicated if the patient is stable and the clinical signs are not progressive.

a) *The patient should be monitored closely for signs of respiratory distress, as the leakage of air may produce pneumothorax.*

b) *The external wound should be clipped and cleaned, and a light occlusive bandage with antibiotic ointment should be placed over the neck wound to prevent continued absorption of air.*

2) If respiratory distress is evident or clinical signs are persistent or progressive, surgical repair of the laceration will be necessary.

3) The patient should be stabilized prior to surgery with thoracocentesis to relieve the pneumothorax if present.

4) The owners should be warned that tracheal tear or rupture may stabilize initially but that severe respiratory distress may occur several days later as a result of tracheal stenosis from the granulation tissue at the rupture site.

9. Tracheal collapse

a. Collapse of the tracheal lumen may occur in the cervical region only but more often involves the thoracic portion as well and can extend into the bronchi.

b. It results from a deficiency of the tracheal cartilage organic matrix of glycoprotein and glycosaminoglycan. As a result, the cartilage rings cannot maintain their shape and therefore collapse.

c. Clinical signs

1) Tracheal collapse is generally recognized in middle-aged to aged toy and small-breed dogs but may occur at any age. It occurs rarely in cats.

2) Collapse most commonly occurs in the dorsoventral direction. The dorsal tracheal membrane prolapses into the lumen of the trachea.

3) Most dogs have a chronic history of a "honking" dry cough, although some dogs may present in extreme respiratory distress without any chronic history of coughing.

4) The cough is often elicited during exercise or excitement. Excitement is often what precipitates the acute respiratory distress.

5) Some animals have a history of syncope when coughing.

6) The respiratory distress can range from mild to life threatening.

7) Mucous membrane color may be normal or cyanotic.

8) Body temperature may sometimes be very high, reflecting the animal's inability to cool itself through the respiratory tract.

9) Cardiac sounds may be normal, although many of these dogs have associated mitral insufficiency.

10) Respiratory sounds vary from mild referred upper airway sounds to rattling, wheezing, and expiratory grunts. A snapping or clicking sound can sometimes be auscultated when the animal exhales. This is the result of the opposing tracheal walls slapping together.

11) Hepatomegaly has been noted in a large percentage of these patients.

d. Diagnosis

1) Obtain dorsal/ventral and lateral radiographs of both the cervical and thoracic areas.

2) Take lateral radiographs of the cervical and thoracic portions of the trachea during maximum inspiration and expiration. On inspiration the cervical trachea may collapse and the intrathoracic trachea may dilate. On expiration the intrathoracic trachea may collapse and the extrathoracic trachea may dilate.

3) Avoid extreme flexion or extension of the head and neck during radiographic procedures to avoid iatrogenic narrowing of the trachea.

4) The clinician must be careful to differentiate true narrowing of the trachea (>50% decrease in lumen size during respiration or coughing) from superimposition of the esophagus and soft tissues of the shoulder giving a false appearance of tracheal narrowing.

5) Fluoroscopy will demonstrate the dynamic collapse of the trachea. Also obtain fluoroscopic images of the trachea during coughing, to demonstrate the full extent of the collapse of the intrathoracic airways.

6) Bronchoscopy will also show the dynamic collapse of the trachea and airways. The disadvantage of this technique is that it requires general anesthesia. The excitement phase during recovery from general anesthesia can exacerbate the tracheal collapse and can be life threatening.

e. Treatment

1) Immediately stabilize patients with extreme respiratory distress.

a) Provide supplemental oxygen immediately. Anesthesia and intubation may be required in severely affected patients that do not improve with oxygen therapy alone or in patients that present in a semicomatose/comatose state.

b) The immediate goals are to minimize stress, provide oxygenation, relieve inflammation, and decrease body temperature if it is increased.

c) As anxiety is relieved with correction of the hypoxia, the trachea is less likely to collapse.

d) Stress may be alleviated by administration of acepromazine (30-50 μg/kg IV or IM). Avoid this in patients with concurrent seizure disorders or hypotension.

e) Other sedatives that may be administered include butorphanol (0.05–1 mg/kg SC q4–6h) or morphine (0.25–0.5 mg/kg SC, IM as needed).

f) Antiinflammatory doses of glucocorticoids will decrease mucosal swelling, inflammation, and irritation.

g) Terbutaline (0.01 mg/kg IV or SC) will help dilate lower airways if they are affected.

h) Administer cooling measures if the patient's body temperature is >40.5°C (105°F). Discontinue cooling measures once the body temperature reaches 39.5°C (103°F).

2) Long-term therapy

a) Treat any underlying conditions that exacerbate the problem, including obesity, pulmonary infections, and heart disease. Use of a harness instead of a collar is also recommended.

b) Judicious use of anti-inflammatory doses of corticosteroids and cough suppres-

sants. Corticosteroids should be administered for short term only, to avoid side effects such as weight gain, immune suppression, and panting.

c) Bronchodilators may be helpful in patients with lower airway collapse by minimizing small airway obstruction and therefore reducing intrathoracic pressure. This, in turn, decreases the tendency of the larger airways to collapse.

1. Terbutaline (1.25–5 mg/dog, BID-TID)

2. Albuterol (50 μg/kg TID)

3. Theo-Dur tablets (20 mg/kg BID)

4. Slo-bid Gyrocaps (20–25 mg/kg BID)

d) Cough suppressants will reduce coughing and therefore help alleviate airway irritation.

1. Hydrocodone (0.22 mg/kg PO BID to QID)

2. Butorphanol (0.55–1.1 mg/kg PO BID to QID)

3. Dextromethorphan (in over-the-counter cough medications such as Robitussin DM, 2 mg/kg q8h)

4. Adjust doses on the basis of the frequency and severity of the cough, and taper as the cough subsides.

e) Antibiotics

1. Dogs with collapsing trachea are prone to upper respiratory infections because of tracheal irritation and reduced clearance.

2. A 2- to 3-week course of broad-spectrum antibiotics (cephalosporins, potentiated sulfa drugs) may benefit dogs with acute exacerbation of cough.

3. Perform culture and sensitivity testing if there is a fever, evidence of pneumonia, or productive cough with mucopurulent exudate.

f) Combination therapy

At Auburn University, an elixir that combines a sedative, an antihistamine/decongestant, bronchodilators, and an expectorant has been used for 25 years in the medical management of these cases. (See box below.) Owners seem pleased with results, and dogs have been successfully managed for years.

ISUPREL COMPOUND ELIXIR FOR MEDICAL MANAGEMENT OF COLLAPSING TRACHEA

Phenobarbital Elixir 96 mg (24 mL)
Isoproterenol 1 mg injectable (5 mL)
Ephedrine 200 mg (4 mL of 50 mg/mL or 8 mL
  of 25 mg/mL); either injectable or capsule
Theophylline 720 mg (135 mL)
SSKI (potassium iodide) 2,400 mg (2–4 mL)

Karo Syrup 60 mL
  Dilute with water to 240 mL
  Dose: 0.1–0.2 mL/lb q8h as needed
*Monitor heart rate so that it does not exceed
160.

---

g) Surgical options have met with varied results.

1. Chondrotomy
2. Plication of the dorsal membrane
3. Resection and anastamosis of the affected segment
4. Application of intraluminal or extraluminal prostheses

10. **Infectious tracheobronchitis** (kennel cough)
    a. Usually a self-limiting disease lasting 1–2 weeks
    b. Commonly there has been exposure to other dogs within the last 2–10 days.
    c. The larynx, trachea, and bronchi are frequently affected. Rarely, the pulmonary interstitium is affected.
    d. Many bacteria and viruses have been implicated as causative agents. The most common are *Bordetella bronchiseptica* and canine parainfluenza virus.
    e. *B. bronchiseptica* adheres to the respiratory cilia, causing ciliostasis, compromising local immune responses, and facilitating colonization of the respiratory tract epithelium by other organisms.
    f. Other organisms less commonly implicated include mycoplasmas, canine adenoviruses and herpesvirus, reovirus, and canine distemper virus.
    g. Clinical signs
       1) Characteristic "honking" cough in an otherwise healthy dog
       2) Retching or gagging may occur at the end of a coughing episode as a result of expulsion of respiratory secretions.
    h. Physical examination
       1) In most dogs the results of physical examination are relatively unremarkable, although a cough is often easily elicited from tracheal palpation. Mild rhinitis and conjunctivitis may be present as well.
       2) Rarely, patients will develop bronchopneumonia with pulmonary parenchymal disease and signs of systemic illness.
       3) Patients with laryngeal paralysis or collapsing trachea may have respiratory distress.
    i. Diagnosis
    Primarily made on history, clinical signs, and physical examination findings
    j. Treatment
       1) Uncomplicated cases are often treated with antimicrobials despite the self-limiting nature of the disease and the potential role of viruses in this disease.
       2) Antibiotics that are effective against *B. bronchiseptica* include tetracycline (22 mg/kg PO TID for a minimum of 7 days) and trimethoprim-sulfonamide (15 mg/kg PO BID for 1–2 weeks). Avoid tetracycline in pregnant females during the last 3 weeks of gestation and in puppies less than 2 months old, because of potential tooth discoloration in the puppies.
       3) Antimicrobial therapy has not been shown to decrease the duration of clinical disease or decrease therapy.
       4) Antiinflammatory doses of corticosteroids may help decrease respiratory epithelial inflammation (prednisolone 0.25–0.5 mg/kg BID for 5–7 days).
       5) Cough suppressants (hydrocodone 0.22 mg/kg q4–8h PO or butorphanol 0.55–1.0 mg/kg PO BID to QID). Avoid cough suppressants in patients with complicated infectious tracheobronchitis (pneumonia) or patients with a productive cough.

III. PLEURAL SPACE DISEASE

A. Clinical signs

1. Clinical signs will vary depending upon the underlying cause of the pleural space disease. Clinical signs of pleural space disease may vary from mild tachypnea to life-threatening respiratory distress. Signs of respiratory distress will be typical of any patient with respiratory compromise. Signs consistent with pleural space disease include short, shallow respirations with intermittent attempts at deep inspirations and are typical of most patients with pleural effusions. Paradoxical respirations may be noted in patients with diaphragmatic hernia.

2. Physical examination
   a. The most striking finding is diminished airway sounds on auscultation. With fluid occupying the pleural space the airway sounds tend to be the quietest in the ventral area. With pneumothorax, air accumulates in the dorsal portion of the pleural space, causing the most muffled areas to be dorsal. With extremes of pleural effusion or pneumothorax, airway sounds may be diminished over all aspects of the thorax. Auscultatory findings tend to be symmetric, although in the minority of cases pleural effusions and pneumothoraces can be unilateral, creating asymmetry. Diaphragmatic hernia may be only on one side, creating asymmetrical auscultatory findings.
   b. Palpate the cranial thorax of cats with suspected pleural space disease. Decreased compressibility of this area of the thorax suggests a space-occupying mass as a cause of the pleural space disease. Normal, but very old cats have very brittle ribs and may not be as compressible as younger cats.
   c. Abdominal palpation may indicate a paucity of organs, suggesting a diaphragmatic hernia.
   d. Perform a thorough full-body examination of any animal with suspected pleural space disease to look for an underlying cause.
   e. Subcutaneous emphysema, fractured ribs, evidence of chest wall trauma, tachypnea, and weak pulses in a trauma patient should prompt the clinician to suspect pneumothorax.

3. Diagnosis
   a. A pleural space disease is primarily recognized by physical examination and thoracic radiographs.
   b. Thoracic radiographs
   If pleural effusion or pneumothorax is the cause of the respiratory distress, then radiographic detection should be relatively obvious. Thoracic ultrasound is sometimes required when pleural fluid is locculated. Diaphragmatic rupture must be considered in any patient when the crura of the diaphragm cannot be clearly discerned. Often bowel loops or cranial displacement of abdominal organs is noted with diaphragmatic hernia, although secondary pleural effusion can obscure the structures. Widening of the mediastinum may suggest a mediastinal mass or mediastinal fluid accumulation. If possible with pleural effusion, determine the size and shape of the cardiac silhouette; cardiac failure or pericardial effusion may be a cause for pleural effusion.
   c. Thoracocentesis (see p. 130) is both diagnostic and therapeutic in patients with suspected pleural space disease.

B. Causes/differential diagnosis

1. Pleural effusion
   a. Pleural effusion results from increased vascular permeability, increased hydrostatic pressure within the capillaries or lymphatics, decreased intravascular oncotic pressure, trauma, coagulopathies, vessel erosion from neoplasia, or pleuritis.
   b. Specific causes include idiopathic chylous effusion, lymphatic obstruction leading to chylous effusion, pleural inflammation due to bacterial infection or sterile inflammation, hemorrhage (due to bleeding disorders, neoplasia, or trauma), thoracic duct abnormalities (due to trauma, congenital abnormalities, or neoplasia), congestive heart failure, heartworm disease, *Aleurostrongylus* spp., mediastinal lymphosarcoma, pericardial disease including pericardioperitoneal and pleuroperitoneal hernias, lung lobe torsion, parenchymal bacterial infections, pulmonary thromboembolism, feline infectious peritonitis, peritonitis from pancreatitis or infection, systemic inflammation, and hypoalbuminemia.
   c. Fluid analysis of the pleural fluid is one of the most important steps in identifying the underlying cause of the fluid accumulation.
   d. Types of pleural effusions are listed in *Table 9-1.*

TABLE 9.1
TYPES OF PLEURAL EFFUSIONS

Fluid Type	Color	Turbidity	Total Protein (g/dL)/(cells/μL)	Triglyceride	Bacteria (bacteria may be present and not seen)	Cell Types	Possible Causes
Transudate	Colorless, pale yellow	Clear	<2.5/<1500	None	None	Relatively acellular, occasional red blood cells, mesothelial cell	Hypoproteinemia
Modified transudate	Yellow or pink	Clear, slightly cloudy	~3.0/1500–5000	None	None	Moderately cellular: some rbcs, macrophages, and mesothelial cells	Long-standing transudate; congestive heart failure; pericardial effusion; diaphragmatic hernia; neoplasia
Exudate	Yellow to red brown	Cloudy	>3.0/>5000	None	Not present, aseptic exudate	Predominantly nondegenerate to degenerate neutrophils	**Nonseptic inflammation:** chronic chylothorax; feline infectious peritonitis; fungal infection, neoplasia, SIRS, pancreatitis
					Not present, exudate		**Septic inflammation:** Ruptured esophagus; penetrating chest wound; foreign body inhalation; ruptured infected tumor; parapneumonic spread; ruptured pulmonary abscess; bacterial hematogenous spread
Chylous	Milky white	Turbid	2.5 or above (turbidity may give high protein reading on refractometer)/500–20,000	Present, triglyceride content exceeds the concentration in blood, cholesterol: triglyceride ratio <1	Absent	Mature lymphoctyes, neutrophils, and macrophages	Mediastinal mass; trauma; heartworm; cardiomyopathy; lung lobe torsion, idiopathic
Hemorrhage	Red	Cloudy	>3.0/similar to peripheral blood if recent or active	None	None	Similar to peripheral blood	Trauma; coagulopathy; neoplasia; lung lobe torsion; thymic hemorrhage

2. Pneumothorax causes include trauma (blunt or penetrating chest wounds), severe coughing (cats), tracheal disruption, esophageal perforation, iatrogenic (jugular puncture, transtracheal wash), ruptured bullae, and gas-forming bacteria in a pyothorax.

3. Diaphragmatic hernia causes
   a. Trauma
   b. Congenital

C. Procedures

1. Thoracocentesis
   a. Indications
   Thoracentesis is indicated when the presence of air or fluid within the pleural space causes respiratory distress. Removal of the air or fluid in these conditions often results in rapid resolution of the respiratory distress if the fluid or air is the only cause for the distress.
   b. Contraindications
   Avoid thoracocentesis in the presence of a bleeding disorder, although if the hemorrhagic pleural effusion is causing significant respiratory distress, then the benefits of therapeutic thoracocentesis outweigh the risks of potential hemorrhage that might occur from the procedure. If possible, correct the bleeding disorder with a plasma transfusion and vitamin K administration before attempting thoracocentesis.
   c. Equipment
   Clippers, material for sterile skin preparation, sterile 18- to 22-gauge needle or butterfly needle, sterile IV extension tubing, sterile three-way stopcock, sterile 20- to 60-mL syringe.
   d. Setup and procedure (sedation or local anesthesia is rarely necessary, as patients tolerate this procedure well as long as supplemental oxygen is provided during the procedure)
      1) The three-way stopcock should be attached to the end of the syringe, and the IV extension tubing should be attached to the three-way stopcock. The needle should be attached to the opposite end of the extension tubing. All connections should be checked for leaks. A leak in any of the connections may give the false impression of pneumothorax when aspirating (typically, condensation occurs inside the extension tubing as the warm air from the pleural space contacts the cooler tubing).

      2) To expedite removal of fluid, an 18- to 21-gauge needle is preferred. Smaller-gauge needles may significantly prolong therapeutic aspiration time.
      3) Both sides of the thorax should be prepared and tapped if the extent or location of the pleural fluid or air is unknown. The area to be tapped should be clipped and sterilely prepared. The seventh or eighth intercostal space is the location for needle placement. Place the needle more dorsally if pneumothorax is suspected or ventrally if fluid is thought to be the primary problem (just above or below the costochondral junction).
      4) Needle placement should be in the caudal aspect of the intercostal space just cranial to the rib, to avoid the blood vessels and nerves that run along the caudal aspect of the ribs.
      5) Ideally, one person should hold the syringe and be ready to start aspirating as another person places the needle into the pleural space and holds it steady.
      6) The bevel of the needle should be facing dorsally as the needle enters the pleural space. As the needle punctures the pleural space a slight "pop" will be felt, and resistance to passage of the needle will suddenly decrease. As soon as the needle enters the pleural space, the needle should be manipulated so that its long axis parallels the thoracic wall (*Fig. 9-3*). This will minimize the chances of iatrogenic trauma to the lungs. As the needle is directed parallel to the thoracic wall, the beveled opening of the needle tip should be facing the lungs. In this position the needle can be rotated like the hands of clock around a 360° circumference while the long axis remains parallel to the thoracic wall and the beveled opening continues to face the lungs.
      7) If the patient is tolerating the procedure well, remove as much of the fluid or air as possible. This will be noticed when a vacuum is reached. Avoid aggressive aspiration, to prevent aspiration of lung tissue into the needle. A 20-mL syringe is used for cats, and a 60-mL syringe for dogs.
         a) Multiple areas of the thorax may need to be aspirated to ensure maximal removal of the fluid or air. If the respiratory signs are due to pleural effusion or air, then

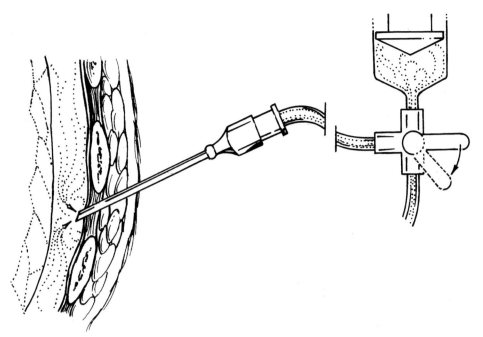

FIGURE 9.3   Thoracocentesis. Note how the bevel is facing dorsally and how the needle can be manipulated so that the bevel faces the lung tissue, avoiding trauma to the lung from the needle tip. (From Crowe DT, Devey JJ. Thoracic drainage. In Bojrab MJ, Ellison GW, Slocum B, eds. Current techniques in small animal surgery. Baltimore: Williams & Wilkins, 1998:403-417.)

signs should resolve immediately upon removal. If signs do not abate, then either more fluid or air is present or another problem exists.

b) In general, significant respiratory signs may be seen with 50 mL of fluid or air in the cat or >20 mL/kg in the dog.

c) Monitor animals with pneumothorax closely for recurrence of clinical signs. Repeat thoracocentesis in 20–30 minutes or sooner in animals showing signs of distress. If significant amounts of air are aspirated three times or more, placement of a thoracic drain is indicated.

  e. Complications

    1) Pneumothorax

This is usually very mild.

    2) Lung trauma

Lung laceration may occur causing hemorrhage or air leakage and pneumothorax.

    3) Laceration of the intercostal blood vessels or internal thoracic artery may result in severe hemothorax and hypovolemia.

    4) Complications are rare when the procedure is done properly.

2. Placement of thoracic drains

  a. Indications

Chest tubes are placed when there is an ongoing requirement for aspiration of fluid, air, or both from the pleural space.

  b. Procedure

    1) Equipment: Scalpel blade, clippers, preparation solution, local block, curved carmault forceps, thoracic drain tube, needle holders, suture material, tape. It is best to use commercially available thoracic drains because red rubber tubes tend to collapse or clog easily with blood or fibrin clots. Commercial chest tubes also are marked with radiopaque lines that allow the clinician to determine easily if placement is adequate (Argyle trocar catheter with sentinel eye, Argyle Division of Sherwood Medical, St. Louis, MO 63103).

    2) Chest tubes may be placed with just local anesthesia, but it is best to place them with the patient under general anesthesia. The lateral chest walls where the chest tube will be placed should be clipped and partially prepared prior to induction of

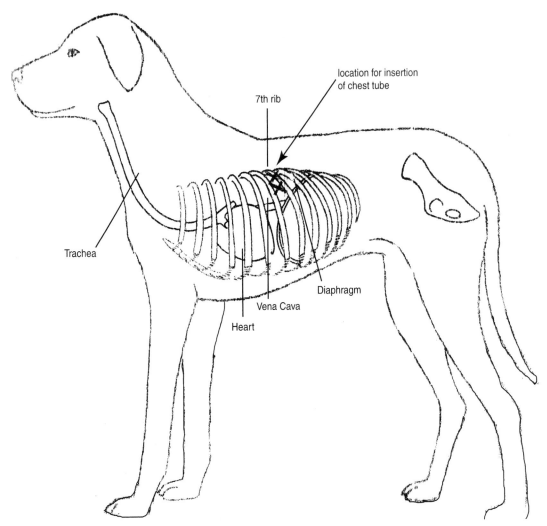

FIGURE 9.4   Location for chest tube placement. This is also a good area for thoracocentesis when aspirating a pneumothorax. (From Crowe DT, Devey JJ. Thoracic drainage. In Bojrab MJ, Ellison GW, Slocum B, eds. Current techniques in small animal surgery. Baltimore: Williams & Wilkins, 1998:403-417.)

anesthesia (*Fig. 9-4*). In patients with pneumothorax, more air will accumulate within the pleural space upon intubation and positive-pressure ventilations. Careful monitoring of the patient is warranted during this dynamic period. If tension pneumothorax develops, perform a rapid incision into the pleural space to allow air to escape.

3) Make a skin incision at the tenth intercostal space. An assistant grasps the thoracic skin of the patient and pulls it cranially until the skin incision rests over the seventh or eighth intercostal space (*Fig. 9-5*). The chest tube should enter the thoracic cavity at the seventh or eighth intercostal space, avoiding the intercostal artery that runs caudal to each rib. (If an assistant is not available, the clinician uses blunt dissection to form a tunnel from the tenth rib to the seventh intercostal space). If the chest tube has a trocar, the trocar is used to tunnel under the skin and is "tapped" into the pleural space. The tube and trocar are elevated perpendicular to the chest and grasped tightly, just above the skin to ensure that the trocar does not penetrate too deeply and lacerate the

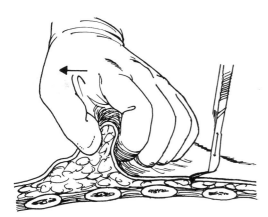

FIGURE 9.5 Advancement of thoracic skin for chest tube placement. An assistant grasps the skin over the thoracic wall and pulls it cranially so that the skin incision sits over the seventh or eighth intercostal space. (From Crowe DT, Devey JJ. Thoracic drainage. In Bojrab MJ, Ellison GW, Slocum B, eds. Current techniques in small animal surgery. Baltimore: Williams & Wilkins, 1998:403-417.)

lung tissue when it is tapped into the pleural space. Alternatively, for entrance of the tube into the pleural space, the intercostal muscles may be bluntly dissected into the pleural space to facilitate passage of the chest tube. This latter technique provides easier control of the chest tube as it enters into the pleural space and decreases the chances of lung tissue laceration (Fig. 9-6). All tube fenestrations must be in the pleural space (Fig. 9-7), and the end of the thoracic drain must be clamped off to prevent entry of air into the pleural space. The skin incision is closed with a pursestring suture, and the tube is fastened in place with a "Chinese finger trap" suture pattern. Anchor the tube by creating a butterfly with white tape and suturing it to the skin. Placing the anchoring suture through the periosteum of a rib will provide a more stable anchor (see Fig. 9-7). Aspirate the tube until a negative pressure of 3–5 cm³ is achieved. Avoid extreme negative pressures to prevent lung damage.

4) After the pleural space is completely emptied, a clamp may be placed across the tube to close it or closure may be achieved by placement of a syringe adaptor and three-way stopcock; 18-gauge wire is used to wire the two pieces together, and the ports of the three-way stopcock are covered with catheter caps to prevent contamination or introduction of air into the thoracic cavity.

5) Cover the incisions with antibiotic ointment and a sterile nonadherent pad. A circumferential wrap can then be placed around the chest, covering the incisions.

6) Thoracic radiographs will provide objective information regarding chest tube positioning and provide a baseline for future reference should the tubes stop functioning and subsequent thoracic radiographs be performed.

  c. Maintenance of chest tubes

1) The skin incisions should be treated and monitored like any other surgically created wound. Check the chest tube bandage daily and evaluate the skin incisions for infection (purulent discharge, excessive redness or pain, swelling, subcutaneous emphysema).

2) If periodic aspiration is being performed, record the volumes obtained at each aspiration in the medical record.

3) If available, continuous suction can be achieved with a pleurovac unit (Pleur-Evac.-Deknatel, Division of Howmedica, Queens Village, NY 11429).

4) Exercise extreme caution to prevent animals from chewing at the tubes or prematurely dislodging them.

5) The end of the tube can be clamped off, fitted with a stopcock, attached to continuous suction, submerged under water, or fitted with a Heimlich valve (Heimlich Chest Drain Valve, Becton Dickinson, Franklin Lakes, NJ 07417.) A Heimlich valve is not recommended for very small patients (i.e., cats) or for patients with hemorrhage, as clots may impair the function of the valve or allow air to enter the chest.

  d. Complications of chest tubes

1) Direct trauma to the pulmonary tissue during placement.

2) Disconnection of the chest tubes can be life threatening. Patients with chest tubes in place should be monitored constantly.

3) A sudden decrease in the volume aspirated compared with previous times may indicate chest tube dysfunction. Clinical signs and auscultation suggest significant air or effusion, yet nothing can be obtained during aspiration. Flushing the chest tubes

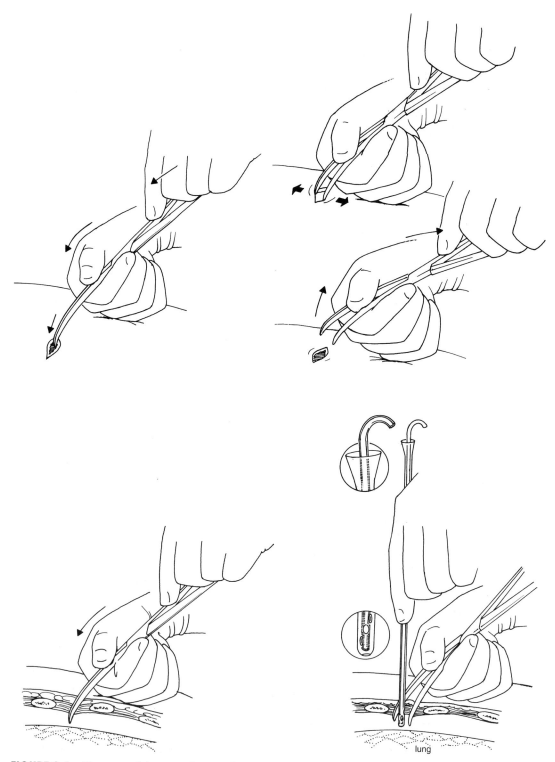

FIGURE 9.6   Placement of thoracic tube into pleural space. Blunt dissection through the intercostal musculature eases placement of the thoracic tube. (From Crowe DT, Devey JJ. Thoracic drainage. In Bojrab MJ, Ellison GW, Slocum B, eds. Current techniques in small animal surgery. Baltimore: Williams & Wilkins, 1998:403-417.)

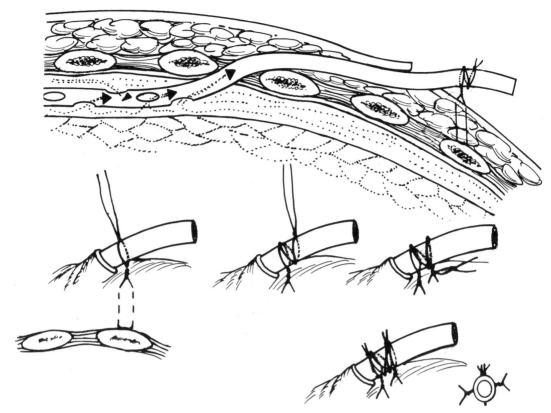

FIGURE 9.7   Thoracic tube in place. Note that all fenestrations are within the pleural space. Also note how previously pulling the skin forward has created a subcutaneous tunnel for the tube to pass through. A tighter suture anchor is achieved by passing the suture through the periosteum of the underlying rib. (From Crowe DT, Devey JJ. Thoracic drainage. In Bojrab MJ, Ellison GW, Slocum B, eds. Current techniques in small animal surgery. Baltimore: Williams & Wilkins, 1998:403-417.)

with sterile saline to check for patency, repositioning the tubes or patient to facilitate aspiration, and taking thoracic radiographs to assess chest tube positioning are the most common ways to troubleshoot chest tube function problems.

   e. Chest tube removal
   1) Chest tubes should be removed when the underlying disease process has resolved and fluid or air is no longer accumulating.
   2) Cytology and culture of the pleural fluid can be used to monitor an infectious disease process and its resolution.
   3) The presence of the chest tube itself generates 2 mL/kg/day of fluid.
3. Continuous-suction drainage
   a. Indications
   When large amounts of fluid or air are being produced, continuous drainage is indicated.

   b. Underwater seal and suction drainage is an effective method for continuous-suction drainage.
   c. Closed chest suction is available through Argyle Division of Sherwood Medical Products, St. Louis, MO 63103.
   d. The most commonly used method is the three-bottle system connected in series (Fig. 9-8). The first bottle acts as a trap for fluid that is drained from the chest. The second bottle in series is the underwater seal and provides unidirectional flow of air. The last bottle is where the suction is applied, and it acts as a negative pressure regulator. Water is added to this last bottle and the depth of the water determines the amount of negative pressure that is applied. For example, a depth of 15 cm of water limits the amount of negative pressure that can be applied to the pleural space at 15 cm of wa-

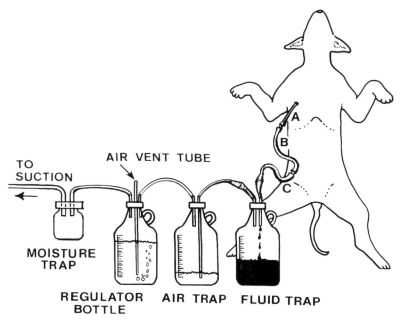

TO SUCTION

AIR VENT TUBE

MOISTURE TRAP

REGULATOR BOTTLE   **AIR TRAP**   **FLUID TRAP**

FIGURE 9.8   Three-bottle suction drainage system. A, Distal end of the chest tube exiting from the bandaged thorax; B, gum-rubber tubing (approximately half inch in diameter, ~ 3 feet in length); C, polyvinyl chloride "bubble" tubing. (From Crowe DT, Devey JJ. Thoracic drainage. In Bojrab MJ, Ellison GW, Slocum B, eds. Current techniques in small animal surgery. Baltimore: Williams & Wilkins, 1998:403-417.)

ter. Commercially available underwater seal suction kits exist but can be quite expensive.

4. Pleuroperitoneogram
  a. Indications
  When diaphragmatic hernia is suspected but not definitively diagnosed.
  b. Technique
    1) An area on the midline of the abdomen at the umbilicus or just caudal to it is clipped and sterilely prepared. Sterile iodonated contrast material is mixed to a concentration of 25% and 2 mL/kg of this solution is injected into the peritoneal space at the umbilicus or just caudal to it on the midline. Avoid injecting the material into the falciform fat, as this will inhibit the contrast material from distributing throughout the peritoneal space. If possible, the animal should be slightly tilted so that the cranial half of the body is lower than the caudal half. After 5 minutes, obtain lateral chest and abdominal radiographs. If contrast material has entered the chest cavity then a rent in the diaphragm is present (Fig. 9-9).

    2) Complications
    As with any abdominocentesis.

C. Management of specific conditions

1. Pneumothorax
  a. The most life-threatening aspect of pneumothorax is its effect on oxygenation of the blood and, in cases of tension pneumothorax, diminished tissue perfusion as a result of the high pressure within the thorax impeding venous return to the heart. Tension pneumothorax will result in progressive signs of shock—tachycardia, weak pulses, pale membranes—as tissue perfusion worsens and respiratory distress becomes more pronounced.
  b. Emergency therapy
    1) If tension pneumothorax is present (often recognized by extreme distress, poor tissue perfusion, barrel chest appearance, muffled lung sounds, and resonant sounds on percussion of the chest), a small incision entering into the thorax will rapidly relieve the high pressure in the pleural space and its physiologic effects. Once the

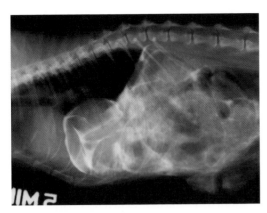

FIGURE 9.9 Pleuroperitoneogram. Note the positive-contrast material, initially injected into the abdomen, entering the chest of this dog with a partial diaphragmatic hernia.

air is released the incision should be covered with a sterile occlusive bandage, and a chest tube should be placed.

2) If cardiac arrest occurs in an animal exhibiting signs of progressive tension pneumothorax, initiate open-chest CPR without delay.

3) In most instances of traumatic pneumothorax, thoracocentesis is often effective in stabilizing the patient on a short-term basis. Remove air until a negative pressure is achieved on aspiration. If a negative pressure is not achieved (check all connections to be sure there is no leak in the apparatus), then place a chest tube and apply continuous suction. Both sides of the thorax should be aspirated if the patient does not respond to aspiration from one side. Record the amount of air removed in the medical record.

4) The patient should stabilize immediately if the pleural space is evacuated. If the patient is not stable, then all the air has not been removed or other underlying problems exist and further investigation is necessary.

5) After stabilization, the patient should be constantly monitored for signs of reoccurrence of the pneumothorax. If substantial amounts of air continue to accumulate and cause clinical compromise, then perform thoracocentesis. If substantial amounts of air are obtained after each aspiration within hours of presentation then place a chest tube.

6) The animal with pneumothorax should be hospitalized with constant monitoring of perfusion and respiratory parameters. The degree of monitoring should reflect the severity of the patient compromise.

7) As a general rule, most traumatically induced pneumothoraces require thoracocentesis only once or twice. Spontaneous pneumothoracies (without history of trauma) tend to be much more severe and generally continue to accumulate air within the pleural space. In those instances, chest tube placement with continuous suction is warranted, and surgical lobectomy may be required.

c. Diagnostic evaluation

　1) Spontaneous pneumothorax

　　a) Underlying causes of spontaneous pneumothorax include bacterial pneumonia, neoplasia, dirofilariasis, paragonimiasis, uremic pneumonitis, blastomycosis, thromboembolism, bullous emphysema, and idiopathic. Bullous emphysema is by far the most common cause of spontaneous pneumothorax.

　　b) Once the patient is stable, obtain thoracic radiographs to assess for underlying pulmonary disease. Emphysematous bullae are commonly observed in dogs with spontaneous pneumothorax.

　　c) Further diagnostic evaluation should include a complete blood count (CBC), chemistry profile, dirofilarial examination, fecal floatation and sediment examination, tracheal wash with cytology and culture or bronchoalveolar lavage, and abdominal ultrasound if metastatic neoplasia is possible.

　2) Traumatic pneumothorax

　　a) Once the patient is stable, obtain thoracic radiographs.

　　b) Full-body assessment for other injuries should be evaluated in patients with traumatic pneumothorax.

d. Further therapy

　1) Treat the underlying cause of the pneumothorax.

　2) In patients with ongoing pleural air accumulation, place a chest tube with continuous or intermittent suction if quantification of air accumulation is required. If, after 24–48 hours, air continues to leak into the pleural space, it is unlikely that this therapy will be effective, and exploratory thoracotomy for potential lung lobectomy or laceration repair should be considered.

3) Perform exploratory thoracotomy if non-invasive measures have failed to identify an underlying cause (and air continues to accumulate) or if the identified underlying cause needs to be surgically repaired.

4) Warn owners that pneumothorax may recur, particularly if the underlying cause was not found and definitively treated.

2. Hemothorax

a. Hemothorax is diagnosed when cell counts, packed cell volume, and total protein content of the pleural effusion are at least 50% of those of peripheral blood values.

b. The most common cause of spontaneous hemothorax in a young dog is coagulopathy. (Spontaneous acute thymic hemorrhage of unknown cause has also been reported in young dogs.)

c. Hemothorax also may occur with trauma and neoplasia.

d. Emergency therapy

1) The two major problems with substantial hemothorax are respiratory compromise and poor tissue perfusion due to hypovolemia. If hemothorax has resulted in hypovolemia, then substantial pleural effusion must be present.

2) Approach should be as with any patient in respiratory distress.

3) Perform thoracocentesis if respiratory compromise is severe.

4) Administer intravenous volume replacement with balanced electrolyte solutions, colloids (caution with coagulopathies), and blood products.

5) Treat the underlying cause of the hemothorax.

e. Diagnostic approach

1) Perform fluid analysis, including assessment of packed cell volume, total solids, cell counts, and cytologic analysis. Consider fluid culture if fluid analysis suggests infection as an underlying cause.

2) If there is no history of trauma, a coagulation screen including prothrombin time (PT), partial thromboplastin time, platelet count, and fibrin split products should be evaluated. Obtain a thorough history including specific questions regarding exposure to rodenticide anticoagulants. Measurement of PIVKA (proteins induced by vitamin K antagonism) may also be performed (Thrombotest, Burroughs-Welcome).

3) Further diagnostics that should be considered in spontaneous hemothorax include buccal bleeding time, CBC, serum chemistry profile, and urinalysis. Venipuncture should be performed carefully and held off well with pressure in patients with coagulation disorders. Cystocentesis should not be performed in patients with coagulation or platelet disorders. Collect urine via free catch or catheterization if necessary.

4) Thoracic radiographs after thoracocentesis will help identify the presence of masses as the cause of the hemothorax. Thoracic ultrasound may be helpful as well in patients with significant pleural effusion.

5) Obtain thoracic radiographs in any patient with traumatic hemothorax. Total body assessment for other traumatic injuries should be done as well.

f. Further therapy

1) Treat the underlying cause.

2) Only in very rare cases with traumatic hemothorax will surgery be required to control the hemorrhage. Stabilization with thoracocentesis, administration of fluid and blood products, and treatment of other trauma-associated injuries generally suffices.

3) Fresh or fresh-frozen plasma transfusions (10–15 mL/kg), packed red blood cells, and vitamin K_1 (5 mg/kg SC initially, DO NOT GIVE IM or IV) are indicated for patients with rodenticide anticoagulant intoxications (see "Rodenticide anticoagulant intoxication"). If blood component therapy is not available, then use fresh whole blood in anemic patients, NOT stored blood, because it does not contain active clotting factors. After completion of plasma transfusion, assess coagulation to evaluate the efficacy of the plasma administration. If coagulation parameters are still prolonged, administer more plasma.

3. Chylothorax

a. Chylothorax is the accumulation of chyle within the pleural space. A true chylous effusion has a cholesterol concentration that is less than or equal to that of serum and a triglyceride concentration that exceeds that of serum. True chylous effusions will clear with ether.

"Pseudochylous" effusions often occur with neoplasia; the fluid is very cellular, resulting in the opacity.

b. Causes of chylothorax include cardiomyopathy, mediastinal masses, heartworm disease, pericardial effusions, trauma, fungal granulomas, venous thrombi, and idiopathic (most common).

c. Emergency management

1) The most common acute life-threatening result of chylothorax is respiratory distress as a result of the pleural effusion or constrictive pleuritis.

2) Thoracentesis and removal of the effusions should immediately relieve the respiratory compromise. If it does not, then more pleural fluid is present, constrictive pleuritis is present, or other pulmonary problems exist.

d. Diagnostic evaluation

1) Routine fluid analysis, including total protein concentration, specific gravity, evaluation for chylomicrons, total white blood cell count, cytology, triglyceride and cholesterol concentrations (compare with those of simultaneously collected serum). Also, culture pleural fluid.

a) Triglyceride concentration may vary depending upon when the animal last ate. Ideally, postprandial triglyceride concentration of pleural fluid will optimize diagnosing chylothorax.

b) Cytology may vary depending upon the chronicity of the pleural fluid. Generally, the predominant cell types are small lymphocytes or neutrophils, with smaller numbers of lipid-laden macrophages.

2) Thoracic radiographs after removal of pleural fluid may reveal cardiac abnormalities, vascular irregularities, or masses that may be the underlying cause of the chyle accumulation.

3) Thoracic ultrasound with the pleural fluid still present may facilitate identification of a mediastinal mass or identification of cardiac abnormalities.

4) Other diagnostic tests should include CBC, serum chemistry profile, heartworm test (occult), and viral serology in cats (FeLV and FIV).

e. Further therapy

1) Longer-term therapy usually includes feeding a low-fat diet supplemented with medium-chain triglycerides and intermittent thoracentesis to control respiratory compromise. Conservative therapy should be continued for 2 weeks if traumatic rupture of the thoracic duct is suspected. Most traumatic ruptures heal within this period of time.

2) Fibrosing pleuritis is a potential long-term sequela to chronic chylothorax. Decortication of the visceral lung pleura may be necessary in these patients (although prognosis is poor if diffuse lung involvement is present).

3) For idiopathic chylothorax not responsive to conservative therapy, surgical options include thoracic duct ligation, passive pleuroperitoneal shunting, active pleuroperitoneal or pleurovenous shunting, and pleurodesis.

4) Pursue aggressive investigation for a treatable underlying cause because of the long-term effects of chylothorax (fibrosing pleuritis) and the ineffectiveness of most nonspecific treatments.

5) Electrolyte abnormalities including hyponatremia and hyperkalemia have been reported in animals with chylothorax, particularly when thoracentesis and fluid removal have been done repeatedly.

6) Rutin is a product available from health food stores that has been used in the medical management of chylothorax to improve fluid resorption and decrease fibrosis (50 mg/kg PO TID).

4. Hydrothorax

a. The fluid that characterizes a hydrothorax is a transudate with a total protein content less than 3 g/dL, which is relatively acellular.

b. Causes of hydrothorax include heart failure, hypoalbuminemia, pulmonary thromboembolism (may have a transudate or exudate), and diaphragmatic hernia (may be transudate or exudate). The pleural effusion associated with thromboembolism is relatively minor in volume.

c. Emergency management

1) Thoracocentesis as with any pleural effusion that causes respiratory compromise

2) Treat the underlying cause.

3) Tube thoracostomy is not needed with hydrothorax.

d. Diagnostic evaluation
  1) Perform pleural fluid analysis.
  2) Thoracic radiographs
  3) CBC and serum chemistry evaluation
  4) Coagulation evaluation if pulmonary thromboembolism and loss of antithrombin III are suspected
  5) Cardiac ultrasound if cardiac disease is suspected
  6) Abdominal ultrasound and radiographic contrast studies if diaphragmatic hernia is suspected
  7) Rule out causes of hypoproteinemia:
    a) Liver—bile acids, serum ammonia, BUN, glucose, liver enzymes
    b) Renal loss—urine protein:creatinine ratio >1 indicates excessive protein loss in urine in the face of a non-remarkable sediment
    c) GI loss—fecal examination, serum B_{12}, folate, Trypsin-like immunoreactivity (TLI) assessment may indicate malabsorption, maldigestion, bacterial overgrowth, or parasites
e. Further therapy

  1) *Treat the underlying disease process.*
  2) *Administer colloid therapy (10–20 mL/kg/day) to patients with low oncotic pressure until the pleural effusion resolves.*
  3) *Multiple thoracenteses may be necessary while the underlying disease process is being treated.*

5. Feline infectious peritonitis
  a. Pleural effusion due to FIP may be moderate to severe in volume.
  b. Emergency management
  Thoracentesis, as in any pleural effusion causing respiratory compromise
  c. Diagnosis
    1) Diagnosis is based on an accumulation of information including history, physical examination, laboratory findings, serology, and pathology. FIP may cause signs of liver disease, renal disease, CNS disease, GI disease, or ocular disease.
    2) Cats with FIP commonly are purebred cats originally from a multiple-cat household (either kittens or older cats), and they have a fever that does not respond to antibiotics.
    3) Findings more specific for FIP include hyperproteinemia characterized by hyperglobulinemia, pleural fluid findings of an exudate with very high total protein, and

cytologic findings of a mixed population of nondegenerate neutrophils and macrophages. The fluid is often tenacious, cloudy, and yellow with fibrin clumps present. It may clot on exposure to air.
    4) FIP antibody titers are nonspecific, as cross reactivity with other coronaviruses occurs. A negative titer is not useful in ruling out FIP, because negative titers have been found in confirmed cases of FIP. A very high FIP titer (>1:2500) in the presence of hyperglobulinemia, lymphopenia, and ophthalmic lesions (uveitis, retinal granulomas, hypopion, keratic precipitates) strongly suggests FIP.
    5) Further therapy
      a) There is no known therapy that cures FIP. Immunosuppressive agents such as prednisolone and cytotoxic agents (cyclophosphamide, phenylalanine mustard, melphalan) have been suggested.
      b) Anecdotal reports suggest beneficial results from low-dose oral interferon-α (30 IU PO q24h, daily for 7 days every other week). See Box for preparation instructions (p 141).
      c) In catteries where FIP has been diagnosed, kittens should be weaned early and separated from the queen and other adult cats at 4–5 weeks of age. They are hand raised until they are 7–8 weeks old. This practice prevents spread of the virulent FIP virus to young kittens.

6. Pyothorax
  a. Pleural effusion can be mild to severe in volume.
  b. Animals may be compromised not only from the effects of the pleural fluid but also from the severe infection.
  c. Emergency management
    1) Many patients will be severely dehydrated as well as septic; institute therapy for these problems if they are present.
    2) Perform thoracentesis and remove as much of the fluid as possible to relieve the respiratory distress and decrease the bacterial and inflammatory load of the patient. Submit fluid for Gram staining, aerobic and anaerobic culture, and sensitivity testing. Because the fluid is often thick and contains clumps of bacteria and fibrin, it may be impossible to drain the thorax effectively without performing tube thoracostomy.

INTERFERON PREPARATION

Intron A 3 million units
Dilute 3,000,000 units in 1,000 mL of saline =
3,000 units/mL*
Add 1.5 mL of 3,000 units/mL (4,500 units) dilution and add to 150-mL bag of saline to make
30 units/mL*

Dosage
  1 mL qd PO × 7 days
  Stop 7 days
  Repeat
*Dilutions may be frozen and stored for up to
2 years.

3) Administer intravenous antibiotics with broad-spectrum coverage. Antibiotics included should be a penicillin (22 mg/kg IV q8h) and an aminoglycoside (gentamicin 2 mg/kg IV q8h or 6 mg/kg IV q24h). Anaerobic coverage may be increased by the addition of metronidazole (25 mg/kg PO or IV q12h). Avoid aminoglycosides if renal perfusion is compromised or renal disease is present. A second-generation cephalosporin (cefoxitin, 30 mg/kg IV q8h) or Enrofloxacin (5 mg/kg IM q12h) may be substituted.

4) As soon as possible perform tube thoracostomy with continuous-suction drainage or intermittent flush and drainage. Place chest tubes on both sides of the thorax to facilitate complete removal of the septic fluid.

d. Diagnosis

1) Diagnosis is confirmed by pleural fluid analysis demonstrating a septic effusion. Rarely, bacteria are not noted on pleural fluid cytologic evaluation but confirmed by positive culture.

2) Aerobic culture and sensitivity and anaerobic cultures should be performed on pleural fluid.

3) Pyothorax in cats most commonly results from bite wounds and contamination of the pleural space with anaerobic bacteria. The hair should be clipped and the skin examined for bite wound scars. Anaerobic bacteria commonly cause a thick purulent fluid that looks like tomato soup and has a foul odor.

4) Obtain thoracic radiographs after pleural drainage, to rule out the presence of any underlying problems.

5) Perform feline serology including evaluation for FeLV and FIV.

6) Perform CBC, chemistry profile, and urinalysis to assess for associated diseases or organ dysfunction.

e. Further therapy

1) Perform continuous-suction drainage until fluid drainage is 2 mL/kg or less per 24 hours and the cytologic evaluation demonstrates resolution of the septic process. This is confirmed by decreasing numbers of degenerate neutrophils with an absence of bacteria. Culture of pleural fluid will help confirm control of the infection, but the standard 2-day delay of bacterial culture results will unnecessarily delay removal of the chest tubes. Continuous-suction drainage can be combined with intermittent flushing of the pleural space (below) to liquefy secretions and promote removal.

2) If continuous-suction drainage is not available, then intermittent flushing of the pleural space will be effective. Warm (body temperature) sterile saline (10–20 mL/kg) should be flushed into the pleural space and drained. Perform this flushing in each chest tube until the effluent is relatively clear. This procedure should initially be performed TID. Tapering of the frequency of flushing may be guided by the appearance of the effluent from the first flush. If the effluent from the first flush is clear, then the frequency may be decreased by one time per day. If the effluent from the first flush is consistently clear after three separate flush procedures, removal of the chest tubes should be considered by the above criteria.

3) Administer antibiotics on the basis of the culture and sensitivity results, for 6 weeks.

4) Reevaluate with thoracic radiographs prior to discontinuation of the antibiotics to confirm complete resolution of the pleural effusion and to check for atelectatic lung lobes and/or possible pulmonary abscesses. Sometimes surgical removal of diseased lung tissue is required to prevent recurrent infections.

7. **Diaphragmatic hernia**
   a. The degree of respiratory distress with diaphragmatic hernia may vary from mild to severe.
   b. Pleural effusion may obscure the diagnosis of diaphragmatic hernia.
   c. Emergency therapy
      1) Therapy for other problems such as hypotension, lung contusion, and other intraabdominal injuries is often necessary.
      2) Thoracocentesis may be necessary in patients with substantial pleural fluid accumulation.
      3) Gastric dilation with the stomach in the chest can cause substantial pulmonary compression and respiratory distress. Thoracocentesis with trocarization of the stomach and air removal may be necessary.
      4) Once the animal is stabilized, surgical therapy and definitive repair should be performed because of the potential for bowel compromise or organ ischemic damage. Some authors recommend 12–24 hours of medical stabilization prior to surgery. If the patient cannot be stabilized medically, institute surgical therapy as soon as possible. The presence of the stomach within the thorax is an indication for immediate surgery after short-term stabilization.
      5) In some cases, respiration may improve if the animal is held under the elbows in an upright position and gently shaken to promote displacement of abdominal organs from the pleural space.
   d. Diagnosis
      1) Thoracic radiographs form the basis of the diagnosis. Consider diaphragmatic hernia in any instance in which the complete outline of the diaphragm cannot be delineated. The presence of abdominal contents in the thoracic cavity confirms the diagnosis. Often, pleural effusion obscures the diagnosis, and contrast studies are required.
      2) Upper gastrointestinal contrast radiography will confirm the diagnosis if a portion of the stomach or intestinal contents is present within the thoracic cavity.
      3) Injection of 2 mL/kg of 25% iodinated contrast material into the peritoneal cavity followed by abdominal and thoracic radiographs may facilitate a diagnosis of diaphragmatic rupture. The presence of contrast material within the thoracic cavity indicates a defect in the diaphragm.
      4) Ultrasound can sometimes be helpful in the diagnosis of diaphragmatic hernia, but diagnosis via this method is difficult for even the most experienced ultrasonographers.
   e. Therapy
      1) Surgical reduction of the hernia and correction of the diaphragmatic tear is the only treatment.
      2) Chronic diaphragmatic hernia is more difficult to repair because of adhesions and scar tissue.
      3) In chronic cases, shock or hypotension may occur when compromised organs are "untwisted" and replaced to their normal positions, resulting in toxemia and reperfusion injury. The surgeon must be prepared to support blood pressure with aggressive fluid therapy and pressor agents if needed.

8. **Flail chest**
   a. Flail chest results from the fracture of two or more consecutive ribs in two places (ventral and dorsal). The diagnosis is confirmed with observation of the paradoxical motion of the chest wall during respiration.
   b. The degree of respiratory distress may vary, depending upon the severity of the chest trauma that caused the flail chest. Respiratory distress occurs as a result of pendulous movement of air, pulmonary contusions, pain, and pleural space problems.
   c. Emergency therapy
      1) Most veterinary patients respond reasonably to conservative therapy including oxygen supplementation, conservative intravenous fluid management, and administration of analgesics.
      2) Use fluid therapy cautiously in patients with flail chest because of concomitant pulmonary contusions. Colloidal solutions may be necessary (see fluid therapy section, p. 58).
      3) Mechanical ventilation may be necessary in patients refractory to oxygen supplementation.

4) Intercostal nerve blocks with 0.25–0.50 mL of 0.5% bupivacaine hydrochloride caudal to the ribs involved in the flail segment as well as one rib cranial and caudal to the segment may provide better ventilation through decreased splinting and atelectasis.

5) Intrapleural 0.5% bupivacaine (1.5 mg/kg) may provide adequate analgesia.

6) Surgical stabilization may not be necessary if respiration is adequate and the patient is responding well to medical therapy.

7) Short-term stabilization may be achieved with placement of towel clamps around the affected ribs and elevation of the flail segment (sedation or anesthesia will likely be required).

8) Long-term stabilization may be achieved with internal stabilization with wires or external splinting using aluminum rods or malleable plastic frames. The splint should remain in place for 2–4 weeks.

9. **Pneumomediastinum**

   a. Defined by the presence of air within the mediastinum

   b. Air may enter the mediastinum by penetrating wounds to the head, neck, and cranial thorax (including venipuncture), or air from abdominal surgery or viscus rupture may move from the abdomen and retroperitoneum. Air may also accumulate in the mediastinum secondary to esophageal perforation. The most frequent cause of pneumomediastinum is airway or alveolar rupture. Particularly consider tracheal disruption when pneumomediastinum occurs after intubation.

   c. Pneumomediastinum can progress to pneumothorax, but pneumothorax does not progress to pneumomediastinum.

   d. Emergency therapy

   1) Pneumomediastinum rarely causes problems by itself, although one report exists of a suspected tension pneumomediastinum. Tension pneumomediastinum can result in hypotension and respiratory failure.

   2) Many patients are asymptomatic, although subcutaneous emphysema can sometimes be severe, especially in cases of tracheal lacerations from intubation or trauma. Severe subcutaneous emphysema is

not life threatening by itself, but aggressive investigation for the cause is warranted.

   3) Treat pneumothorax as mentioned above.

   4) Clinical signs may be a result of the underlying disease process rather than pneumomediastinum.

   e. Diagnosis

   1) Pneumomediastinum is diagnosed by the ability to visualize mediastinal structures not routinely seen on plain thoracic radiographs such as aorta, vena cava, esophagus, and azygous vein.

   2) It may take 10–20 days for the mediastinal air to be reabsorbed.

   3) Search for underlying cause of the air leak is warranted.

10. **Penetrating chest wound**

   a. Penetrating chest wounds may result from animal bites, projectiles, knife stab wounds, and other trauma such a motor vehicle accidents or falling from a height.

   b. Clinical signs vary, depending upon the amount of tissue trauma and specific organ damage. Penetrating wounds may lacerate large arteries, resulting in severe hypotension from blood loss and respiratory distress from hemothorax. Open chest wounds may result in pneumothorax, or pneumothorax may be a result of airway damage. Pulmonary parenchymal trauma may also cause respiratory compromise.

   c. Emergency therapy

   1) Severity of compromise will vary, depending upon what has been damaged.

   2) Perform thoracentesis for pneumothorax or hemothorax if they are causing respiratory compromise (see treatment for pneumothorax, p. 136).

   3) Treat hypotension and poor tissue perfusion with intravenous fluids, colloids, or blood (see "Hypovolemia" pp. 61–62) and relief of tension pneumothorax if present.

   4) Exploratory thoracotomy may be necessary with severe chest trauma or continued inability to stabilize the patient medically.

   5) Immediately cover open, sucking chest wounds with an occlusive dressing and evacuate air from the chest via thoracentesis.

   d. Diagnosis

   1) Usually confirmed by physical examination of the wound.

2) Thoracic radiographs may demonstrate free air in the pleural space and pulmonary parenchymal changes.

IV. LOWER AIRWAY DISEASE

A. Clinical signs

1. Signs are similar to those of most diseases of the respiratory tract.
2. Respiratory distress may vary from mild to severe.
3. Airway disease is often characterized by coughing.
4. Lower airway disease often manifests itself with expiratory dyspnea, though with fixed intrathoracic obstruction difficulty may be noticed on both inspiration and expiration.

B. Diagnosis

1. Clinical signs, history, thoracic radiographs, bronchoscopy, transtracheal wash, bronchoalveolar lavage, and lung biopsy form the basis of diagnosis of lower airway disease.
2. Clinical signs, history, thoracic radiographs, and transtracheal wash (cytology and culture) are the most common diagnostic tools used to arrive at a diagnosis.

C. Causes/differential diagnosis

The most common causes include feline allergic bronchitis (asthma), canine infectious tracheobronchitis, and compression of the mainstem bronchus secondary to atrial enlargement from congestive heart failure. Other causes include canine allergic bronchitis, chronic bronchitis, bronchiectasis, bronchoesophageal fistulas, bronchial foreign bodies or parasites, bronchial neoplasia, and chronic obstructive pulmonary disease.

D. Procedures

1. Nebulization
  a. Adequate airway hydration is essential for normal airway clearance mechanisms because airway drying increases the viscosity of secretions and decreases ciliary function.
  b. Nebulization is no substitute for systemic hydration.
  c. Nebulizers create water droplets ranging from 0.8 to 6.0 μm. Saline is generally the agent nebulized for airway humidification.

  d. The aerosols are administered via mask, enclosed cage, or oxygen cage.
  e. Nebulization should be administered for 30 minutes every 4–12 hours, depending upon the requirements of the patient.
  f. Coupage is often administered (see below) after nebulization to stimulate coughing and mobilization of airway debris and secretions.
  g. Complications with nebulization include overhydration, overheating, transmission of infection from one patient to the next, airway irritation, and bronchospasm. These complications are rare, and most patients tolerate this procedure well.
  h. Adding antibiotics to the nebulization solution is generally not indicated, because there is no advantage over the systemic administration of antibiotics. However, in very young puppies with pneumonia, renal toxicity can generally be avoided by administering gentamicin via nebulization rather than parenterally; 50 mg gentamicin is added to 2–3 mL of saline and nebulized for 10 minutes q12h.
  i. Albuterol has been used as a bronchodilator for asthmatic cats. To nebulize, 0.5 mL of 0.083% solution is added to 4 mL saline and administered for 10–20 minutes q6h.

2. Transtracheal wash
  a. Indications include chronic coughing, undiagnosed lower airway disease, and pulmonary parenchymal disease.
  b. Equipment required includes local anesthetic (lidocaine), sterile nonbacteriostatic saline, 5- to 10-mL syringes, sterile 16- to 18-gauge over-the-needle intravenous catheters or a 19-gauge 8- or 12-inch long catheter/needle unit (Intracath, Becton Dickinson, Sandy, Utah), culture tubes/culturettes, material for surgical scrub, and #15 scalpel blade.
  c. Procedure (Fig. 9-10)
    1) The animal should be backed into a corner in a sitting position and the head raised by an assistant. Some animals are too fractious for this procedure to be done without sedation.
    2) This procedure should not be performed on animals with severe respiratory distress. General anesthesia with intubation may be necessary to obtain tracheal wash samples from these patients (see below).
    3) Shave the ventral neck from cranial to the larynx, to the proximal cervical trachea. Locate the cricothyroid ligament by palpation

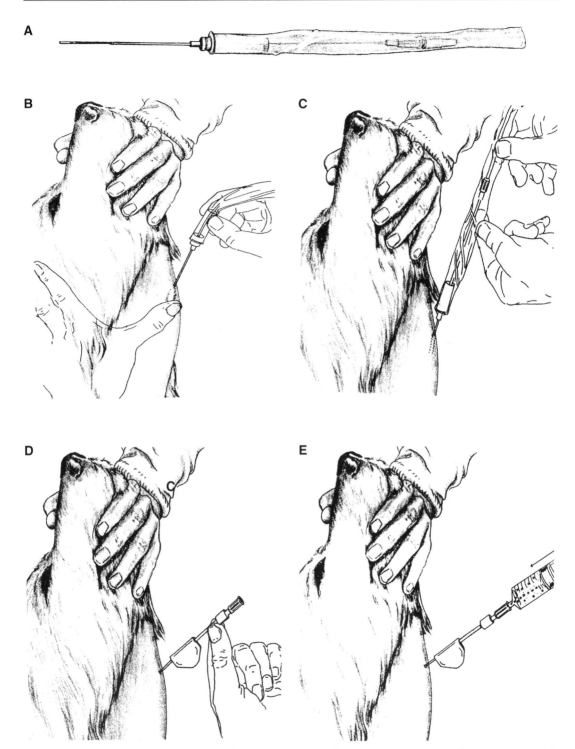

FIGURE 9.10   Transtracheal wash using a through-the-needle catheter (Intracath, Becton Dickinson, Sandy, Utah.) A, Through the needle cather. B, Puncturing tracheal or cricothyroid membrane. C, Threading the catheter through the needle into the tracheal lumen. D, Withdrawal of the needle from the tracheal lumen and attachment of the needle guard. E, infusing sterile saline through the catheter.

(continued)

F

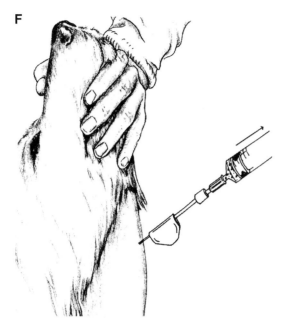

FIGURE 9.10   (continued) F, Apirating tracheal fluids through the catheter. (From Crow SE, Walshaw SO. Manual of clinical procedures in the dog, cat, and rabbit, 2nd ed. Philadelphia: Lippincott Williams & Wilkins, 1997.)

of a triangular depression just cranial to the cricoid cartilage. This and the surrounding area should be sterilely scrubbed. Inject local anesthetic over the area of the cricothyroid ligament, make a small relief hole in the skin over this area for passage of the catheter, and then perform a final sterile scrub over the area. While wearing sterile gloves, pass the needle with the catheter through the relief hole and through the cricothyroid ligament (a small "pop" should be felt as the needle passes through the ligament). The needle should be passed with the bevel facing down or caudally. Once the needle has entered the tracheal lumen, the catheter should be fed into the trachea and the needle withdrawn. Generally the animal begins to cough when the catheter enters the lumen of the trachea. A syringe is then attached to the catheter and aspirated. If no material is obtained, then the sterile, bacteriostatic saline is injected (5-10 mL) and then reaspirated. The presence of cloudy aspirate or mucous plugs is adequate for cytology and culture. The injection of saline and aspiration may be repeated several times if insufficient material has been obtained (up to approximately 1.0–1.5 mL/kg of saline may be used in total). Once the specimen has

been obtained, then withdraw the catheter and apply pressure with a gauze sponge to the area for several minutes. It is sometimes difficult to obtain a sample from large dogs using the transtracheal method because the catheter is not long enough to reach the bronchi.

4) Alternatively, general anesthesia may be induced and specimens obtained by passing a long catheter through a sterile endotracheal tube. A polyurethane or red rubber sterile male urinary catheter works well, but care must be taken not to perforate the airway. The catheter is gently passed through the sterile endotracheal tube until slight resistance is felt as the bronchus narrows. The catheter is then withdrawn several centimeters and 5–30 mL of sterile saline is rapidly injected and immediately aspirated. The animal should cough during the procedure. A total dose of up to 5 mL/kg can be injected if necessary to obtain adequate samples.

5) Evaluate obtained samples cytologically and perform aerobic and anaerobic cultures and sensitivity.

3. Bronchoalveolar lavage (BAL)

a. Equipment: Bronchoscope, 50 mL of warm sterile saline, ice

b. Procedure

1) Anesthetize animal as for routine bronchoscopy.

2) Perform bronchoscopic examination of all airways. For lavage, pick the most affected lobes as determined by radiography and visual examination.

3) Pass scope into main airway of affected lobe. Pass until the end of the bronchoscope fits snugly with the airway walls.

4) Inject 25 mL (for cats inject 5 mL/kg body weight) of warmed sterile saline through the biopsy channel into the airway. Aspirate immediately after injection. The goal is to obtain 40–80% of the sterile saline that was injected.

5) Place the aspirated sample on ice and repeat the injection/aspiration of 25 mL of sterile saline and place on ice.

6) Repeat the lavage procedure for each affected lobe.

7) After completion of BAL, gently inflate the lungs several times and allow the animal to breath 100% oxygen until extubation.

8) Continuously monitor the animal with a pulse oximeter to avoid hypoxemia. If it occurs, supplement with oxygen.

E. Management of specific conditions

1. Allergic bronchitis/feline bronchial asthma syndrome

a. The cause of feline asthma is unproven but is believed to involve a type 1 hypersensitivity reaction to inhaled allergens. In endemic areas, feline dirofilariasis may be the underlying cause.

b. Most cats are young middle age to middle age.

c. Clinical signs

1) Most cats have had respiratory signs for several weeks or months prior to presentation. The signs tend to be recurrent, although some cats can present with acute onset of respiratory distress without any prior signs.

2) Coughing may be paroxysmal and vary in intensity. Vomiting or retching may occur following the coughing. Some clients may complain that their cat is vomiting rather than coughing.

3) Respiratory distress may range from just tachypnea to severe dyspnea.

d. Physical examination

1) Inspiratory and expiratory loud airway sounds (rhonchi) may be auscultated. Duration of expiration is generally much greater than that of inspiration. An end-expiratory grunt may be heard as well as abrupt cessation of airflow near end expiration. Expiratory wheezes are also very common findings on auscultation. Inspiratory crackles may occur as well. Cats may have a combination of loud respiratory sounds, wheezes, and crackles.

2) Rarely, lung sounds may be quiet because of severe air trapping within the lungs or, on rare occasion, spontaneous pneumothorax.

e. Diagnosis

1) History and physical examination findings often provide the most information for diagnosis. Careful auscultation for heart murmurs or arrhythmias is necessary to differentiate cardiac disease from respiratory conditions.

2) Thoracic radiographic findings range from normal to increased bronchial and/or increased bronchial and interstitial patterns with or without alveolar densities. The classic finding is peribronchial infiltrate that appears as "donuts" on the VD view and "railroad tracks" on the lateral view. Lung hyperinflation with flattening of the diaphragm is also common. Although some studies have found that the severity of the radiographic findings parallels the severity of the clinical signs, this is not always the case. Collapse of the right middle lung lobe has also been noted as well as collapse in other lung lobes. On rare occasions pneumothorax may occur in cats with severe coughing.

3) CBCs may reveal increased numbers of circulating eosinophils. This finding is inconsistent but has been noted in up to 60% of cats in some studies.

4) Bronchial cytology is variable, with predominant cell types including eosinophils, neutrophils, and macrophages. In one study eosinophils were the predominant cell type in only 18% of the cats. Eosinophils can be found in normal cat airways.

5) In endemic areas, dirofilariasis (feline heartworm disease) can cause allergic lung disease. Thoracic radiographs reveal enlarged caudal lobar arteries, and serology may be positive for antibodies or heartworm antigen. Low worm numbers may cause false negative results, however.

f. Treatment

1) Emergency therapy

a) Provide oxygen supplementation to any patient with signs of respiratory distress.

b) Antiinflammatory doses of corticosteroids will decrease airway inflammation.

1. Prednisone sodium succinate (50–100 mg/ cat IV or IM)

2. Prednisone (0.5–1.0 mg/kg IM q8–12h)

3. Dexamethasone sodium phosphate (0.1–0.25 mg/kg IV or IM q12h)

4. Flovent inhaler—2 puffs are administered into a pediatric breathing chamber (Aerochamber, Forest Pharmaceuticals, Inc., St. Louis, MO 63405), and the cat is allowed to take 10–12 breaths.

c) Bronchodilators

1. Aminophylline (5 mg/kg orally or slowly IV). Intravenous aminophylline may cause hypotension.

2. Terbutaline (0.1 mg/cat IV, IM, or SC)

3. Epinephrine (0.1 mg IM or SC).

Epinephrine should be reserved for extreme cases of respiratory distress with this condition, as epinephrine is arrhythmogenic, particularly with myocardial hypoxia.

4. Terbutaline is the author's bronchodilator of choice in the patient with acute distress. Signs of improvement are often noted within 15–30 minutes after the injection. Hypotension and tachycardia are potential side effects, especially with IV administration.

5. Bronchodilators can also be administered via inhalation. Albuterol (0.5 mL of the 0.083% solution in 2 mL saline) can be administered by nebulization. Commercially available inhalers (terbutaline, albuterol, cromolyn) can be administered through a pediatric breathing chamber or cardboard toilet paper roll (two puffs, with the cat taking 10–12 breaths). Hypokalemia may occur with albuterol inhalation therapy.

d) Oxygen, corticosteroids, and bronchodilators are the mainstays of emergency therapy. Many cats may be removed from oxygen supplementation after several hours, although rare patients may require more than a day to respond adequately.

2) Long-term therapeutic considerations

a) Eliminate any underlying inciting cause by treating parasitic diseases, changing or eliminating litter, cleaning house vents, replacing or cleaning furnace or heater filters, eliminating cigarette smoke, evaluating for infectious causes, etc.

b) Taper initial antiinflammatory doses of corticosteroids to the lowest dose sufficient to control clinical signs. In some instances higher doses may be required.

c) Once clinical signs are controlled, administer the corticosteroid dose every other evening at the lowest dose sufficient to control clinical signs.

d) Methylprednisolone acetate (a long-acting corticosteroid), 2.0–4.0 mg/kg IM q2–4 weeks or as needed to control clinical signs may be used in cats when oral administration is not possible. Fortunately, cats are

more resistant to side effects from prolonged corticosteroid administration than dogs.

e) Administration of oral bronchodilators may decrease the dose of corticosteroid necessary to control clinical signs. There is some argument that corticosteroids should be administered despite resolution of clinical signs because of ongoing airway inflammation that may cause irreversible damage. This argument has not been resolved in cats with this condition.

1. Theophylline (4 mg/kg PO q8–12h). Blood theophylline concentration can be measured at human hospitals (5–20 μg/mL is considered the therapeutic range).

2. Aminophylline (5 mg/kg PO q8–12h)

3. Theo-Dur Tablets (25 mg/kg PO q24h)

4. Slo-Bid Gyrocaps (25 mg/kg PO q24h)

5. Terbutaline (one-eighth to one-quarter of a 2.5-mg tablet PO q12h). Hypotension, tachycardia, tremors, and excitability are potential side effects. Dosage may be increased if signs persist and no adverse effects are present.

6. There is some evidence that cyproheptadine, a serotonin antagonist (2 mg/cat q12h PO), may prevent bronchoconstriction in cats with asthma.

7. In cats with recurrent bouts of emergency respiratory distress, the owners could be taught to give terbutaline SC or IM (0.01 mg/kg) when respiratory difficulty develops. (Owners could be taught in a manner similar to that used to teach owners of diabetic cats to give insulin.)

8. In very resistant asthmatic cats, when all drugs seem to be failing to alleviate the signs or when extremely high doses are required and the owner is considering euthanasia, cyclosporine may be considered. An initial dose of 10 mg/kg PO q12h is recommended. Absorption varies between individuals; therefore, cyclosporine levels should be measured weekly until a steady dose is achieved that maintains a trough blood level of 500–1000 ng/mL.

9. Another drug that may alleviate bronchoconstriction in cats is cyropheptadine (2 mg/cat q12–24h). This drug is a serotonin antagonist, and it is thought that bronchoconstriction in cats is mediated, at least in part, by serotonin.

10. Cats vary in their response to the various combinations of drugs and doses, and therapy should be tailored to the individual patient.

2. **Tracheobronchitis** (see above, "Infectious tracheobronchitis")

3. **Compression of the mainstem bronchus** (see "Congestive Heart Failure," pp. 167–170)
   a. Some dogs with mitral valve endocardiosis develop compression of the left mainstem bronchus as a consequence of severe left atrial enlargement.
   b. The primary clinical sign is excessive coughing, especially during stress, exercise, or excitement.
   c. In addition to managing the heart failure, a cough suppressant is usually needed (hydrocodone, 0.22 mg/kg q4–8h or butorphanol, 0.55 mg/kg PO q6–12h).
   d. Hydralazine is a potent arterial dilator that may reduce the regurgitant fraction, resulting in a smaller left atrium and decreased coughing. Initial dosage is 0.5 mg/kg q12h, titrated up to 2.2 mg/kg q12h. Monitor for tachycardia and hypotension as unwanted side effects.

4. **Smoke inhalation**
   a. Involves injury to both airways and lung parenchyma as a result of thermal injury, chemical injury, inhalation of foreign body particulate mater, and asphyxia.
   b. Clinical signs
      1) Smoke odor, soot, burns, singed hair and whiskers.
      2) Respiratory signs may include any of the following: normal presentation; respiratory stridor; soft, moist cough; tachypnea; and dyspnea.
      3) Mucous membranes may be cherry red or cyanotic.
      4) Nasal and ocular discharge are often present as a result of mucosal irritation.
      5) Clinical signs often worsen for the first 48 hours after presentation.
   c. Diagnosis is based on history and clinical signs.
      1) Thoracic radiographs may be normal initially and progress to a peribronchial

infiltrative pattern followed by an alveolar pattern with air bronchograms if pneumonia occurs.
      2) Arterial blood gas determinations may reveal hypoxemia and metabolic acidosis.
      3) Pulse oximetry is unreliable with carbon monoxide poisoning.
   d. Treatment
      1) Initially, 100% oxygen should be administered to promote carbon monoxide elimination and prevent tissue hypoxia.
      2) Inspired O_2 concentration should be weaned to the lowest level that will maintain the $PaO_2 > 60$ mm Hg. Humidification is very important.
      3) Fluid therapy is needed to maintain hydration and provide support to burn patients. Colloids are often required in burn patients that develop hypoproteinemia.
      4) Bronchodilators:
         a) *Terbutaline 0.01 mg/kg SQ TID-QID*
         b) *Albuterol 0.02–0.04 mg/kg PO BID-TID*
      5) Corticosteroids
      Not indicated unless significant upper airway edema is contributing to dyspnea
      6) Diuretics
      Avoid if possible, because pulmonary edema is noncardiogenic. They may result in dehydration and inability to cough up secretions.
      7) Saline nebulization can help keep the airways moist and facilitate clearance of respiratory secretions.
      8) Coupage and walking will stimulate coughing and help clear secretions and particulate matter.
      9) Antibiotics
         a) *Pneumonia is a common sequela that occurs 2–3 days after smoke inhalation.*
         b) *Do culture and sensitivity testing of animals exhibiting clinical signs of pneumonia to aid in antibiotic selection.*
      10) Animals with smoke inhalation often get worse over the initial 24–48 hours, and then gradual improvement begins in those that recover, or ARDS develops in those that die.

5. **Chronic obstructive pulmonary disease**
   a. Chronic bronchitis results most commonly from bronchial irritation from environmental pollutants (smoke, toxic fumes, paint, dust, etc.) or allergens.

b. Bronchiectasis is an irreversible dilation of the bronchi, usually secondary to chronic airway disease and inflammation. It is rare in cats but common in dogs with severe chronic bronchitis.

c. Emphysema is the abnormal enlargement of air spaces distal to the terminal bronchioles that occurs secondary to destruction of alveolar walls. Pulmonary changes are irreversible and lead to air trapping and airflow resistance, primarily during expiration.

d. Clinical signs may include dry or productive coughing and gagging, tachypnea, and exercise intolerance.

e. Diagnosis radiographs:

  1) Thoracic radiographs:

   a) *Peribronchial infiltrates, atelectasis, consolidation—chronic bronchitis*

   b) *Increased size of bronchial lumen—bronchiectasis*

   c) *Hyperinflation of lung fields—flattened diaphragm, attenuated vessels (emphysema)*

  2) Bronchoscopy can confirm the presence of dilated bronchi, bronchial irritations, and secretions.

  3) Cytology can be helpful in choosing therapy. Eosinophils suggest an allergic cause that would require corticosteroid treatment, whereas bacteria and neutrophils warrant culture and sensitivity testing and antibiotic treatment.

d. Treatment

  1) Dogs with chronic obstructive pulmonary disease often have chronic respiratory changes that are incurable. Exacerbation of signs often results from secondary bacterial infection.

  2) Although long-term prognosis is usually poor, short-term improvement can be achieved by early recognition of infections, identification of the infective agent, and appropriate therapy for at least 3 weeks.

  3) Oxygen is administered initially to stabilize the patient if needed.

  4) Antibiotic choices are based on culture and sensitivity testing. Commonly used antibiotics include enrofloxacin or trimethoprim/sulfa or amoxicillin–clavulanic acid.

  5) Percussion/coupage may help to loosen bronchial secretions.

  6) Long-term corticosteroids are the mainstay of treatment for animals with allergic bronchitis. Initial prednisone dosage is 1 mg/kg PO BID for 10–14 days, tapered to a maintenance dose of 0.1–0.25 mg/kg PO every other day, or the lowest effective dose to control signs.

  7) Bronchodilators may be helpful

   a) *Albuterol (dog): 0.02 mg/kg initially, increasing to 0.05 mg/kg PO SID-TID. Transient side effects may include hyperactivity and tremors.*

   b) *Theo-Dur tablets:*

    Dog: 20 mg/kg PO BID
    Cat: 25 mg/kg PO at night

   c) *Terbutaline (cat): 0.625 mg/cat PO BID*

  8) A weight-loss program is recommended for obese patients.

  9) Surgery can be considered in animals with localized disease or bullous cysts that might result in spontaneous pneumothorax.

V. PARENCHYMAL DISEASE

A. Clinical signs

1. Respiratory signs may range from mild tachypnea to severe distress.

2. Coughing may or may not be present. It is usually a soft, moist cough.

3. Signs consistent with the underlying disease process may be evident.

4. Auscultation usually reveals labored breathing with pulmonary crackles and wheezes.

5. The clinician should check for underlying heart disease—pulse quality, arrhythmias, heart murmur, tachycardia, or gallop rhythm in cats.

6. In puppies with acute onset of dyspnea, do a thorough oral examination to check for evidence of electric cord burn.

B. Diagnosis

1. Diagnosis is obtained via clinical signs, history, physical examination, thoracic radiographs, transtracheal wash, bronchoscopy, BAL, and lung aspirate or biopsy.

2. An interstitial/alveolar pattern on thoracic radiographs suggests pulmonary parenchymal disease.

C. Causes/differential diagnosis

General causes include edema, hemorrhage, infection, neoplasia, eosinophilic diseases, inflammatory diseases, trauma, thromboembolism, lung lobe torsion, hypersensitivity reactions, parasites, and atelectasis.

D. Procedures

1. Lung aspirate

    a. Indications

Aspiration of discrete lung lesions, guided by ultrasound, fluoroscopy, plain radiographs, or computerized tomography (CT) imaging in patients that cannot tolerate surgical open lung biopsy or that have diffuse lung disease, when other methods of diagnosis have failed to obtain diagnostic samples (e.g., transtracheal wash, BAL).

    b. Procedure

    1) This is often a low-yield procedure.

    2) Bleeding and coagulation disorders should be corrected prior to this procedure.

    3) Fluoroscopy or ultrasonography will facilitate accurate placement of the needle for discrete lung lesions. The skin site is clipped and sterilely prepared. A local anesthetic is infiltrated at the skin and subcutaneous areas. A 19- to 23-gauge needle or spinal needle with a stylet is used for the procedure. The needle is advanced to the appropriate depth as determined previously by radiographs or simultaneously with fluoroscopy or ultrasonography. The stylet is removed and a 12- to 20-mL syringe with extension tubing is attached. Aspiration is applied to the syringe barrel, and the needle is moved back and forth over approximately 0.5 to 1.0 cm (similar to a lymph node aspirate). Samples obtained should be evaluated cytologically and cultured if indicated.

    4) The animal should be under general anesthesia when the aspirate is performed. The lungs are fully inflated to prevent spontaneous breathing and movement of the lungs while the aspiration sample is obtained. After the needle is withdrawn from the thorax, the lungs are allowed to deflate.

    5) Complications include hemoptysis, hemorrhage, pneumothorax, and rupture of an abscess and pyothorax. Monitor animals closely for 24 hours for these complications.

2. Coupage

    a. Indications

To loosen secretions and stimulate coughing in patients with lower airway secretions (e.g., pneumonia, smoke inhalation). It is generally performed after nebulization of airways.

    b. Procedure

The palm of the hand is partially cupped to create a hollow area between the palm and the chest wall when the hand strikes the chest. The frequency of percussion is similar to clapping during applause. The strength of the percussion should be similar to that of clapping as well. Coupage over all affected areas of the lungs. Coupage should last 5–10 minutes and is generally performed after nebulization. Coupage is sometimes uncomfortable for some patients.

E. Management of specific conditions

1. Pneumonia

    a. Pneumonia may vary in its effects from relatively minimal signs to severe life-threatening respiratory distress, hypotension, and sepsis.

    b. The large surface area of the lungs provides opportunity for absorption of inflammatory mediators and endotoxin in the systemic circulation as well as bacterial access. Hence, animals with bacterial pneumonia should be treated aggressively.

    c. Diagnosis

    1) History, clinical signs, physical examination, and thoracic radiography form the primary basis for diagnosis. Transtracheal wash with cytology and culture or BAL confirm the diagnosis of bacterial pneumonia.

    2) Radiographs usually demonstrate a ventral and cranial distribution of alveolar pattern. Aspiration pneumonia is most commonly diagnosed in the right middle lung lobe *(Fig. 9-11)*. Embolic pneumonia (relatively rare compared with aspiration pneumonia) has a more generalized and patchy alveolar pattern. Radiographic signs may lag 12–24 hours behind clinical signs of deterioration or improvement.

    3) Cytologic findings of transtracheal wash most typically reveal an acute inflammatory reaction with a mixed population of bacteria.

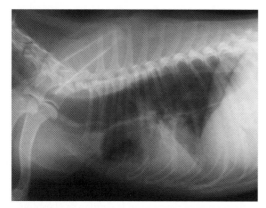

FIGURE 9.11 Left lateral thoracic radiograph of aspiration pneumonia in a dog with megaesophagus. Note the alveolar pattern in the right middle lung lobe and the dilated esophagus.

4) Bacterial pneumonia is usually a secondary problem, and a search for an underlying cause is warranted (e.g., megaesophagus, laryngeal paralysis, heartworm disease, severe leukopenia, immunosuppression, vomiting due to another underlying cause).

5) Fungal pneumonia (blastomycosis, histoplasmosis, coccidioidomycosis, aspergillosis) can usually be confirmed by serology or by finding the organism in a cytologic sample obtained by tracheal washing.

d. Treatment

1) Principles of treatment of respiratory distress should be applied to the patient with pneumonia in distress.

2) Perform nebulization and coupage three to four times daily initially.

3) Encourage animals to do some mild exercise to help mobilize and clear respiratory secretions. Recumbent animals with pneumonia are very difficult to treat.

4) Maintain systemic hydration.

5) If possible, obtain cytologic evaluation and culture of respiratory secretions prior to administration of antibiotics.

6) Initially administer broad-spectrum antibiotics (preferably intravenously). A combination of metronidazole (25 mg/kg IV BID), ampicillin (22 mg/kg IV TID), and gentamicin (2 mg/kg IV TID) can be used to provide coverage against gram-positive, gram-negative, and anaerobic bacteria while awaiting culture results. When using an aminoglycoside, be sure the animal is well hydrated and renal

perfusion is adequate. Alternatively, fluoroquinolones may be used instead of aminoglycosides.

7) Fungal pneumonia is most commonly treated with itraconazole (5–10 mg/kg PO BID) continued for 1 month after resolution of clinical signs.

8) When the animal is eating and drinking on its own and respiration has stabilized and can be maintained by the animal, it may be discharged. Antibiotics should be administered for a total of 4–6 weeks (based on initial culture and sensitivity). Discontinuation of antibiotics should be based on absence of signs of infection and radiographic appearance.

2. Noncardiogenic pulmonary edema

a. Noncardiogenic pulmonary edema is due to an increase in permeability of the pulmonary vessels rather than a increase in hydrostatic pressure as seen in cardiogenic pulmonary edema.

b. The most distinct entity of noncardiogenic pulmonary edema in small animals is neurogenic pulmonary edema.

c. The four most common causes of neurogenic pulmonary edema in dogs and cats are seizures, upper airway obstruction, head trauma, and electrocution.

d. Clinical signs of neurogenic edema generally appear within minutes of the CNS insult (head trauma, electrocution, and seizures) or of the upper airway obstruction.

e. Upper airway obstruction may be relatively transient and still cause severe pulmonary edema.

f. Diagnosis

1) History, clinical signs, physical examination and thoracic radiographs are the mainstay of diagnosis.

2) Typical clinical history is rapid onset of respiratory distress within minutes to an hour of the inciting event.

3) Respiratory signs may range from mild to severe. Caudorsal distribution of interstitial/alveolar pattern is characteristic of neurogenic pulmonary edema *(Fig. 9-12)*.

a) In severe cases, alveolar pattern may be present in all quadrants of the lungs.

b) If the caudorsal quadrant is not involved, it is unlikely that neurogenic pulmonary edema is the problem.

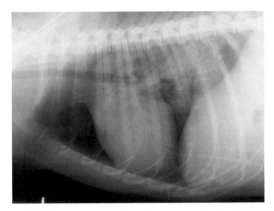

FIGURE 9.12 Lateral thoracic radiograph of a dog with neurogenic pulmonary edema. Note the caudodorsal distribution of the alveolar pattern, which is characteristic of neurogenic pulmonary edema.

    g. Emergency therapy
      1) Therapy as for any patient in respiratory distress
      2) Furosemide (dogs, 2 mg/kg IV or IM; cats, 1 mg/kg IV or IM)
      3) Some patients may require positive-pressure ventilation to maintain oxygenation.
      4) Some patients lose so much high-protein fluid into the lungs that they become hypovolemic and require intravenous synthetic colloid supplementation.
      5) Patients that require positive-pressure ventilation and/or colloid support generally have a poor prognosis.

3. Cardiogenic pulmonary edema

See Cardiac emergencies section, p. 160.

4. Parasitic lung diseases
    a. Rarely result in significant respiratory distress
    b. The most common respiratory sign is coughing.
    c. Most signs result from the inflammatory reaction to the parasite.
    d. Parasites to be considered include *Capillaria aerophila*, *Aelurostrongylus abstrusus* (cat lungworm), *Paragonimus kellicotti* (lung fluke), *Filarioides hirthi* (dogs), *Oslerus osleri* (dogs), *Andersonstrongylus milksi* (dogs), *Crenosoma vulpis* (dogs), and intestinal parasite migration of such as *Toxocara canis*, *Strongyloides stercoralis*, and *Ancylostoma caninum*.
    e. Diagnosis
      1) A definitive diagnosis is based on identification of the parasite or its characteristic eggs or larvae via tracheal wash, fecal floatation, or Baermann technique.
      2) CBC may show eosinophilia.
      3) Radiographic appearance varies, depending upon the type of parasite and the severity of the inflammatory response.
    f. Treatment
      1) Ivermectin (400 μg/kg PO once) is the most effective anthelmintic for most parasitic lung diseases and is safe except in collie-type dogs.
      2) *Paragonimus* infections can be treated with praziquantel (Droncit) at a dosage of 25 mg/kg PO TID for 3 days.
      3) A variety of other anthelmintics have been recommended, depending upon the type of parasite infection.
      4) Prednisone (0.5–1 mg/kg PO BID) should be given concurrently because death of the parasites may cause a significant pulmonary inflammatory response.

5. Pulmonary thromboembolism
    a. Any condition that causes vascular endothelial cell injury, venous stasis, or hypercoagulability of the blood can induce thromboembolic disorders.
    b. Cardiac disease, neoplasia, hyperadrenocorticism, pancreatitis, protein-losing nephropathy, orthopaedic trauma or surgery, disseminated intravascular coagulation, sepsis, and immune-mediated hemolytic anemia are common diseases associated with pulmonary thromboembolism.
    c. Clinical impression suggests that there are two general courses of pulmonary thromboembolism in veterinary patients: sudden onset of respiratory distress that stabilizes and does not progress or sudden onset of respiratory distress that progresses rapidly despite aggressive therapy.
    d. Clinical signs and physical examination
      1) Clinical signs may be very mild or absent in mild cases. The most common clinical signs reported in veterinary medicine include respiratory distress, tachypnea, and depression. Respiratory signs are often sudden in onset.
      2) Backward and forward heart failure and sudden collapse and death have been infrequently reported.
      3) Physical examination findings are variable but may include pulmonary crackles

(rales), tachycardia, and split second heart sound.

e. Diagnosis

1) Consider pulmonary thromboembolism in any patient with sudden onset of respiratory signs that has an associated disease process.

2) Thoracic radiographic findings are variable, but the two most common findings in dogs are hypovascular lung regions and alveolar infiltrates, best visualized on dorsoventral or ventrodorsal projections. Pulmonary infiltrates may be solitary or multiple and most commonly occur in the right and caudal lung lobe regions. Right-sided cardiomegaly, main pulmonary artery segment enlargement, and pleural effusion may sometimes be seen as well.

3) Thoracic radiographs may appear completely normal despite severe respiratory distress.

4) The most common arterial blood gas findings include decreased PaO_2 and increased alveolar–arterial oxygen concentration difference, and decreased $PaCO_2$. Normal blood gas findings do not rule out pulmonary thromboembolism.

5) Pulmonary scintigraphy and pulmonary angiography are the best tests to confirm pulmonary thromboembolism, but these are not routinely performed in veterinary medicine.

f. Therapy

1) Apply general treatment for respiratory distress. Institute short-term anticoagulant therapy with heparin–initial intravenous dose of 200 IU/kg, followed by 100–200 IU/kg SC q6h or a constant intravenous rate of infusion of 15–20 IU/kg/h. The goal of therapy is to prolong the activated partial thromboplastin time (APTT) to 1.5–2.0 times normal or prolong the activated clotting time by 15–20 seconds (not as accurate as APTT). Do not use heparin if the APTT is already prolonged. Heparin therapy should be slowly tapered to avoid a hypercoagulable state. Antithrombin III must be present for heparin to be effective. Administration of fresh frozen plasma may be necessary in some patients that are hypoproteinemic.

2) Warfarin may be used for long-term anticoagulant therapy, but it requires 2–7 days to become effective. Overlapping with heparin therapy prevents the initial hypercoagulable state observed at the start of warfarin ther-

apy. Warfarin dose is 0.2 mg/kg initially, followed by 0.05–0.10 mg/kg daily. The goal of therapy is to prolong PT to 1.5–2.0 times normal. Evaluate PT daily until a consistent PT is achieved and then twice weekly. Continue treatment until the underlying disease process is resolved.

3) Heparin or warfarin will not dissolve an existing clot but may prevent formation of additional thrombi. Dissolution of pulmonary thromboemboli may be attempted with fibrinolytic drugs such as streptokinase or tissue plasminogen activator (TPA). The effectiveness of these drugs in naturally occurring pulmonary thromboembolism in dogs has not been evaluated.

4) Mini-dose aspirin (0.5 mg/kg PO q12h—dog) has been used to suppress platelet activity and may slow the progression of further thrombus formation. In cats, a dose of 81 mg PO three times weekly has been used.

5) Low molecular weight heparins (LMWH) are expensive and their use has not been well documented in animals. They are considered safe anticoagulants and do not require close hemostatic monitoring. Proposed doses are:

    a) *Enoxaparin (Lovenox)—1 mg/kg SC q12h.*

    b) *Dalteparin (Fragmin) 100 IU/kg SC q12–24h.*

6) Newer anticoagulants used in humans to inhibit platelet function have not been studied in animals (ticlopidine, clopidogrel, lamifiban).

7) We have had some clinical success with streptokinase in dogs with pulmonary thromboembolism. The initial dose is 90,000 IU IV followed by 45,000 IU/h for 3 hours. If the patient remains dyspneic, the infusion can be continued for another 3–6 hours. This therapy should be initiated as soon as pulmonary thromboembolism is suspected or diagnosed.

8) The dosage for TPA is 1–2 mg/kg/h followed by 0.25–1.0 mg/kg/h with heparin (200–400 U/kg IV followed by 150 U/kg SC q6h). There is little clinical experience with this drug in dogs because it is very expensive.

9) The main complication with anticoagulant and fibrinolytic drugs is hemorrhage, and therefore patients should be monitored diligently for this complication.

Streptokinase may also cause hypersensitivity reactions (urticaria, hives, facial edema) that may be relieved with diphenhydramine or corticosteroids.

6. **Pulmonary contusions**

   a. Pulmonary contusion can be mild and associated with few clinical signs or it can result in severe respiratory compromise and hypoxemia.

   b. Lesions tend to worsen over the first 24–36 hours, and therefore the severity may not be evident until after presentation.

   c. Diagnosis

   1) Based on history of trauma, physical examination findings of harsh respiratory sounds or crackles/rales on thoracic auscultation. Physical signs may vary from mild respiratory compromise manifested by tachypnea to severe dyspnea and open-mouth breathing. A soft cough at presentation usually represents severe pulmonary contusions. Signs may not be evident immediately at presentation, and thus serial evaluations should be performed.

   2) Radiographically, pulmonary contusions appear as diffuse or patchy areas of alveolar/interstitial patterns. These lesions may not be evident until 4–6 hours after the insult.

   3) Rib fractures are almost always accompanied by pulmonary contusions, although severe pulmonary injury may occur in the absence of rib fractures.

   d. Treatment

   1) Pulmonary contusion is rarely an isolated injury. The patient should be thoroughly assessed and treated for other injuries.

   2) If resuscitation for shock is necessary, fluid therapy should be conservative if possible, to avoid exacerbation of pulmonary edema. A mixture of crystalloids (10–20 mL/kg) and colloids (5–20 mL/kg) often suffices to restore blood pressure without worsening pulmonary signs.

   3) General principles of treatment are as for any animal in respiratory distress.

   4) Primary therapy for pulmonary contusions is mainly supportive. Provision of supplemental oxygen and cage rest are most important.

   5) Corticosteroid therapy is controversial, and no definitive advantages have been demonstrated in its use for pulmonary contusions.

   a) *If corticosteroids are used, they should be administered shortly after injury, as continued therapy may be harmful.*

   b) *Corticosteroid therapy for pulmonary contusions is not used in our hospitals.*

   6) Bronchodilators are unlikely to provide much benefit to patients with pulmonary contusions.

   7) If rib fractures are present, administration of analgesics such as butorphanol (0.2–1.0 mg/kg in dogs and 0.1–0.4 mg/kg in cats; IV, IM, SC q2–4h as needed) or buprenorphine (0.005–0.02 mg/kg in dogs and 0.005–0.01 mg/kg in cats; IV, IM q4–12h as needed) will afford the animal more comfort in breathing and the ability to take deeper breaths.

   8) Diuretics are not recommended and should be avoided in patients with hypovolemia.

   9) Prophylactic antibiotic therapy is not indicated and should only be used when bronchopneumonia has developed.

   10) Improvement is generally noted within 3–7 days in severe cases. Mild cases may take less time for improvement.

VI. CYANOSIS

1. Cyanosis indicates reduced hemoglobin within the capillaries (generally >5 g/dL of reduced hemoglobin, which may not be evident in anemic, hypoxic patients).

2. High concentrations of methemoglobin also impart a cyanotic appearance to the mucous membranes.

3. Cyanosis generally is not detected in a nonanemic dog until the PaO_2 is < 50 mm Hg and therefore represents severe hypoxemia when observed.

4. Cyanosis is more difficult to detect under fluorescent lighting and in poorly illuminated environments.

5. Causes

   a. Any condition that causes hypoxemia and desaturation of oxygen from hemoglobin

1) Congenital heart disease with right-to-left shunt—e.g., PDA, tetralogy of Fallot
2) Pulmonary disease
   a) Upper airway obstruction—e.g., laryngeal paralysis, nasopharyngeal polyp, foreign body, neoplasia
   b) Obstructive lower airway disease—e.g., asthma
   c) Alveolar disease—pneumonia, pulmonary edema, atelectasis
   d) Restrictive disease—pleural fibrosis, pleural space disease
   e) Pulmonary thromboembolism
   f) Decreased inspired oxygen concentration
3) Chemical or drug exposure resulting in methemoglobinemia or sulfhemoglobinemia—e.g., nitrites, nitrates, fertilizer, acetaminophen (cats)

b. Respiratory compromise is the most common cause of cyanosis.

c. Poor tissue perfusion or slow passage of blood through tissues, allowing maximal extraction of oxygen from the hemoglobin can cause enough desaturation of hemoglobin to produce cyanosis—e.g., shock, hypothermia, low-output heart failure.

d. Peripheral cyanosis occurs when there is poor circulation to an area—e.g., saddle thrombus in cats resulting in cyanosis of distal limbs, footpads, and nail beds.

6. Treatment
   a. Oxygen supplementation and treatment of the underlying cause
   b. A typical diagnostic workup includes PCV/TS (to check for polycythemia secondary to chronic hypoxia), arterial blood gas determinations (to document hypoxemia), thoracic radiographs (to check for heart or lung disease), echocardiography (to check for cardiac defects), and history (to rule out toxins).

VII. MECHANICAL VENTILATION

A. Indications

1. Patients with ventilatory failure determined by arterial blood gas determination with a $PaCO_2$ of 50 mm Hg or above and an arterial pH < 7.3. This may result from alteration of central respiratory control (severe brain disease or general anesthesia), impaired neuromuscular function such as peripheral neuropathies (myasthenia gravis, tick paralysis, polyradiculoneuropathy, botulism), or cervical disk disease or trauma, mechanical function damage (chest wall trauma, diaphragmatic hernia), or respiratory muscle fatigue.

2. Patients that have a $PaCO_2$ < 50 mm Hg despite 100% oxygen supplementation or patients that require prolonged periods of high inspired oxygen concentrations (>50% for more than 12–24 hours) to maintain a PaO_2 > 50 mm Hg (e.g., severe aspiration pneumonia, severe neurogenic pulmonary edema, acute respiratory distress syndrome)

B. Types of ventilators

1. Pressure-cycled ventilators

Termination of inspiration is determined by a preset peak airway pressure regardless of the duration of the breath or the volume administered.

2. Volume-cycled ventilators

Termination of inspiration is determined by a preset tidal volume regardless of the pressure necessary to achieve that volume.

3. Modes of ventilation
   a. Control
   Both the ventilator rate and pressure or volume are preset on the ventilator by the operator. This mode is used in patients that cannot initiate ventilation on their own (anesthetized patients, patients with respiratory muscle and diaphragm paralysis) or when complete control of ventilation is required (hyperventilation in the treatment of increased intracranial pressure).
   b. Assist control
   Both ventilator rate and pressure or volume are preset by the operator, but the patient may increase the rate of ventilation.
   c. Intermittent mandatory
   Both ventilation rate and pressure or volume are preset by the operator, but the patient may be able to breathe spontaneously at its own pressures or tidal volumes.
   d. Synchronized intermittent mandatory
   Both ventilator rate and pressure or volume are preset by the operator, but the ventilator's breaths are synchronized with the patient's inspiratory efforts. This prevents "stacking" of a mechanical breath on top of a spontaneous inspiration.

4. Positive End-Expiratory Pressure (PEEP)
   a. Defined as the maintenance of positive airway pressure at the end of expiration
   b. PEEP can improve lung compliance, oxygenation, and shunt fraction and decrease the work of breathing while allowing for lower inspired oxygen concentrations.
   c. PEEP is used primarily in patients with hypoxic pulmonary failure.
   d. High levels of PEEP (10–15 cm H_2O) can cause hemodynamic compromise. Increased intrathoracic pressure decreases venous return to the heart and lowers cardiac output.

5. Positive-pressure ventilation requires 24-hour nursing care with veterinary nurses and doctors who are familiar with this mode of therapy. The decision to ventilate a patient mechanically should take into account the reversibility of the disease process.

C. Monitoring the respiratory system

1. **Pulse oximetry**
   a. Provides a noninvasive way to estimate arterial oxyhemoglobin saturation by transmitting light through a skin fold (or tongue). It senses the difference between light absorption during pulsations (arterial) and the background between pulses (venous blood and tissue). Measurement thus requires adequate perfusion to the tissue where the probe is placed.
   b. The pulse oximeter gives a continuous readout of percentage saturation of hemoglobin with oxygen and also a pulse rate.
   c. Common areas for probe placement include the tongue, lip, ear, axillary skin fold, inguinal skin fold, metacarpals, gastrocnemius, and the digits. Rectal probes are also available. A rectal probe may also be used in the prepuce or vagina if necessary.
   d. As a rule of thumb, if the heart rate reading on the pulse oximeter and the heart rate of the animal are similar, it is likely that the hemoglobin saturation reading is accurate. A good pulse waveform and a strong auditory signal in addition to matching heart rates also lend confidence to the hemoglobin saturation reading.
   e. Movement, respiratory artifact, poor tissue perfusion, and skin pigmentation may affect readings. Also, oxygen saturation determined by pulse oximetry is unreliable in patients with carbon monoxide intoxication or methemoglobinemia.
   f. A hemoglobin saturation of 90% corresponds to an approximate PaO_2 of 60 mm Hg. Therefore a pulse oximeter reading of 90% is the minimal acceptable reading. Administer therapy to improve oxygenation when hemoglobin saturation is less than 90%.

2. **End-tidal CO_2**
   a. These monitors continuously aspirate gas from plastic tubing placed in airways and analyze the CO_2 concentration. The plateau of the end-tidal carbon dioxide measurement for each breath theoretically reflects alveolar CO_2. Since CO_2 is readily diffusible, this measurement is proposed to reflect arterial P_{CO_2}.
   b. Veterinary studies have found that end-tidal CO_2 measurements alone do not reflect Pa_{CO_2} reliably. End-CO_2 can be used to identify hypoventilation in nonpanting patients (panting makes the measurement inaccurate). For example, if the monitor says that the PCO_2 is high, this can reliably be interpreted to mean that the patient is hypoventilating, but it does not necessarily accurately reflect the exact $PaCO_2$ concentration.

3. **Arterial blood gases**
   a. The body tries to maintain a blood pH of 7.4. With primary metabolic disturbances, the body tries to compensate with respiratory changes and vice versa. An important principle to remember when interpreting acid/base changes is that the body never overcompensates.
   b. Evaluation of acid/base status from arterial blood gas determination
      1) Determine the pH change.
         a) pH > 7.4 indicates alkalemia
         b) pH < 7.4 indicates acidemia
      2) Determine the changes in bicarbonate concentration and $PaCO_2$.
         a) A high $PaCO_2$ indicates respiratory acidosis.
         b) A low $PaCO_2$ indicates respiratory alkalosis.
         c) A high bicarbonate concentration indicates metabolic alkalosis.
         d) A low bicarbonate concentration indicates metabolic acidosis.
      3) Compare the pH change and the $PaCO_2$ and bicarbonate concentration changes (keeping in mind that the body NEVER overcompensates) to determine which is the primary change and which is the compensatory change.

a) For example: pH >7.4 indicates alkalemia. If the $PaCO_2$ indicates alkalosis, then the primary abnormality is respiratory alkalosis. If the bicarbonate concentration is high, it is primary metabolic alkalosis.

b) Another example: pH <7.4 indicates acidemia. If the $PaCO_2$ is high, primary respiratory acidosis is present. If the bicarbonate concentration is low, there is primary metabolic acidosis.

c) Normal dog values

pH: 7.40 ± 0.05
PaO_2: 100 ± 10 mm Hg
$PaCO_2$: 34 ± 8 mm Hg
HCO_3 : 21 ± 3 mEq/L
Base excess: -1 ± 2 mEq/L

d) Normal cat values

pH: 7.38 ± 0.07
PaO_2: 103 ± 7 mm Hg
$PaCO_2$: 33 ± 7 mm Hg
HCO_3: 19 ± 2 mEq/L
Base excess: -2 ± 3 mEq/L

Values for the dog and cat are approximate, and values will vary depending upon the machine used.

4) Determining what primary process is causing the pH change is the most important information to obtain from the blood gas analysis. The next step to refine the information is to determine if the compensatory change is normal or not.

a) Expected respiratory compensation for primary metabolic acidosis:

Expected $PaCO_2$
 = Normal $PaCO_2$ − [Change in bicarbonate from normal) × 0.8

If the measured value and expected value differ by more than 2 mm Hg, a mixed metabolic and respiratory disturbance is present.

b) Expected respiratory change for primary metabolic alkalosis:

Expected $PaCO_2$
 = [Change in bicarbonate concentration from normal)
 × (0.7)] + Normal $PaCO_2$

If the measured value and expected value differ by more than 2 mm Hg, then a mixed

metabolic and respiratory disturbance is present.

c) Expected bicarbonate concentration compensatory change in response to a primary acute respiratory acidosis:

Expected bicarbonate concentration
 = [(Change in $PaCO_2$ from normal) × (0.15) + Normal bicarbonate concentration

If the measured and expected bicarbonate concentrations differ by more than 2 mEq/L, then a mixed metabolic and respiratory disturbance is present.

d) Expected bicarbonate concentration compensatory change in response to a primary chronic respiratory acidosis:

Expected bicarbonate concentration
 = [(Change in $PaCO_2$ from normal)]
 × (0.37)] + Normal bicarbonate concentration

If the measured and expected bicarbonate concentrations differ by more than 2 mEq/L, then a mixed metabolic and respiratory disturbance is present.

e) Expected bicarbonate concentration in response to a primary acute respiratory alkalosis:

Expected bicarbonate concentration
 = Normal bicarbonate
 − [(Change in $PaCO_2$)] × (0.2)

If the measured and expected bicarbonate concentrations differ by more than 2 mEq/L, then a mixed metabolic and respiratory disturbance is present.

f) Expected bicarbonate concentration in response to a primary chronic respiratory alkalosis:

Expected bicarbonate concentration
 = Normal bicarbonate
 − [(Change in $PaCO_2$)] × (0.55)

If the measured and expected bicarbonate concentrations differ by more than 2 mEq/L, then a mixed metabolic and respiratory disturbance is present.

g) Note: When calculating expected compensatory bicarbonate changes, the clinician must try to determine if the primary respiratory disorder is chronic or acute be-

cause metabolic compensatory changes take a few days to develop.

5) After acid/base assessment of the arterial blood gas analysis is completed, the oxygenation assessment should be performed.

   a. PaO_2 should be evaluated in light of the $PaCO_2$, to determine if hypoventilation is the cause of the hypoxemia.

   b. If PaO_2 is < 80 mm Hg, correct hypoventilation if present, treat the underlying cause, and provide oxygen supplementation.

   c. A useful calculation in veterinary medicine is determining the alveolar:arterial oxygen gradient (A–a gradient). In normal patients this gradient should not exceed 10 mm Hg. Gradients steeper than this suggest a defect in oxygenation, most likely caused by ventilation/perfusion mismatch or shunting.

   1. A—a gradient = PAO_2
      (Alveolar O_2) − PaO_2 (arterial O_2)
   2. PAO_2 = (Barometric pressure −47)FiO_2 − 1.2 ($PaCO_2$)

   At sea level, with the patient breathing room air, one can use the approximate formula

   PaO_2 = 150 mm Hg − 1.2 ($PaCO_2$)

   3. Once the PAO_2 is calculated, the measured PAO_2 is subtracted to compute the A–a gradient. Valves exceeding 10–15 mm Hg are consistent with ventilation/perfusion mismatch or shunting.

   4. Calculation of the A–a gradient is unreliable with oxygen supplementation. The patient should be breathing room air during the measurements and calculation.

   d. PaO_2/FIO_2 *Ratio.*

   1. This ratio is useful for assessing respiratory function in animals receiving supplemented oxygen.
   2. The PaO_2 is the partial pressure of oxygen dissolved in arterial blood as measured by blood gas analysis in mm Hg.
   3. The FiO_2 is the fractional percentage of inspired oxygen (eg, room air = 0.21, nasal O_2 = 0.4)
   4. Normal PaO_2/FiO_2 ratios are 400–500. Values less than 300 indicate severe lung injury, and values < 200 are consistent with ARDS (acute respiratory distress syndrome).

4. **Respiratory rate and auscultation**

   a. Monitoring respiratory rate, effort, and thoracic auscultation is essential in monitoring the patient with respiratory disease.

   1) All patients should be assessed at presentation to set a baseline and then monitored serially for changes in physical respiratory parameters. Measurements of arterial blood gases, pulse oximetry, and end-tidal CO_2 cannot be assessed in isolation from the physical examination findings. There is no substitute for physical examination of the respiratory system.

   2) Determine the frequency of monitoring respiratory rate and effort and thoracic auscultation by the severity of the patient's compromise and the dynamics of the disease process. Frequent monitoring initially to establish a trend will help the clinician to determine the optimal monitoring intervals.

CHAPTER 10

CARDIAC EMERGENCIES

I. CLINICAL SIGNS

Look for clues in the physical examination and history that will differentiate cardiac disease from respiratory disease in dyspneic patients.

A. Dogs with cardiac disease commonly have a history of coughing (moist, nocturnal), exercise intolerance, labored breathing, cachexia, and sometimes collapse.

B. Cats rarely have a history of coughing with cardiac disease. Coughing is more commonly seen with bronchial asthma and other pulmonary diseases of cats.

C. Breed predispositions:

> Small breeds—mitral valve disease
> Large/giant breeds—dilated cardiomyopathy
> Boxers—heart base tumors, boxer myocarditis
> Cats—prone to pleural effusion secondary to cardiomyopathy

D. Pulmonary crackles and wheezes are heard with pulmonary edema.

E. Percussion can be used to detect dull areas where there is pleural effusion.

F. Breathing is often labored, exhibiting both inspiratory and expiratory dyspnea, and the respiratory rate is increased.

G. Mucous membranes may be injected, pale, or cyanotic. Animals with cardiac disease may have an increased hematocrit from chronic hypoxia, resulting in injected membranes. Pallor can be seen with poor perfusion secondary to cardiogenic shock. Cyanosis indicates hypoxemia, secondary to pulmonary edema.

H. Cats with congestive heart failure are often hypothermic, and they sometimes have a slow heart rate (100–120) with weak pulses.

I. Dogs with congestive heart failure are often tachycardic at rest or develop an increased heart rate with mild exercise.

J. Absent pulses and posterior paralysis can be seen in cats with cardiomyopathy and distal aortic thromboembolism.

K. Pulse deficits (lack of a detectable pulse with each auscultable heart beat) can indicate atrial fibrillation, premature beats, or ventricular tachycardia.

L. Most animals in heart failure have weak pulses secondary to decreased stroke volume and increased peripheral vascular resistance.

M. If pulses seem to get weaker during inspiration, pericardial effusion with pulsus paradoxus should be suspected.

N. Signs of right-sided heart failure include jugular venous distension, ascites, pleural effusion, and hepatosplenomegaly. These signs are particularly prominent in dogs with pericardial disease but can also be seen in dogs with biventricular failure secondary to dilated cardiomyopathy or pure right-sided failure associated with congenital heart defects or heartworm disease.

II. DIAGNOSIS

Confirmed with physical examination, cardiac auscultation, electrocardiogram, echocardiogram, thoracic radiographs, and sometimes Holter monitoring.

III. DIAGNOSTIC AND MONITORING PROCEDURES

A. Auscultation

1. Listen for murmurs, gallop rhythm, or arrhythmias

2. Lack of murmur or tachycardia in a small-breed dog generally rules out congestive heart failure as the cause of dyspnea.

3. Always feel pulses simultaneously with auscultation to check for pulse deficits that may indicate arrhythmias.

4. Point of maximum intensity varies with murmur

    a. Pulmonic valve: 3rd intercostal space on left, low

    b. Aortic valve: 4th intercostal space on left, high

    c. Mitral valve: 5th intercostal space on left, low

    d. Patent ductus arteriosus (PDA): 3rd intercostal space on left, high

    e. Tricuspid valve: 4th intercostal space on right side

    f. Ventricular septal defect (VSD): 3rd intercostal space on right side

    g. Murmurs in cats are often heard best low along the sternal border

B. Electrocardiography

1. Animal should be in right lateral recumbency if possible. If animal is dyspneic, a standing electrocardiogram (ECG) rhythm strip can be obtained.

2. Electrodes are attached just proximal to the elbows and stifles and wet with alcohol or electrode gel.

3. If a continuous ECG is needed, steel sutures can be placed at the sites of electrode attachment for placement of alligator clips, or commercially available ECG pads can be used.

4. ECG wave forms (*Figs. 10-1, 10-3*)

    a. The **P wave** reflects atrial depolarization. Left atrial enlargement causes a wide, notched P wave. Right atrial enlargement causes a tall P wave.

    b. The **PR interval** represents the conduction of the impulse from the SA node to the AV node. It is measured from the beginning of the P wave to the beginning of the QRS. Prolongation of the PR interval constitutes first-degree heart block and is seen with digitalis toxicity and other conduction disturbances.

    c. The **QRS complex** represents ventricular depolarization. A wide QRS indicates slowed conduction and can be seen with left ventricular hypertrophy, bundle branch block, or ventricular ectopic beats.

        1) QRS amplitude >3.0 mV indicates ventricular enlargement.

        2) QRS amplitude <0.5 mV may indicate pericardial or pleural effusion.

    d. The **T wave** represents repolarization. It can be positive or negative and should not be taller than one-quarter the amplitude of the R wave.

    e. The **ST segment** is measured from the end of the S wave to the beginning of the T wave. Elevation or depression of the ST segment from baseline may signify myocardial ischemia, electrolyte imbalance, or underlying disease.

    f. ECG analysis: Use lead II at 50 mm/sec; calibration 1 cm = 1 mV (*Figs. 10-2*) (*Tables 10-1 and 10-2*)

        1) Calculate heart rate (multiply the number of QRS complexes in 30 boxes—1.5 seconds—by 20 to obtain beats/min). A quick way to approximate this is with the "Bic pen

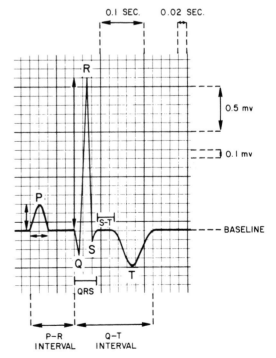

FIGURE 10.1 Close-up of a normal canine lead II P-QRS-T complex with labels and intervals, P, 0.04 sec by 0.3 mv; P-R, 0.1 sec; QRS, 0.05 sec by 1.7 mv; S-T segment and T wave, normal; Q-T, 0.18 sec. (From Tilley LP. Essentials of canine and feline electrocardiography. Philadelphia: Lea & Febiger, 1992.)

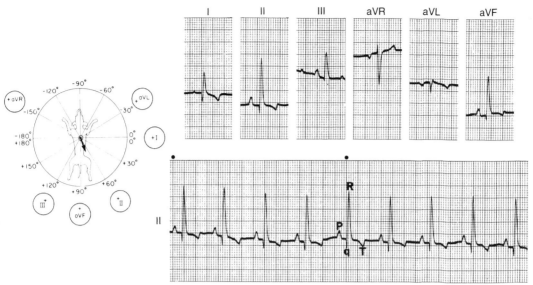

FIGURE 10.2   Normal canine electrocardiogram. Heart rate, 165 beats/min. Heart rhythm, normal sinus. Complexes and intervals: P, 0.04 sec by 0.3 mv; P-R, 0.08 sec; QRS, 0.05 sec by 1.9 mv; S-T segment and T wave, normal; Q-T, 0.16 sec. Mean electrical axis, +70E. (From Tilley LP. Essentials of canine and feline electrocardiography. Philadelphia: Lea & Febiger, 1992.)

technique." Count the number of complexes that occur in the length of a standard writing pen and multiply by 20 to obtain the heart rate.

2) Evaluate rhythm—normal sinus or irregular, paroxysmal or sustained
3) Identify P waves—is atrial activity regular?

4) Identify QRS complexes—Are they supraventricular (narrow QRS) or ventricular (wide QRS)?

a) For very rapid rates, press on the ocular globes while recording ECG, to help determine source of arrhythmia; atrial tachyarrhythmia will usually slow, ventricular will not.

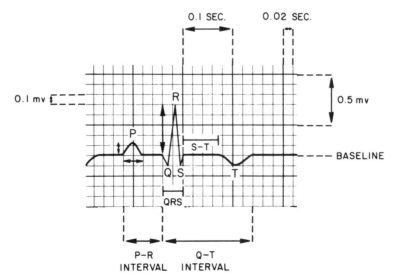

FIGURE 10.3   Close-up of a normal feline lead II P-QRS-T complex labels and intervals. (From Tilley LP. Essentials of canine and feline electrocardiography. Philadelphia: Lea & Febiger, 1992.)

TABLE 10.1
NORMAL CANINE ELECTROCARDIOGRAPHIC VALUES

Rate
  70 to 160 beats/min for adult dogs
  60 to 140 beats/min for giant breeds
  Up to 180 beats/min for toy breeds
  Up to 220 beats/min for puppies

Rhythm
  Normal sinus rhythm
  Sinus arrhythmia
  Wandering SA pacemaker

Measurements (lead II, 50 mm/sec, 1 cm = 1 mv)
  P wave
    Width: maximum, 0.04 sec (2 boxes wide)
         maximum, 0.05 sec ($2^1/_2$ boxes wide) in giant breeds
    Height: maximum, 0.4 mv (4 boxes tall)
  P-R Interval
    Width: 0.06 to 0.13 sec (3 to $6^1/_2$ boxes)
  QRS complex
    Width: maximum, 0.05 sec ($2^1/_2$ boxes) in small breeds
         maximum, 0.06 sec (3 boxes) in large breeds
    Height of R wave*: maximum, 3.0 mv (30 boxes) in large breeds
                    maximum, 2.5 mv (25 boxes) in small breeds
  S-T segment
    No depression: not more than 0.2 mv (2 boxes)
    No elevation: not more than 0.15 mv ($1^1/_2$ boxes)
  T wave
    Can be positive, negative, or diphasic
    Not greater than one-fourth amplitude of R wave; amplitude range $\pm$0.05–1.0 mv ($^1/_2$ to
      10 boxes) in any lead
  Q-T interval
    Width: 0.15 to 0.25 sec ($7^1/_2$ to $12^1/_2$ boxes) at normal heart rate; varies with heart rate (faster rates
      have shorter Q-T intervals and vice versa)

Electrical axis (frontal plane)
  +40° to +100°
Precordial chest leads (values of special importance)
  CV_5RL (rV_2): T wave positive, R wave not greater than 3.0 mv (30 boxes)
  CV_6LL (V_2): S wave not greater than 0.8 mv (8 boxes), R wave not greater than 3.0 mv (30 boxes)[a]
  CV_6LU (V_4): S waves not greater than 0.7 mv (7 boxes), R wave not greater than 3.0 mv (30 boxes)[a]
  V_{10}: negative QRS complex, T wave negative except in Chihuahua

[a]Not valid for thin deep-chested dogs under 2 years of age.

---

5) Determine relationship between P waves and QRS complexes. Is there a P wave for every QRS? Note premature/ectopic beats.

6) Classify arrhythmia—supraventricular vs. ventricular, tachycardia vs. bradycardia, ectopic/premature beats vs. escape beats

7) Determine whether treatment is indicated—are there any clinical signs associated with the arrhythmia?

C. Echocardiography

  1. 2-D echocardiography records a planar image of the heart; useful for identifying masses, evaluating valves, and assessing wall motion

---

TABLE 10.2
NORMAL FELINE ELECTROCARDIOGRAPHIC VALUES

Rate
 Range: 120 to 240 beats/min
 Mean: 197 beats/min

Rhythm
 Normal sinus rhythm
 Sinus tachycardia (physiologic reaction to excitement)

Measurements (lead II, 50 mm/sec, 1 cm = 1 mv)[a]
 P wave
  Width: maximum, 0.04 sec (2 boxes wide)
  Height: maximum, 0.2 mv (2 boxes tall).
 P-R Interval
  Width: 0.05 to 0.09 sec ($2^1/_2$ to $4^1/_2$ boxes)
 QRS complex
  Width: maximum, 0.04 sec (2 boxes)
  Height of R wave: maximum, 0.9 mv (9 boxes)
 S-T segment
  No depression or elevation
 T wave
  Can be positive, negative, or diphasic; most often is positive
 Maximum amplitude: 0.3 mv (3 boxes)
 Q-T Interval
  Width: 0.12 to 0.18 sec (6 to 9 boxes) at normal heart rate (range 0.07 to 0.20 sec, $3^1/_2$ to 10 boxes);
   varies with heart rate (faster rates, shorter Q-T intervals; and vice versa)

Electrical axis (front plane)
 0 to ±160° (not valid in many cats)

Precordial chest leads
 CV_6LL (V_2): R wave <1.0 mv (10 boxes)
 CV_6LU (V_4): R wave not greater than 1.0 mv (10 boxes)
 V_{10}: T wave negative; R/Q <1.0

[a]From the Animal Medical Center. Computed by adding and subtracting 1.96 times the standard deviation from the mean for the axis (P < .05 or 95% of the observations) and 1.645 times the standard deviation for widths and heights of waves and intervals (P < .10 or 90% of the observations). Numbers are rounded off to the nearest whole.

---

2. M-mode records an "ice-pick" view.
 a. Measurements of chamber dimensions and wall thicknesses are made best with M-mode.
 b. Functional indices are calculated through dimension measurements.

3. Simultaneous ECG is recorded for timing.
 a. Diastolic measurements are taken at the onset of the Q wave.
 b. Systolic measurements are taken at the point of maximum septal wall excursion.

4. Ultrasound frequencies: Lower frequencies provide deeper penetration but less definition.
 a. Large animals: 5.0- to 7.5-MHz probe
 b. Small animals: 7.5-MHz probe

5. For image enhancement
 a. Clip hair on thorax.
 b. Apply coupling gel liberally to provide air-free contact.
 c. Image from the underside, with the patient in lateral recumbency on a "cutout" table.
 d. Place transducer at the precordial impulse (4th or 5th intercostal space) and adjust probe

to obtain clear visualization of the heart (best acoustic window).

6. Chemical restraint can be used if necessary.
Dogs: buprenorphine 0.0075–0.1 mg/kg IV with acepromazine 0.03 mg/kg IV
Cats: hydromorphone 0.5 mg/kg IV or butorphanol 0.1 mg/kg IV with midazolam 0.2 mg/kg IV

7. Use right parasternal short axis view to obtain M-mode measurements. Visualize the heart on 2-D and place the cursor at the level of the chordae tendinae just below the mitral valve. Do not include papillary muscles.

8. Measurements are made from leading edge to leading edge of the septum and left ventricular free wall during systole and diastole.
   a. The shortening fraction (FS) is calculated and is commonly used as an index of left ventricular (LV) function.

   b. $FS = \dfrac{LVIDd - LVIDs}{LVIDd} \times 100$

      1) LVIDd is the internal diameter measured at onset of QRS complex.
      2) LVIDs is the internal diameter measured at peak IVS posterior motion or peak anterior motion of LV free wall.
      3) FS is increased with early mitral insufficiency, hypertrophic cardiomyopathy, thyrotoxic heart disease, and hypertension.
      4) FS is decreased with dilated cardiomyopathy, PDA, infarction, and other causes of cardiac failure (severe mitral valve regurgitation).

9. Measurements of the aortic root and left atrium are obtained.
   a. Aortic root—end-diastole
   b. Left atrium—maximum systole
   c. Ratio should be 1:1. (left atrium: aortic root)
      1) Normal dog: 0.83–1.13
      2) Normal cat: 0.99–1.39

10. Echocardiographic features of common diseases
    a. Feline myocardial disease
       1) Hypertrophic cardiomyopathy
          a) Diastolic thickness of IV septum or LV free wall >5–5.6 mm
          b) Thickened papillary muscles, reduced LV lumen
          c) Enlarged LA
          d) Normal to increased fractional shortening
       2) Feline restrictive CM
          a) Endomyocardial fibrosis causes a bright endocardial surface.
          b) Increased LA size
    b. Dilated cardiomyopathy
       1) Dilation of left and right chambers
       2) Poor systolic wall and septal motion
       3) Increased LV dimensions
       4) Decreased fractional shortening
       5) Increased mitral valve E point to septal separation
    c. Mitral valve insufficiency
       1) Thick, knobby-appearing valves
       2) Ruptured chordae tendineae cause paradoxical valve motion or flailing.
       3) Marked left atrial enlargement
       4) Increased fractional shortening, normal E point septal separation, exaggerated septal motion prior to myocardial failure
    d. Pericardial effusion
       1) Appears as echo-free space between the bright pericardium and the epicardium
       2) Most of the fluid surrounds the apex of the heart rather than the base.
    e. Bacterial endocarditis—aortic valve
       1) Bright densities—vegetation
       2) Diastolic fluttering indicates insufficiency

D. Holter monitor

1. Continuously records ECG on cassette tape for 24 hours
2. Computer reads the tape and produces a record of cardiac rhythm during the recording period.
3. Method of choice for evaluating response to antiarrhythmic therapy and for determining frequency of arrhythmias.
4. Cost is about $150 per 24-hour study if done through a commercial service. (Lab Corp, Ambulatory Monitoring Services Division, Burlington, NC: 800-289-4358)
5. The Holter monitor weighs 400 g and may be too bulky for small patients.
6. Useful for evaluating causes of syncope and correlating arrhythmias with clinical signs
7. Does not require owner participation

E. Event-based recorders

1. Used for infrequent symptomatic arrhythmia evaluation
2. Smaller than Holter monitor; weighs 100 g

3. Must be triggered by owner when event occurs

4. The recorder has a 5-minute memory; five intermittent 1-minute segments can be recorded by the client.

5. Event-based recorders cost the veterinarian about $95 for 1 week or $280 for 1 month.

F. Nonselective angiogram

1. Sedation is usually required.

2. Less precise than selective angiography, but adaptable to private practice

3. Place an 18- to 20-gauge catheter in the right jugular, cephalic, or saphenous vein.

4. With animal in left lateral recumbency, inject 1 mL/kg of iothalamate or iohexal as rapidly as possible.

5. The first film is taken just before completion of the injection. Subsequent films can be taken as rapidly as possible (if a rapid film changer is not available).

6. A film taken 6–8 seconds after the injection usually provides a good left ventricular study. Severe heart failure will result in prolonged circulation times, however.

7. This technique can be used to differentiate dilated and hypertrophic cardiomyopathy in cats if echocardiography is not available. A lateral radiograph of the abdomen taken 10–15 seconds after contrast administration can be used to detect aortic thromboemboli.

8. Dilated chambers, wall thickness, and obstructive lesions (aortic stenosis, pulmonic stenosis) can be detected with this procedure.

G. Cardiac catheterization and selective angiography.

1. Provides assessment of pressures, oxygen tension, and cardiac output and shunt quantitation

2. Requires specialized equipment
  a. Monitor with ECG and pressure channels
  b. Recorder
  c. Fluoroscopic capabilities
  d. Pressure transducer
  e. Catheters
  f. Rapid film changer
  g. Video recorder
  h. Cardiac output computer

3. May require general anesthesia

4. For right-sided catheterization, a Swan-Ganz catheter is fed into the right jugular vein. Pressures are recorded as each chamber is entered. When the characteristic pressure wave of the right ventricle is seen (20/0 mm Hg), the balloon is partially inflated so that the catheter is flow-directed to the pulmonary artery. The catheter is directed further into the pulmonary artery and pressures are recorded. WARNING: Never "wedge" the catheter and then inflate the balloon, as rupture of the pulmonary artery can occur.)

5. The pulmonary wedge pressure is used to estimate left atrial pressure when the balloon is fully inflated and wedged in the pulmonary capillary.

6. Left-to-right shunts can be identified by noting increased oxygen tensions on the right side.

7. Abnormal pressure gradients can be seen with valvular stenosis or shunts.

8. Selective angiography allows evaluation of valvular regurgitation, septal defects, and other shunts as well as wall thickness and chamber size.

9. Following the procedure, the jugular vein (or the carotid) can be ligated without consequence if necessary to stop hemorrhage.

10. Diagnostic cardiac catheterization procedures have largely been replaced by noninvasive color flow Doppler imaging and echocardiographic bubble studies. It is still used for patients requiring therapeutic valvuloplasty.

TABLE 10.3
NORMAL PRESSURE AND OXYGEN SATURATION IN THE HEART CHAMBERS OF DOGS

Chamber	Pressure (mm Hg)	O_2 Saturation (%)
Vena cava	5/–1, mean 3	75
Right atrium	5/–1, mean 3	75
Right ventricle	20/0, end-diastolic 3	75
Pulmonary artery	20/10, mean 15	75
Pulmonary artery wedge	12/6, mean 8	98
Left atrium	14/5, mean 8	98
Left ventricle	120/0, end-diastolic 6	98
Aorta	120/80, mean 100	98

IV. MANAGEMENT OF SPECIFIC CONDITIONS

A. Congestive heart failure (AV valve degeneration)

1. Mitral regurgitation is the most common cause of congestive heart failure (CHF) in dogs; 30% of small-breed dogs >10 years old are affected.

2. Predisposed breeds include Cavalier King Charles Spaniels, Poodles, Miniature Schnauzers, Chihuahuas, Fox Terriers, Cocker Spaniels, Boston Terriers, and Dachshunds.

3. This is a degenerative disease in which the valve leaflets become knobby and thickened. Regurgitant blood causes progressive enlargement of the left atrium and left ventricle.

4. Progression of disease may take years. Signs range from asymptomatic murmur, to exercise intolerance, to total decompensation with severe dyspnea at rest.

5. Although contractility remains normal until late in the disease, increased left atrial pressure results in pulmonary venous congestion and pulmonary edema.

6. Acute decompensation can occur if chordae tendinae rupture resulting in increased regurgitant fraction, elevated left atrial pressure, and fulminant pulmonary edema.

7. In severe cases, acute decompensation also can occur with an atrial tear and bleeding into the pericardial sac, causing cardiac tamponade.

8. Physical examination findings:
  a. Holosystolic murmur, low on left 5th intercostal space.
  b. Tachypnea, harsh lung sounds, inspiratory crackles progressing to crackles and wheezes throughout respiration.

9. Radiographic findings
  a. Left atrial enlargement—bulging of dorsocaudal border of the heart on the lateral view; compression of left mainstem bronchus; bulge at 2–3 o'clock on the VD view signifies left auricular enlargement.
  b. Left ventricular enlargement can be verified using Buchanan's measurement scale for dogs.
    1) A blank paper is placed on the radiograph and the long axis of the heart is measured from the base to the apex and marked.
    2) The paper is then turned perpendicularly, the short axis measurement of the heart is added to the first measurement, and a second mark is placed on the paper.
    3) The paper is then held up to the vertebrae beginning at T4, and the vertebrae are counted for the length of the measurement to the second mark.
    4) Measurements >10.5 vertebrae are consistent with cardiomegaly.
  c. Assessment of pulmonary edema
    1) Earliest sign of CHF is pulmonary venous congestion seen best in the cranial lobar veins on the lateral view. Veins are ventral; sequence is artery–bronchus–vein (from top to bottom). The vein should not be larger than the artery.
    2) In dogs, pulmonary edema is perihilar then dorsocaudal, then bilaterally symmetrical with progressive fluid buildup.
    3) Mild pulmonary edema initially results in increased interstitial markings, progressing to peribronchial cuffing. More-severe pulmonary edema causes fluffy opacities and air bronchograms.

10. Echocardiographic findings
  a. Wide P waves (>0.04 sec) are consistent with left atrial enlargement.
  b. Tall R waves (>3 mV in lead II) suggest left ventricular enlargement.
  c. Atrial arrhythmias can be seen with severe left atrial enlargement.

11. Echocardiographic findings
  a. Mitral valve leaflets appear hyperechoic and thickened. Flailing can be observed with ruptured chordae tendinae.
  b. Left atrial enlargement results in a left atria:aorta ratio >1:1.
  c. Shortening fraction is usually normal to increased.
  d. Ventricular wall motion is good, indicating normal contractility.

12. Treatment
  a. Class I: Murmur present, no other clinical signs
    1) No treatment indicated. Reevaluate every 6 months.
    2) Avoid high-salt foods.
  b. Class II: Still asymptomatic, but radiographs reveal marked left atrial enlargement and pulmonary venous congestion.
    1) Avoid strenuous exercise
    2) Feed a moderately salt restricted diet. Use diets formulated for geriatric dogs or dogs with renal disease. These diets are generally more palatable than diets with

marked sodium restriction that are formulated for heart failure patients. Weight loss is encouraged for obese dogs.

3) Begin administering enalapril (0.5 mg/kg q24h). Increase dosage to q12h if response is inadequate. Decrease dosage to 0.25 mg/kg q24h if weakness, hypotension, or azotemia develop.

4) Marked left atrial enlargement can cause compression of the left mainstem bronchus and a chronic dry, hacking cough. Treatment involves a cough suppressant (hydrocodone 0.22 mg/kg q6–12h PO or butorphanol 0.5–1 mg/kg PO q8–12h) and an arterial vasodilator to reduce the regurgitant fraction (hydralazine 0.5–2 mg/kg PO q12h)

c. Class III: Clinical signs of pulmonary congestion and weakness exacerbated by exercise and activity

1) Moderate sodium restriction

2) Restrict exercise.

3) Initiate enalapril treatment at 0.5 mg/kg q24h.

4) Diuretic therapy is provided at the lowest dose to control pulmonary congestion and edema. Initial doses may be higher and then tapered down.

a) Furosemide: 1–2 mg/kg q8–48h

b) Spironolactone: 2 mg/kg PO q24h— This is a potassium-sparing diuretic that can improve long-term response to treatment if given early in the course of therapy by limiting the neurohumoral compensatory responses that lead to volume overload (primarily through the inhibition of aldosterone)

5) Digoxin is indicated if there is marked left ventricular enlargement, tachycardia, atrial arrhythmias, systolic dysfunction as determined by echocardiography, or persistence of clinical signs despite diuretic and vasodilator therapy.

a) Digoxin reduces sympathetic stimulation of the heart by stabilizing baroreceptor function. It also improves contractility and slows the heart rate by decreasing AV conduction.

b) Dosage

i) Small-breed dogs: 0.0055–0.011 mg/kg q12h PO
Large breed dogs: 0.22 mg/m^2 q12h PO
ii) Digoxin elixir is absorbed more readily than the tablet form. If the elixir

is used, 80% of the calculated dose should be administered to avoid toxicity.
iii) Generic formulations of digoxin are not recommended.

c) Avoid toxicity

i) Rule out azotemia, hypokalemia, and hypothyroidism before administering digoxin.

ii) Base dosage on lean body weight. Reduce dose with renal disease, thyroid dysfunction, ascites, cachexia, or concurrent quinidine therapy.

iii) To dose dogs with chronic renal disease, either divide the dose by the serum creatinine level and administer on schedule or multiply the dosage interval by the serum creatinine level and decrease the frequency of dosing accordingly. For example, if the creatinine level is 2.0, the dosage interval (12 h) would be increased to 24 h (2 × 12), or the dose would be decreased by one-half every 12 hours.

iv) Serum digoxin levels should be checked 7 days after initiating therapy, 8 hours after the last dose. The therapeutic range for most laboratories is 0.8–2.2 mg/mL. If values are not in the therapeutic range, the dosage should be adjusted accordingly.

v) Signs of digoxin toxicity include anorexia, vomiting, diarrhea, lethargy, and arrhythmias. If these signs occur in a patient receiving digoxin, take a blood sample and discontinue giving digoxin until the results are available.

vi) For severe digoxin toxicity, digoxin-binding antibodies (Digibind) can be given to lower the digoxin concentration rapidly, but the cost is very high, limiting the use of this treatment in veterinary medicine.

d. Class IV: Severe pulmonary edema with clinical signs of tachypnea, cyanosis, and labored breathing at rest. Aggressive therapy is indicated.

1) Give oxygen supplementation immediately by face mask or "flow by" during initial examination and treatment.

2) Place an intravenous catheter and administer furosemide. A dosage of 4–8 mg/kg q1–4h is used for fulminant pulmonary edema and 2–4 mg/kg q8–12h for maintenance. Try to avoid excessive doses that can result in dehydration, hypovolemia, hypokalemia, and alkalosis. Cats are more sensitive to these side effects, and an initial dosage not to exceed 2–4 mg/kg IM, IV or SC q8–12h is recommended.

3) Topical nitroglycerine (0.25–1 inch q4–6h) is applied to a shaved or hairless area to induce venodilation. If the ears are warm, indicating good perfusion, apply the paste there. Otherwise, use a shaved area on the flank or the inguinal or axillary region. This effect is very rapid. As venous capacitance is increased through vasodilation, pulmonary venous congestion and preload are decreased, resulting in less pulmonary edema.

4) If significant improvement is not seen within 30 minutes following initiation of therapy with oxygen, furosemide, and nitroglycerine, initiate a nitroprusside drip.

a) The dosage is 0.5–10 μg/kg/min administered as a constant-rate infusion (CRI)

b) Make up the drip in 5% dextrose and water at an initial dosage of 2 μg/kg/min using the following formula:

$$M = \frac{(D)\,(W)\,(V)}{(R)\,(16.67)}$$

where M is mg of nitroprusside to add to solution

D is the dose in μg/kg/min (in this case, 2)

W is the dog's body weight in kilograms

V is the volume of solution (5% dextrose)

R is the delivery rate in mL/h. This should be set at no more than half maintenance (1 mL/kg/h maximum).

c) The dog is initially given the nitroprusside drip at a dosage of 2 μg/kg/min. If there is no improvement in 20–30 minutes, the CRI dosage is increased by 1 μg/kg/min by adding half of the initial volume of nitroprusside to the drip solution. This process is repeated every 20–30 minutes until the respiratory rate decreases and fewer crackles and wheezes are ausc!ted. The effective dosage for most dogs is 5–8 μg/kg/min. The drip can be continued for 48–72 hours at the effective dosage until the patient has stabilized (Table 10-4).

d) Discontinue therapy with nitroglycerine if a nitroprusside drip is administered.

e) Monitor blood pressure during initial therapy to avoid hypotension.

f) Nitroprusside is metabolized to cyanide. To avoid toxicity, the CRI should be discontinued by 72 hours.

TABLE 10.4
NITROPRUSSIDE CRI

Example: 10 yo MC Poodle, 5 kg
Fulminant CHF secondary to chronic mitral regurgitation with acute ruptured chordae tendinae

PE findings: T, 100; P, 186; R, 90 (labored with crackles and wheezes)

Initial treatment: Oxygen and furosemide

Nitroprusside drip: (see text) Begin at 2 μg/kg/min

$$M = \frac{DWV}{R(16.67)} = \frac{(2\,\mu g/kg/min)(5\,kg)(250\,mL)}{(5)(16.67)} = 30 \text{ mg of nitroprusside}$$

Nitroprusside is 50 mg/mL, so 30/50 = 0.6
Add 0.6 mL of nitroprusside to 250 mL of 5% dextrose
Administer at 5 mL/h

Monitoring: Auscult thorax, check mm color, CRT, HR, RR q20–30 min. If no improvement, increase dose by 1 μg/kg/min (add 0.3 mL of nitroprusside to drip). Marked improvement is usually seen within 1–3 hours. The respiratory rate should decrease, and respiratory efforts will appear less labored. Once the target dose is reached, the dog is maintained on nitroprusside CRI at that dosage until clinical signs stabilize (up to 72 hours).

g) *The nitroprusside CRI can be discontinued 30 minutes after oral dosing with enalapril. (dog: 0.5 mg/kg PO q12–24h; cat: 0.25–0.5 mg/kg PO q12–24h)*

h) *The nitroprusside bag and tubing must be protected from light. Cover all exposed tubing with tape or other wrap.*

5) Initiate maintenance therapy with digoxin. If the dog is already receiving digoxin, check serum levels to make sure they are in the therapeutic range.

6) Decrease the furosemide dosage to 2 mg/kg q8–12h and add spironolactone (2 mg/kg q12–24h) as soon as the pulmonary edema is under control.

7) Check blood for serum digoxin level, BUN, and electrolytes 7 days after discharge. Azotemia generally requires reduction of the diuretic dose.

8) When dogs become refractory to treatment, adjustments can be made to increase the enalapril to BID or to increase the diuretic dose.

9) Morphine (0.1–0.2 mg/kg SC) can be given as initial therapy to dogs that are very anxious and excited. It is anxiolytic, causes mild pulmonary venodilation, and reduces tachycardia.

10) Severe pulmonary edema may be relieved by nebulization. A mixture of 2–3 mL of ethyl alcohol, 1 mL saline, and 1–2 drops of 5% metaproterenol sulfate (Alupent Inhalation Solution, Boehringer-Ingelheim) can yield significant improvement in some animals but must be discontinued if tachycardia occurs.

B. Canine dilated cardiomyopathy (DCM)

1. Occurs primarily in Doberman Pinchers, "giant" breeds, and other large dogs. Also can be seen in Springer Spaniels and American Cocker Spaniels. More common in males than females.

2. Clinical signs include dyspnea, tachypnea, exercise intolerance, weight loss, cachexia, abdominal distension (ascites), and syncope.

3. Signs—especially weight loss—can be dramatic and sudden, occurring over 2–4 weeks.

4. Physical examination findings include

   a. Tachycardia, weak pulses, ± pulse deficits, soft mitral or tricuspid murmurs secondary to stretching of the annular ring, and inability of valve leaflets to close.

   b. Muffled heart and lung sounds are noted with pleural effusion, and inspiratory crackles are ausculted with pulmonary edema.

   c. Hepatomegaly, splenomegaly, ascites, peripheral edema ("stocking up" of rear limbs), and jugular venous distension are signs of right-sided heart failure.

5. Boxers have their own breed-specific form of cardiomyopathy, characterized primarily by severe ventricular arrhythmias and sudden death. If arrhythmias are controlled, the dogs can live 1–3 years before classic signs of DCM (cardiomegaly, systolic dysfunction, CHF) become evident.

6. Thoracic radiographs usually reveal severe cardiomegaly with marked dilation of all four chambers and diffuse pulmonary edema. Sometimes cardiomegaly is so prominent that it must be differentiated from the globoid appearance of the heart shadow seen with pericardial effusion. Cardiomegaly is not always seen in Boxers with myocarditis. In Dobermans, left atrial enlargement is a prominent finding.

7. Common electrocardiographic findings include

   a. Tachycardia with tall, wide QRS complexes (helps rule out pericardial effusion, which has small complexes)

   b. Atrial fibrillation is the most common arrhythmia seen in large-breed dogs with DCM.

   c. Dobermans and Boxers often have ventricular arrhythmias—premature ventricular contractions (PVCs) or paroxysmal ventricular tachycardia.

8. Draw blood for CBC, chemistries, electrolytes, and free T4. Rule outs include bacterial endocarditis, congenital cardiac disease, neoplastic disease, and primary valvular disease.

9. Many large-breed dogs are hypothyroid (especially Doberman Pinchers). Although thyroid supplementation does not improve myocardial function, it is necessary to prevent digitalis toxicity.

10. Echocardiography reveals dilation of atrial and ventricular chambers, thinning of the myocardium, and decreased contractility evidenced by poor wall motion and decreased fractional shortening.

11. The antineoplastic drug doxorubicin causes progressive myocardial degeneration secondary to toxic effects of cumulative doses. Dogs should be evaluated for underlying cardiac disease prior to treatment and monitored closely during therapy, especially after the fourth treatment. If DCM occurs, it is treated according to clinical signs, and doxorubicin therapy must be discontinued.

12. Treatment

a. Dogs presented as emergencies should receive supplemental oxygen during initial examination and hospitalization.

b. Place an intravenous catheter, and if there is evidence of CHF (tachypnea, inspiratory crackles, tachycardia, heart murmur), give **furosemide** immediately (2–4 mg/kg IV).

c. Diagnostic work-up should include blood sampling, ECG, thoracic radiographs, and echocardiography as soon as the patient has stabilized.

d. Dogs with severe systolic dysfunction and cardiogenic shock may benefit from immediate **positive inotropic support**.

1) Dobutamine is the drug of choice for providing immediate positive inotropic effects for short-term management of severe myocardial failure.

   a) There is evidence in humans with CHF that dobutamine infusion can result in a sustained improvement in myocardial function even after the drip is discontinued, because of replacement of myocardial catecholamines.

   b) The dosage is 5–20 μg/kg/min (see Appendix E, "Constant Rate Infusions" for help in setting up the drip).

   c) Start at 10 μg/kg/min. If tachycardia or exacerbation of atrial fibrillation occurs, the dosage can be decreased. If there is no improvement in pulse quality, mucous membrane color, or capillary refill time, the dosage can be increased.

   d) The drip rate should not exceed 1 mL/kg/h because patients with CHF tend to be volume overloaded.

2) Dopamine is also a positive inotrope, and it is cheaper than dobutamine. Unfortunately, it is more likely to cause arrhythmias and tachycardia and should be monitored closely during infusion.

   a) The recommended dosage is 2–20 μg/kg/min. The best dosage for positive inotropic effects is 5–7 μg/kg/min. Dosages of 10–20 μg/kg/min can cause marked peripheral vasoconstriction resulting in increased afterload for the failing heart. Low dosages (2–3 μg/kg/min) have little effect on the heart and primarily act to dilate renal and mesenteric arteries.

   b) It is best to start at a dosage of 5 μg/kg/min and cautiously increase the dosage if necessary.

3) Amrinone is a positive inotrope that has not been heavily investigated for veterinary use. It is both a positive inotrope and a vasodilator.

   a) The dose is 1–3 mg/kg IV bolus followed by 10–100 μg/kg/min CRI titrated to effect.

   b) At high dosages it can cause tachycardia and hypotension. It can also exacerbate atrial fibrillation.

   c) It is incompatible with solutions containing dextrose.

4) Digoxin should be started at an oral maintenance dose concurrently with the intravenous positive inotrope because it will take 3–5 days for digoxin to take effect.

   a) Large-breed dogs generally require less digoxin on a per weight basis than small-breed dogs. It should be dosed according to body surface area: 0.22 mg/ m² q12h. In general, the dosage should not exceed 0.015 mg/kg/day for large dogs.

   b) Doberman Pinchers are particularly sensitive to digitalis toxicity. A maximum dose of 0.375 mg/day is recommended for this breed.

   c) For rapid atrial fibrillation, a double dose can be given for the first 24–48 hours.

   d) If ventricular arrhythmias are severe, avoid digoxin until they are controlled. If quinidine is used, reduce the digoxin dose by 50%.

   e) Check serum digoxin levels 5–7 days after initiating treatment. The therapeutic range is 0.8–2.2 ng/mL 8 hours after dosing.

5) Procainamide is the drug of choice for ventricular arrhythmias.

   a) Procainamide can cause severe hypotension if given rapidly IV. In emergency situations, administer 2 mg/kg IV over 3–5 minutes and follow with 20–50 μg/kg/min CRI.

   b) For most other situations, procainamide can be given IM or PO, 8–20 mg/kg q6h. The sustained-release form is given q8h.

   c) Other drugs that have been effective in managing chronic ventricular tachy-

cardia include tocainide (10–20 mg/kg q8h PO), mexiletine (5–8 mg/kg q8h PO), or sotalol (2 mg/kg q12h PO)

6) For **atrial fibrillation**, add a β-blocker or diltiazem 72–96 h after beginning digoxin. The dose is titrated upward until the resting heart rate is 100–150 bpm.

a) Diltiazem: 1.0–1.5 mg/kg q8h.

b) Atenolol: 0.25–1.0 mg/kg PO q12–24h.

c) Always start at the low end of dosage to avoid excessive negative inotropic effects.

d) This treatment generally does not convert atrial fibrillation to normal sinus rhythm, but it slows the ventricular rate enough to allow adequate diastolic filling.

e) Very rapid atrial fibrillation with ventricular rates >260/min, warrants more-aggressive treatment. Intravenous digitalization (0.02–0.04 mg/kg total dose; give 25% hourly for up to 4 hours combined with oral diltiazem (0.5 mg/kg) started 3 hours into the digitalization protocol) will usually bring the heart rate down.

7) Vasodilators are indicated to aid the failing heart.

a) In emergency situations, intravenous nitroprusside should be considered only after positive inotropic therapy has been implemented and only in animals that cannot be stabilized with oxygen, diuretics, and positive inotropic therapy.

b) Enalapril 0.25–0.5 mg/kg q12–24h PO (titrated to effect) is indicated to provide balanced vasodilation.

c) If azotemia or hypotension develops, lower the diuretic dose.

8) Diuretics—use lowest effective dosage

a) Furosemide: 1–4 mg/kg q8–12h

b) Spironolactone: 1–2 mg/kg q12h

9) Coenzyme Q-10 (Nutramax: 800-925-5187) has yielded beneficial effects in people with dilated cardiomyopathy and has no adverse effects other than cost. Recommended dosage is 2–5 mg/kg q8–12h.

10) Supplementation with **carnitine** and **taurine** is recommended in American Cocker Spaniels with DCM, and there is some evidence to suggest that Golden Retrievers with DCM may also be taurine deficient.

a) L-Carnitine (Now Foods, Inc: 800-283-3500): 50 mg/kg PO q8h. There are

no bad side effects, but the cost is high, and there is no guaranteed benefit.

b) Taurine (Twinlab, 800-645-5626): 20–25 mg/kg PO q12h.

11) Recent studies in humans suggest a beneficial effect of chronic administration of β-blockers in patients with DCM.

12) The prognosis for dogs with DCM is variable. Dobermans rarely live >6 months past the time of diagnosis. Up to 40% of other breeds may exceed 6 months survival time with appropriate therapy. Lifespan rarely exceeds 18 months.

C. Digoxin toxicity

1. Toxicity is common because of the narrow therapeutic index (0.8–2.2 ng/mL)

2. Clinical signs include lethargy, anorexia, vomiting, and diarrhea.

3. ECG signs include sinus bradycardia, first- and second-degree AV block, sinus arrest, conduction abnormalities, junctional rhythms, and ventricular arrhythmias.

4. To avoid toxicity

a. Reduce dose for fat or fluid (ascites) Dose on the basis of lean body weight.

b. Reduce dose by 10–15% if using elixir, to account for better absorption.

c. Dose large dogs at 0.22 mg/M^2 q12h. Do not exceed 0.375 mg/day in Doberman Pinchers or 0.015 mg/kg/day for large-breed dogs.

d. Reduce the dose in animals with renal insufficiency. Divide dosage by the serum creatine level or increase the dosage interval by multiplying by the serum creatinine level.

e. Measure electrolytes and correct hypokalemia, as it predisposes to digitalis toxicity.

f. Check thyroid status. If hypothyroidism is present, correct and use a lower dosage of digoxin.

g. Avoid drugs that can increase serum digoxin levels: quinidine, verapamil, cimetidine.

h. Monitor serum digoxin concentration 7–10 days after initiating therapy and periodically thereafter.

i. Warn owners to discontinue digoxin and call the veterinarian if the animal exhibits depression, anorexia, vomiting, and/or diarrhea while receiving digoxin therapy.

5. Treatment

a. For mild signs, discontinue digoxin for 24–48 hours and reinitiate treatment at $^1/_2$ dose. Check the digoxin level in 7 days.

b. Dogs with more-severe signs require veterinary attention.

   1) Draw blood for serum digoxin determination.

   2) Consider antiarrhythmic agents.

      a) Atropine for bradyarrhythmias

      b) Lidocaine for ventricular arrhythmias

      c) Dilantin (phenytoin) has been recommended for emergency treatment of refractory digitalis-induced arrhythmias: 1.0 mg/kg/min IV for a total of up to 6 mg/kg.

   3) Supportive care with oxygen and judicious fluid therapy may also be indicated.

D. Pericardial disease

1. Causes of pericardial effusion in dogs: neoplasia, infectious disease, pericardial cysts, peritoneopericardial diaphragmatic hernia, left atrial tear (secondary to mitral regurgitation), trauma, coagulopathy, foreign body, idiopathic.

2. Clinical signs

  a. Prominent signs of right heart failure: hepatosplenomegaly, ascites, pleural effusion, jugular venous distension and jugular pulses

  b. Muffled heart sounds

  c. Weakness, collapse, syncope, sudden death

  d. Pulsus paradoxus—pulse intensity weakens during inspiration

3. Cardiac tamponade occurs when enough fluid accumulates in the pericardial sac to limit ventricular filling and cardiac output.

  a. Rapid fluid accumulation can cause cardiac tamponade at relatively low volumes (100–200 mL)

  b. Slow fluid accumulation allows the pericardium to stretch, resulting in a large volume of fluid (up to 2000 mL) before compromise is noted.

  c. With constrictive pericarditis, the pericardium lacks distensibility because of fibrosis. Small fluid volumes can result in significant impairment of cardiac function.

4. Thoracic radiography often reveals a globoid heart. The caudal vena cava appears enlarged on lateral view.

5. Electrocardiography reveals small QRS complexes, sinus tachycardia, and (sometimes) electrical alternans (changing amplitude of QRS complexes

associated with cardiac "swinging" in the pericardial fluid)

6. Echocardiography provides the definitive diagnosis of pericardial fluid. The pericardium appears as a bright line with a hypoechoic fluid space separating it from the left ventricular free wall. Careful examination may reveal cardiac or pericardial masses. Collapse of the right ventricle may also be evident.

7. Evaluation of fluid:

  a. Pericardial fluid can be differentiated from blood because

   1) It should not clot.

   2) Hematocrit of fluid is usually less than the patient's hematocrit.

  b. Cytology is often not helpful.

   1) Reactive mesothelial cells can look neoplastic but are not.

   2) Neoplastic cells are rarely found, because hemangiosarcoma and chemodectoma do not tend to exfoliate.

  c. The pH of the fluid can be checked. Neoplastic effusions tend to be more alkaline (7.0–7.5) than inflammatory effusions (6.5–7.0), but overlap makes this test fairly inaccurate.

8. Treatment—Pericardiocentesis

  a. Clip and prepare right side of dog from the 3rd to the 8th rib, sternum to midthorax.

  b. Monitor the ECG during procedure. If ventricular arrhythmias occur, withdraw catheter until they abate.

  c. Use a 14- to 16-gauge over-the-needle catheter with extra side holes.

  d. Decide where to enter the thorax on the basis of thoracic radiographs or ultrasound—usually between the 4th and 6th ribs at the costochondral junction. Avoid the intercostal artery caudal to each rib.

  e. Apply a local block with lidocaine, making sure to include the pleura. Sedation is often not required.

  f. Pericardiocentesis is usually performed with the dog in lateral recumbency, which allows the heart to fall away from the centesis needle, but it could be done with the patient in sternal or even standing as long as no movement occurs.

  g. Use a no. 11 scalpel blade to prick the skin; then direct the needle and catheter into the pleural space and then the pericardium. If pleural fluid is present, it is often pale yellow, while the pericardial fluid is usually hemorrhagic.

h. As soon as you enter the pericardial sac, remove the needle and continue advancing the catheter. Extension tubing, stopcock, and syringe are attached to the catheter.

i. Drainage of the pericardial fluid generally results in significant improvement of cardiac function. Complexes increase in size on the ECG, pulses improve, and heart rate slows.

j. Diuretics and vasodilators are not indicated, as removal of the fluid restores normal cardiac function. High doses of these drugs could cause hypotension and dehydration.

k. Pericardiocentesis is curative in approximately 50% of cases of idiopathic pericardial effusion. A course of corticosteroids (1 mg/kg prednisone q12h PO tapered down over 3 weeks) has been recommended to decrease inflammation, fibrosis, and adhesion formation.

l. The most common neoplasms are hemangiosarcoma, chemodectoma, mesothelioma, and thyroid carcinoma.

   1) Hemangiosarcoma has a poor prognosis because metastasis to the liver, spleen, and lungs has usually already occurred at the time of diagnosis. Perform abdominal ultrasound as part of the continuing workup of these patients to check for other tumor sites.

   2) For other tumor types—especially chemodectoma—pericardectomy can provide more long-term benefit, because these tumors are slower to grow and metastasize.

m. After pericardiocentesis, pericardial effusion may return in several days to weeks. Recurrent clinical signs warrant subtotal pericardectomy, which can be curative for idiopathic cases or can prolong life—at least temporarily—in patients with neoplastic disease.

E. Canine heartworm disease

1. Emergencies associated with canine heartworm disease include right-sided heart failure and pulmonary hypertension associated with chronic disease, caval syndrome associated with heavy worm burden, or acute pulmonary thromboembolism usually following adulticide treatment.

2. Clinical signs include coughing, respiratory distress, lethargy, exercise intolerance, cachexia, ascites, ± hemoptysis.

   a. Animals with caval syndrome also have icterus, hemoglobinuria, bilirubinuria, and pale mucous membranes.

   b. Auscultation may reveal a systolic murmur over the tricuspid valve, a gallop rhythm, splitting of the second heart sound due to pulmonary hypertension, and harsh lung sounds.

3. Thoracic radiographs of patients with advanced heartworm disease reveal right-sided heart enlargement; enlargement, truncation, and tortuosity of the caudal lobar arteries; enlargement of the pulmonary artery segment; and pulmonary infiltrates or granulomas.

4. Blood work usually reveals eosinophilia, basophilia, elevated liver enzymes, and azotemia. Thrombocytopenia with subclinical disseminated intravascular coagulation (DIC) may also be present.

5. Diagnosis

   a. Knott's test may reveal microfilaria.

   b. Many chronic cases are occult.

      1) ELISA test result will be positive for heartworm antigen.

      2) Strength of positive test reaction roughly correlates with worm number.

   c. In caval syndrome or severe infections with a large worm burden, echocardiography can be used to identify worms in the right heart chambers and/or pulmonary artery. Inability to visualize worms does not rule out dirofilariasis.

6. Dogs presented as an emergency would likely be placed in class 3—severe heartworm disease. These animals have a strong positive antigen test reaction and obvious clinical signs.

7. Treatment

   a. Dogs in severe respiratory distress should receive supportive care with oxygen and cage rest.

      1) Prednisone 0.5–1 mg/kg q12h tapered over 2–3 weeks can significantly reduce pulmonary eosinophilic infiltrates or granulomatous inflammation associated with dying heartworms.

      2) Weigh the pros and cons of using corticosteroids.

         a) They can significantly improve respiration through effective treatment of allergic lung disease.

         b) They may promote thromboembolism.

         c) They may make the patient more susceptible to bacterial pneumonia.

         d) Corticosteroids can make worms more resistant to adulticide, thereby reducing the kill rate. (In severely infected dogs with a *large worm burden, a reduced kill rate may actually be safer.)*

3) Another controversial recommendation is aspirin (5–7 mg/kg q24h) or heparin (75 mg/kg SC q8h) given 1–3 weeks before treatment and continued until 3 weeks after treatment. This treatment may reduce platelet aggregation and proliferative arteritis but may enhance bleeding tendencies.

b. The primary time to expect hemoptysis and respiratory distress secondary to pulmonary thromboembolism from dying heartworms is 1–3 weeks postadulticide.

1) Dogs should have strict confinement for 6–10 weeks postadulticide.

2) Bronchoalveolar lavage can be done to obtain samples for culture and sensitivity testing and cytology if the dog is febrile or secondary bacterial pneumonia is suspected.

3) Antibiotics (cephalexin, trimethoprim-sulfa) can be administered concurrently with the steroids.

c. Dogs with caval syndrome (worms evident in vena cava and right atrium, acute hemolytic syndrome) require physical elimination of heartworms as soon as possible.

1) A local block is applied over the jugular vein, and it is isolated. It can be ligated permanently or temporarily occluded with umbilical tape above the venotomy site.

2) A no. 11 scalpel blade is used to perform a venotomy, and either long straight alligator forceps or an endoscopic basket retrieval device is passed down the jugular vein to the vena cava and right atrium. Worms are grasped and removed through the venotomy site.

3) In most cases, the jugular vein is permanently occluded with ligatures, with minimal side effects. Alternatively, the venotomy site can be closed with vascular sutures.

4) Further adulticide therapy can be accomplished at a later date after the animal has stabilized.

5) If worm removal is impossible through the jugular vein, a thoracotomy can be performed and the worms removed through an incision in the right auricle.

6) A large worm burden can be life threatening in a small dog, and often the dog's only hope is surgical extraction of the worms, even though the procedure can be dangerous.

d. Adulticide therapy can be administered after dyspneic animals have been stabilized with cage rest, oxygen, corticosteroids, and antibiotics.

1) Melarsomine HCl (Immiticide) should only be administered to dogs with severe disease according to the split-dosing schedule (not the rapid 2 day/2 dose schedule).

a) *Rapid kill-off of worms may cause severe pulmonary compromise or death.*

b) *One injection is given (2.5 mg/kg IM) and then two more are administered 24 hours apart after waiting 30 days.*

c) *Strict confinement must be enforced for 8–10 weeks.*

d) *Injections must be given deep IM in the lumbar muscles according to the manufacturer's recommendations. Pain at the injection site is a common complication.*

2) The other option for adulticide therapy is thiacetarcemide sodium (Caparsolate), but it is difficult to find.

a) *Dogs are given 2.2 mg/kg IV 6–8 hours apart BID for 2 days. The overnight interval must not exceed 16 hours.*

b) *This drug has more potential for renal and hepatotoxicity. If anorexia, vomiting, or icterus develops during treatment, it should be discontinued and the full series repeated in 30 days.*

c) *Caparsolate is less effective than melarsomine. Female worms are most resistant to treatment and another course of adulticide therapy may be needed to clear the infection.*

d) *Successfully treated dogs will have a negative heartworm antigen test result 20–24 weeks posttreatment.*

e. Microfilaria should be eliminated to reduce the possibility of infection of other pets by mosquito transmission.

1) Ivermectin at a dose of 50 μg/kg PO or SC is microfilaricidal. It can be repeated in 10 days if microfilaria are still present.

a) *An allergic shock–like reaction can occur in dogs with large numbers of microfilaria. Administration of prednisone (1 mg/kg 1 hour before and 6 hours after treatment) should prevent severe reactions.*

b) *The prophylactic dose of milbemycin (500 μg/kg PO) is also microfilaricidal. This is the preferred treatment for Collies.*

f. Dogs with right-sided heart failure also will benefit from the following treatments.
   1) Furosemide, 1 mg/kg q12h
   2) Enalapril, 0.5 mg/kg q12–24h
   3) Digoxin, 0.22 mg/m^2 PO q12h
   4) Dietary sodium restriction
   5) Strict exercise limitation
g. Some dogs with severe disease are not good candidates for treatment, especially older animals with underlying renal or hepatic disease, and small dogs with a large worm burden. Owners should be advised of the inherent risks of treatment and cautioned on the importance of cage confinement postadulticide.

F. Feline heartworm disease

1. Although less common in cats than dogs, feline heartworm disease has been reported in all heartworm endemic areas.
2. Clinical signs include coughing, intermittent dyspnea, vomiting, lethargy, weight loss, unthrifty haircoat, and sudden death.
3. Auscultation may reveal a gallop rhythm, harsh lung sounds, or muffled heart and lung sounds secondary to pleural effusion (often chylous).
4. Radiographs reveal enlargement and tortuosity of the pulmonary caudal lobar arteries and peribronchial or interstitial infiltrate.
5. Most infected cats are occult and do not have circulating microfilaria. Antigen or antibody tests are used to confirm the diagnosis.
   a. Low worm numbers, all male infection, or immature stages may result in a false-negative antigen test result.
   b. A positive heartworm antigen test result is consistent with infection.
   c. A negative antibody test result rules out heartworm disease as the cause of dyspnea and weight loss.
   d. A positive antibody test result indicates exposure only. An active infection may or may not be present.

6. Heartworms can often be visualized with echocardiography as parallel lines in the pulmonary artery.
7. Most investigators do not recommend adulticide treatment because of the risk of sudden death from thromboembolic disease. There is also some evidence that suggests heartworms have a shorter lifespan in the cat than in the dog. Symptomatic treatment may allow time for the heartworms to

die naturally over a period of several years. If adulticide therapy is used:
   a. Melarsomine is not approved for use in cats and there is little information available documenting its safety or efficacy in cats.
   b. Thiacetarsamide sodium has been used at the same dosage as in dogs.
     1) 0.22 mL/kg IV q6–8h BID for four treatments given on 2 days, with the overnight interval not to exceed 16 hours
     2) Complications include sudden death, hemoptysis, hepatic or renal toxicity, and perivascular sloughing or cellulitis following poor injection technique.

8. Most cats are treated as cats with chronic asthma.
   a. Prednisone, 1–2 mg/kg q12h during periods of dyspnea and then tapered to the lowest effective dose
   b. Bronchodilators
     1) Theo-Dur, 25 mg/kg PO q24h at night
     2) Terbutaline, 0.625 mg/cat PO q12h or 0.01 mg/kg SC or IM (can be administered at home by the owner in response to an asthmatic crisis)

G. Feline cardiomyopathy

1. There are three primary types
   a. Dilated cardiomyopathy
     1) Associated with taurine deficiency. It should be suspected in any cat with heart disease that is not eating a standard commercial feline diet (e.g., eating dog food or "people food")
     2) This type is now fairly uncommon because commercial feline diets have been supplemented with taurine since 1989.
     3) Taurine deficiency also causes retinal lesions that can be seen on ophthalmic examination. These appear as sharply delineated, highly reflective lesions in the area centralis of the retina.
     4) Thoracic radiographs may reveal generalized cardiomegaly or left atrial and ventricular enlargement. Signs of CHF include pulmonary venous distension, patchy pulmonary edema, and pleural effusion.
     5) Echocardiography
       a) Dilated left atrium (>16 mm)
       b) Dilated left ventricle (>12 mm end-systole, >21 mm end-diastole)

c) Decreased fractional shortening (<25–30%)

6) The primary dysfunction with DCM is systolic—decreased inotropy, weak pulses, CHF.

7) Dilatative CHF can also occur in the later stages of congenital valvular disease, endocarditis, or other causes of heart failure.

b. Hypertrophic cardiomyopathy

1) Occurs most commonly in male middle-aged cats in good body flesh with acute onset of signs. Familial hypertrophic cardiomyopathy occurs in Maine Coon Cats.

2) Concentric hypertrophy of the left ventricular free wall and interventricular septum results in increased myocardial stiffness and decreased lumen size.

3) Decreased ventricular compliance requires higher filling pressures. This is primarily a diastolic dysfunction.

4) Hypertrophic obstructive cardiomyopathy (HOCM) occurs when thickening of the interventricular septum causes obstruction of ventricular outflow. Mitral regurgitation can also occur when papillary muscle hypertrophy causes systolic anterior motion of the septal mitral valve leaflet (SAMS). Signs of heart failure worsen with stress and tachycardia.

5) Thoracic radiographs

a) Classically, the heart is "valentine" shaped because of left and right atrial enlargement, and the apex point is maintained and shifted toward the midline. This does not always occur. Sometimes there is generalized cardiomegaly or the heart shadow may appear normal.

b) Definitive diagnosis of the type of cardiomyopathy cannot be made from survey radiographs.

6) Echocardiography

a) Thickened interventricular septum and/or left ventricular free wall (>6 mm at end-diastole). Thickening may be segmental.

b) Left atrial enlargement (>16 mm), left atrium:aorta ratio >1.2.

c) Systolic function is normal unless secondary mitral regurgitation is severe.

d) Ventricular lumen size is decreased because of concentric hypertrophy of ventricle.

7) A potentially reversible form of hypertrophic cardiomyopathy can occur secondary to hyperthyroidism and/or hypertension.

a) These conditions must be ruled out, especially in cats ≥10 years old.

b) Hypertension most commonly occurs secondary to chronic renal disease.

c) Perform blood tests for BUN, creatinine, and serum T4 as well as urinalysis and blood pressure measurement as part of the diagnostic workup.

c. Restrictive cardiomyopathy

1) In this condition, there is a marked decrease in ventricular compliance, caused by myocardial fibrosis resulting in impaired filling and diastolic dysfunction.

2) Cats are usually middle-aged or older.

3) The etiology is unknown.

4) Cats with restrictive cardiomyopathy are predisposed to thromboembolism because of stagnation of blood in the dilated left atrium and inflammation of the endocardial surface.

5) Thoracic radiographs cannot be used to differentiate from the other types of cardiomyopathy.

6) Echocardiography

a) The left atrium is usually markedly dilated (>16 mm, often >20 mm) in the absence of mitral valve disease.

b) The left ventricular diameter is normal (<12 mm at end-systole and <21 mm at end-diastole).

c) The heart is not hyperkinetic. Shortening fraction is usually normal to slightly decreased.

d) A bright, hyperechoic endocardium is evidence of endocardial fibrosis.

e) The left ventricular lumen may appear irregular because of variable wall thickness and fibrosis.

2. Clinical signs

a. The underlying type of cardiomyopathy cannot be determined by clinical presentation.

b. Most cats exhibit marked respiratory distress (open-mouth breathing, cyanosis, tachypnea) that is exacerbated by stress.

c. Signs of pleural effusion may be present: muffled heart and lung sounds; rapid, shallow respirations; tachypnea.

d. Careful auscultation will detect abnormalities in up to 80% of cats with cardiomyopathy. Auscult carefully in a quiet place.

    1) Tachycardia, gallop rhythm (S_3 heart sound)

    2) Systolic murmur

    3) Arrhythmias and pulse deficits can occur in all types, but are most commonly seen in restrictive CM.

    4) Pulmonary crackles and wheezes secondary to pulmonary edema

e. Very weak or absent pulses; stiffened hind limbs; and pale, cold footpads may indicate distal aortic thromboembolism. (See p. 179.)

f. Cats with hyperthyroid heart disease or hypertension are usually thin, older cats with tachycardia ± arrhythmias.

g. Cats with hypertrophic CM are often middle-aged (4–9 years) male cats. The apex beat may be quite prominent.

h. Cats with severe CHF may have relative bradycardia, hypotension, and hypothermia.

3. Diagnosis

a. Thoracic radiographs are usually necessary to differentiate cardiac disease from primary respiratory disease. The cat must be stabilized initially before radiographs are attempted.

b. Echocardiography is generally necessary to differentiate the type of cardiomyopathy and to evaluate systolic function. If the cat is too unstable to be placed in lateral recumbency, standing echocardiography can be done.

4. Treatment

a. Dyspneic cats are very fragile. The cat must be handled very carefully and stabilized as much as possible before stressful diagnostic procedures are performed.

    1) Administer **supplemental oxygen**. (See p. 115–117.)

    2) Place an **intravenous catheter**.

    3) Perform **thoracocentesis** (see p. 130–131) if physical examination findings are consistent with pleural effusion. Pleural fluid may be clear, serosanguineous, or chylous in cats with CM.

    4) Differentiate cardiac and respiratory disease.

        a) *Heart murmur, gallop rhythm, pulmonary crackles or pleural fluid, wide or tall QRS complexes on electrocardiogram, arrhythmias, and no history of cough tend to rule in cardiac disease.*

        b) *History of cough, expiratory dyspnea with abdominal press, harsh lung sounds (rhonchi) tend to rule in feline bronchial asthma (see p. 147).*

b. Dyspneic cats should be given **1–2 mg/kg of furosemide IV** and allowed to stabilize in an oxygen-rich environment for 20–30 minutes before further diagnostic tests are performed.

c. Cats with fulminant pulmonary edema may benefit from **2% nitroglycerine ointment**, $\frac{1}{4}$–$\frac{1}{2}$ inch applied to a hairless area. This can cause immediate improvement in pulmonary congestion by increasing venous capacitance through venodilation and allowing the blood to be redistributed from the pulmonary circulation.

d. Sedation may be needed for **radiographs and echocardiography**.

    1) It may be possible to avoid sedation by supplying oxygen and using minimal restraint with a calm, reassuring manner.

    2) If sedation is used, be prepared for complications.

        a) *Ketamine/valium combination can sometimes cause respiratory arrest, laryngeal spasm, and bradycardia in cats with hypertrophic CM. Do not administer to stressed or excited cats, and be prepared to intubate and ventilate if necessary. This anesthetic protocol is generally not recommended in cats suspected to have hypertrophic CM.*

        b) *Propofol can sometimes cause hypotension and myocardial depression (bradycardia, arrhythmias) in cats with CM. Do not overdose, and do not give repeated doses.*

        c) *Butorphanol/valium is a fairly safe combination but may cause hypotension and bradycardia.*

        d) *Atropine can cause refractory tachycardia and arrhythmias and should probably be avoided in cats with CM unless bradycardia is a problem.*

e. If the cat is sedated, draw blood for **baseline blood work** (CBC, chemistries, electrolytes, T4, ± toxoplasmosis, feline leukemia virus [FeLV] and feline immunodeficiency virus [FIV] titers).

f. Once the underlying type of cardiac disease is diagnosed, therapeutic recommendations can be made.

    1) Dilated CM

        a) *Furosemide* can be given at a dosage of 1–2 mg/kg q8h until breathing has improved. Once the cat has stabilized, decrease the dosage to 1–2 mg/kg PO SID–BID.

b) Digoxin, $^1/_4$ of a 0.125 mg tablet PO (0.0312 mg/cat) q24–48h

   i) Serum digoxin levels should be tested in 10–14 days.

   ii) Serum digoxin concentration should be 1.0–2.0 ng/mL 8 hours after the last dose.

   iii) Cats usually do not like the elixir, and toxicity is more likely with the elixir because absorption is greater than with the tablet.

c) Taurine supplementation should be given until a deficiency has been ruled out (250–500 mg PO BID). Send whole blood or plasma to University of California, Davis, Diagnostic Laboratory (530-752-0168).

d) Enalapril, 0.25–0.5 mg/kg PO q24–48h

e) Aspirin, 25 mg/kg PO q72h

f) In cases of severe fulminant CHF (bradycardia, hypothermia, hypotension), an intravenous positive inotrope can be given.

   i) Dobutamine, 2.5–5 μg/kg/min (see Appendix E for instructions for preparing CRI drip). Higher doses can cause seizures in cats.

   ii) Dopamine, 5–7 μg/kg/min

g) 2% Nitroglycerine ointment is useful during the first 48 hours of treatment to relieve pulmonary edema; $^1/_4$–$^1/_2$ inch is reapplied every 6 hours.

h) Monitor renal function, hydration status, serum potassium concentration, blood pressure, and serum digoxin concentration during hospitalization and 7–10 days after discharge to avoid problems with medication toxicity.

2) Hypertrophic CM

a) Furosemide is administered at a dosage of 1 mg/kg IV q8–12 h initially. It is important **NOT** to overdose diuretics in cats with hypertrophic CM (HCM). Avoid dehydration and hypotension to ensure that an adequate preload is available to allow for ventricular filling. As soon as pulmonary edema has resolved, decrease the diuretic dose to the lowest possible dose (1 mg/kg q12–48h).

b) Diltiazem is a calcium channel blocker that has a lusiotropic effect (relaxes the heart), a mild negative chronotropic effect, a mild negative inotropic effect, and a mild vasodilatory effect. It is available in regular or sustained-release preparations. Dosage interval varies with the preparation.

   i) Cardiazem (30-mg tablet), give $^1/_4$ tablet (7.5 mg) q8h

   ii) Dilacor SR is available in 240-mg capsules containing four 60-mg tablets in each capsule. The dosage is 30 mg ($^1/_2$ tablet) q12h.

   iii) Cardiazem CD is available in various capsule sizes. The dosage is 10 mg/kg q24h.

c) Cats with persistent tachycardia, dynamic outflow obstruction, arrhythmias, or hyperthyroidism should be treated with β-blockers instead of calcium channel blockers. These drugs are generally more effective in reducing very rapid heart rates but also have more of a negative inotropic effect. Begin giving **atenolol** at a dosage of 6.25–12.5 mg PO q24h ($^1/_4$–$^1/_2$ of a 25-mg tablet). Increase to BID if heart rate is >160 bpm.

d) Enalapril can be added in cases of refractory heart failure. It is important to begin at a low dosage because even mild hypotension can be devastating to cats with HCM. A high filling pressure is required to fill the stiff ventricle. The dosage is 0.25–0.5 mg/kg q24–48h.

e) Aspirin, 25 mg/kg q72h to prevent thromboembolism

3) Restrictive cardiomyopathy

a) Treatment is the same as for HCM, except that **digoxin** is added for systolic dysfunction at a dosage of 0.0312 mg/cat PO q24–48h ($^1/_4$ of a 0.125-mg tablet)

b) Serum digoxin levels should be checked 10–14 days after beginning therapy. Therapeutic levels are 1–2 ng/mL 8 hours after the last dose.

H. Feline thromboembolism

1. Thromboembolism has been found in 25–48% of cats with cardiomyopathy at the time of necropsy.

2. Predisposing factors

   a. Atrial or ventricular endothelial lesions

   b. Stagnation of blood in dilated left atrium; inability to empty into small, stiff ventricle

   c. Feline platelets are highly reactive.

3. Most common site is the aortic trifurcation but it can also occur in renal, mesenteric, or brachial arteries.

4. Clinical signs depend on degree of heart disease and location of thromboembolism.

   a. It is often the first evidence of cardiac disease, but sometimes cats will show severe signs of CHF: dyspnea, cyanosis, open-mouth breathing.

   b. The classic presentation is a lateralizing posterior paresis with weak or absent pulses in the rear limbs. Gastrocnemius and anterior tibial muscles can become rock hard by 10–12 hours postembolization because of ischemic myopathy. Foot pads are pale, and the toenail will not bleed when cut to the quick.

   c. Renal thrombosis causes lumbar pain, vomiting, and progressive azotemia. Mesenteric thrombosis causes acute vomiting, diarrhea, abdominal pain, and shock. Thromboembolism to the brain can cause seizures, coma, acute vestibular signs, or death. Prognosis is poor for all of these conditions.

   d. Careful auscultation will detect heart murmurs or gallop rhythm in most cats. Echocardiography may confirm heart disease or identify a thrombus in the left atrium.

   e. Diagnosis is usually made on the basis of physical examination findings, but the presence of a thrombus can be confirmed with abdominal ultrasound or nonselective angiography.

   f. Cats with renal or mesenteric thromboembolism, extreme pain, rock-hard rear limb muscles, or severe CHF should probably be euthanatized because of their very poor prognosis.

   g. Surgical treatment (embolectomy) is not recommended, as the cats are at high risk and commonly die during the procedure or reembolize postsurgery.

   h. Aggressive thrombolytic therapy may be tried if the clinician feels the thrombus is recent (<2–4 hours) and the heart disease is manageable. Prognosis is guarded.

     1) Streptokinase, 90,000 IU/cat over 30 minutes followed by 45,000 IU/cat/h for 3 hours

       a) *Life-threatening hyperkalemia commonly occurs secondary to massive muscle damage.*

       b) *Reperfusion injury is common.*

       c) *Bleeding can occur, since streptokinase results in systemic fibrinolysis.*

     2) Tissue plasminogen activator

       a) *Dissolves clot but does not cause systemic bleeding*

       b) *Very expensive*

       c) *High percentage of fatal reactions due to hyperkalemia and shock (from reperfusion injury)*

       d) *No proven benefit in survival over conservative medical therapy*

i. Conservative medical therapy

     1) Manage heart failure as above. Provide cage rest and oxygen therapy.

     2) Provide analgesia.

       a) *Butorphanol, 0.15–0.2 mg/kg IM in cranial lumbar muscles q8h*

       b) *Acepromazine (0.05–0.1 mg/kg SC q8h) may promote vasodilation as well as calm the cat.*

     3) Prevent enlargement of thrombus.

       a) *Heparin, 200 IU/kg IV followed by 150–200 IU/kg SC q8h*

       b) *This will not dissolve the existing thrombus.*

       c) *Development of collateral circulation may occur over 2–5 days.*

     4) Monitor serum potassium and creatinine. Be prepared to treat acute hyperkalemia (p. 238).

     5) The cat can be discharged for continued nursing care at home if there is perfusion of distal limbs.

       a) *Continue acepromazine orally 1–2 mg/kg PO q12h for 7–10 days.*

       b) *Discontinue heparin (taper) and administer aspirin 25 mg/kg q72h (one 81-mg baby aspirin or $1/4$ of a 5-grain tablet)*

     6) Return of function is gradual over 7–14 days and is complete by 6–8 weeks. Residual paresis is common.

j. Maintenance therapy

     1) Aspirin can be continued 25 mg/kg q72h for the rest of the cat's life.

       a) *In vitro studies show that it is effective in decreasing feline platelet aggregation.*

       b) *Unfortunately, reembolization is not uncommon, even if cats are receiving aspirin prophylaxis.*

     2) Warfarin (coumadin) can be used instead of aspirin, but monitoring is much more intense, and side effects (bleeding) more common.

   a) *The dose must be titrated to prolong the prothrombin time to 1.5–2 times the baseline.*
   b) *Usual cat dosages range from 0.25 mg/cat q48h to 0.5 mg/cat q24h.*
   c) *The most accurate way to assess warfarin therapy is to standardize the prothrombin time (PT) with the international sensitivity index (ISI), which is provided by the manufacturer for each batch of thromboplastin used for the PT assay. Using this information, an international normalizing ratio (INR) of 2–3 should be the target range according to the following formula:*

$$INR = (\text{patient PT} \div \text{control PT})^{ISI}$$

I. Bacterial endocarditis

1. Colonization of heart valves or endocardial surface by bacteria (most common are *Staphylococcus* spp., *Streptococcus* spp., *Pasteurella* spp., *Escherichia coli, Pseudomonas* spp., and *Erysipelothrix* spp.)
2. Bacteremia may result from intravenous or urinary catheterization, dental procedures, infections of the skin, mouth, prostate, etc. Immunosuppressed animals with invasive procedures are at increased risk.
3. Vegetative masses of platelets and thrombin can form thrombi that can embolize to yield multiple infarcts in various organs.
4. Clinical signs are variable.
   a. Recurrent fever, shifting lameness, hematuria, polyarthritis, diskospondylitis (back pain, paresis), signs of CHF.
   b. A diastolic murmur at the left heart base and bounding pulses are noted with vegetative lesions of the aortic valve.
5. Blood for cultures should be drawn in suspect cases.
   a. Three blood samples for culture are taken with sterile technique 30 minutes to 1 hour apart.
   b. Unless the animal is small, each blood sample should be 10 mL to increase bacterial yield and improve the chances of obtaining a positive culture. A negative blood culture does not rule out bacterial endocarditis.
   c. A urine sample can also be submitted for culture.

6. Echocardiography may reveal a hyperechoic vegetative mass and abnormal valve motion. Valves most commonly affected are the mitral and aortic.
7. Treatment
   a. Therapy with broad-spectrum intravenous bactericidal combination antibiotics is given until culture results are available.
      1) Cephalosporin or penicillin for gram-positive organisms
      2) Aminoglycoside or fluoroquinolone for gram-negative organisms
      3) Metronidazole or clindamycin for anaerobes.
   b. Parenteral therapy is administered for the first week. Further antibiotic therapy is based on results of culture and sensitivity testing and should be continued for at least 6–8 weeks.
8. The prognosis is guarded for cases involving the mitral valve. The prognosis is poor when the aortic valve is infected because of the high incidence of disseminated arterial thrombi.
9. Anaerobic and gram-positive bacterial infections have a better prognosis than gram-negative infections.

J. Syncope

1. Syncope is a short period of unconsciousness that results from cerebral dysfunction because of reduced cardiac output.
2. Cardiovascular causes include
   a. AV blocks, atrial standstill (rule out hyperkalemia)
   b. Abnormal pacemaker—sick sinus syndrome, ectopic beats
   c. Supraventricular and ventricular tachyarrhythmias may occur secondary to other diseases.
   d. Congenital heart disease, especially tetralogy of Fallot, subaortic stenosis
   e. Acquired heart disease—heartworm disease, cardiomyopathy, chronic valvular disease, pericardial effusion

3. Common breeds that have sinus node dysfunction include Miniature Schnauzers, Dachshunds, Cocker Spaniels, and brachycephalic breeds. Dobermans and Pugs can have AV conduction defects.
4. Syncope can result from other causes
   a. Severe anemia or hemorrhage causing hypotension

b. Vasovagal reflex can be seen in brady-cephalic dogs with enhanced vagal tone and is especially aggravated by vomiting.

c. Violent coughing spasms or severe tracheal collapse can lead to hypoxia and syncope.

d. Hypoglycemia can also result in collapsing episodes.

e. Drugs that cause vasodilation can result in syncope or collapse from hypotension. These drugs include α-blockers (acepromazine) diuretics, and vasodilators (angiotensin-converting enzyme [ACE] inhibitors, calcium channel blockers, hydralazine, nitrates)

5. Syncope must be differentiated from seizure.
  a. Seizures usually have an aura, tonic–clonic convulsions, and postictal behavior and are accompanied by urination and defecation.
  b. Syncope often occurs following exercise or excitement, lasts a very short time (seconds), and is not accompanied by postictal disorientation. Opisthotonus, crying, rigidity, and urination may occur, causing the episode to resemble a true seizure.

6. Physical examination often reveals evidence of underlying cardiovascular disease: heart murmur, gallop rhythm, cyanosis.

7. Diagnosis may require 24-hour Holter monitoring (see p. 165).
  a. ECG, thoracic radiographs, and echocardiogram are warranted to evaluate the heart.
  b. Other tests that should be performed in dogs with a history of collapsing include hematocrit, serum glucose, serum electrolytes, blood gases, blood ammonia, serum calcium, heartworm test, and endocrine testing for adrenal and thyroid function.

8. Treatment depends on correction of the underlying problem or disease.
  a. Paroxysmal arrhythmias can be treated with antiarrhythmic agents (see below).
  b. Dogs with sinus bradycardia or AV block can have a test dose of atropine (0.02–0.04 mg/kg IM) while the heart is being monitored with an ECG. If the arrhythmia improves, oral treatment with propantheline bromide may be effective. (Dosage: small dogs, 7.5 mg q8h PO; medium dogs, 15 mg q8h PO; large dogs, 30 mg q8h PO). Adverse effects include constipation, dry mucous membranes, urine retention, and tachycardia.

c. Temporary improvement may be obtained in some dogs with terbutaline 2.5–5.0 mg/dog PO.

d. Permanent pacemaker implantation is usually required in dogs with complete AV block, symptomatic atrial standstill, and sick sinus syndrome associated with bradycardia–tachycardia.

e. Pacemaker implantation is usually performed at a specialty referral hospital.

f. Emergency stabilization of life-threatening bradycardia can be accomplished with temporary transvenous pacing. Required equipment includes a pacing generator, a pacing lead, and a percutaneous introducer sheath to allow insertion of the pacing lead into the right jugular vein. The lead is advanced through the right atrium and tricuspid valve into the right ventricle where it is wedged into the myocardium near the apex. The ECG should document capture of the heart rhythm when the electrode is properly placed. The position of the lead can also be confirmed with fluoroscopy.

g. An alternative method for temporary stabilization of patients with life-threatening bradycardia is transthoracic pacing. This method requires an external pacer (Lifepak 10/10c, Physiocontrol Corp., Redmond, WA 98703) and Quik-Pace external pacing electrodes, also from Physiocontrol. The animal must be under general anesthesia. The chest wall is shaved and electrodes are placed directly over the heart on the right and left hemithorax just above the sternum. After the electrodes are in position, the pacemaker is turned on and the desired heart rate is set. The current is increased until the ventricle is captured and an arterial pulse is palpated. If a syncopal episode has resulted in loss of consciousness, analgesia or anesthesia will be necessary if transthoracic pacing is continued.

K. Life-threatening arrhythmias

1. Supraventricular tachyarrhythmias (*Fig. 10-4*)
  a. Sinus tachycardia
    1) HR >140 (large dogs), >180 (small dogs), or >200 (cats)
    2) Regular rate, P wave for every QRS complex, narrow QRS
    3) No response to vagal maneuver
    4) Tachycardia caused by excessive catecholamine release.

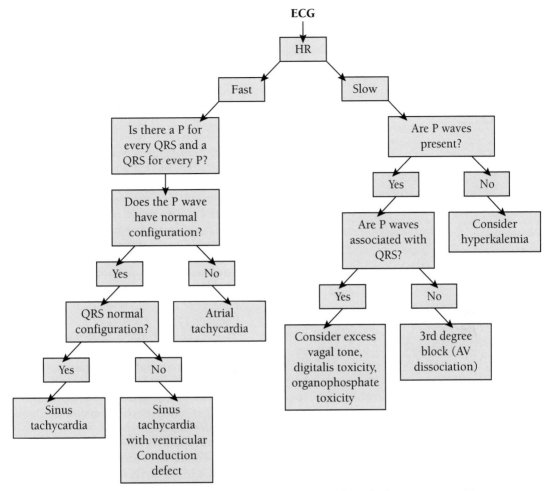

FIGURE 10.4 Approach to supraventricular arrhythmias.

5) Treatment: Correct underlying condition (pain, fever, hypovolemia, anxiety, fear, CHF)

b. Atrial tachycardia, junctional tachycardia, atrial flutter

1) Regular rhythm, narrow complex QRS (unless there is a conduction defect or bundle branch block)

2) Rate decreases with vagal maneuver (apply firm pressure to eyeballs or carotid arteries, and monitor heart rate).

3) Most commonly, these arrhythmias are associated with severe underlying structural heart disease with marked left atrial enlargement.

4) Treatment choices

   a) Intravenous digoxin: Draw up 0.01–0.02 mg/kg and give $^1/_4$ dose q30min up to 4 times.

   i) *This is the only positive inotrope that is a negative chronotrope.*

   ii) *If the arrhythmia is secondary to myocardial failure, this may be the drug of choice.*

   b) Diltiazem: 0.25 mg/kg IV over 2 minutes. Repeat 2 times q15min to effect. This is a calcium channel blocker with mild negative chronotropic, inotropic, and vasodilatory effects.

   c) Verapamil: 0.05 mg/kg IV slowly. Repeat up to 2 times to effect.

   i) *This is another calcium channel blocker that has been shown effective in reversing rapid supraventricular tachyarrhythmias. Caution: It can predispose patient to digitalis toxicity and should probably not be used concurrently. Also,*

QUICK FORMULA FOR CALCULATING CONSTANT RATE INFUSIONS:

Dosage (μg/kg/min) $\times$ (kg BW) = mg of drug to place in 250 mL of fluids at a rate of 15 mL/h.

---

it is a more potent vasodilator and negative inotrope than diltiazem.

ii) *Effective in abolishing reentrant tachycardia*

d) *Esmolol: 0.05–0.1 mg/kg boluses q5min to a maximum dosage of 0.5 mg/kg*

i) *This is a very short acting β-blocker specific for beta 1 receptors (cardioselective).*

ii) *If the initial boluses are effective, esmolol can be administered as a CRI at a dosage of 25–200 μg/kg/min.*

iii) *Esmolol can be a potent negative inotrope and hypotensive agent, but used cautiously, it is an excellent drug for treating arrhythmias induced by excessive sympathetic tone or sensitization of the myocardium to catecholamines.*

iv) *Response to esmolol can be used to predict the effectiveness of*

longer-acting oral β-blockers, such as atenolol.

e) *DC cardioversion*

i) *In an emergency situation, a precordial thump to the chest may convert atrial tachycardia.*

ii) *If there is no response to vagal maneuvers or digitalis, DC cardioversion can be attempted.*

a) *Narcotic analgesia is followed by ECG-gated DC shock at 1 J/kg.*

b) *Electrical cardioversion can be repeated up to three times.*

c) *Place the animal on a lidocaine drip (25–80 μg/kg/min) following cardioversion, because ventricular arrhythmias are common.*

c. Atrial fibrillation

1) ECG reveals irregular R-R intervals, no discernible P waves, and an oscillating baseline (*Fig. 10-5*).

2) Common arrhythmia in dogs with dilated cardiomyopathy, chronic valvular disease, or untreated congenital heart disease.

3) In dogs, atrial fibrillation is usually a symptom of serious underlying heart disease, and conversion to normal sinus rhythm is not likely.

4) The goal of therapy is usually to slow AV conduction enough so that the ventricular rate is <160 bpm, thereby allowing improved filling and stroke volume.

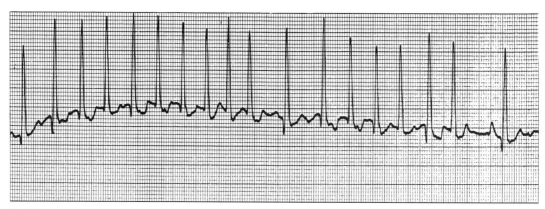

FIGURE 10.5   Atrial fibrillation in an Irish Wolfhound with a 2-week history of weight loss and exercise intolerance. Note lack of discernible P waves, irregular R-R intervals, and rapid rate (240–260 bpm). (From Tilley LP, Miller MS, Smith FWK Jr. Canine and feline cardiac arrhythmias: self-assessment. Philadelphia: Lea & Febiger, 1993.)

a) Digoxin—slow maintenance oral dose unless resting HR is >240 bpm. For rapid HR, use IV digitalization protocol under atrial tachycardia above (p. 183).

b) After 3–4 days, if the resting heart rate is >160 bpm, cautiously add diltiazem (0.5 mg/kg PO q8h, gradually increased to 1.5 mg/kg PO q8h) or propranolol. (Begin treatment at 0.2–0.3 mg/kg PO and gradually increase to a maximum dosage of 1.0 mg/kg q8h).

c) Other drugs for CHF (furosemide, spironolactone, and enalapril) are also indicated in most dogs with atrial fibrillation.

5) Occasionally animals can develop acute atrial fibrillation after trauma, anesthesia, or surgery in the absence of organic heart disease.

a) In these patients, conversion should be attempted with quinidine gluconate 6–20 mg/kg IM q6h for up to 4 doses.

b) Once conversion to normal sinus rhythm occurs, oral antiarrhythmic therapy can be continued for 2–3 weeks and then tapered off. It can be reinitiated if the arrhythmia returns.

c) Other drugs that may be effective in converting acute atrial fibrillation are verapamil and diltiazem (see above under "Atrial Tachycardia") (p. 183).

2. Ventricular arrhythmias

a. Premature ventricular contractions

1) Usually secondary to an underlying condition—hypoxemia, trauma, GDV, sepsis, splenic disease, drugs

2) Isolated PVCs are not life threatening. They serve as a marker for underlying disease.

3) Treatment: Give oxygen, treat underlying disease, pursue diagnostic tests to determine cause.

b. Ventricular tachycardia, ventricular flutter

1) ECG appearance

a) Regular rhythm—no relation to P waves

b) Wide, bizarre QRS complexes—multifocal or unifocal

c) Look for fusion beats and capture beats (Fig. 10-6)

2) May occur 12–48 hours after shock, trauma, or GDV as a result of myocardial ischemia or contusions.

3) Need for treatment

a) Antiarrhythmic therapy is not always indicated when abnormalities are noted on the ECG. Side effects, especially proarrhythmic effects, can be dangerous.

b) Antiarrhythmic therapy is indicated in the following situations:

　i) Frequent PVCs (>30/min) can cause hypotension.

　ii) Paroxysmal ventricular tachycardia with a rate of >140 bpm can impair hemodynamics.

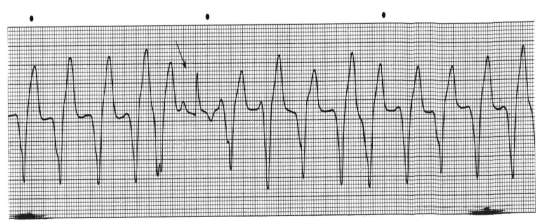

FIGURE 10.6 Ventricular tachycardia is characterized by wide, bizarre QRS complexes, capture beats, and fusion beats. The marked complex represents a capture beat (normal P-QRST) and the one directly following it is a fusion beat. (From Tilley LP, Miller MS, Smith FWK Jr. Canine and feline cardiac arrhythmias: self-assessment. Philadelphia: Lea & Febiger, 1993.)

iii) *Multiform (multifocal) QRS complexes imply irritated myocardium.*
iv) *R on T phenomenon—the VPCs occur at the apex of the previrus T wave during a vulnerable period when ventricular fibrillation can be initiated*
v) *Clinical signs of weakness, depression, or syncope indicate decreased cardiac output.*

4) Idioventricular tachycardia
   a) *Resembles ventricular tachycardia, but rate is slow enough to maintain adequate ventricular filling and perfusion.*
   b) *Ventricular rhythm < 130 bpm.*
   c) *Usually clinically benign and does not require treatment—normal pulse pressure, spontaneous remission within 24–48 h*

c. Treatment for ventricular arrhythmias
   1) Lidocaine bolus: Give 2–8 mg/kg slowly IV (over 2 min) to effect. Monitor ECG tracing. Arrhythmia should convert to normal sinus rhythm within minutes.
   a) *Minimal hemodynamic effects but can be hypotensive if given rapidly.*
   b) *Neurotoxic effects occur at high doses but are readily controlled by intravenous diazepam (2–10 mg).*
   c) *For cats, use approximately ONE-TENTH OF THE DOG DOSE (0.25–0.75 mg/kg slowly IV), as felines are prone to toxicity.*
   2) If the lidocaine bolus is effective, make up a CRI (25–75 µg/kg/min).
   3) Lidocaine is rapidly cleared from the plasma by the liver, and repeat boluses of 2 mg/kg may be needed q20–30min until a steady-state concentration is reached with the CRI (this usually takes 4–6 hours).
   4) The most common signs of lidocaine overdosage include nausea, vomiting, disorientation, depression, twitching, and convulsions. If these signs occur, reduce the dosage. Drugs such as cimetidine, which suppress hepatic metabolism, should be avoided in patients receiving lidocaine.
   5) Lidocaine CRI is usually continued for 48–72 hours and then tapered off while monitoring the ECG. Long-term control can usually be obtained if necessary with oral quinidine or procainamide (6–20 mg/kg PO q6–8h).
   6) If lidocaine is ineffective, the following drugs can be considered:
   a) *Magnesium sulfate: 25–30 mg/kg diluted in 5% dextrose in water or magnesium chloride (0.15–0.3 mEq/kg) administered IV over 5–10 minutes. If effective, add same dosage to IV fluids to be administered over 12–24 hours. Magnesium deficiency can occur in critically ill patients with anorexia, gastrointestinal (GI) losses, or polyuria and can result in refractory ventricular arrhythmias.*
   b) *Procainamide is usually the second-line drug if lidocaine is ineffective. Intravenous boluses are avoided because severe hypotension can result, but in urgent situations up to ten 2 mg/kg IV boluses can be given in a 30-minute period.*
   i) *Intramuscular injections are rapidly absorbed: 6–15 mg/kg IM q4–6h.*
   ii) *Procainamide can also be delivered by CRI: 20–50 mg/kg/min.*
   iii) *Maintenance therapy is continued with sustained-release procainamide 8–20 mg/kg PO q8h.*
   c) *Esmolol is an ultrashort-acting β-adrenergic blocking drug that has a very short half-life (9 minutes).*
   i) *An initial IV bolus (0.5 mg/kg) can be given slowly IV to slow or eradicate the arrhythmia.*
   ii) *IV bolus can be followed by CRI: 25–200 µg/kg/min.*
   d) *For severe refractory ventricular tachycardia or ventricular fibrillation, consider bretylium 5–10 mg/kg IV. (Not readily available.)*

7) If there is NO RESPONSE to treatment
   a) *Reevaluate ECG, repeat vagal maneuver to rule out the possibility of supraventricular tachycardia with aberrant conduction causing wide-appearing QRS.*
   b) *Check serum potassium. Administer oxygen.*

8) The therapeutic endpoint is not complete eradication of the arrhythmia from the ECG tracing. Ideally, the heart rate should be <140 bpm, and hemodynamic improvement (improved color, CRT, pulse strength) should be seen.
   a) *Most acute ventricular arrhythmias secondary to shock, trauma, pain, etc. resolve within 72 hours.*
   b) *Some acute arrhythmias may persist for 10 days or longer.*

3. Bradyarrhythmias
   a. Sinoatrial arrest
      1) A pause >2 R-R intervals is seen on the ECG tracing (Fig. 10-7).

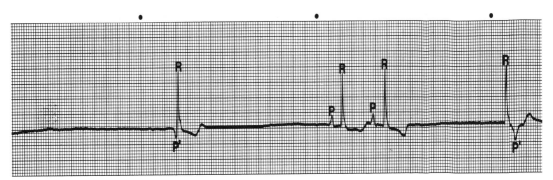

FIGURE 10.7   A pause >2 R-R intervals is consistent with sinoatrial arrest and may result in clinical signs of syncope. (From Tilley LP. Essentials of canine and feline electrocardiography. Philadelphia: Lea & Febiger, 1992.)

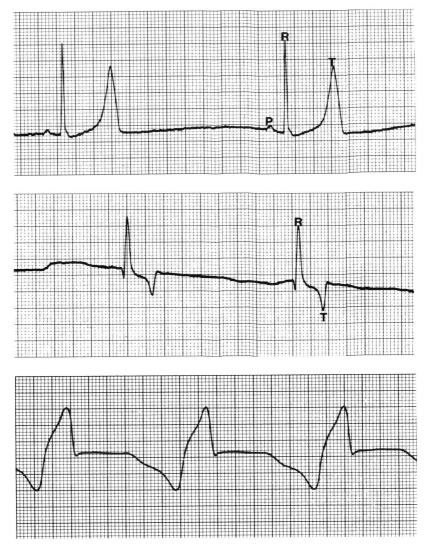

FIGURE 10.8   Hyperkalemia can cause the following ECG abnormalities. A, Mild: Peaked T wave. B, Moderate: Flattened P wave, slow heart rate. C, Severe: Wide QRS, sinoventricular rhythm. (From Tilley LP. Essentials of canine and feline electrocardiography. Philadelphia: Lea & Febiger, 1992.)

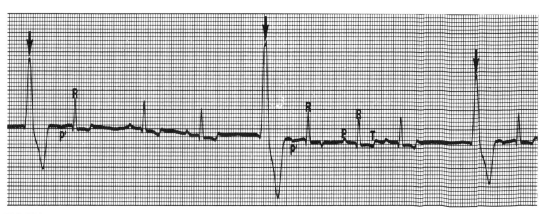

FIGURE 10.9   Ventricular escape beats appear as wide bizarre complexes after a pause. These should never be suppressed with anti-arrhythmic therapy. (From Tilley LP. Essentials of canine and feline electrocardiography. Philadelphia: Lea & Febiger, 1992.)

2) This condition may be associated with increased vagal tone (brachycephalic dogs) or sick sinus syndrome and often manifests clinically as recurrent episodes of syncope.
3) Treatment
    a) An atropine response test is performed in the hospital with the animal on a heart monitor—0.04 mg/kg IM.
    b) If atropine is effective, oral anticholinergic therapy is attempted with propantheline bromide 3.75–7.5 mg PO q8–12h.
    c) If medical therapy is ineffective in controlling symptoms, pacemaker implantation is indicated.
b. Atrial standstill
  1) The ECG tracing reveals absence of P waves.
  2) The most common cause is hyperkalemia (*Fig. 10-8*; hypoadrenocorticism in dogs and urethral obstruction in cats).
  3) Treatment for life-threatening hyperkalemia involves one or all three of the following.
    a) 10% calcium gluconate, 0.2–0.5 mL/kg IV
    b) Insulin/dextrose, 0.25 U/kg regular insulin plus 0.5 g/kg dextrose IV
    c) Sodium bicarbonate, 1–2 mEq/kg slowly IV to effect

c. Ventricular escape beats (*Fig. 10-9*)
  1) Appear as wide bizarre complexes after a pause
  2) These represent the ventricular pacemaker activity and should not be suppressed with lidocaine or other antiarrhythmic drugs or cardiac arrest will result.
d. Sinus bradycardia
  1) Causes include organic heart disease, endocrinopathies, hypothermia, drug administration, and increased vagal tone.
  2) Most cases resolve with treatment of the underlying disorder. Normal cardiac output can be achieved with rates as low as 40–50 bpm.
  3) Rule out hypoglycemia, hypothermia, hyperkalemia, and hypothyroidism. Reverse narcotic analgesics/sedatives and discontinue inhalation anesthesia.
  4) Treatment is atropine (0.02 to 0.04 mg/kg IM, IV, SC or glycopyrolate 0.005 to 0.01 mg/kg IV, IM, SC).
  5) Naloxone (0.02–0.1 mg/kg IV) can be given to reverse opioid induced bradycardias.

CHAPTER 11

GASTROINTESTINAL EMERGENCIES

I. CLINICAL SIGNS, DIAGNOSIS

A. Differentiate between vomiting and regurgitation

1. Regurgitation is the passive expulsion of a food bolus from the pharynx or esophagus. It occurs abruptly without retching or abdominal contractions. The food bolus is often tubular.

    a. Thoracic radiographs may reveal megaesophagus and aspiration pneumonia.

    b. Fluoroscopic studies are used to evaluate esophageal motility.

2. Vomiting is the forceful expulsion of gastric contents through the mouth.

B. Differentiate between large bowel and small bowel diarrhea.

1. Small bowel diarrhea is characterized by increased volume of watery feces, digested blood (melena), steatorrhea, and weight loss.

2. Large bowel diarrhea is characterized by mucus, fresh blood, tenesmus, and increased frequency of small quantities with each defecation.

3. Parasites should be ruled out with fecal examination and therapeutic deworming trial before more invasive diagnostics are done.

II. DIAGNOSTIC AND MONITORING PROCEDURES

A. Abdominal auscultation

1. Should precede palpation to avoid examination-induced changes in bowel sounds

2. Borborygmus is increased with acute enteritis, acute obstruction, or toxicity.

3. Borborygmus is decreased with peritonitis, ileus, chronic obstruction, or free peritoneal fluid.

4. Ectopic bowel sounds may indicate diaphragmatic, body wall, or inguinal herniation.

B. Abdominal palpation

1. Methodical approach from cranial to caudal and superficial to deep ensures optimum results.

2. Excessive pressure may cause animal to tense abdominal muscles making thorough palpation difficult.

3. Elevating forequarters may aid in detecting cranial abdominal abnormalities; especially intussusception in young dogs.

4. Examine for organomegaly, masses, foreign bodies, intussusception, mesenteric lymphadenopathy (cats), free fluid, and pain.

5. Abdominal pain may originate from hepatobiliary, gastrointestinal (GI) tract (including mesentery and mesenteric lymph nodes), pancreatic, splenic, urogenital, or peritoneal abnormalities. Pain results from displacement, distention/obstruction, inflammation/infection, perforation, or ischemia.

C. Abdominal radiographs

1. Survey abdominal radiographs, ventrodorsal and lateral views, may show decreased serosal detail, organ enlargement, masses, ileus, radiodense foreign bodies or uroliths, diaphragmatic or body wall hernia, and prostatic or uterine abnormalities (*Fig. 11-1*).

2. Lack of serosal detail may indicate free peritoneal fluid (ascites, hemorrhage, feline peritonitis

(FIP), septic peritonitis, neoplasia) or loss of intraabdominal fat (cachexia, neonates).

3. Pneumoperitoneum, most readily identified as gas density between diaphragm and liver, indicates hollow viscous rupture and is an indication for emergency laparotomy.

    a. Nonsurgical causes of pneumoperitoneum include open-needle abdominocentesis or recent (within 18 days) abdominal surgery. Rarely, severe pneumomediastinum pneumothorax can result in pneumoperitoneum.

4. Right lateral projection is preferred for detecting gastric dilatation/volvulus in which pylorus is distended and displaced craniodorsal to fundus and appears as "double bubble" (two gas shadows separated by band of soft tissue) (*Fig. 11-4*).

5. Pancreatitis may cause loss of serosal detail in right cranial abdomen and/or lateral displacement of gas-filled duodenum (sentinel loop sign).

6. Retroperitoneal space abnormalities, (e.g., urine leakage, or hemorrhage, may cause streaking of soft tissues ventral to lumbar vertebrae, depressed psoas line, or ventral displacement of the descending colon.

D. Abdominocentesis

1. Indications

    a. Loss of serosal detail on survey radiographs

    b. Blunt trauma with abdominal injury, multiple injuries, progressive anemia, or refractory shock

    c. Acute abdominal pain of unknown cause

    d. Postoperative complications potentially caused by leakage from enterotomy or anastomotic site, for example

2. Not indicated with penetrating abdominal injury—exploratory surgery is necessary

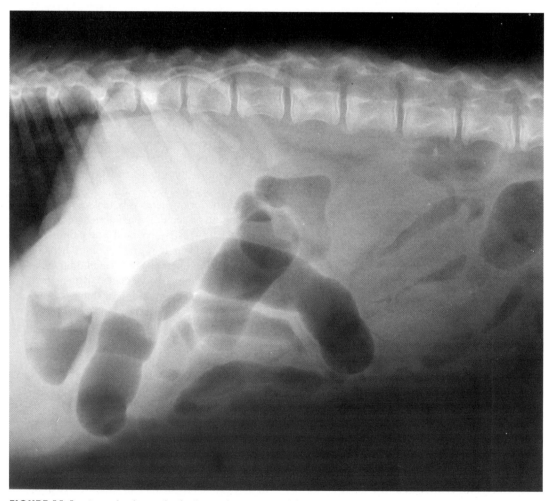

FIGURE 11.1   Lateral radiograph of a dog with an intestinal foreign body reveals marked gaseous distension of the small bowel.

3. Precautions include coagulopathy, adhesions caused by prior abdominal surgery, organomegaly, and pyometra.

4. Procedure

   a. Skin of ventral abdomen is clipped and prepared using standard aseptic technique with the patient in lateral recumbency.

   b. Sedation or local anesthetic is usually not necessary.

   c. One or two at a time, 20- to 22-gauge needles without syringe are inserted, into the four quadrants of the abdomen.

   d. Any fluid retrieved is collected in a lavender-top tube for fluid analysis, cytology, ± culture/sensitivity, and biochemical analysis as indicated (see below, E.5).

5. Advantages

   a. Quick, inexpensive, no special equipment

   b. High specificity

6. Disadvantages

   a. Main disadvantage is low diagnostic accuracy rate caused by false negative results in approximately 50% of cases. Accuracy can be improved with ultrasound-guided aspiration.

   b. Large volumes (5.2–6.6 mL/kg) of peritoneal fluid are necessary for detection via abdominocentesis.

   c. Applying suction via syringe increases the likelihood of a false-negative result by causing omentum or viscera to occlude the needle.

E. Diagnostic peritoneal lavage (DPL)

1. Indications

   a. Same indications as abdominocentesis (see above) after obtaining a negative result using 4-quadrant abdominocentesis.

2. Contraindications and precautions as for abdominocentesis (see above)

   a. DPL should be used with caution in patients with respiratory distress because instilled fluid may put pressure on the diaphragm.

   b. DPL should be used with caution or not at all in patients with diaphagmatic hernia.

3. Procedure

   a. Skin of the ventral abdomen is clipped and prepared using standard aseptic technique.

   b. Local anesthetic is infiltrated in skin, subcutaneous tissue, and linea alba just caudal to the umbilicus on the ventral midline.

   c. An 18- to 20-gauge over-the-needle catheter is inserted into the abdomen in a caudodorsal direction through a stab incision just caudal to the umbilicus on the ventral midline.

     1) Additional side holes can be created within 1 cm of the tip of the catheter using a no. 15 scalpel blade to facilitate drainage.

     2) Commercial peritoneal lavage catheters (Stylocath), without the trocar, can be used.

   d. If no fluid is retrieved, 22 mL/kg of warmed sterile saline is instilled, dispersed throughout the abdomen by gentle massage or rocking the patient from side to side, and drained into a sterile collection system. Failure to retrieve significant fluid is common with peritoneal inflammation. Instillation using 1/2 the initial fluid volume can be repeated.

   e. Fluid is analyzed as for abdominocentesis.

4. Advantage

   a. Primary advantage of DPL is higher diagnostic accuracy because of a lower false-negative rate than with abdominocentesis.

     1) Less fluid is required for detection, 1.0–4.4 mL/kg for DPL vs. 5.2–6.6 mL/kg for abdominocentesis.

     2) Localized lesions may be identified because of dispersal of lavage fluid throughout abdomen.

   b. Disadvantages are few with experience; this is somewhat more technically challenging than abdominocentesis.

5. Interpreting results of abdominocentesis and DPL

   a. Hemoperitoneum—free blood does not clot (clotting blood indicates penetration of spleen, liver, or blood vessel)—most common with trauma, with ruptured splenic tumor or as complication of ovariohysterectomy, or coagulopathy.

     1) PCV/TS of abdominal fluid compared to that from peripheral vein may indicate severity or acuity of hemorrhage.

     2) Increasing PCV/TS of abdominal fluid with serial assessment indicates ongoing hemorrhage and may dictate emergency laparotomy.

   b. Toxic or degenerate neutrophils with intracellular bacteria indicate septic peritonitis; this finding mandates an emergency laparotomy.

   c. In cases of suspected urinary leakage, creatinine and potassium concentrations will be significantly higher in abdominal fluid than in serum.

d. Similarly, in pancreatitis, amylase and lipase values will be higher in abdominal fluid than serum.

e. Abdominal effusion in animals with peritonitis has higher lactate and lower glucose than serum.

f. Abdominal effusion due to bile peritonitis will have higher bilirubin concentrations in the abdominal fluid compared to peripheral blood.

F. Abdominal ultrasound

1. More sensitive than radiography for detecting small volumes of free fluid and characterizing lesions within solid organs

2. Experienced operator may identify bowel lesions including thickened/edematous bowel walls, intussusception, foreign body, or mass.

3. Most sensitive method for diagnosing pancreatitis, especially in cats

4. Useful in emergency setting for evaluating patients with acute abdomen or hemoperitoneum, and may help determine the need for exploratory laporotomy.

5. Facilitates aspiration of abdominal fluid or masses and urinary bladder

G. Specific blood tests

1. TLI

a. Low values indicate exocrine pancreatic insufficiency in dogs and cats.

b. High values may indicate acute pancreatitis (usefulness questionable in cats).

1) Elevated values may also be seen in normal animals, renal disease, inflammatory bowel disease, and postprandially.

2. Cobalamin (vitamin B_{12})/folate

a. Used in conjunction with TLI to assess absorptive capacity of small bowel and bacterial overgrowth

b. Low serum concentrations of cobalamin and folate indicate malabsorption from ileum and proximal jejunum, respectively (e.g., inflammatory bowel disease (IBD)).

c. Small intestinal bacterial overgrowth is characterized by increased serum folate (produced in lumen by bacteria and absorbed into circulation) and decreased serum cobalamin (bound by luminal bacteria).

1) Pattern of increased folate/decreased cobalamin has nearly 100% specificity for SIBO; sensitivity is low (5%), however.

3. Bile acids

a. Sensitive but nonspecific indicator of liver dysfunction

b. Paired samples, fasting and 2-hour postprandial, preferred.

c. Both pre- and postprandial values are 2–5 times the reference range in most forms of significant liver disease.

d. Milder elevations are common with hyperadrenocorticism.

e. Congenital or acquired portocaval shunts are characterized by a postprandial value significantly higher than the fasting value.

f. Fasting value is higher than the postprandial level with interdigestive gall bladder contraction and generally indicates normal liver function.

g. Ursodeoxycholic acid (Actigall) may interfere with certain bile acid assays; the medication should be withheld for 2–7 days before determining bile acids in these patients.

4. Albumin/globulin concentration

a. Decreased concentrations of both (panhypoproteinemia) in the absence of hemorrhage indicates severe small bowel disease (i.e., protein-losing enteropathy).

b. Low albumin with high globulin concentration may be seen with liver disease or immunoproliferative enteropathy of Basenji dogs.

c. GI diseases associated with increased globulin levels include IBD, extramedullary plasmacytoma, and FIP.

d. Increases in both albumin and globulin levels indicate dehydration.

H. Endoscopy

1. Widely used for diagnosing mucosal disorders of GI tract, (e.g., IBD)

2. Multiple mucosal biopsies of stomach and duodenum are taken regardless of gross appearance because significant histopathologic lesions may exist with no visible mucosal abnormalities.

3. Performing biopsies of the esophagus may be difficult and often is not done.

4. Biopsy of deep ulcers should be avoided to prevent perforation.

5. Other uses include foreign body retrieval and percutaneous gastrostomy tube placement.

I. Esophagram (barium swallow)

1. Indications
   a. To assess swallowing function with fluoroscopy
   b. To confirm megaesophagus
   c. To demonstrate esophageal foreign bodies or stricture

2. Procedure
   a. Fast animal 6–24 h.
   b. Obtain survey radiographs of neck and thorax.
   c. Mix barium paste in canned dog food.
   d. If perforation is suspected, use 5–15 mL of iodinated contrast instead of barium.

J. Upper/lower gastrointestinal study

1. Indications
   a. To identify suspect foreign body mass or obstruction not seen on survey films
   b. To confirm abnormal location of GI organs (hernias)
   c. To evaluate GI motility

2. Procedure
   a. Fast 12–24 h.
   b. Obtain right lateral and VD survey radiographs.
   c. Pass lubricated orogastric tube through oral speculum or roll of tape.
      1) Measure from tip of nose to last rib and mark tube.
      2) Verify placement before administering contrast. Aspirate for fluid, blow in tube, palpate neck.
   d. Administer 12 mL/kg of liquid barium (use 2–4 mL/kg iodinated contrast if perforation suspected).
   e. Radiographs are taken immediately and at 0.5, 1, 3, 5, and 24 hours

3. Possible findings
   a. Normal gastric emptying time: 2–3 h (dog) or 1–2 h (cat)
   b. Most of the barium is in the colon by 3–5 h (dog) or 2–3 h (cat).
   c. Rapid transit is common in enteritis.
   d. Delayed transit—mechanical or functional obstruction

   e. Filling defect—foreign body, neoplasia, mucosal disease
   f. Linear foreign body, intestinal plication
   g. Hernias, diverticulum

K. Barium enema

1. Indications
   a. To evaluate colon in animals with large bowel diarrhea
   b. To demonstrate intussusception or intraluminal neoplasia

2. Procedure
   a. Colon must be empty of fecal material.
      1) Feed low-residue diet.
      2) Fast 24 h.
      3) Administer cathartics and warm water enemas as needed.
   b. General anesthesia is preferred.
   c. Place lubricated Foley catheter in rectum and inflate bulb.
   d. Fill colon with 7–14 mL/kg liquid barium and clamp tube. (Use iodinated contrast if perforation is suspected.) Do not overfill.
   e. Obtain radiographs (increase kVp by 5–10 for improved technique).
   f. A double-contrast study can be performed by removing the barium and filling the colon with air.

3. Findings
   a. The normal colon is smooth and nonsacculated.
   b. Intussusception, neoplasia, polyp, mucosal ulceration, or foreign body may appear as filling defects.
   c. Annular neoplasia or scar may appear as a stricture.

L. Pneumocolonography
1. This is a simple procedure that may help diagnose ileocecal intussusception.
2. The colon must be empty.
3. Sedation or general anesthesia is required.
   a. Butorphanol (0.2–0.4 mg/kg) with diazepam (0.2 mg/kg) or acetylpromazine (0.025–0.05 mg/kg) IV—dog
   b. Ketamine 4–6 mg/kg with diazepam 0.2 mg/kg IV—cat
4. Air, carbon dioxide, or nitrous oxide (7–14 mL/kg) is used to fill the ascending, transverse, and descending colon and cecum.

5. An ileocecal intussusception will appear as an intraluminal mass in the cecum.

M. Fecal examination (rectal examination)

1. A rectal examination should be done in animals with acute GI signs.
  a. The prostate should be palpated to check for pain, enlargement, or abnormal consistency.
  b. The character of the feces should be noted.
    1) Mucous and fresh blood indicate colonic disease.
    2) Bone fragments or sharp objects could indicate intestinal perforation/peritonitis in animals with shock.
    3) Dark, tarry stool indicates bleeding from the upper GI tract.
    4) Orange feces can be seen with hemolytic disease.
    5) Gray (acholic) stool is seen with bile duct obstruction.
    6) Evidence of a linear foreign body is sometimes found on rectal examination.

2. Microscopic evaluation
  a. *Trichuris* sp. (whipworm) eggs are brown, bioperculated and football shaped.
  b. *Entamoeba histolytica* is an amoeba often acquired from human sources that may be seen as motile trophozoites in direct fecal smears stained with new methylene blue.
  c. *Balantidium coli* is another amoeba parasite that can infect dogs, usually after exposure to swine.
  d. *Cryptosporidium parvum* oocysts are thick walled and 5 μm in diameter and can be detected on fecal flotation or enzyme-linked immunosorbent assay (ELISA) on the feces for *Cryptosporidium* antigen.
  e. Coccidian oocysts may be seen on fecal floatation and are common in young puppies and kittens.
  f. *Giardia* spp. can be identified as motile trophozoites from a direct smear or as cysts following zinc sulfate centrifugal flotation technique.
  g. *Pentatrichomonas* spp. may be seen on direct smear or saline preparation of feces.
  h. Hookworm, roundworm, or tapeworm ova are commonly found in fecal samples from young animals.
  i. Baermann's apparatus may be necessary to detect *Aelurostrongylus* and *Strongyloides* larvae.

j. Direct-stained fecal smear may reveal large numbers of eosinophils (eosinophilic gastroenteritis) or fungal organisms (histoplasmosis).
k. Animals with maldigestion have high fecal fat (orange droplets with Sudan III stain), high fecal starch (blue granules with Lugol's stain), and increased number of striated muscle fibers on microscopic fecal examination.
l. Spores of *Clostridium* spp., neutrophils, and bacteria can be seen in dogs with clostridial diarrhea. Spores are oval structures with "safety pin" appearance.

III. MANAGEMENT OF SPECIFIC CONDITIONS

A. Regurgitation

1. Clinical signs
  a. Passive retrograde evacuation of undigested food, often in "tube" shape
  b. No abdominal press as seen with vomiting; occurs abruptly without retching
  c. Sign of esophageal disease
  d. Frequency and timing related to meals are variable.
  e. Coughing, cyanosis, tachypnea, and fever are seen with aspiration pneumonia.
  f. History of recent anesthesia may suggest gastric reflux esophagitis.
  g. Horner's syndrome, noncompressible cranial thorax in cats may indicate mediastinal mass causing esophageal obstruction.
  h. May occur in young puppies
    1) Congenital inherited—Miniature Schnauzer, Wire-haired Fox Terrier, German Shepherd Dog, Great Dane, Irish Setter, Labrador Retriever, Shar Pei
    2) Vascular ring anomaly—German Shepherd dog, young puppies following weaning
  i. Adult onset
    1) Rule out hypothyroidism, hypoadrenocorticism, myasthenia gravis, esophagitis, systemic lupus erythematosus (SLE), polymyositis, botulism, dysautonomia, thallium, lead, cholinesterase inhibitors

2. Diagnosis
  a. Dilated air/fluid/ingesta-filled esophagus on thoracic radiographs
  b. Retention of contrast material

c. Abnormal motility on fluoroscopy

d. Alveolar opacities, air bronchograms with aspiration pneumonia

e. Endoscopy may reveal esophagitis, esophageal stricture, foreign body, mass lesions, or gastroesophageal intussusception.

3. Treatment

a. Rule out the underlying cause. Megaesophagus may resolve with treatment for hypothyroidism, hypoadrenocorticism, myasthenia, esophagitis, or polymyositis.

b. Vascular ring anomaly—surgical ligation and resection of the restricting vessel followed by upright feeding. The dilated portion of the esophagus may not regain normal motility.

c. Idiopathic—medical therapy

1) Feed in elevated or vertical position and maintain erect posture for 10–15 min after feeding.

2) High-calorie diet in small, frequent (4–6/day) meals. Canned food pressed into "meatballs" is often easiest to swallow.

3) Gastrostomy tube can be placed if per os feeding is not successful.

a) *Consider low-profile gastrostomy device for long-term feeding.*

4) Prokinetic drugs (e.g., metoclopramide) are generally ineffective.

5) Broad-spectrum antibiotics are indicated if concurrent aspiration pneumonia is present.

B. Esophagitis

1. Reflux esophagitis

a. May occur following anesthesia, vomiting, ingestion of irritant, hiatal hernia, or anticholinergic therapy. Reflux may also occur with a nasogastric or esophagostomy tube.

1) Fast animal prior to anesthesia.

2) Do not position with head down if possible.

3) Use nasoesophageal rather than nasogastric tubes to avoid crossing gastroesophageal sphincter and promoting reflux.

b. Clinical signs: hypersalivation (ropey, blood-tinged), anorexia, painful swallowing, regurgitation

c. Best diagnosed with endoscopy—erosions, mucosal erythema

d. Treatment

1) Sucralfate suspension (1 g/10 mL of warm water). Give 5–10 mL PO TID–QID.

2) Omeprazole (2 mg/kg q24h PO)—best way to decrease gastric acidity with severe esophagitis (proton pump inhibitor)

3) Histamine H_2 receptor antagonists can be used instead of omeprazole:

a) *Ranitidine 2 mg/kg PO or IV q8–12h*

b) *Famotidine 0.5–1 mg PO q12–24h*

c) *Cimetidine 5–10 mg/kg PO q8h*

4) Metoclopramide (0.2–0.4 mg/kg TID PO) increases gastroesophageal sphincter tone; give 30 min prior to feeding.

2. Toxic irritants

a. Neutralize acids with milk of magnesia, 5–10 mL/kg q4–6h PO.

b. Neutralize bases with diluted vinegar or lemon juice (1:4 dilution).

c. Suction and remove gastric contents after neutralization.

d. Contact poison control (217–333-2053)

3. Nutrition

a. Withhold food for 24–48 hours.

b. Diet: Low-fat, high-protein diet increases lower esophageal sphincter tone and decreases gastric acid secretion. Continue bland diet for 3–4 weeks.

c. For severe damage, place a gastrostomy tube.

4. Prognosis

a. Most cases improve with medical management.

b. In severe cases, esophageal motility disorders or strictures may develop.

C. Esophageal foreign body (FB)

1. Common foreign bodies include balls, toys, bones, fishhooks, needles, sticks, walnuts, chestnuts, acorns, pecans, and corncobs.

2. Clinical signs include hypersalivation, dysphagia, persistent gulping or swallowing, regurgitation, anorexia, and respiratory distress.

3. Physical examination

a. Palpate cervical esophagus (left side of neck): may palpate object or mass.

b. Auscult lungs: Crackles and wheezes are noted with aspiration pneumonia.

c. Examine oral cavity and under base of tongue

4. Diagnosis
   a. Thoracic radiographs
      1) Gas or fluid accumulation cranial to obstruction
      2) Pneumomediastinum, pneumothorax can occur with perforation (indication for surgery).
      3) Most common sites are thoracic inlet, heart base, and diaphragm.
   b. Endoscopy
      1) Can evaluate mucosal lesions surrounding foreign body
      2) Can attempt removal
   c. Observation of foreign body ingestion followed by clinical signs of esophageal disease.

5. Treatment
   a. Distal objects can be pushed into the stomach and removed via gastrostomy if they are not digestible or are considered too sharp to pass safely. Most bone foreign bodies can be left in the stomach to dissolve without requiring surgical removal.
   b. Rigid or flexible scope and large grasping forceps can be used to remove foreign bodies.
   c. Evaluate mucosa endoscopically following removal. Give antibiotics if perforated or severe mucosal necrosis/ulceration is present.
   d. Institute therapy for esophagitis (p. 195).
   e. Surgery (thoracotomy) is needed if you cannot dislodge the foreign body or if thoracic drainage is required (perforated esophagus with pneumothorax or pneumomediastinum on thoracic radiographs).
   f. Antiinflammatory doses of corticosteroids, 0.5–1.0 mg/kg/day, may reduce risk of stricture (i.e., 180° or more, deep mucosal ulceration).

6. Complications
   a. Esophageal stricture
      1) Fibrosis can occur 1–3 weeks following mucosal damage.
      2) Diagnosis—endoscopy or barium esophagram. (If perforation is suspected, use iodinated contrast material.)
      3) Balloon dilation (Rigiflex Dilators, Microvasive Inc, Medford, MA) repeated at 1- to 2-week intervals until stricture is resolved.
      4) Follow with medical therapy for esophagitis (p. 195.)
      5) Prednisone may prevent further fibrosis and stricture formation (0.5–1 mg/kg q12h tapered over 14 days).

      6) Surgical resection has a guarded prognosis. Restricture is common following surgery.
   b. Esophageal perforation—mediastinitis

D. Gastric foreign body
1. Clinical signs
   a. May present with chronic intermittent vomiting if in fundus, or acute onset of protracted, projectile vomiting if in pylorus
2. Diagnosis
   a. Endoscopy, barium study, or double-contrast gastrogram to detect radiolucent objects.
   b. Electrolytes/blood gases
      1) May reveal metabolic alkalosis from loss of HCl through vomitus
      2) Hypokalemia, hyponatremia are common.
3. Treatment
   a. Difficult to see with plain radiographs unless radiodense object
      1) Fishing sinkers, batteries, and lead objects should be removed to prevent lead toxicity (central nervous system (CNS), GI signs, anemia).
      2) Coins (pennies) should be removed to prevent zinc toxicity (hemolytic anemia).
   b. Correct electrolyte/blood gas imbalances.
   c. IV fluid therapy 0.9% NaCl with potassium supplementation is the fluid of choice for metabolic alkalosis.
   d. Endoscopic removal or gastrostomy when stable enough to tolerate general anesthesia

E. Intestinal obstruction

1. Intraluminal foreign body is the most common cause (tumors, polyps, foreign bodies, and intussusceptions). Extraluminal compression (adhesions, strangulation, volvulus, incarceration in a hernia), intramural thickening (mycotic disease, FIP, neoplasia), and intraluminal neoplasia also occur. Strangulation, incarceration, and volvulus cause obstruction associated with pain and shock.

2. Clinical signs
   a. Proximal obstruction is more acute and severe than distal.
      1) Protracted vomiting, rapid progression to dehydration
      2) Severe electrolyte imbalances, $\downarrow Na^+$, $\downarrow K^+$, $\uparrow HCO_3^-$, $\downarrow Cl^-$

3) Metabolic alkalosis, with or without aciduria

4) Secondary gut stasis can lead to bacterial translocation, endotoxemia, and septic shock.

b. Distal obstruction

   1) More gradual onset

   2) Weight loss, vomiting, anorexia

   3) Palpable intestinal mass

c. Partial obstruction: Animals with distal partial obstruction (i.e., ileocecal intussusception) can present for chronic weight loss, anorexia, intermittent vomiting, and scanty stool. Bloody diarrhea is common.

d. Perforation, compromised vascular integrity (i.e., thrombosis, volvulus, strangulation)

   1) Peritonitis, endotoxemia, sepsis, and severe shock occur with volvulus, incarcerated bowel or thrombosis.

   2) Abdominal pain is common in these patients. They may exhibit panting or "praying" position.

3. Diagnosis

a. Abdominal palpation—mass, painful with direct palpation

b. Plain abdominal radiographs

   1) Fluid- or gas-filled loops of bowel proximal to obstruction (*Fig. 11-1*).

   2) Linear foreign bodies—pleated bowel, sacculation, bubbles with tapered ends (*Fig. 11-2*). Sublingual string is common in

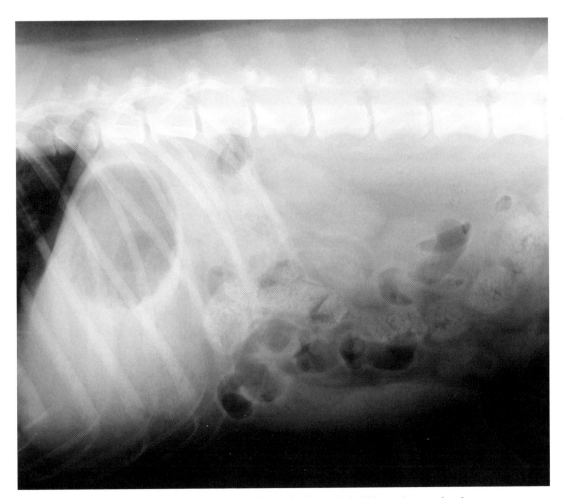

FIGURE 11.2. Lateral view of a dog with a linear foreign body reveals bubbles with tapered ends and sacculated appearance to the intestines.

cats and occasionally dogs with linear foreign bodies.
  3) Horizontal beam may show gas-fluid interface at different levels with complete obstruction.
  c. Positive-contrast radiographs
    1) Delayed gastric emptying and transit time
    2) Adherence of contrast material to linear foreign body.
    3) Avoid barium if suspect perforation; use iodine contrast agents (Gastrografin) instead.
  d. Abdominal ultrasound—classic 6-layered appearance to intussusception

4. Treatment
  a. Correct fluid and electrolyte imbalances prior to anesthesia.
  b. Begin giving broad-spectrum parenteral antibiotics.
    1) Cefazolin 22 mg/kg IV q8h
    2) Ampicillin 10–20 mg/kg IV q8h and gentamicin 6.6 mg/kg IV q24h
    3) Can substitute enrofloxacin (5 mg/kg q12h IV) for aminoglycoside; especially in patients with dehydration or hypotension
  c. Resect devitalized portions of bowel and perform anastomosis. Preserve ileum and ileocecal junction whenever possible.
  d. To facilitate removal of linear foreign body, tie to stylet or catheter, thread into bowel, then perform enterotomy.
  e. To prevent reoccurrence of intussusception, perform plication following reduction.
  f. Consider placing feeding tube in debilitated patients.
  g. Monitor hypoproteinemic animals for dehiscence.
  h. Maintain colloid oncotic pressure >15, total protein >3.5 g/dl and serum albumin >1.5 g/dl with plasma and/or synthetic colloid administration.

F. Gastric erosion/ulceration

1. Predisposing factors: nonsteroidal antiinflammatory drugs (NSAIDs), corticosteroids, shock, hypotension, mast cell tumor, pancreatic tumor, renal failure, liver disease, gastric foreign body, Helicobacter spp., hyperadrenocorticism, hypoadrenocorticism, sepsis, trauma, major surgery, heatstroke, intervertebral disk disease
2. Clinical signs
  a. Vomiting is the most common sign. "Coffee grounds" or frank blood indicate gastric hemorrhage.
  b. Melena may be present, indicating digested blood.
  c. Animals with significant anemia may exhibit pale mucous membranes and weakness.
  d. Acute weakness and abdominal pain may occur with perforation. Tachycardia and signs of shock are also evident.
  e. Animals with uremic gastritis secondary to renal disease will have oral ulcerations and uremic breath.

3. Diagnosis
  a. Microcytic, hypochromic anemia can occur secondary to iron deficiency with chronic GI blood loss.
  b. Regenerative anemia is seen 3–5 days after acute blood loss.
  c. Contrast radiography—use iodide instead of barium if perforation is suspected.
  d. Buffy coat smear, lymph node and splenic aspirates, and evaluation of any skin masses may help identify mast cell tumors.
  e. Endoscopy is the most definitive means of diagnosis.
    1) Punctate hemorrhagic lesions are seen along greater curvature, pyloric antrum, and duodenum.
    2) Obtain biopsy specimens (avoid center of ulcer); look for invasive spirochetes (request silver stains), neoplasia, and pythiosis.
  f. Coagulopathies (e.g., thrombocytopenia, disseminated intravascular coagulation (DIC), anticoagulant rodenticide toxicity, severe liver disease) should be ruled out as a cause of melena/GI bleeding.
  g. Routine CBC/chemistries and UA should be done to rule out underlying metabolic causes, such as renal and liver disease.

4. Treatment
  a. H_2 receptor blockers (choose one)
    1) Cimetidine, 5–10 mg/kg PO, SC, IV q8h
    2) Ranitidine, 2 mg/kg PO, SC, IV q8–12h
    3) Famotidine, 0.5–1 mg/kg PO, IV q12–24h
  b. Proton pump inhibitor: omeprazole, 0.7 mg/kg PO SID, is the most potent gastric acid secretion inhibitor. Indicated in patients refractory to treatment with H_2 receptor blockers and sucralfate or patients with nonresectable gastrinoma
  c. Mucosal protectant: sucralfate, 0.5–1 g PO TID; suspension may be more effective than pill (1 g/10 mL of warm water, 5–10 mL PO q6–8h).

d. Synthetic prostaglandin to protect against NSAIDs: misoprostol 3–5 μg/kg PO q8–12h

e. Treatment for *Helicobacter* spp. (usually 2–3 weeks)

    1) Amoxicillin, 22 mg/kg PO q12h

    2) Metronidazole, 15–20 mg/kg PO q12h

    3) Pepto-Bismol, 1.0 mL/kg PO q12h

f. Promotility agent(s): metoclopramide 0.2–0.4 mg/kg PO q8h

g. Antiemetics

    1) Chlorpromazine, 0.5–4 mg/kg q6–8h SC, IM, IV

    2) Prochlorperazine 0.1–0.5 mg/kg q6–8h SC, IM, IV, PO

h. Severe GI blood loss may require blood transfusion or administration of Oxyglobin. Ferrous sulfate or iron dextran is indicated if anemia is microcytic and nonregenerative.

i. Oral intake should be discontinued until vomiting subsides. IV fluids are administered to maintain hydration.

j. Duration of therapy depends on response to treatment. Severe cases can be treated for 6–8 weeks and monitored with repeat endoscopy.

G. Acute vomiting

1. Etiology

a. Direct stimulation of vomiting center in medulla

    1) CNS inflammation—neoplasia, granulomatous disease

    2) Increased cerebrospinal fluid (CSF) pressure—head trauma, neoplasia, hydrocephalus

b. Stimulation of chemoreceptor trigger zone—uremia, drugs, acidosis, endotoxemia, vestibular stimulation

c. Direct stimulation of vagal and sympathetic fibers in the GI tract, liver, pancreas, peritoneum, urinary tract and heart. Stretch receptors, chemoreceptors, and osmoreceptors provide afferent stimulation to the vomiting center in the medulla through the vagus nerve.

d. Stimulation of vestibular apparatus (motion sickness, vestibular syndrome) can also stimulate the vomiting center.

2. Diagnosis

a. Characterize vomiting

    1) "Coffee grounds"—gastric ulcer

    2) Projectile—pyloric obstruction (more common in Boston Terriers, Boxers, and other brachycephalic dogs)

    3) Bile, food >6 hours after eating—delayed emptying

    4) Ascarids

    5) Plant material—possible toxin

    6) Miscellaneous—dietary indiscretion, foreign body, toxin

b. Laboratory work

    1) CBC, blood smear, or fecal ELISA test to rule out parvoviral enteritis or feline panleukopenia

    2) PCV, TS to evaluate for dehydration

    3) Serum electrolytes

        a) Hypokalemia, hyponatremia, hypochloremia are common.

        b) Hyponatremia, hyperkalemia with Addison's disease

    4) Amylase and lipase are elevated with pancreatitis, renal disease (not useful in cats).

    5) BUN, creatinine, urinalysis to rule out renal failure

    6) Glucose, urinalysis to rule out diabetes mellitus

    7) Blood gases

        a) Metabolic alkalosis with high obstruction or severe pancreatitis

        b) Metabolic acidosis secondary to dehydration, lactic acidosis, ketoacidosis, ethylene glycol toxicity, salicylate toxicity

    8) Fecal examination—ascarids, whipworms commonly associated with vomiting

        a) Physaloptera *(dog stomach worm)—may see ova on fecal flotation*

        b) Ollulanus tricuspis *(cats)—may see parasite larvae in vomitus*

c. Abdominal radiographs—serial films or barium series to rule out obstruction, foreign body

d. Endoscopy is useful for identifying gastric erosions or ulceration, neoplastic or fungal disease, gastric foreign bodies, and some parasites

e. Abdominal ultrasound may reveal evidence of pancreatitis, abdominal mass, bowel thickening, foreign body, or intussusception.

3. Treatment

a. Search for and correct underlying cause.

b. Supportive care: Dietary indiscretion is the most common cause of acute gastroenteritis and usually responds to symptomatic care within 48 hours.

1) Fluid therapy
   a) *For metabolic alkalosis—0.9% NaCl*
   b) *Add 14–20 mEq/L of KCl*
   c) *For animals with dehydration or metabolic acidosis, use buffered balanced electrolyte solution.*
2) Nothing per os for 24 hours
3) Ice cubes or small amounts of water
4) Begin bland low-fat diet—boiled chicken or boiled hamburger and rice, small amounts fed frequently
5) Antiemetics
   a) *Avoid masking signs of foreign body or obstruction. Use only after establishing diagnosis.*
   b) *Phenothiazine tranquilizers are often most effective antiemetics, but may cause hypotension in dehydrated animals—rehydrate before using. May cause sedation. Avoid in animals with epilepsy—has been reported to lower seizure threshold.*
      i) *Chlorpromazine, 0.5 mg/kg IM, SC or 0.05–0.1 mg/kg IV q6–8h*
      ii) *Prochlorperazine, 0.1–0.5 mg/kg IM, SC q6–8h*
   c) *Metoclopramide has antiemetic effects and promotes gastric emptying to prevent gastric atony and ileus. Add to fluids for CRI: 1–2 mg/kg/24 h or give 0.2–0.4 mg/kg PO or SC q6–8h*
   d) *For vomiting due to vestibular stimulation*
      i) *Dramamine (Dimenhydrinate)— dog, 4–8 mg/kg PO, IM, IV q8h; cat, 12.5 mg/cat IV, IM, PO q8h*
      ii) *Bonine (meclizine HCl)—dog, 25 mg (4 mg/kg) l h before travel, one per day; cat, 12.5 mg/cat once daily*
   e) *For blocking the chemoreceptor trigger zone: trimethobenzamide (Tigan)— 3 mg/kg IM, PO, q8h, dogs only*
   f) *For vomiting associated with chemotherapy: ondansetron (Zofran) 0.5–1.0 mg/kg IV or PO 30 min prior to chemotherapy drug*
c. Anthelmintics for parasites that may cause vomiting
   1) Ascarids—pyrantel pamoate, 5–10 mg/kg PO
   2) Physaloptera (dogs)—pyrantel pamoate, 5 mg/kg PO
   3) Ollulanus *tricuspis* (cats)—pyrantel pamoate, 20 mg/kg PO
   4) Trichuris vulpis (dogs)—fenbendazole, 50 mg/kg PO q24h × 3 days
   5) *Giardia*
      a) *Fenbendazole, 50 mg/kg PO q24h × 3 days*
      b) *Metronidazole, 25 mg/kg PO q12h × 5–7 days*

H. Acute diarrhea

1. General considerations
   a. Abrupt onset, short duration
   b. Common problem
      1) Easily resolved
         a) *Intestinal parasitism (whipworms, roundworms, hookworms, strongyloides, coccidia, Giardia, Pentatrichomonas, entamoeba, balantidium, tapeworms)*
         b) *Dietary indiscretion (abrupt changes, overfeeding, garbage ingestion, ingestion of abrasive or indigestible material.*
         c) *Drug or toxin (NSAIDs, corticosteroids, antimicrobials, anthelmintics, heavy metals, insecticides, antineoplastic agents)*
      2) Life threatening
         a) *Parvoviral enteritis*
         b) *Hemorrhagic gastroenteritis (HGE)*
         c) *Any diarrhea associated with severe hemorrhage, dehydration, hypoproteinemia, endotoxemia, or acid–base/electrolyte abnormalities*
   c. Differentiate large bowel vs. small bowel diarrhea
      1) Large bowel–tenesmus, mucus, frank blood, increased frequency, small amounts, increased urgency
      2) Small bowel–weight loss, liquid, melena, increased fecal volume, steatorrhea, flatulence
      3) Diffuse disease (inflammatory bowel disease, lymphocytic–plasmocytic enterocolitis, eosinophilic enterocolitis, lymphosarcoma, histoplasmosis) may cause signs of both small and large bowel diarrhea.

2. Before in-depth diagnostics, a symptomatic approach is warranted.
   a. Rule out systemic disease with minimum database.
      1) Hemoconcentration ($\uparrow$PCV)—dehydration, HGE.
      2) Leukopenia—parvoviral enteritis, overwhelming sepsis, feline panleukopenia, endotoxemia

3) Hypoproteinemia—malabsorption, maldigestion, protein losing enteropathy

4) Anemia—GI blood loss, (RBC microcytosis–iron deficiency)

5) Thrombocytopenia—predominant clinical sign may be bloody diarrhea.

6) Azotemia—dehydration, renal disease, hypoadrenocorticism; ↑BUN/creatinine ratio with GI hemorrhage

7) Hyperkalemia/hyponatremia—hypoadrenocorticism, whipworms

8) Fecal examination—*Giardia, Coccidia,* hookworms, roundworms, whipworms, clostridia, trichomonads, campylobacter spp., salmonella spp.

9) Hyperthyroidism is a common cause of diarrhea in cats over 10. Palpate neck for thyroid nodules and check serum T4 levels.

b. Animals with bloody diarrhea, painful abdomen, dehydration, shock, weakness, collapse, or other signs of systemic disease should be hospitalized for further diagnostics and supportive care.

1) Intravenous fluid therapy, antibiotics, correct electrolyte and acid–base imbalances

2) Complete blood count, serum chemistries; urinalysis; electrolytes; blood gases; amylase and lipase; B_{12}, folate, trypsin-like immunoreactivity test (TLI); fecal examination

3) Abdominal radiographs, ultrasound, GI contrast studies

4) Exploratory surgery, GI biopsies, endoscopy

c. Symptomatic treatment for acute diarrhea

1) Withhold food for at least 24 hours to "rest" the GI tract; water free choice

2) When feeding is resumed, use a low-fat, high-carbohydrate diet fed in small amounts frequently. Commercial prescription diets can be used, or feed boiled rice, potatoes, or pasta combined with boiled skinless chicken, yogurt or low-fat cottage cheese

a) Cats may not require protein restriction or tolerate excessive carbohydrates. Use commercial feline diet

b) A low-fat, high-fiber diet may help to firm up the stool.

3) The regular diet can be gradually reintroduced after the diarrhea has resolved. If inflammatory bowel disease or dietary hypersensitivity is suspected, a dietary trial with a restricted diet is warranted.

4) For mild diarrhea, particularly in neonates that are not dehydrated, oral electrolyte solutions (Entrolyte, Beecham) can be used to balance GI losses.

5) Symptomatic treatment for giardiasis and trichuriasis is often warranted before pursuing invasive and expensive diagnostics because of intermittent shedding of parasites.

a) Metronidazole, 10–25 mg/kg PO BID × 8 days

b) Fenbendazole, 50 mg/kg PO SID × 3 days (repeat in 3 weeks and 3 months)

c) Repeated infestation with Trichuris can be eliminated by administering a monthly heartworm preventative that also prevents intestinal parasites.

6) *Clostridium perfringens* enterotoxin can cause stress-related large bowel diarrhea with blood, mucus, and foul odor.

a) Fecal ELISA for enterotoxin analysis (TechLabs, Blacksburg, VA) is positive.

b) Fecal cytology reveals large numbers of clostridial spores (>5/hpf oval structures with "safety pin" appearance).

c) Response to treatment is usually rapid (within 48 hours) with appropriate antibiotic therapy (ampicillin, amoxicillin, metronidazole, tylosin, clindamycin).

7) Symptomatic treatment of diarrhea may be warranted for short-term use but may mask ability to gauge response to treatment.

a) Opioids impede bowel transit time and reduce intestinal fluid loss by enhancing segmental contractions and decreasing peristalsis (probably the most effective symptomatic treatment for diarrhea).

   i) *Diphenoxylate (Lomotil), 0.1–0.2 mg/kg PO q8–12h (dog) or 0.05–0.1 mg/kg PO q12h (cat)*

   ii) *Loperamide (Imodium), 0.1 mg/kg q12h PO*

b) Antiprostaglandins have antiinflammatory, antisecretory effect

   i) *Bismuth subsalicylate (Pepto-Bismol), 0.25–2.0 mL/kg PO q6–8h (dog)*

   ii) *Sulfasalazine, 10–20 mg/kg PO q8h (dog)—for colitis. Use with caution in cats due to potential salicylate toxicity; 10 mg/kg PO q12–24h (cat).*

c) Antispasmodic agents may potentiate ileus by reducing gut motility, but may aid in decreasing urgency and discomfort of colitis.

    i) Aminopentamide (Centrine), 0.01–0.03 mg/kg IM, SC, PO q8–12h (dog); 0.1 mg/cat IM, SC, PO q8–12h (cat)

    ii) Isopropamide/prochlorperazine (Darbazine), 0.14–0.22 mg/kg SC q12h

I. Acute pancreatitis

1. Risk factors

a. Dog—middle age/older, obesity, disorders of lipid/triglyceride metabolism (diabetes mellitus, hyperadrenocorticism, hypothyroidism, familial hyperlipidemia), drugs (anticonvulsants, azathioprine, ±glucocorticoids), prior GI disease, breed (Yorkshire Terrier, Schnauzer, Miniature Poodle, Cocker Spaniel), hypercalcemia

b. Cat—trauma, infectious disease (e.g., toxoplasmosis), possibly concurrent liver disease (cholangiohepatitis, hepatic lipidosis) and/or inflammatory bowel disease. Siamese cats may be predisposed.

2. Clinical signs vary from mild localized inflammation responsive to supportive therapy to severe systemic inflammation leading to systemic inflammatory response syndrome and refractory shock.

a. Vomiting—common in dogs, but not in cats

b. Cranial abdominal pain—reluctant to move, arched posture (dogs)

c. Diarrhea—may be bloody

d. Cats—signs variable and vague, most often lethargy, anorexia, weight loss, dehydration, and hypothermia

3. Physical examination

a. Severe cases may present with signs of hypovolemic or septic shock (i.e., fever, dehydration, hypotension, collapse).

b. Abdomen is painful, tense, and distended—free fluid if peritonitis present.

c. Cranial abdominal mass effect in some cases is due to enlarged pancreas or adhesions.

d. Fever is common in dogs. Hypothermia or fever can be seen in cats.

e. Icterus is common in cats and occurs occasionally in dogs. Biliary stasis secondary to edema near the common bile duct or ascending

cholangitis can result in icterus as can hepatic lipidosis in cats.

f. Signs of DIC, petechial/ecchymotic hemorrhage, epistaxis, and rectal bleeding have been reported in severe cases.

4. Diagnosis: Currently no single test confirms the diagnosis of acute pancreatitis (other than biopsy).

a. Clinical signs and physical examination (vomiting and cranial abdominal pain) are highly suggestive in dogs.

b. History of recent ingestion of fatty food in some cases

c. Elevated amylase/lipase variable in dog and not useful in cat

    1) Normal amylase and lipase do not rule out pancreatitis.

    2) Amylase and lipase are elevated with renal disease.

    3) There is no correlation between the magnitude of enzyme increase and the severity of pancreatitis.

d. Increased trypsinlike immunoreactivity is more specific for pancreatitis, but normal levels do not rule it out.

    1) Prolonged turnaround time limits usefulness.

    2) Send to GI Lab, Texas A&M University, College Station, TX 77843

e. Other laboratory changes (nonspecific)

    1) PCV may be increased (dehydration) or decreased (coagulopathy, concurrent disease)

    2) WBC count is commonly increased with a left shift, but may be decreased with overwhelming infection/inflammation. Toxic neutrophils are common.

    3) Liver enzyme activities and bilirubin are high with concurrent hepatobiliary disease or biliary obstruction.

    4) Hypocalcemia secondary to saponification of peripancreatic fat occurs in some cases (up to 45% of cats).

    5) Hyperglycemia may occur because of concurrent diabetes mellitus or stress.

    6) Hypoglycemia (especially in cats) can be seen with sepsis or endotoxemia. Bacterial translocation is common in cats with pancreatitis because they have higher bacterial counts in the upper small intestine than dogs.

    7) Hypercholesterolemia/hypertriglyceridemia is found in 26–50% of dogs with acute pancreatitis.

8) Evidence of coagulopathy/DIC—low platelets, prolonged PT, PTT, ACT, increased fibrin degradation products, decreased AT III levels—occur in severe cases.

f. Radiographic signs—increased soft tissue density (mass effect) or loss of visceral detail in right cranial quadrant ("ground glass" appearance), displacement of gas-filled descending duodenum to right ("sentinel loop" sign), caudal displacement of transverse colon

1) Normal abdominal radiographs do not rule out disease.

2) Chest radiographs may reveal pleural effusion, aspiration pneumonia, or diffuse infiltrates (e.g., acute respiratory distress syndrome).

g. Ultrasonography

1) More sensitive than radiography

2) Nonhomogeneous hypoechoic mass in acute cases

3) Cyst or abscess formation may occur as sequela of previous episodes of pancreatitis

4) Useful for evaluating hepatobiliary structures

h. Abdominocentesis

1) Exudative fluid (protein >2.5; specific gravity >1.020) with nondegenerate neutrophils and no bacteria

2) High amylase plus lipase values >serum in abdominal fluid

5. Treatment

a. Restore fluid and electrolyte balance using isotonic crystalloid solutions (shock dose if indicated) supplemented with potassium to replace GI losses.

b. Nothing per os for 2–4 days or until vomiting has ceased for ~24 hours.

1) Attempt to feed cats a low-fat diet within 48 hours if possible. Prolonged anorexia in cats can lead to hepatic lipidosis.

2) Do not force the animal to eat if it is not interested in food.

c. Broad-spectrum antibiotics—some question use

1) Recommended if the animal is febrile or has a left shift and toxic neutrophils on the hemogram

2) Recommended in all cats with pancreatitis. Cats have a higher bacterial count in the duodenum than dogs, and bacterial translocation is common.

3) Used to prevent sepsis or pancreatic abscess formation

a) Enrofloxacin, 2.5–5 mg/kg IV, IM q12h

b) Trimethoprim-sulfa, 14 mg/kg SQ q12h

c) Cefazolin, 22 mg/kg IV q8h

d) Combination therapy for severe infections (e.g., enrofloxacin with ampicillin 22 mg/kg IV q8h)

d. Reintroduce water 1–2 days after vomiting has stopped, followed by a low-fat, moderate-protein diet (rice, pasta, boiled potatoes). Never force-feed if animal is not interested in eating as it may result in food aversion.

e. Additional therapy for severe cases

1) Fresh frozen plasma transfusion, 5–20 mL/kg IV through filtered line, or daily administration of 50–250 mL until improvement is noted, to replenish α_2-macroglobulin and other antiproteases

2) Dextran 70 or hetastarch, 4–6 mL/kg IV bolus during resuscitation, 20 mL/kg/day IV maximum to restore oncotic pressure and improve pancreatic microcirculation. Oxyglobin could also be used to improve oxygen delivery to the ischemic pancreas.

3) Antiemetics are indicated if vomiting is intractable.

a) Metoclopramide, 0.2–0.4 mg/kg IM or SC q8h or 1–2 mg/kg/24h as a constant rate infusion (CRI) with IV fluids

b) Chlorpromazine 0.5 mg/kg IM, SQ q6–8h

4) Analgesic therapy for severe abdominal pain

a) Butorphanol, 0.2–0.4 mg/kg IV, SQ, IM q4–8h

b) Oxymorphone or hydromorphone, 0.1–0.2 mg/kg IV, SQ, IM q4–8h

c) Epidural narcotic analgesia—see p. 52–53

5) Nutritional support

a) Partial parenteral nutrition (see Chapter 8) is indicated if oral feedings must be withheld beyond 3–4 days.

b) Total parenteral nutrition or jejunostomy tube feeding should be considered in severe cases with prolonged hospitalization beyond 1 week. Lipid content should be restricted

c) Enteral feeding can be given via nasoesophageal tube using low-fat diet in anorectic patients with no vomiting (cats).

6) Remove or correct inciting cause whenever possible.

7) Miscellaneous medical therapies

a) Selenium, 0.1 mg/kg IV q24h

b) Aprotinin (Trasylol, Bayer)—a protease inhibitor—250 mg by IP injection q6–8h

c) Heparin, 250 U/kg SQ q8h, to prevent DIC (controversial)

d) Oral pancreatic enzymes (Viokase) can be added to food to decrease pancreatic enzyme secretions via negative feedback.

8) Indications for surgery include the following:

a) Drainage of a pancreatic abscess

b) Lavage and drainage of septic peritonitis

c) Debridement of necrotic pancreatic tissue

d) Placement of a jejunal feeding tube

e) Obstruction of the common bile duct

9) Potential complications of severe pancreatitis include

a) Acute renal failure—maintain systolic blood pressure >80 mm Hg and mean blood pressure >60 mm Hg.

b) Diabetes mellitus—may need to treat with regular insulin drip (1–2 U/kg/24 h) to maintain glucose <250 mg/dL, especially if PPN or TPN are given.

c) DIC may occur because of vasculitis from circulating proteolytic enzymes. (Treat with plasma 10–20 mL/kg incubated with 75 U/kg heparin to activate antithrombin III.)

d) Acute respiratory distress syndrome may occur in severe cases when proteolytic enzymes and vasoactive substances damage alveolar membranes (monitor blood gases, respiration, and thoracic radiographs).

e) Cardiac arrhythmias (ventricular) have been reported. (Monitor ECG in severe cases.)

f) Pancreatic inflammation may cause bile duct obstruction.

  i) May require cholecystoduodenostomy

  ii) Vitamin K-responsive coagulopathy can occur because of inability to absorb fat-soluble vitamins. Vitamins A, D, E, and K can be given IM.

J. Hemorrhagic gastroenteritis (HGE)

1. Clinical signs

a. Caused by peracute loss of GI tract mucosal integrity, possibly due to immune-mediated reaction against mucosal elements; role of *Clostridium perfringens* is unclear

b. Typically affects small or toy breeds of middle age with no known garbage or toxin exposure. Most common breeds include Schnauzer, Dachshund, Yorkshire Terrier, and Miniature Poodle.

c. Acute vomiting is usually the first sign, with rapid progression to bloody diarrhea, dehydration, and hypovolemic shock.

d. Bloody diarrhea—raspberry jam appearance due to mucus and sloughed mucosal epithelium.

e. Bacterial translocation through the damaged mucosa may result in septic or endotoxic shock.

2. Diagnosis

a. History, signalment, and clinical signs

b. PCV ≥60 (as high as 80) with normal TS

c. Other laboratory findings and stool examination are negative for parasites but may show clostridial spores on fecal cytology. Glucometer reading may be falsely low because of hemoconcentration; serum blood glucose is usually in the normal range.

d. Dogs may be bright, alert, and not clinically dehydrated in the early stages of disease.

3. Treatment

a. Aggressive fluid therapy is required to normalize the hematocrit.

  1) Lactated Ringer's solution at 20–90 mL/kg in first hour, followed by 2–4 mL/kg/h until the PCV is ~50%

  2) KCl 20–40 mEq/L should be added to the fluids once the patient has been rehydrated or treated for shock.

  3) Serial assessment of PCV/TS and electrolytes is necessary to guide fluid therapy.

b. Broad-spectrum antibiotics

  1) Ampicillin 22 mg/kg IV q8, plus

  2) Enrofloxacin 5 mg/kg IV or IM q12h

c. Nothing per os until vomiting resolves; then gradual reintroduction of water followed by bland diet

d. Recovery usually complete after 2–4 days of supportive care. Relapses can occur.

K. Gastric dilatation—volvulus

1. Etiology unclear

a. Delayed gastric emptying of solid particles possibly associated with abnormal electrical activity of gastric smooth muscle

b. Increased length/laxity of hepatoduodenal and hepatogastric ligaments allows dynamic movement of the stomach following ingestion of food or water or aerophagia.

c. Possible risk factors include large/giant breed, deep narrow chest conformation, single meal/day feeding schedule, nervous fearful demeanor, rapid ingestion of food accompanied by aerophagia, exercise after ingesting large amount of food or water.

d. Small-breed dogs and cats can be affected (rare). Common breeds include German Shepherds, Great Danes, St. Bernards, Rottweilers, Labrador Retrievers, Alaskan Malamutes, Doberman Pinchers, Irish Setters.

2. Pathophysiology

a. Gastric distention (alone or resulting from malposition) results in decreased venous return to the heart because of compression of the caudal vena cava and portal vein.

   1) Gastric distention is caused by swallowed air, fluid, or food.

   2) Volvulus occurs when the distended stomach twists on its long axis and occludes the esophageal hiatus and pylorus, thereby trapping the stomach contents.

   3) Clockwise rotation (as viewed from caudal to cranial with the dog in dorsal recumbency) is most common.

      a) Less or more rotation (up to 360°) can occur.

      b) The pylorus and duodenum are displaced ventrally and toward the left side, across the midline and ending dorsal to the cardia on the left side.

   4) The spleen commonly rotates with the stomach (attached by gastrosplenic ligaments) to the right ventral abdomen.

      a) Congestion and splenomegaly are common.

      b) Splenic infarction or thrombosis may occur.

      c) Serious complications include splenic torsion or avulsion of splenic vessels.

   5) Increased gastric wall pressure causes ischemia to the gastric mucosa. Infarction and necrosis may result, especially along the greater curvature of the stomach.

   6) The distended tympanic stomach, in addition to impairing venous return to the heart, causes congestion of the splanchnic vessels, which may result in breakdown of the gut mucosal barrier, bacterial translocation, activation of systemic inflammatory mediators, and DIC.

3. Diagnosis

a. Clinical signs

   1) Large, deep-chested dog with distended, tympanic abdomen and an acute history of nonproductive retching is the classic common presentation. Ptyalism with thick, ropey saliva is also common. Abdominal distention may be minimal initially because the stomach is hidden by the ribs.

   2) Shock—tachycardia, hypotension, prolonged capillary refill time. Mucous membranes may be blue-gray with profound hypoperfusion/hypotension or sepsis. They may be hyperemic with early shock.

   3) Hypersalivation and agitation due to abdominal pain may be present in some patients.

   4) Vague signs of lethargy and anorexia may be the only presenting complaints.

b. Abdominal radiographs are indicated to differentiate between gastric dilation volvulus (GDV) and gastric distension without torsion (*Figs. 11-3 and 11-4*).

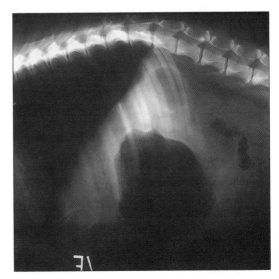

FIGURE 11.3 Left lateral view of a dog with gastric dilation volvulus reveals severe distension but no evidence of torsion.

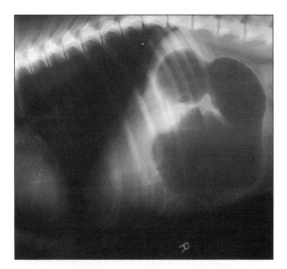

FIGURE 11.4   Right lateral radiograph of the same dog reveals the classic "Popeye arm" seen in dogs with gastric dilation volvulus when both the fundus and pylorus are distended with air. The right lateral view is preferred for diagnosing GDV.

1) GDV—Right lateral view reveals classic "double bubble" gas pattern with compartmentalization signs. A soft tissue fold can be seen separating the displaced pylorus from the distended fundus with volvulus.

2) Gastric dilation—The stomach is distended with air and may occupy nearly the entire abdominal cavity.

3) VD or DV projection reveals distended pylorus to the left of midline.

4) The position of the fundus can be confirmed if necessary by outlining rugal folds with 10–20 mL of barium.

5) Free air in abdominal cavity (most readily seen between the liver and diaphragm) indicates stomach rupture.

4. Treatment

a. Obtain emergency database (PCV/TS, glucose, BUN, blood gases, electrolytes, platelet count, activated clotting time).

b. Treat hypovolemic shock.

1) Shock and circulatory compromise should be treated immediately, before decompression is attempted and before diagnostic tests (e.g., radiographs) are performed.

2) Lactated Ringer's solution or other isotonic crystalloid at 90 mL/kg/h during first hour using two large-bore peripheral catheters in forelimbs only (Rear limb infusion is ineffective because of compromised venous return to the heart.)

a) *Subsequent volume to be administered is determined by response: use CVP, PCV/TS, BP, and urine volume to assess perfusion.*

b) *Potassium (20–40 mEq/L) or dextrose (2.5–5%) may need to be added to subsequent fluids once the shock has been treated.*

3) Hypertonic saline (7% NaCl in 6% dextran) or hetastarch (4–6 mL/kg IV over 5–10 min) can be used to rapidly restore intravascular volume in critical patients. It should be followed with 10–30 mL/kg crystalloid fluids.

4) Dexamethasone sodium phosphate 4 mg/kg IV or prednisolone sodium succinate 15–30 mg/kg IV can be considered to stabilize membranes, treat endotoxemia, improve cardiovascular stability, and prevent reperfusion injury, but the use of corticosteroids is controversial and generally avoided by the authors (see pp. 29–33).

c. Gastric decompression

1) Should not be attempted until after fluid therapy has begun

2) Pass well-lubricated, premeasured (from nose to last rib) and marked orogastric tube.

a) *Oxymorphone or hydromorphone, 0.1–0.2 mg/kg IV, and diazepam, 0.1 mg/kg IV, can be given if sedation is necessary.*

b) *Change animal's position (side to side, sitting) or gently rotate the tube if necessary to facilitate passage.*

c) *Avoid excessive force to reduce risk of perforation.*

d) *Multiple warm water gastric lavage infusions (20–50 mL/kg) can be administered to fully evacuate the stomach once the tube is passed.*

3) Gastrocentesis (trocarization) can be used if the patient is critical and the orogastric tube cannot be passed.

a) *Clip and aseptically prepare an area behind the last rib on the right side.*

b) *Confirm the location by ausculting a "ping" and avoid the spleen*

c) *Use a 16- to 18-gauge needle as a trocar.*

d) *An orogastric tube can usually be passed after decompression has been achieved.*

d. Surgery

1) Ideally performed as soon as patient is hemodynamically stable. Stabilization is usually achieved within 2–4 hours.

2) Prompt surgery may minimize gastric necrosis and/or splenic congestion/thrombosis.

3) Gastric decompression can be maintained using a nasogastric tube if surgery is delayed.

4) Incisional gastropexy or belt loop gastropexy are the most commonly performed procedures.

  a) *For incisional gastropexy, incisions are made in the right abdominal wall and gastric antrum and are sutured together.*

  b) *For the belt-loop gastropexy, a tongue-shaped flap is created in the gastric mucosa of the antrum and passed under two slits in the transversus abdominus muscle on the right body wall before reattaching the flap to the antrum.*

  c) *Gastropexy reduces recurrence rates from as high as 80% to as low as 3–5%.*

5) Resection of necrotic stomach may be necessary.

  a) *The most common area of the stomach affected is the greater curvature and gastric fundus.*

  b) *Blue-gray, black, or greenish appearance, lack of fresh blood when cut, and lack of peristalsis are indications for resection.*

  c) *Dark red serosa is usually reversible. Suspicious areas can be evaluated after the stomach is repositioned.*

  d) *A partial gastrectomy can be performed rapidly using a stapling device to remove necrotic devitalized areas of the stomach.*

  e) *An inverting suture pattern can be used to invaginate devitalized tissue if the area is not extensive and time is a factor.*

6) Splenectomy should be performed if perfusion does not return after the stomach is decompressed and repositioned. Splenic necrosis results from vessel infarction or avulsion. Partial or total splenectomy may be required.

e. Postoperative care

1) Identify and treat life-threatening complications.

2) ECG—Ventricular arrhythmias are common, especially 12–36 hours postoperatively, and are treated with lidocaine 2% 2–4 mg/kg IV bolus, then 50–75 μg/kg/min by CRI when indicated.

  a) *Indications for treatment of ventricular arrhythmias include*

    i) *Clinical signs associated with decreased cardiac output*

    ii) *More than 20–30 ventricular premature contractons (VPCs) per min*

    iii) *Multifocal/multiform VPCs*

    iv) *R on T phenomenon*

    v) *Failure to resolve with correction of acid–base or electrolyte abnormalities or hypoxic conditions*

  b) *Arrhythmias usually resolve within 72 hours.*

3) Broad-spectrum antibiotics are indicated if sepsis is suspected or the gut mucosal barrier is compromised.

  a) *Cefoxitin. 30 mg/kg IV q6–8h or*

  b) *Cefazolin (22 mg/kg IV q8h) plus enrofloxacin (5 mg/kg IV q12h).*

4) Vital signs and blood pressure are monitored q1–4h immediately postoperatively.

5) PCV, TS, electrolytes, and acid–base status should be determined 1–4 times daily until the animal is stable.

6) Blood glucose concentration, BUN/creatinine, platelet count, ACT, PCV/TS are monitored to permit early detection of complications such as sepsis, oliguria (usually due to inadequate fluid therapy), or DIC.

7) Provide analgesia

  a) *Butorphanol, 0.2–0.4 mg/kg SQ, IM, or IV q4–6h*

  b) *Oxymorphone, 0.1–0.2 mg/kg IV q4–6 h*

8) Food and water are introduced 12–24 h postsurgery. Delay refeeding for 1–2 days if gastric resection is performed.

L. Acute stomatitis/oral ulcers

1. Clinical signs

  a. Dysphagia—may drop food from mouth

  b. Reluctance to eat—may show interest in food but pain prevents eating

  c. Ptyalism, blood-tinged saliva, pawing at mouth, and complete anorexia in severe cases

  d. More common in cats (calicivirus, eosinophilic granuloma complex (EGC), lymphocytic–plasmacytic stomatitis) than dogs (immune-mediated most common)

2. Diagnosis
   a. Consider electrical cord burn, ingestion of caustic substance, linear foreign body around base of tongue, or ingestion of irritating plant material as possible underlying causes.
   b. Lesions vary from superficial erosions to deep ulcers.
   c. Gingival hyperplasia may be present.
   d. Lesions are located on the gingival mucosa, buccal mucosa, glossopalatine arch (faucitis), pharynx, or hard palate.
   e. Sedation or general anesthesia may be required if pain prevents thorough oropharyngeal examination.
   f. Biopsy helps differentiate eosinophilic granuloma complex (EGC), lymphocytic/plasmacytic stomatitis, squamous cell carcinoma, lymphosarcoma, or immune-mediated disease.
   g. CBC is usually unremarkable but may reveal absolute eosinophilia in cats with EGC.
   h. Biochemical profile may reveal hyperglobulinemia in dogs with immune-mediated disease, cats with lymphocytic–plasmacytic stomatitis, or uremia in animals with renal failure.
   i. Proteinuria with high protein/creatinine ratio suggests immune-mediated disease with glomerulonephritis.
   j. Feline leukemia virus (FeLV) and feline immunodeficiency virus (FIV) serology may indicate an underlying immunosuppressive disorder.
   k. Dental radiographs are taken in cats to identify alveolar bone loss, root lesions, or incomplete root extractions.

3. Treatment
   a. Identify and correct underlying disease (e.g., uremia).
   b. Antibiotics with good anaerobic activity
      1) Clavamox, 12.5–25 mg/kg PO q12h
      2) Clindamycin—dog, 11mg/kg PO q12h; cat, 5.5 mg/kg q12h
      3) Metronidazole, 10–15 mg/kg q12h
   c. Corticosteroids—primarily cats with EGC or lymphocytic–plasmacytic stomatitis and dogs with immune–mediated or idiopathic stomatitis
      1) Cat—methylprednisolone acetate, 10–20 mg/cat IM q3–6 weeks; oral prednisone is less effective.
      2) Dog—prednisone 2–4 mg/kg/day PO for 2–3 weeks, then taper dose
   d. Other immunosuppressive drugs may be considered in refractory cases.
      1) Azathioprine, 0.3 mg/kg PO q48h, cats; 1–2 mg/kg q24–48h, dogs
      2) Chlorambucil, 0.25–0.33 mg/kg PO q72h, cats; 1–2 mg/m² PO q48 h, dogs
   e. Gold salts, aurothioglucose, may have beneficial immunosuppressive properties but are not commonly used (1 mg/kg IM weekly for 10–20 weeks, then monthly).
   f. Dental care—scaling/polishing, periodontal treatment, or extraction—is useful in cats with stomatitis.
      1) Extracting all teeth may be necessary and is well tolerated.
      2) Used as a last resort in cats with recurrent, nonresponsive disease. Removes the source of chronic antigenic stimulation.

M. Large bowel diarrhea—colitis

1. Clinical signs
   a. Tenesmus, mucus, frank blood, increased frequency, small amounts
   b. Causes include diet (e.g., indiscretion, allergy), parasites, bacteria or bacterial toxins (e.g., *Clostridium* spp.), and viral infection.
   c. Acute colitis is usually self-limiting and not associated with signs of systemic illness. Anorexia and lethargy are seen in severe cases.
   d. Vomiting may precede diarrhea with dietary indiscretion or toxin ingestion.

2. Diagnosis
   a. Clinical signs and history
   b. Physical examination usually normal—abdominal pain in severe cases
   c. Rectal examination may reveal mucus, fresh blood, little or no stool, and pain.
   d. Fecal examination
      1) Flotation/direct smear—whipworms, *Giardia*
      2) Stained fecal smear—clostridial spores, >3–5/oil immersion field (look like "safety pins")
      3) Serial examinations may be necessary.
   e. Further diagnostics (i.e., laboratory work, radiographs, fecal culture) are reserved for severe or refractory cases.
   f. Definitive diagnosis is by colonic biopsy.

3. Treatment
   a. Withhold food for 12–24 hours. Not necessary to withhold water
   b. High-fiber diet
     1) Commercial diets—w/d, r/d (Hills)
     2) Add psyllium (Metamucil) 1–4 tsp/meal, wheat bran 1–2 tbsp/meal, or pumpkin pie filling 1–4 tbsp/meal
     3) Chronic inflammatory colitis may improve with a hypoallergenic diet.
   c. Antibiotics
     1) Tylosin, 10–15 mg/kg PO q12h × 7 days)—*Clostridium, Campylobacter* spp.
     2) Amoxicillin, 22 mg/kg PO q12h—*Clostridium* spp.
     3) Metronidazole 10–15 mg/kg PO q12 h—inconsistent against *Clostridium* spp.
   d. Sulfasalazine—dog, 25–40 mg/kg PO q8–12h for 2–4 weeks; cat, 5–10 mg/kg q24h for 2 weeks
     1) Reserve for chronic cases
     2) Consider immunosuppressive drugs (prednisone and azathioprine) for eosinophilic colitis or lymphocytic–plasmacytic colitis nonresponsive to sulfasalazine.
   e. Antiparasitic drugs
     1) *Trichuris, Ancylostoma, Giardia*—fenbendazole (50 mg/kg PO q24h × 3 days; repeat in 3 months)
     2) *Giardia, Entamoeba, Balantidium, Trichomonas*—metronidazole (25 mg/kg PO q12h × 5–7 days)

N. Constipation/obstipation/megacolon

1. Definitions
   a. Constipation—difficult defecation, stool retention in colon
   b. Obstipation—severe, prolonged constipation with inability to defecate
   c. Megacolon—dilation/hypomotility of large bowel because of chronic constipation/obstipation

2. Clinical signs
   a. Tenesmus
   b. Small amount of liquid stool may pass around impaction. Owners may present pet for diarrhea.
   c. Idiopathic megacolon in cats is the most common presentation (middle-aged to older cats). Abnormal colonic smooth muscle function is the probable cause.

   d. Other causes in dogs and cats—dietary (hair, bones, plant material), colorectal neoplasia/polyp, painful defecation (perineal fistula, anal sac abscess), neurologic disease (dysautonomia, spinal cord disease, sacral nerve trauma), pelvic fracture, dehydration (chronic renal disease), prostatomegaly, perineal hernia, and rectal or colonic strictures.

3. Diagnosis
   a. Abdominal palpation may reveal a distended abdomen with firm stool in the colon.
   b. Digital rectal examination: Look for foreign material, perineal hernia, prostatomegaly, etc.
   c. Neurologic examination: Lower motor neuron signs of rear limbs, anus, or perineum may be present indicating spinal cord or sacral nerve involvement.
   d. Abdominal radiographs—colon distended with feces, foreign material. Evaluate for pelvic canal stenosis due to prior fracture, prostatomegaly, sublumbar lymphadenopathy, or other abnormality.

4. Treatment
   a. Constipation
     1) Rehydrate if necessary—balanced electrolyte solution IV
     2) Warm water enema—repeat as necessary
     3) Use low-residue diet in most patients. Addition of Metamucil or pumpkin pie filler may improve colonic function.
     4) Lactulose, 1 mL/4.5 kg PO q8–12h, can be used as a stool softener.
     5) If available, cisapride improves colonic motility—dogs, 0.1–0.5 mg/kg PO q8–12h; cats, 2.5–10 mg q8–12h
     6) Identify and correct underlying disease
     7) Docusate sodium can be used as a stool softener instead of lactulose. Hairball laxatives are usually ineffective.
   b. Obstipation
     1) Digital evacuation under general anesthesia. Use gloved finger to break up hard impactions.
     2) Repeated procedures may be necessary using warm water enemas and water-soluble K-Y jelly.
     3) Gentle manipulation to avoid tearing friable colon
     4) Hospitalize for 12–24 hours for rehydration prior to deobstipation.

5) Fiber and lactulose are indicated as with constipation.

  c. Megacolon

    1) Treat constipation or obstipation as necessary.

    2) Subtotal colectomy if medical management fails

    3) Lifelong lactulose postsurgery

O. Acute hepatic failure

1. Etiology—see *Table 11-1*

  a. Toxin exposure and infectious disease are the most common causes in the dog and cat.

  b. The inciting cause may not be evident at the time of presentation.

  c. Hepatic necrosis is a common result regardless of cause.

  d. The large functional reserve and regenerative capacity of the liver improve the chance of full recovery if the animal survives the acute stage.

  e. Prior liver disease increases the likelihood of permanent and/or progressive liver damage.

2. Clinical signs

  a. Anorexia, vomiting, icterus, diarrhea, and lethargy are common clinical signs.

  b. Onset of signs is usually rapid.

  c. Weight loss, chronic vomiting, or diarrhea suggest prior illness.

  d. Dehydration due to vomiting, diarrhea, and anorexia may be severe.

  e. Shock, hypovolemic and/or septic in critical patients, may be associated with acute liver failure.

  f. Epistaxis, petechiae/ecchymoses, and bloody diarrhea may indicate a coagulopathy or DIC.

  g. Altered mentation, stupor/coma, or seizures are seen with hepatic encephalopathy.

TABLE 11.1
ACUTE HEPATITIS

Toxins	**Infectious Disease**
Drugs/anesthetics	Bacterial
Acetaminophen	Abscess
Carprofen	Cholangiohepatitis—acute, suppurative
Diazepam (cat)	Leptospirosis
Diethylcarbamazine-oxibendazole	Sepsis/bacteremia
Glipizide (cat)	Viral
Griseofulvin (cat)	Infectious canine hepatitis
Halothane	Feline infectious peritonitis
Imidocarb diprorionate (dog)	Fungal/protozoal/parasitic
Ketoconazole	Toxoplasmosis
Mebendazole (dog)	Systemic fungal infections
Methimazole	Heartworm—caval syndrome
Methoxyflurane	
Tetracycline	**Metabolic disorder**
Thiacetarsamide (dog)	Acute pancreatitis
Trimethoprim-sulfadiazine (dog)	Hepatic lipidosis
Plants/chemicals	
Aflatoxin	**Trauma,** other
Amanita spp. (mushroom)	Hit by car
Blue-green algae	Heatstroke
Cycad palm seed	Liver lobe torsion
Chinaberry tree	
Heavy metals, solvents	
Pennyroyal oil	

3. Diagnosis
   a. History and clinical signs: Question owner regarding toxin exposure, mushroom (*Amanita* spp.) ingestion, medications (e.g., carprofen, phenobarbital), and over-the-counter drugs (e.g., acetaminophen).
   b. Laboratory findings
   1) Dramatic increases in serum alanine aminotresterase (ALT), alkaline phosphatase (ALP), and gamma-glutanyl transferase (GGT). GGT may be normal or only mildly increased in cats with lipidosis and acute hepatic failure.
   2) Hyperbilirubinemia
   3) Elevated fasting and postprandial bile acids
   4) Hyperammonemia
   5) Hypoglycemia common—impaired gluconeogenesis, glycogen depletion, sepsis
   6) Anemia—hemorrhage, coagulopathy, DIC
   7) Electrolyte changes—Hypokalemia is common in liver disease; hyponatremia reflects GI loss; hyperaldosteronism can result in hypernatremia and hypokalemia.
   8) WBC may be high (stress), have a left shift (infection) or be low (overwhelming sepsis).
   c. Coagulation assessment
   1) Coagulation abnormalities (prolonged PT, PTT, ACT) can occur with liver dysfunction and/or DIC.
   2) Mild-to-moderate thrombocytopenia can occur with peripheral consumption due to hemorrhage or DIC. Leptospirosis also commonly results in thrombocytopenia.
   3) High FDPs, D-dimer, or low AT III are consistent with DIC. FDPs may be high because of impaired hepatic clearance.
   d. Abdominal radiographs are usually normal with acute liver disease.
   1) Mild hepatomegaly is possible.
   2) Microhepatia suggests chronic disease (fibrosis) or portosystemic shunt.
   3) Ascites or hemorrhage result in loss of abdominal detail.
   4) Intrahepatic gas suggests a possible infarction (abscessation with clostridial overgrowth).
   e. Abdominal ultrasound
   1) Generalized hypoechogenicity with diffuse necrosis
   2) Hyperechogenicity is seen in cats with hepatic lipidosis.
   3) A mixed pattern is consistent with chronic disease—fibrosis, neoplasia, cholangiohepatitis.

4. Treatment
   a. Immediate restoration of intravascular volume—crystalloids, colloids if necessary (hypoproteinemia, ascites)
   1) Fluids with acetate (not lactate) buffer preferred, e.g., Plasmalyte, Normosol-R
   b. Supplement potassium—14–40 mEq KCl/L
   c. Correct hypoglycemia
   1) Bolus 50% dextrose, 0.5–1.0 mL/kg IV, dilute 1:4 if given through peripheral vein
   2) Add 2.5–5.0% dextrose to IV fluids
   3) Monitor BG q4–12h
   d. Broad-spectrum combination antibiotic therapy
   1) Amikacin (30 mg/kg IV q24h), gentamicin (6 mg/kg IV q24h), or enrofloxacin (2.5–5 mg/kg q12–24h)with
   2) Ampicillin (22 mg/kg IV q8h) or cefazolin (22 mg/kg q8h IV)
   e. Packed RBC, fresh whole blood, or FFP if anemia or coagulopathy; heparin 150–250 units/kg SQ q8h for DIC—contraindicated in bleeding patients (controversial)
   f. Nutritional support if anorexia for >2–3 days
   1) Clinicare (Pet Ag) or Peptamen (Baxter) via nasoesophageal tube initially
   2) More permanent esophagostomy, gastrostomy or jejunostomy (if vomiting) if support needed beyond 4–7 days of NE feeding
   g. Remove inciting cause, discontinue potential toxic medication, or give antidote when possible.
   1) Acetaminophen toxicity—N-acetylcysteine, vitamin C, cimetidine (see p. 387)
   2) Penicillin G, 1×10^6 units/kg IV infusion on 2 subsequent days (based on human recommendation), is a possible antidote for *Amanita* spp. ingestion.
   3) Leptospirosis—Treat with penicillin, 40,000 U/kg IM or IV, or ampicillin, 20 mg/kg IV, to clear leptospiremia (see pp. 242–243).

P. Hepatic encephalopathy (HE)

1. Etiology
   a. Neurologic signs are due to impaired hepatic clearance of products of protein or bacterial metabolism from the GI tract.

b. Putative toxins include ammonia, altered neurotransmitters (e.g., γ-aminobutyric acid (GABA), glutamate, serotonin), mercaptans, phenols, short-chain fatty acids, bile salts, and possibly increased benzodiazepine receptors or sensitivity. The concentration of aromatic amino acids increases, while branched chain-amino acids decrease, allowing the generation of false neurotransmitters.

c. Portosystemic shunts (PSS), cirrhosis/fibrosis, and (less commonly) fulminant acute liver failure may result in HE.

2. Clinical signs

    a. Neurologic

        1) Dog—depression, stupor, coma

        2) Cat—more likely to exhibit aggression or seizures

        3) Both—blindness, ataxia

    b. Hypersalivation and discolored iris (copper) in cats

    c. Stunted growth is seen in animals with congenital portosystemic shunts.

    d. Vomiting, diarrhea, anorexia may mimic GI disease.

    e. Enlarged symmetrical kidneys are sometimes seen as a result of portal hypertension. Trophic factors, such as insulin-like growth factor, are not cleared by the abnormal liver.

    f. Pu/Pd more common in dogs than cats

    g. Lower urinary tract signs—stranguria, pollakiuria, hematuria—can occur with urate urolithiasis. Ammonium urate stones can be formed when there is severe liver disease such as cirrhosis or portosystemic shunt.

    h. Hemorrhage and coagulopathy are most common with fulminant acute liver failure.

3. Diagnosis

    a. Clinical signs and history

    b. Neurologic signs may be worse after meals.

    c. High resting NH_3. Ammonia tolerance test is contraindicated if there are neurologic signs.

    d. Increased pre- and especially postprandial bile acids

    e. Abnormal liver function on chemistry panel as evidenced by hypoalbuminemia, low BUN, hypocholesterolemia, ± hypoglycemia. Hyperbilirubinemia is uncommon.

    f. Anemia with microcytosis is common with portosystemic shunt because of altered iron metabolism.

    g. Abdominal radiographs

        1) Microhepatia is seen with PSS or cirrhosis.

        2) Ascites is rare with PSS. It may occur if there is hypoalbuminemia or portal hypertension (fibrosis).

    h. Ultrasonography may reveal small liver, vascular anomaly, or changes due to fibrosis, etc.

    i. Coagulation abnormalities or evidence of DIC may include prolonged PT, PTT, with increased FDPs. Schistocytes and thrombocytopenia are present with DIC.

4. Treatment

    a. The primary goals are to maintain fluid and electrolyte balance, prevent absorption and production of gut-derived neurotoxins, and prevent or treat complications known to exacerbate HE.

    b. Fluid and electrolyte balance

        1) Crystalloids with an acetate buffer (Normosol, Plasmalyte) are administered at a rate and volume to restore and maintain intravascular volume. If alkalosis is present, the fluid of choice is 0.9% NaCl. If hypoglycemia, hypernatremia, or ascites is present, the fluid of choice is 2.5% dextrose in 0.45% saline.

        2) Colloids are indicated if hypoalbuminemia is present.

        3) Packed RBCs, fresh whole blood, or fresh frozen plasma is given as indicated for anemia or coagulopathy. Avoid stored blood because of high NH_3 levels.

        4) Supplement potassium—12–40 mEq/L as needed. Hypokalemia increases renal production of NH_3 and transfer of nonionized NH_3 (via alkalosis) across the blood–brain barrier

    c. Decreased absorption or production of gut-derived neurotoxins

        1) Lactulose causes an osmotic diarrhea, acidifies the colon by decreasing the absorption of NH_4^+, and provides a nonprotein substrate for bacterial metabolism.

        a) Retention enema causes a rapid improvement in neurologic signs.

          i) *Dilute lactulose 1:3 with water and instill 5–10 mL/kg as high in colon as possible using a Foley catheter. Can add neomycin (22 mg/kg).*

          ii) *Dwell time: 15–20 min*

          iii) *Repeat q6h as needed.*

        b) Oral lactulose is used for stable patients or maintenance.

i) *1–2 mL/10kg PO q12h*

ii) *The dose should be titrated to achieve a semiformed stool. (Overdose causes diarrhea.)*

2) Antibiotics with activity against colonic anaerobes help to lower ammonia production by colonic bacteria.

a) Ampicillin, amoxicillin, 10 mg/kg q12h PO

b) Metronidazole, 7.5 mg/kg q8h PO

c) Neomycin, 10–20 mg/kg q8–12h PO or per rectum

d. Precipitating factors

1) Avoid alkalosis and hypokalemia (see above) and coagulopathy.

2) GI hemorrhage should be treated because digested blood proteins exacerbate hyperammonemia.

a) GI ulceration is common because of elevated gastrin/histamine levels in patients with liver failure.

b) H$_2$ blockers (famotidine, ranitidine), omeprazole, misoprostol, and/or Carafate are indicated to prevent or treat GI ulceration.

c) Avoid NSAIDs and corticosteroids because they can cause GI bleeding.

3) Constipation increases the absorption of toxins. Lactulose usually controls it, but fiber and enemas can be added if necessary.

4) Avoid methionine (common in supplements, "liver pills"). It is metabolized to mercaptans, which are synergistic with ammonia in causing hepatoencephalopathy.

e. A high-quality protein-restricted diet is recommended, with carbohydrates as the main source of calories. Commercial diets or home-cooked recipes are available.

1) Vitamin supplements (without methionine) are recommended because of impaired absorption and metabolism.

2) Consider arginine (250 mg PO q12h) and carnitine (250 mg PO q12h) in cats with HE secondary to hepatic lipidosis.

f. Seizure control: Patients with HE may have increased sensitivity to barbiturates and benzodiazepines via increased GABA receptor sensitivity.

1) Decrease dose 25–50% and titrate to effect.

2) Lactulose enemas may prevent further seizures.

3) Monitor blood glucose.

4) Propofol may control seizures.

5) Give KBr in rare instances when maintenance anticonvulsant treatment is necessary.

Q. Rectal prolapse

1. Clinical signs

a. An everted tubular portion of rectum is seen protruding through the anus.

b. Tenesmus is the primary sign.

c. Rectal prolapse is most common in animals <4 months of age associated with inflammation caused by endoparasites.

d. It can occur at any age in association with colonic neoplasia, cystitis, perineal hernia, urolithiasis, constipation, dystocia, prostatitis, or foreign body.

e. Manx cats may be predisposed.

2. Diagnosis

a. Typical clinical signs—hyperemic, edematous, necrotic (if chronic) tubular structure protruding from the anus with tenesmus

b. Must differentiate from prolapsed intussusception

1) Lubricated blunt probe or thermometer cannot be advanced between rectal wall and prolapsed tissue with rectal prolapse; it will contact the fornix. If the probe passes easily, a prolapsed intussusception should be suspected.

2) Signs of GI obstruction (vomiting, anorexia) may occur with prolapsed intussusception.

3. Treatment

a. Replace prolapsed tissue. Animals with mild cases exhibit hyperemic, edematous tissue that bleeds easily.

1) Lavage with warm isotonic fluids.

2) Lubricate and gently massage tissue until reduced. If extreme edema makes reduction impossible, 50% dextrose solution can be applied to reduce edema.

3) Apply loose purse string suture in anus. This can be tightened around a syringe barrel to allow an opening for the passage of stool.

4) Feed low-residue diet and give stool softener (Lactulose, 1 mL/4–5 kg q8–12h to effect, or docusate sodium—cat, 50 mg PO q12–24h; dog, 50–200 mg PO q8–12h).

5) Identify and correct underlying cause.

6) Remove purse string in 10–14 days.

7) Continue stool softener for an additional 2–3 weeks.

b. Resection and anastomosis are required in severe cases with necrotic/devitalized tissue. Nonviable tissue is purple to black, is ulcerated, and exhibits dark, cyanotic blood on cut surface.

c. A colopexy is performed if prolapse recurs; 4–5 mattress sutures using nonabsorbable suture material are used to anchor the descending colon to the left body wall, with slight cranial traction to prevent future recurrences.

R. Intussusception

1. Etiology and clinical signs

a. It is due to invagination ("telescoping") of a segment of bowel into an adjacent segment.

b. It results in complete or partial bowel obstruction.

c. The ileocolic junction is the most common location.

d. It occurs primarily in animals less than 1 year old.

e. It is more common in dogs than cats.

f. Clinical signs vary with location. High intussusceptions have an acute onset of vomiting, abdominal discomfort, and collapse. Low intussusceptions have a more chronic presentation including weight loss, bloody or mucoid diarrhea, scanty stool, and tenesmus.

g. Occasionally, ileocolic intussusception protrudes through the anus.

h. Predisposing factors include endoparasites, gastroenteritis (viral, other), linear foreign body, intestinal surgery, tumors, and adhesions.

1) Signs may be intermittent and/or mild, especially with low or "sliding" intussusceptions.

2) Vomiting, diarrhea, abdominal pain, lethargy, and anorexia are common.

i. Gastroesophageal intussusception occurs most commonly in German Shepherd dogs.

2. Diagnosis

a. A tubular segment of bowel is present on abdominal palpation.

b. Palpation may be normal with an intermittent or "sliding" intussusception.

c. Abdominal radiographs may reveal a tubular soft tissue density, an obstructive pattern, or no abnormalities.

d. Ultrasonography reveals a classic multiple concentric ring pattern on the cross-sectional view. This is highly specific for intussusception.

e. Barium upper GI series (obstructive pattern) or enema (colonic filling defect with ileocolic intussusception) may aid in diagnosis by outlining the intussusception, but may delay therapy.

f. Gastroesophageal intussusception can be identified on thoracic radiographs by viewing a tissue-dense mass in the caudal aspect of an air-filled, dilated esophagus. Endoscopy is also diagnostic.

3. Treatment

a. Surgical reduction of intussusception should be followed by bowel plication to prevent recurrence.

b. Resection and anastomosis are recommended if reduction is not possible or if the bowel segment is nonviable. Viability is assessed by color, pulsation, intestinal contractions, or demonstration of fluorescence with a Wood's lamp following IV injection of fluorescein dye.

c. Deworming and other treatment for any underlying disease may help prevent recurrence; 20–30% of patients that do not receive enteroplication exhibit recurrence within 2–3 days.

d. Gastroesophageal intussusception is treated by performing a gastropexy of the fundus to the left abdominal wall following reduction.

S. Intestinal volvulus

1. Description/predisposing factors

a. Rotation of intestine at mesenteric root causing occlusion of cranial mesenteric artery

b. Results in ischemic necrosis of bowel from distal duodenum to proximal descending colon

c. German Shepherd, medium-to-giant breeds, and male dogs are predisposed; it is rare in cats.

d. Colonic and cecocolic volvulus are less common.

e. The etiology is unknown. The roles of diet, activity in relation to eating, prior or current GI disease, exocrine pancreatic insufficiency, and trauma are unclear.

2. Clinical signs
   a. Acute to peracute onset of vomiting, hematochezia, abdominal pain/distention
   b. Hypovolemic or septic shock occur rapidly.
   c. Tenesmus and lack of feces occur with ceco-colic volvulus.
   d. Weight loss or chronic vomiting and diarrhea may precede the acute signs and reflect concurrent disease (e.g., IBD).

3. Diagnosis
   a. Acute onset of severe GI signs—acute abdomen
   b. The abdomen is distended and *painful*.
   c. Hypovolemic or septic shock
   d. Radiographs reveal generalized small bowel ileus. Free fluid due to venous/lymphatic obstruction, torn splenic or mesenteric vessels, or peritonitis may be present.
   e. Diagnosis is confirmed during emergency exploratory laporotomy.
   f. Unfortunately, the diagnosis is often made at necropsy because of the acute onset and rapid deterioration.

4. Treatment
   a. Immediate surgical correction of volvulus with resection of nonviable or necrotic intestine is the only treatment.
   1) Removal of entire small bowel may be necessary; short bowel syndrome results.

   2) Most cases are fatal because of extensive ischemic necrosis.
   3) Survival has been reported with closure after derotation and with complete bowel resection and pancreatic enzyme supplementation.
   b. Postoperative care
   1) Hypoproteinemia is common; colloids are usually necessary.
   2) Broad-spectrum combination antibiotics—aminoglycoside or enrofloxacin with ampicillin or cefazolin is commonly used
   3) Nutrition—enteral route preferred (nasogastric tube or surgically placed jejunostomy tube) using Clinicare to promote health of enterocytes. Partial parenteral nutrition (PPN) or total parenteral nutrition (TPN) may be necessary if >4–5 days nutritional support is needed; strict asepsis is critical in these debilitated patients.
   4) Analgesia—injectable narcotic and/or fentanyl patch

T. Protein-losing enteropathy (PLE)

1. Definition/etiology
   a. This is a general term for severe small intestinal disease that results in protein leakage into the gut lumen (*Table 11-2*).
   b. The two general causes of protein leakage are increased mucosal permeability or impaired lymphatic drainage.

TABLE 11.2
CAUSES OF PROTEIN-LOSING ENTEROPATHY

Inflammatory conditions causing increased permeability
Lymphocytic/plasmocytic enteritis
Eosinophilic gastroenteritis
Small intestinal bacterial overgrowth
Histoplasmosis, pythiosis
Gluten enteropathy (Irish Setters)
GI parasites—young animals
Chronic intussusception or foreign body
GI neoplasia (e.g., lymphosarcoma)
GI blood loss—ulcerative disease, NSAIDs, parasites, neoplasia, thrombocytopenia

Obstructive conditions with reduced lymphatic drainage
Lymphangiectasia—congenital (Norwegian Lundehund)
Neoplasia obstructing lymphatic drainage
Cardiovascular disease

c. Nonintestinal diseases (e.g., congestive heart failure, portal hypertension) uncommonly cause PLE.

d. There is a breed disposition in the Yorkshire Terrier, Lundenhund, soft-coated Wheaton Terrier, Shar Pei, Irish Setter, Basenji, and Rottweiler.

e. PLE is uncommon in cats and is usually caused by GI lymphoma.

2. Clinical signs
   a. Diarrhea—not always present
   b. Vomiting—variable, often absent
   c. Weight loss—often severe, including poor body condition and dull haircoat
   d. Ascites, pleural effusion, peripheral edema due to decreased oncotic pressure
      1) Small breeds (Yorkshire Terrier)—ascites
      2) Large breeds—peripheral edema (limbs)
   e. Thromboembolic disease due to GI loss of AT III is occasionally seen. Distal aorta is the most common site.

3. Diagnosis
   a. Physical examination often reveals extreme cachexia, edema, or ascites and/or muffled heart and/or lung sounds if pleural effusion.
   b. Laboratory
      1) Panhypoproteinemia
         a) Albumin <1.5 g/dL associated with edema
         b) Globulins may be high in immunoproliferative enteropathy of Basenjis or histoplasmosis, but are low with most other causes of PLE.
         c) Rule out glomerular disease (urinalysis, urine P/C ratio) and liver disease (bile acids) as cause of low protein. Globulins remain normal to high in renal or hepatic causes of hypoalbuminemia.
      2) Hypocalcemia
         a) Ionized calcium is the preferred test and is most often normal, although total serum calcium measurements will be low because of hypoalbuminemia.
         b) Normal total calcium with severe hypoalbuminemia should raise suspicion of lymphoma.
      3) Hypomagnesemia
         a) Severe depletion may cause refractory hypokalemia and cardiac arrhythmias (see p. 330).
      4) Hypocholesterolemia, lymphopenia due to loss of plasma and lymph (chyle) is common

in animals with lymphangiectasia and reduced fat absorption.

      5) Serial fecal flotations and direct smears to detect parasites/ova should be performed to look for whipworms, coccidia, and hookworms.
      6) Blood for serum TLI, cobalamin, and folate to detect exocrine pancreatic insufficiency and small intestinal malabsorption can be submitted to the GI Diagnostic Lab, Texas A&M University, College Station, TX 77843.
      7) Increased fecal α_1-protease inhibitor (molecular weight similar to that of albumin) confirms PLE when the concentration exceeds 6 µg/g of feces. If the test cannot be run within 36 hours, the fecal sample can be stored at 4°C for up to 7 days. This test is species specific and can only be run in laboratories with canine reagents.

   c. Radiography
      1) Abdominal radiographs are often normal.
         a) Loss of detail with ascites
         b) Mass/organomegaly, foreign body, lymphadenopathy, and thickened intestines may be seen.
      2) Chest radiographs are evaluated for pleural effusion, metastatic disease, or hilar lymphadenopathy (fungal disease).

   d. Abdominal ultrasound is more sensitive than radiographs but still often normal.
      1) May show lymphadenopathy, thickened intestines
      2) Especially useful when ascites is present

   e. Intestinal biopsy is required for definitive diagnosis.
      1) Full-thickness biopsy specimens from multiple sites (stomach, jejunum, ileum, mesenteric lymph node, and possibly liver) taken at the time of exploratory surgery is the preferred method of diagnosis but carries increased risk.
         a) Grossly dilated lymphatics and yellow–white nodules may be seen in animals with lymphangiectasia. Diffuse thickening of the intestines and lymphadenopathy can be seen with granulomatous or neoplastic disease.
         b) Biopsy specimens must be obtained whether or not gross lesions are identified.
         c) Hypoalbuminemia increases postoperative morbidity and delays healing.

Preoperative stabilization with colloids combined with careful surgical technique using nonabsorbable suture material will minimize potential complications.

2) Endoscopic mucosal biopsy

a) Less risk of dehiscence in severely hypoproteinemic patients, but greater chance of missing the diagnosis than with full-thickness biopsy

b) May miss lymphoma, lymphangiectasia, or lesions distal to proximal/midduodenum.

4. Treatment

a. Plasma or colloids should be given to maintain oncotic pressure in patients with severe ascites or pleural effusion or to stabilize patients prior to surgery (5 mL/kg/h × 4 hours of plasma, hetastarch, or dextran 70).

b. Diuretics can be considered if effusions are severe enough to cause respiratory distress (pleural fluid/tense ascites) or abdominal discomfort (ascites).

1) Lasix, 1–2 mg/kg q12h

2) Spironolactone, 1–2 mg/kg q12h

3) The effective circulating volume is decreased in these patients because of low oncotic pressure; avoid overzealous diuretic use.

c. Perform thoracentesis to relieve respiratory distress due to severe pleural effusion.

1) Supplemental O_2 is recommended as needed.

d. Abdominocentesis is only indicated to improve respiration by relieving pressure on diaphragm caused by tense ascites. Repeated abdominocentesis will only exacerbate hypoproteinemia.

e. Treatment for thromboembolic disease evidenced by acute respiratory distress or acute paresis with lack of detectable pulse. These patients are often hypercoagulable through loss of AT III.

1) Aspirin, 1 mg/kg q8–12h

2) Heparin, 200 units/kg IV, then 75–100 units/kg SC q8h to keep ACT or PTT 1.5 × baseline value

3) Streptokinase, 90,000 units IV by CRI over 30 min, followed by 45,000 U/h for 6–12 hours until pulses return

4) Tissue plasminogen activator (tPA), 1.1 mg/kg IV bolus q1h, 2–10 boluses prn

5) Hemorrhagic complications may occur with streptokinase; fresh whole blood or packed RBCs and FFP should be readily available.

f. Treatment of PLE depends on the underlying cause.

1) Lymphangiectasia is treated with a low-fat diet supplemented with a protein source such as low-fat cottage cheese and medium-chain triglyceride oil (1–2 mL/kg daily in food).

2) Lymphocytic/plasmacytic enteritis, eosinophilic gastroenteritis, and food allergy can be treated with dietary therapy and immunosuppressive therapy (prednisone, 1–2 mg/kg PO q12h × 7–14 days and tapered to lowest effective dose over 2–3 months)

3) Small intestinal bacterial overgrowth can be managed with

a) Tetracycline, 10–20 mg/kg q12h PO × 1 month

b) Metronidazole—dogs, 20–40 mg/kg PO q24h; cats, 10 mg/kg PO q24h

4) Histoplasmosis—itraconazole 5 mg/kg PO q12h with high-fat meal for 2–4 months

g. Intramuscular injection of fat-soluble vitamins (A, D, E, and K) should be given to animals with severe malabsorptive syndromes. Coagulopathy should be ruled out prior to surgical intervention or biopsy.

U. Penetrating abdominal wound

1. Causes

a. Bite wounds most common

b. Gunshot

c. Impalement—metal rod, arrow, knife, fence, etc.

2. Clinical signs

a. Most injuries are readily visible.

b. Hair coat may obscure small wounds, especially cat bite wounds.

c. Abdominal pain is present in most, but not all, cases.

d. Lethargy and collapse are seen with severe injuries that have excessive hemorrhage or peritonitis.

e. Visceral trauma is possible with no external wound present. This is seen with bite wounds—"big dog little dog" syndrome.

3. Diagnosis

a. Usually obvious on the basis of witnessed fight, gunshot, etc.

b. Physical examination reveals skin wound(s) and abdominal pain in most cases.

1) Clip hair coat to identify small wounds or bruising.
2) Wounds to caudal thorax may injure abdominal organs (liver parenchyma, biliary tract, stomach) beneath the rib cage.
3) Omentum or bowel may protrude from wound(s).
4) Hypovolemic (hemorrhage) or septic (bowel perforation, bile leakage) shock may be present.
5) Thorough examination is necessary to detect injury to multiple organ systems.
6) Abdominal radiographs may show disruption of body wall, foreign body (bullet), loss of detail, subcutaneous emphysema, or pneumoperitoneum (most easily seen by detecting air between the liver and diaphragm). Retroperitoneal trauma may appear as streaking, loss of detail, or ventral displacement of the colon.
7) Abdominocentesis or DPL may reveal hemorrhage, bile, urinary tract rupture, peritonitis, or septic peritonitis (WBC with phagocytosed intracellular bacteria).

4. Treatment
  a. Exploratory laparotomy is almost always indicated.
  b. Stable patients with negative DPL may respond to conservative medical therapy if the wound does not actually penetrate the abdominal cavity.
  c. Initial treatment
    1) Stabilize the animal as necessary following guidelines for resuscitating the trauma patient.
    2) Clip hair away from wound and apply a temporary dressing to minimize further contamination.
      a) *Keep any exposed abdominal tissue moist.*
      b) *DO NOT remove impaled objects; stabilize with dressing to limit movement, pending surgical exploration.*
    3) IV antibiotics—cefazolin, 40 mg/kg IV, followed by 20 mg/kg q8h; metronidazole 10–15 mg/kg q8h if hollow viscous perforation
    4) Analgesics as needed for pain
  d. Surgery
    1) Remove blood or fluid and pack off areas that are actively hemorrhaging to aid visualization.

2) Isolate injured organs, but delay repair until a complete systematic exploration of the abdomen has been completed.
3) Injuries should be addressed in the following sequence:
  a) *Stop arterial bleeding via hemostasis or ligation.*
  b) *Ligate or repair venous bleeders.*
  c) *Debride, repair, or resect damaged visceral organs.*
  d) *Address penetrating wounds.*
    i) *Small wounds can be cleaned, debrided, and left to heal by second intention.*
    ii) *Large wounds should be sutured closed, and the herniated tissue replaced.*
4) A sample of abdominal fluid should be obtained for culture and sensitivity testing.
5) Perform abdominal lavage with copious amounts of warm saline (3–30 L).
6) Change gloves and instruments.
7) Consider placing an alimentary feeding tube.
8) For severe contamination, open peritoneal drainage is recommended.
  a) *Close midline with a loose simple continuous pattern using 0 or 1 nonabsorbable suture.*
  b) *Place sterile laparotomy pads over the incision and follow with circumferential wrap.*
  c) *Change bandage using sterile technique q12–24h, depending on the amount of drainage (usually requires sedation or anesthesia).*
  d) *Monitor cytology of abdominal fluid. Repeat lavage if needed.*
  e) *Close abdomen when fluid is clear and bacteria are absent.*
  f) *Complications include hypoproteinemia, dehydration, electrolyte imbalance, sepsis, dehiscence, and pancreatitis.*
  e. Postoperative care
    1) Provide analgesia—injectable or epidural narcotics
    2) Monitor blood pressure, central venous pressure, and urine output in critical patients. Administer fluid support to optimize parameters.
    3) Give colloids or FFP transfusion to maintain oncotic pressure.
    4) Normalize electrolytes, blood glucose, and hematocrit.

5) Give enteral nutritional support with dilute Clinicare beginning 6–12 h postoperatively. PPN or TPN may be indicated if there is vomiting or severe intestinal damage.

6) Patients should be hospitalized for at least 3–5 days postoperatively for monitoring, observation, bandage changes, injectable antibiotics, and pain management.

V. Splenic torsion

1. Clinical signs

   a. Most common in large, deep-chested breeds, e.g., German Shepherd, Great Dane

   b. Can occur with or without gastric dilation volvulus

   c. Acute splenic torsion causes sudden abdominal pain, shock, vomiting, depression, and anorexia.

   d. Chronic splenic torsion causes chronic or intermittent pain, intermittent vomiting, weight loss, abdominal distention, and hemolysis/hemoglobinuria.

2. Diagnosis

   a. Abdominal palpation reveals splenomegaly (may be dramatic) and variable pain.

   b. Abdominal radiographs reveal splenomegaly, displaced abdominal organs, loss of detail, and possibly splenic gas (anaerobic bacteria).

   c. Abdominal ultrasound shows splenomegaly and distended splenic veins.

   d. Laboratory findings

     1) Anemia

     2) Target cells—damage to red blood cells as they traverse the abnormal splenic circulation

     3) Leukocytosis with or without a left shift

     4) Hemoglobinuria is caused by intravascular or intrasplenic hemolysis.

     5) DIC is a common sequela.

3. Treatment

   a. Splenectomy

     1) DO NOT derotate spleen before removal, to avoid release of trapped mediators/toxins/bacteria.

     2) Stabilize patient with fluids, transfusion as necessary prior to surgery.

     3) Consider prophylactic gastropexy at the time of surgery because of the association with gastric dilation volvulus syndrome.

W. Peritonitis

1. Etiology/pathophysiology

   a. Inflammation of peritoneal surfaces increases permeability.

     1) Large surface area leads to dramatic loss of fluid, electrolytes, and protein from vascular compartment into the abdominal cavity.

     2) Conversely, bacteria and other toxic products within abdominal cavity can gain access to the systemic circulation.

     3) The end result is often shock, systemic inflammatory response syndrome (SIRS) and multiple organ dysfunction/failure.

2. Clinical signs/physical examination

   a. Vomiting, diarrhea, lethargy, and anorexia are common, but nonspecific, signs.

   b. Some patients have a history of trauma or recent surgery.

   c. Examination findings vary from mild localized abdominal discomfort to collapse, shock, and extreme pain. Animals with extreme pain may exhibit a classic "praying position" with the front legs outstretched and the rear quarters elevated.

   d. Bruising or penetrating wounds can be seen with trauma.

   e. Icterus may be seen with pancreatitis or biliary tract leakage.

   f. Caudal abdominal pain or mass effect in intact male dogs suggests prostatitis or prostatic abscess.

   g. Intact females with recent estrus should be evaluated for ruptured pyometra.

   h. Uroperitoneum should be considered in animals with a history of difficulty urinating, free abdominal fluid, and/or nonpalpable bladder.

   i. Fever is common with either aseptic or septic peritonitis.

3. Diagnosis

   a. History and examination findings are often nonspecific.

   b. Abdominal radiographs may show masses, fluid density abdomen with loss of visceral detail, free air, or no abnormalities. Free air may persist up to 3 weeks after abdominal surgery.

   c. Laboratory findings:

     1) Neutrophilic leukocytosis with a left shift is seen commonly.

2) Neutropenia may be seen when consumption exceeds bone marrow production or release, as with overwhelming sepsis.

3) Electrolyte abnormalities are also common.

 a) Hyponatremia and hypokalemia are often the result of anorexia and vomiting.

 b) Hyperkalemia may be seen with uroperitoneum.

 c) Occasionally, abdominal effusion may cause hyponatremia and hyperkalemia and should not be confused with Addison's disease.

4) Blood glucose concentration may be high (stress, ±pancreatitis) or low (sepsis).

5) Serum proteins are often low because of third-space loss into the abdominal cavity.

6) Amylase and/or lipase elevation occurs with pancreatitis, small intestinal disease, or impaired renal clearance.

7) Metabolic acidosis is the most common blood gas abnormality.

d. Four-quadrant abdominocentesis/diagnostic peritoneal lavage (DPL)

1) Analysis of retrieved abdominal fluid may aid in diagnosis.

 a) Increased WBC count with intracellular bacteria indicates septic peritonitis— an indication for emergency celiotomy.

 b) Finding large numbers of degenerate neutrophils (vacuolated, toxic granules, swollen nuclei) is another indication for immediate exploratory laparotomy.

 c) Creatinine and potassium levels that exceed corresponding serum values indicate urine leakage.

 d) Amylase/lipase concentrations in the abdominal fluid exceeding serum levels indicate pancreatitis.

 e) High bilirubin indicates rupture of biliary tract.

 f) Elevated alkaline phosphatase concentration may indicate intestinal trauma.

 g) In cats, straw-colored fluid with high protein content and moderate numbers of neutrophils and macrophages is compatible with FIP.

 h) Culture and susceptibility testing of fluid will guide antimicrobial treatment.

e. Abdominal ultrasonography may help to confirm the presence of effusion, localize the lesion, and direct needle aspiration.

4. Treatment

a. Mild localized peritonitis may respond to conservative medical treatment.

1) IV fluids are administered as necessary to maintain hydration, extracellular fluid volume, and tissue perfusion.

2) Broad-spectrum antibiotics—ampicillin, cefazolin for gram-positive spectrum; aminoglycosides, fluoroquinolones for gram-negative spectrum; metronidazole, clindamycin for anaerobes

3) Appropriate monitoring includes frequent serial assessment of vital signs, abdominal palpation, and laboratory parameters (PCV, TS, BG, BUN, and electrolytes). The measured trends are used to determine response to treatment or need for surgery.

b. Surgery is indicated in most cases of generalized peritonitis and all cases of septic peritonitis.

1) Preoperative stabilization

 a) Fluids—large volumes of crystalloids, up to 60–90 mL/kg/h in critical patients. Supplemental potassium is usually required because of peritoneal loss but is not added until the initial rapid fluid bolus has been given to restore perfusion. After that, KCl 15–20 mEq/L can be added to the fluids.

 b) Hetastarch, plasma, or dextran 70 is often necessary because of albumin loss into the abdominal cavity and resultant hypoproteinemia.

2) Surgery—complete exploration of the abdominal cavity is critical.

 a) The source of peritonitis should be isolated from remaining organs with moistened laporotomy pads.

 b) Material (abdominal fluid, necrotic or abscessed tissue) is obtained for culture, cytology, and possibly histopathology.

 c) Following repair, do abdominal lavage with warmed saline (3–10 L).

 d) Adding antiseptic solutions and antibiotics to lavage fluid has no proven benefit and may impair neutrophil function (e.g., povidone iodine).

c. Severe septic peritonitis with extensive contamination of the abdominal cavity is best managed by open peritoneal drainage.
   1) Remove the falciform ligament.
   2) Partially close the linea with continuous monofilament suture leaving a gap of 2–4 cm.
   3) Cover wound with multiple layers of sterile absorbent bandage material.
   4) Change bandage 2–4 times daily or when soaked through, using sedation and sterile technique. Protein and electrolyte loss is expected and may be severe.
   5) The abdomen is closed under general anesthesia after several days, when drainage is decreased and cytology reveals minimal inflammation.
   6) Open peritoneal drainage is not recommended unless 24 hour continuous care is available.
d. Intravenous broad-spectrum antibiotics
   1) Ampicillin or cefazolin
   2) Gentocin/amikacin or fluoroquinolones
   3) Metronidazole or clindamycin can be added to expand anaerobic coverage.
e. Corticosteroids and NSAIDs are controversial and have no proven benefit.
f. Nutritional support is important to replace protein that is lost into the peritoneal cavity and to speed healing.
   1) The enteral route preferred when possible—feed dilute Clinicare (see Enteral nutrition, Chapter 8, p. 102).
   2) A jejunostomy tube can be placed at the time of surgery in patients with proximal intestinal disease, pancreatitis, or persistent vomiting.
   3) PPN or TPN is reserved for patients who cannot tolerate enteral feedings (see Partial parenteral nutrition and total parenteral nutrition, Chapter 8, p. 105).
g. Perioperative analgesia is provided using injectable narcotics and/or a transdermal fentanyl patch.
h. Postoperative complications include
   1) Infection—especially nosocomial infections in patients with open abdomen
   2) Loss of fluid, protein, electrolytes and RBCs through the inflamed peritoneum can cause dehydration, hypotension, hypoalbuminemia, electrolyte imbalance, and anemia.

   3) Possible herniation of abdominal contents can occur in patients with open abdominal drainage.

X. Mesenteric Thrombosis

1. Etiology
   a. Results from changes in blood flow (shock, dehydration, torsions), clotting elements (DIC, hypercoagulable state such as PLE/glomerular disease), or vessel wall damage (vasculitis, heat stroke).
   b. Alterations in blood flow, vessel walls, or coagulability (Virchow's triad) promote thrombosis.
   c. Mesenteric thrombosis may be a sequela.

2. Clinical signs and examination findings
   a. Acute to peracute onset of vomiting, bloody diarrhea, anorexia, and abdominal pain.
   b. Signs or history of chronic illness may precede acute deterioration.

3. Diagnosis
   a. Know the predisposing conditions and maintain a high index of suspicion because this disorder is uncommon.
   b. Physical examination findings of acute abdomen, bloody diarrhea, and shock are suggestive but nonspecific.
   c. Other diagnostic features are similar to those of mesenteric torsion.
   d. Abdominal radiographs may reveal gaseous distension of a single bowel loop.
   e. Abdominal ultrasound may reveal loss of gut motility in a bowel segment and abrupt cessation of blood flow at the site of the thrombus.

4. Treatment
   a. Correcting the underlying disease and maintaining perfusion are the most important aspects of treatment.
   b. Immediate surgery following rapid preoperative stabilization is indicated for resection of the devitalized portion of bowel and abdominal lavage.
   c. Anticoagulant therapy (see Feline thromboembolism, p. 180)
   d. Maintain fluid balance, oncotic pressure, and normal concentrations of serum electrolytes as with any critical patient.
   e. Reperfusion injury may cause sloughing of intestinal mucosa, predisposing to significant protein loss and sepsis.

f. Combination antibiotic therapy to cover gram-negative organisms and anaerobes.
   1) Ampicillin/cefazolin with gentamicin/amikacin
   2) Enrofloxacin can be substituted for aminoglycoside.
   3) Clindamycin or metronidazole may augment anaerobic coverage.

Y. Parvoviral enteritis/canine parvovirus (CPV)

1. Clinical signs
   a. Fever, anorexia, and lethargy are the initial signs.
   b. Vomiting and bloody diarrhea occur within 2–4 days of initial lethargy.
   c. The disease is most common in dogs <6 months old.
   d. There is an increased risk for severe clinical signs in Rottweilers, Doberman Pinschers, and Staffordshire Terriers. The increased risk is possibly due to persistence of maternal antibody and/or an inherited humoral immunity defect.

2. Physical examination findings
   a. Dehydration and poor perfusion (prolonged >2 sec capillary refill time) are commonly seen as a result of vomiting and diarrhea.
   b. Shock, recumbency, and stupor/coma occur in severe cases because of fluid loss, sepsis, and/or hypoglycemia.
   c. Abdominal palpation reveals gas/fluid-filled bowel loops and/or pain. It is important to rule out foreign body or intussusception in these puppies.

3. Diagnosis
   a. Clinical signs with a history of incomplete vaccination status raise the index of suspicion. CPV can occur in well-vaccinated dogs, especially if the last vaccine was given before 4–5 months of age.
   b. Parvoviral, CPV-2, ELISA (CITE, IDEXX), on fresh stool sample.
      1) Rapid "in-house" diagnosis.
      2) Highly sensitive and specific
      3) A weak positive result may occur 5–15 days after vaccination with CPV modified live virus (false positive).
      4) False negative results may occur
         a) *If the test is performed too soon before fecal shedding has begun (usually when the puppy is anorexic, lethargic,*

and vomiting), no viral antigen is detected.
         b) *If there is blood in the stool, humoral antibody can bind the antigen in the feces giving a false-negative result.*
   c. Leukopenia—CBC or peripheral smear will show marked decrease in total WBC in severely affected dogs.
      1) Most dogs develop an initial lymphopenia due to direct lysis during the viremic stage 5–7 days after exposure.
      2) In severely affected dogs, the lymphopenia is followed by profound neutropenia due to peripheral consumption of white cells (GI tract) or stem cell destruction (rapidly divided cells) in the bone marrow.
      3) The total WBC may be normal in some animals on initial presentation but usually drops quite low when severe GI signs develop.
   d. GI loss and decreased intake can result in hyponatremia, hypochloremia, and hypokalemia.
   e. Hypoglycemia is common in young puppies because of immature enzyme systems, sepsis, inadequate glycogen stores, and decreased caloric intake.
   f. Thrombocytopenia, prolonged ACT/PT/PTT, increased FDP/D-dimer, and hemorrhage indicate DIC in severe cases.
   g. Intussusception may be a complication because of changes in intestinal motility.
   h. Fecal floatation/direct smear may reveal concurrent parasites.

4. Treatment
   a. Prompt correction of fluid and electrolyte imbalances is the most important aspect of initial treatment.
      1) Shock doses of crystalloids, up to 90 mL/kg/h, in severe cases
      2) Correct dehydration using the formula Dehydration (%) × BW (kg) = Liters to replace deficit over 4 hours.
      3) Maintenance rate, 2–3 mL/kg/h, plus ongoing losses thereafter
      4) Add potassium 14–20 mEq K/L to correct and maintain serum concentration after resuscitation and rehydration.
   b. Correct hypoglycemia (common) by adding 2.5–5.0% dextrose to crystalloids after rehydration. (Add 50–100 mL of 50% dextrose per liter.)

c. Maintain plasma oncotic pressure if hypoproteinemia, albumin <1.5 g/dL, or total protein <3.5 g/dL.

    1) Plasma/FFP 6–20 mL/kg IV through filtered line over 2–4 hours. Can use whole blood at the same dose if the puppy is anemic.

    2) Hetastarch or dextran 70 at 4 mL/kg IV as part of resuscitation in critical patients followed by ~20 mL/kg/day along with crystalloids.

d. Antibiotics

    1) Aminoglycoside, gentamicin 6.6 mL/kg IV q24h, amikacin 30 mg/kg IV q24h—*after* rehydration, plus ampicillin 22 mg/kg IV q8h or cefazolin 22 mL/kg IV q8h if severe neutropenia (<1500 neutrophils/cm^3) Monitor urine sediment for proteinuria or tubular casts every 2–3 days of aminoglycoside therapy.

    2) Enrofloxacin, 5 mg/kg IV q12h diluted with saline and administered slowly, can be used in place of aminoglycoside to minimize potential nephrotoxicity.

        a) Dilute 1:1 with saline and administer over 5–10 minutes.

        b) Short-term use (3–5 days until leukopenia resolves) is associated with minimal risk of cartilage defect in puppies.

    3) Monotherapy with ampicillin, cephalosporins, or trimethoprim–sulfa (14 mg/kg SC q12h) is adequate in less severe infections with normal WBC.

e. Antiemetics are used to control severe vomiting, minimize fluid/electrolyte derangements, and improve patient comfort.

    1) Metoclopramide, 1–2 mg/kg/24 h CRI, is beneficial because of the promotility effect.

    2) Chlorpromazine, 0.1 mg/kg IV q4–6h or 0.2–0.5 mg/kg IM q6–8h as needed, may cause peripheral vasodilation and hypotension.

    3) Ondansetron (Zofran, Cerenex Pharmaceuticals, Research Triangle Park, NC) 0.1–0.15 mg/kg IV q6–12h. Serotonin antagonist—highly effective and safe but expensive

f. Antiendotoxin, SEPTI- Serum, Immua, Inc, Columbia, MO 75201, 4.4 mL/kg IV diluted 1:1 with crystalloids, given over 30–60 min.

    1) May benefit critical patients by preventing or minimizing endotoxemia.

    2) Give before antibiotics in order to bind endotoxin because antibiotic killoff may release the LPS endotoxin from the gram-negative cell wall, resulting in a massive increase in circulating endotoxin.

    3) Equine origin of antiserum poses risk of anaphylaxis; if repeated dosing is necessary, it should be given within 5–7 days.

g. Recombinant granulocyte colony-stimulating factor (rG-CSF), (Neupogen, Amgen), 5–10 mg/kg SC q24h, may increase WBC in severely leukopenic patients.

    1) WBC generally begins to rise within 24 hours after administration.

    2) Lack of proof of improved survival and expense may limit use.

h. Nutrition

    1) PPN for short-term nutritional support during prolonged illness

        a) Add 300 mL of 8.5% amino acid solution (Travenol, Baxter, Inc) to 700 mL of LRS with 5% dextrose administered at maintenance rate of 60 mL/kg/day.

        b) Administration through a peripheral vein is acceptable, though hypertonicity may cause phlebitis.

    2) Enteral nutrition should be initiated 12–24 hours after vomiting has stopped. Adding glutamine powder at a dose of 0.5 g/kg q12h to drinking water may promote mucosal healing.

    3) Initiate feeding with small amounts of bland, low fat diet. High fat diets may exacerbate diarrhea.

Z. Feline hepatic lipidosis

1. Pathophysiology

    a. Accumulation of fat in the cytoplasm of hepatocytes. Starvation, malnourishment, and diabetes increase mobilization of fatty acids to the liver.

    b. Primary hepatobiliary disease can decrease mitochondrial oxidation of fatty acids.

    c. Disruption of the hepatic urea cycle can interfere with hepatic protein synthesis.

    d. Develops especially in obese cats that have undergone a period of low caloric intake. Actual defect in hepatic metabolism in cats is unknown.

    e. Associated with acute hepatic failure in cats

2. Clinical signs/history

    a. Obese cat, recent stressful event

    b. Icterus

    c. Vomiting, salivation

d. May be associated with concurrent pancreatitis

3. Laboratory abnormalities
   a. Increased bilirubin in serum and urine
   b. Marked increase in serum alkaline phosphatase activity (SAP), moderate increase in serum alanine aminotransferase (SALT).
   c. High ammonia, elevated pre- and postprandial bile acids
   d. Ultrasonography reveals hepatomegaly with diffuse hyperechogenicity of liver ± evidence of pancreatic inflammation.
   e. In severe cases, coagulation tests may be prolonged.

4. Diagnosis
   a. Cytology of liver aspirate—hepatocellular vacuolization and cholestasis
   b. Liver biopsy is diagnostic.
   c. Assess coagulation function before biopsy. Give vitamin K and/or plasma if abnormal prior to biopsy.

5. Treatment
   a. Correct fluid, electrolyte and acid-base disturbances with balanced electrolyte solution with glucose, B vitamins, and potassium.
   b. Provide nutrition.
      1) Nasoesophageal tube can be used for short-term nutrition with liquid diets.
      2) Gastrostomy or esophagostomy tube can be placed for long-term nutritional management in cats with severe disease.
         a) *Anesthesia should be avoided until the patient is stable following IV fluid therapy and nasoesophageal feeding.*
         b) *Use a high-protein feline growth diet made into a gruel.*
         c) *Feed 1/3 of caloric requirement on day 1, 2/3 on day 2, and full amount on day 3. Formula for determining caloric requirement is 30 × body weight (kg) + 70.*
         d) *Refeeding syndrome can occur 12–72 hours after feeding is initiated. Metabolic consumption of phosphorus can result in severe hemolytic anemia. Monitor serum phosphorus and hematocrit. Be prepared to supplement phosphate IV (see p. 331) or transfuse if anemia occurs.*
   c. Gastroprotectants, antiemetics
      1) Famotidine, 0.5–1 mg/kg PO or IV q12–24 h

      2) Metoclopramide, 0.2–0.4 mg/kg PO or SC q8h
   d. Appetite stimulants
      1) Cyproheptadine, 2 mg/kg/day
      2) Avoid benzodiazepines and corticosteroids.
   e. Ancillary treatments—may or may not be effective
      1) Taurine, 500 mg/day
      2) Carnitine, 150–500 mg/day
      3) Thiamine, 100–200 mg/day
   f. When patient can consume adequate nutrition orally, the feeding tube can be removed.

AA. Cholangiohepatitis
1. May be suppurative or nonsuppurative (lymphocytic/plasmacytic infiltration)
2. In cats, commonly occurs with pancreatitis and/or inflammatory bowel disease. In dogs, may be idiopathic or breed related.
3. Clinical signs/history
   a. Usually middle-aged to older cats, any breed
   b. Intermittent vomiting, diarrhea, weight loss, fever, anorexia
   c. Icterus
   d. Occasionally, signs of hepatoencephalopathy (dementia, seizures, salivation)

4. Diagnosis
   a. High bilirubin, liver enzymes, WBC, globulin, ammonia, and bile acids
   b. Low albumin, glucose, BUN
   c. Hepatomegaly on abdominal ultrasonography initially. Microhepatia with chronic disease
   d. Hepatic biopsy
      1) Suppurative—neutrophilic infiltrate, cholestasis
      2) Nonsuppurative—lymphocytic, plasmacytic infiltrate
      3) Biliary cirrhosis and fibrosis
      4) Rule out hepatic neoplasia, hepatic lipidosis, FIP, toxins
   e. Culture biliary aspirate from gall bladder.

5. Treatment
   a. Antibiotics based on culture and sensitivity testing; initial therapy with ampicillin, enrofloxacin, and metronidazole
   b. Correct dehydration and electrolyte and acid–base abnormalities
   c. Nutritional support

1) High-protein diet with added B vitamins
2) Place feeding tube (nasoesophageal, esophagostomy, or gastrostomy) if needed.

d. Choleretic agent—ursodeoxycholate, 10–15 mg/kg q24h PO

e. For lymphocytic/plasmocytic nonsuppurative cholangiohepatitis—prednisone, 1 mg/kg PO BID tapered to 0.25–0.5 mg/kg QUD

f. In dogs, colchicine 0.03 mg/kg PO q24h is used as an antifibrotic agent to prevent cirrhosis.

g. Breed-specific hepatopathies (dogs)
1) Doberman Pinchers—middle-aged females
2) Cocker Spaniels—all ages, primarily males
3) West Highland White Terriers, Bedlington Terriers—often associated with copper accumulation in hepatocytes
4) Skye Terriers

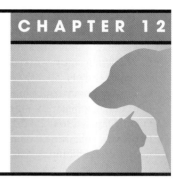

CHAPTER 12

UROLOGIC EMERGENCIES

I. CLINICAL SIGNS, DIAGNOSIS

A. Azotemia refers to the accumulation of nitrogenous wastes (urea, nitrogen, creatinine) in the blood and is characterized by elevated serum BUN and creatinine levels.

1. Prerenal azotemia is secondary to dehydration, shock, hypotension, cardiac failure, hyponatremia, or hypoalbuminemia resulting in decreased renal perfusion.

    a. Urine specific gravity should show a maximally concentrated specimen (>1.035) unless extrarenal factors are present that impair concentrating ability (diabetes insipidus, hyperadrenocorticism, hypoadrenocorticism, osmotic diuresis, or diuretic administration).

    b. Clinical signs associated with prerenal azotemia may include tachycardia, slow capillary refill time, and weak pulses.

    c. Prerenal azotemia is reversible with correction of the perfusion defect.

2. Renal azotemia occurs when >75% of the glomeruli are not functioning.

    a. Renal failure may be either acute or chronic.
      1) Animals with **acute renal failure** are usually in good body flesh, are not anemic, and may have painful kidneys. Acute renal failure is characterized by active urinary sediment (tubular casts, cells) and oliguria (urine output <0.5 mL/kg/h).
      2) Animals with **chronic renal failure** often have anemia, cachexia, poor haircoat, small kidneys, and a history of polydipsia and polyuria (>100 mL/kg/day)

    b. Azotemia can be only partially reversed with fluid therapy.

3. Postrenal azotemia results from reduced excretion of nitrogenous wastes secondary to urinary tract obstruction or rupture.

    a. Clinical signs may include
      1) Large, turgid, painful bladder
      2) Inability to urinate
      3) ±Abdominal pain and distension
      4) ±Fluid-filled abdomen

B. Uremia refers to the constellation of clinical signs and laboratory abnormalities that accompany renal failure—nausea, vomiting, anorexia, oral ulcers, melena, diarrhea, cachexia, metabolic acidosis, nonregenerative anemia, and azotemia.

C. Because signs are variable and nonspecific, urologic disorders must be considered in any critical patient because almost any organ of the body may be affected by urologic dysfunction.

D. Diagnosis of urologic emergencies is made by a constellation of acquired information including clinical signs, clinical history, physical examination, clinicopathology, and imaging procedures.

II. DIAGNOSTIC AND MONITORING PROCEDURES

A. Urethral catheterization

1. Indications
    a. Any patient whose renal perfusion or function is or may be compromised and urine output needs to be monitored
    b. Urethral obstruction
    c. Urethral trauma
    d. To perform urethral or urinary bladder contrast study
    e. To obtain urine for analysis

2. Procedure

   a. The urethral catheter should be placed aseptically.

   b. The hair around the prepuce or vulva should be clipped, and the area should receive a surgical preparation.

   c. The prepuce or vestibule should be flushed with dilute povidone iodine solution.

   d. The prepuce should be retracted, and the penis washed with povidone iodine solution.

   e. The female urethral opening should be visualized by use of a vaginal speculum or otoscope and a head lamp or light. The catheter can sometimes be placed in the female by running the catheter on the ventral midline of the vulva. Palpation of the urethral papilla with a sterilely gloved hand (usually index finger in most dogs) and passage of the catheter ventral to this may also facilitate passage of the catheter without direct visualization.

   f. A long, soft, sterile catheter should be used. The diameter should be estimated by the size of the patient (dogs: 6–12 Fr; cats: 3.5–5 Fr). Use a Foley catheter in female dogs.

   g. The catheter should be lubricated with a sterile lubricant gel and inserted into the urethra until urine is obtained. Passage of too much catheter into the urinary bladder may cause trauma to the bladder mucosa, a knot may form in the catheter, or it may double back on itself.

   h. Once the catheter is placed, a tape butterfly should be placed on the catheter and it should be sutured to the prepuce or labia. If a Foley catheter has been placed, the bulb should be filled with sterile saline to secure the catheter.

   i. The catheter should be attached to a sterile closed drainage system. All connections should be firmly attached to prevent inadvertent disconnection.

   j. The collection system should be placed lower than the urinary bladder to allow drainage by gravity and prevent reflux of urine into the bladder.

   k. Three to 5 mL of 3% hydrogen peroxide or 0.25% acetic acid placed in the urinary collection bag will prevent bacterial growth.

   l. The collection tubing should be taped to the hind leg (female dog or cat) or abdomen (male dog) to prevent traction at the suture anchors. Enough slack should be provided in the collection tubing to allow the patient to move freely without interfering with the collection system and causing patient discomfort.

3. Concerns

   a. The major concern is iatrogenic urinary tract infection.

   1) Prophylactic antibiotics are discouraged because they will allow resistant strains of bacteria to develop. Flushing the catheter with antibiotic solutions is discouraged as well.

   2) The best way to minimize infection is good aseptic placement of the catheter and good management of the catheter and collection system while it is in place.

   3) Perform urine culture and sensitivity testing once the catheter is removed.

   b. Urethral trauma or rupture can be avoided by careful, gentle technique in passing the catheter.

B. Contrast urethrogram/cystogram

1. Indications

   a. Persistent undiagnosed dysuria, pollakiuria, and intermittent chronic hematuria.

   b. Radiographic signs that indicate the need for contrast cystography include increased or decreased opacities that may be associated with the urinary bladder, abnormally shaped urinary bladder, and caudal abdominal masses that may be associated with the urinary bladder.

   c. The most common indication for contrast cystography in emergency medicine is for assessment of the integrity (urinary bladder rupture) of the urinary bladder or urethra.

   1) Inability to visualize the urinary bladder following pelvic trauma in male dogs should prompt the clinician to consider ruptured bladder.

   2) Pitting edema of the rear legs, bruising, and discoloration of the skin suggest urethral tear.

2. Procedure

   a. Ideally, the animal should be fasted for 24 hours and an enema performed prior to performing contrast cystography. This is probably not as important for primarily assessing the integrity of the urinary bladder.

   b. All catheters, contrast media, and equipment should be sterile, and the prepuce or vestibule should be prepared as for urethral catheterization.

c. Equipment necessary for contrast cystography includes a male urethral catheter (appropriate size for the animal), Foley balloon-type catheter (for female dogs), a three-way stopcock, a catheter adaptor for connection of the syringe, a tomcat catheter (for cats), and a large syringe.

  1) Negative-contrast materials include room air, carbon dioxide, or nitrous oxide.

  2) Positive-contrast material can be any organic iodide in a 20% iodine solution. Barium is NOT indicated in positive-contrast cystography.

d. The whole procedure should be performed on the radiograph machine table.

e. The urethra should be catheterized as described above (see urethral catheterization), and the bladder emptied.

f. The volume of contrast material generally injected is approximately 10 mL/kg but may range from 3.5 to 13.1 mL/kg depending upon the species and underlying pathologic process.

  1) Injection of contrast material should be stopped when the bladder feels adequately but not overly distended, if contrast leaks around the catheter, or if back pressure is felt on the syringe.

  2) The bladder must be distended enough to detect small leaks in the urinary bladder, yet one should take care to not rupture the bladder as well.

g. Double-contrast cystography is used to assess the bladder wall and intraluminal filling defects (the bladder should be emptied prior to injection).

  1) Double-contrast cystography is performed by first injecting a small amount of a 20% solution of an organic iodide:

  a) *0.5–1.0 mL/cat*

  b) *1–3 mL for dogs weighing less than 12 kg*

  c) *3–6 mL for dogs weighing more than 35 kg*

  2) The bladder is then distended with negative-contrast (air, carbon dioxide, or nitrous oxide).

h. To fully assess the urinary bladder after contrast injection, four radiographic views should be obtained including ventral dorsal, lateral, and two oblique views. Multiple views are not necessary when assessing for urinary bladder leakage.

i. Ideally, if fluoroscopy is available, contrast injection should be visualized fluoroscopically when looking for leakage. This will allow localization of the site of leakage for surgical repair.

3. Complications

  a. Gas embolization from negative-contrast injection is a very rare but serious complication. This may be prevented by using nitrous oxide or carbon dioxide (these gases are much more soluble in plasma) instead of room air. It is also recommended that the study be performed in left lateral recumbency to minimize the chance of fatal air embolism. In the patients in which this complication has been reported, there was active hemorrhage from the urinary bladder mucosa, and it was assumed that the air entered the low-pressure venous system.

  b. Similar complications may occur as those with urinary catheter placement.

  c. Bladder rupture may occur due to overdistention with injection of contrast material.

C. Contrast urethrogram

1. Indications

  a. Similar to those for contrast cystography; also, for demonstration of the integrity of the urethra

2. Procedure

  a. Preparation of the periurethral area is similar to that for placement of the urinary catheter.

  b. The tip of the urethra is catheterized, and then the distal urethral orifice is squeezed shut around the urinary catheter with sterilely gloved fingers to prevent leakage of contrast material around the urethra.

  c. Five to 10 mL of 20% sterile iodinated positive-contrast material is injected, and a radiograph of the urethra is taken immediately at the end of the injection. Simultaneous fluoroscopy while injecting will facilitate localizing the site of the urethral leakage. With partial urethral ruptures, some contrast material may enter the urinary bladder, but with complete rupture, no contrast material will enter the urinary bladder.

3. Positive-contrast urethrogram and cystograms may be combined by first performing the urethrogram followed by the cystogram.

4. Complications
   a. Similar to those with positive- and negative-contrast cystograms

D. Intravenous urogram

1. Indications
   a. To evaluate the size, shape, and position of the kidneys, ureters, and bladder when the kidneys cannot be identified on plain abdominal radiographs, when their outlines or architecture cannot be fully defined, or some qualitative assessment of renal function is needed
   b. When ureter integrity is questioned or ureteral obstruction is possible

2. Contraindications
   a. Dehydrated patients
   b. Hyperosmolar states

3. Procedure
   a. Ideally, the patient should be fasted for 24 hours.
   b. A cleansing enema should be performed within 2 hours prior to the procedure.
   c. Survey radiographs just prior to injection of contrast material will assure adequate patient preparation.
   d. Injection of 800 mg of iodine/kg body weight of an iodinated contrast material should be given via cephalic or jugular catheter (rapid bolus injection).
   e. Abdominal radiographs should be obtained at the following times postinjection:
      1) Ventrodorsal views: 5–20 sec, 5 min, 20 min, and 40 min
      2) Lateral views: 5 min, 40 min
      3) Oblique views: 3–5 min

4. Complications
   a. Measurement of urine specific gravity within 24 hours of injection of contrast may not be accurate as the contrast media increases the urine specific gravity.
   b. Contrast media in the urine may interfere with growth of bacterial pathogens on culture.
   c. Hypotensive reactions to injection may occur in some sensitized patients. Cardiovascular vital signs should be monitored closely during and after the injection of contrast material.
   d. Emesis commonly occurs following injection of contrast material. The patient should not be muzzled.

   e. Contrast medium induced renal failure has been reported in patients with impaired renal function. The procedure should be followed by fluid diuresis.

E. Urethral hydropropulsion

1. Indications
   a. For passage of urethral catheter when there is an intraluminal obstruction
   b. To dislodge an intraluminal urethral obstruction such as a urolith

2. Technique
   a. This technique is best achieved with general anesthesia or sedation. Anesthesia will also help relax the urethral muscle, facilitating relief of obstruction or passage of the urinary catheter.
   b. In extremely moribund patients, sedation may not be necessary.
   c. A large polyethylene urinary catheter is passed to the site of the obstruction.
   d. A 60-mL syringe is filled with 45 mL of sterile saline and 15 mL of Surgilube and attached to the end of the urinary catheter that has been placed.
   e. Another person then places a gloved finger rectally and the finger is pressed down over the urethra as it runs along the pubic symphysis. Sometimes with urethral obstruction the urethra is distended and easily palpable. Urethral calculi may also be palpable if they are stacked up from the base of the os penis to the urinary bladder.
   f. The tip of the penis is occluded by pinching it between sterile gauze with the thumb and forefinger. The catheter is stabilized with one hand while the saline is injected from the 60-mL syringe with the other hand. Simultaneously, the person with the finger in the rectum presses down on the urethra as it runs over the pubic symphysis, effectively occluding it.
   g. The simultaneous injection and urethral occlusion will dilate the urethra.
   h. Intermittently, the finger occluding the urethra should release, allowing the flush to rush into the bladder, thus (one hopes) dislodging the urethral calculus.
   i. A gentle back-and-forth motion on the catheter with simultaneous injection of the lubricant mixture should allow the obstruction to be dislodged.

j. The above procedure can be repeated several times. One should avoid overdistending the urinary bladder with the flush solution.

k. If the bladder is very distended, back pressure can be relieved by cystocentesis using a needle, stopcock and extension tubing to empty the bladder. Once this has been accomplished, retrograde flushing should be attempted again.

l. Another helpful technique is to try to pass the urinary catheter while flushing and distending the urethra.

m. Sometimes, simultaneously passing a smaller urinary catheter side by side with the primary flush catheter will allow passage of the smaller catheter around the obstruction to allow drainage of the urinary bladder.

n. Once catheter passage is achieved, the urinary catheter should remain in place to prevent reobstruction until cystotomy can be performed to remove cystic calculi.

F. Cystocentesis

1. Indications

    a. To assess urine characteristics free of contamination from the urethra

        1) Helps localize hematuria, pyuria, or bacteriuria

    b. To minimize iatrogenic bacterial infection of urinary bladder compared with urethral catheterization

    c. For therapeutic decompression of the distended urinary bladder due to urethral obstruction when techniques to relieve the urethral obstruction have failed (see below)

        1) A severely distended urinary bladder may have a compromised urinary bladder wall that could easily rupture during puncture.

    d. To remove urine distension prior to hydropropulsion back-flushing techniques

2. Contraindications

    a. Prostatic abscess, pyometra, coagulopathic conditions

3. Procedure

    a. Equipment

        1) Diagnostic cystocentesis: 22-gauge needle (1–1.5 inches long), 2.5–12-mL syringe

        2) Therapeutic cystocentesis: 22-gauge needle (1–1.5 inches long), 20-mL syringe, three-way stopcock, intravenous extension tubing

    b. The skin site where the needle will penetrate should be clipped and cleansed as for a sterile procedure.

    c. The procedure is usually well tolerated, and sedation is generally not necessary.

    d. At least two people are required, with one individual restraining the patient while the other performs the cystocentesis.

    e. Cystocentesis may be performed with the animal standing, in dorsal recumbency, or in lateral recumbency.

    f. The bladder should be gently localized and immobilized with one hand. With the other hand the needle is inserted through the abdominal wall and advanced to the immobilized bladder.

    g. The most common site for cystocentesis is the ventral wall of the bladder, although the ventrolateral and dorsal walls may be used as well.

    h. The needle should enter the urinary bladder at an oblique angle if possible.

    i. While the needle and bladder are immobilized, the urine should be gently aspirated into the syringe.

    j. Once an adequate amount of urine has been obtained, aspiration of the urine should be stopped and the needle backed out of the urinary bladder and abdominal wall.

    k. For therapeutic cystocentesis:

        1) A three-way stopcock should be attached to a 20-mL syringe. The three-way stopcock should then be attached to one end of intravenous extension tubing. The needle for cystocentesis should be attached to the other end of the intravenous extension tubing.

        2) Insertion of the needle is the same as for diagnostic cystocentesis (see above), but ideally, the needle should be placed near the junction of the urethra to the urinary bladder. This will facilitate continued aspiration of urine as the urinary bladder shrinks as it is emptied.

        3) Once the syringe is filled, immobilization of the urinary bladder and needle is maintained while the urine is emptied from the syringe into a bowl via manipulation of the three-way stopcock. Once the syringe is emptied, more urine is then aspirated from the urinary bladder as before. This procedure is repeated until the urinary bladder is empty.

4. Complications
   a. Bladder rupture, penetration of other structures, hemorrhage, peritonitis, tracking of neoplastic cells along the cystocentesis needle tracks, vesicoperitoneal fistulas, contamination of the urine sample with blood, and adhesions

G. Peritoneal dialysis

1. Indications
   a. Acute renal failure nonresponsive to routine treatments (see renal failure), acute decompensation of chronic renal failure, presurgical stabilization of severe uremia secondary to urinary tract leakage, and treatment of certain intoxications
      1) Dialyzable drugs include ethylene glycol, methanol, acetylsalicylic acid, amphetamine, aminophylline, aminoglycosides, cephalosporins, and diphenylhydantoin.
   b. Other indications include treatment of some toxicities (e.g., ethylene glycol), hyperkalemia, hypercalcemia, severe fluid overload, and congestive heart failure.
   c. Severe inflammatory conditions of the peritoneum such as pancreatitis or bacterial peritonitis will sometimes benefit from peritoneal dialysis.
   d. In rare cases of severe hypothermia, peritoneal dialysis can be used to achieve rapid core warming.

2. Contraindications
   a. Abdominal wall trauma, severe ascites, extreme obesity, severe bowel distention, and large abdominal masses may all interfere with catheter placement and so are relative contraindications.
   b. Peritoneal dialysis is an expensive endeavor, and owners should be committed financially. Also, animals with peritoneal dialysis catheters should have 24-hour care and be in a hospital that has individuals experienced with this treatment modality.
   c. Diaphragmatic hernia
   d. Recent abdominal surgery—leakage from the ventral midline incision may lead to peritonitis, delayed wound healing, and leakage of dialysate into subcutaneous tissues and muscle.

3. Procedure
   a. Peritoneal dialysis catheters
      1) The column disk catheter (Lifecath or Vetacath, Quinton Instrument Company, Seattle, WA) is the most efficient and least likely to obstruct of all the peritoneal dialysis catheters. This catheter is no longer readily available and is very expensive. This catheter must also be placed surgically, which can be a disadvantage in severely compromised patients.
      2) Straight, fenestrated tubing catheters such as Parker Peritoneal dialysis cannulas or Tenckhoff catheters (Ash Advantage Peritoneal dialysis catheter, Medigroup, Aurora, IL) are placed without surgery but become more easily obstructed than the column disk-like catheter. Obstruction can be minimized by pulling the omentum through a small midline incision and amputating a portion of it at the time of catheter placement.
   b. Catheter placement
      1) Placement of the straight, fenestrated tubing catheters is clearly described with the insert accompanying the catheter.
         a) Placement should follow strict aseptic technique.
         b) Location on the skin should be on the midline in the area around the umbilicus or just caudal to it.
         c) The catheter should be directed in a caudal-dorsal direction and should end up lying ventrally between the urinary bladder and the ventral abdominal wall.
         d) The catheter should be securely fixed to the skin and attached as directed to the transfer tubing set supplied for peritoneal dialysis (Baxter Health Corporation, Deerfield, IL). All joints should be wrapped with sterile gauze that has been soaked in Betadine solution. The catheter exit site should be covered with sterile gauze pads that have been soaked in Betadine solution. The catheter should be further secured by placing a bandage wrap around the abdomen. This wrap should not kink or occlude the catheter.
   c. Dialysate solutions
      1) Commercially prepared dialysate solutions are available (Dianeal, Baxter Health Care Corp., Renal Division, McGaw Park, IL 60015; Impersol, Fresenius USA, Inc., Walnut Creek, CA 94598; Dialyte, McGaw, Inc., Irvine, CA 92713).
      2) The solutions primarily differ in the concentration of dextrose (1.5–4.25%) and therefore osmolality.

3) Dialysate solution can also be prepared by adding dextrose to lactated Ringers Solution (LRS); 30 mL of 50% Dextrose added to 1 L of LRS will make a 1.5% solution.

  a) *Monitor serum magnesium closely when using this solution because this solution does not contain magnesium. Magnesium can be added to the dialysate at a dosage of 20 mg/L.*

  b) *Commercial solutions are always preferred to homemade because of the possibility of introducing infection from improper handling while mixing.*

4) Solutions containing 1.5% dextrose are generally used for dialysis of solutes, while solutions with higher concentrations of dextrose are reserved for dialyzing volume-overloaded patients.

5) Solutions may be tailored by adding different electrolytes (e.g., sodium, potassium), depending upon the needs of the patient.

6) Add 1000 units of heparin to 2 L of dialysis solution to maintain patency of the catheter fenestrations.

7) The solutions should be warmed to 40°C prior to infusion.

8) The volume administered per exchange is usually between 30 and 40 mL/kg. Abdominal distention, patient comfort, and respiratory status should be monitored, and the infusion volume adjusted accordingly. This volume is infused by gravity drip as fast as possible.

9) Intraabdominal dwell time is about 30 minutes. The fluid should then be gravity drained.

10) Dialysis exchanges should be continuous initially (usually total infusion and drainage time combined is about 1 hour).

  a) *Records of input and drainage volumes should be maintained constantly as well as body weight to avoid overhydration or dehydration.*

  b) *If retrieval volumes are substantially lower than infusion volumes, then*

    i) *The animal may be dehydrated.*
    ii) *The animal should be repositioned.*
    iii) *The catheter should be flushed.*
    iv) *The osmolality of the dialysate may need to be increased.*

11) Once the BUN and creatinine have decreased to reasonable concentrations (BUN, 60–100; creatinine, 4–6; normal potassium, bicarbonate, and phosphorus levels), the frequency of the exchanges can be decreased (usually to every 4–6 hours).

12) Monitor PCV, TS, blood glucose, acid/base status and serum electrolytes including sodium, potassium, magnesium and ionized calcium. Frequency of monitoring should be adjusted to the dynamics of the patient, but a minimum of once per day is recommended.

13) Cytology of the retrieved dialysate solution should be performed daily or every other day to monitor for infection. When infection is present, the fluid will be cloudy.

14) Other monitoring should be adjusted on the basis of the goal of the peritoneal dialysis. For example, BUN and creatinine for treatment of uremia; ethylene glycol concentration; or CVP, body weight, and hydration status for patients that are overhydrated.

15) The catheter site and the area around it should be monitored daily as well as daily bandage changes.

16) Strict adherence to aseptic technique should be maintained at all times when working with the dialysis solutions or the apparatus.

17) Complications

  a) *Catheter obstruction—most common complication*

    i) *Flush with 20 mL of heparinized saline.*
    ii) *Adjust position of catheter or patient to improve drainage.*
    iii) *Placement of a new catheter may be necessary.*
    iv) *Removal of omentum may be necessary.*
    v) *Heparin 100–500 U/L is added to the dialysate to prevent fibrin occlusion of the catheter.*

  b) *Laceration of bowel, bladder, or vessel during catheter placement*
    i) *Empty urinary bladder before placing dialysis catheter.*

  c) *Leakage of dialysate subcutaneously*
    i) *Commercial catheters have a Dacron cuff that helps prevent dialysate from leaking out of the peritoneal cavity.*

d) *Peritonitis*
  i) *Perform culture and sensitivity testing if fluid is cloudy and has large numbers of neutrophils ± bacteria on cytology.*
  ii) *Antibiotics can be added to the dialysate—cephalothin 1 g/L and tobramycin 100 mg/L.*

e) *Electrolyte imbalances*
  i) *Potassium, calcium, magnesium, or bicarbonate can be added to the dialysate fluid if needed.*

f) *Overhydration*
  i) *Elevated CVP, pitting edema, pleural effusion, and pulmonary edema may occur.*
  ii) *Use 4.25% dextrose dialysate, as the hyperosmolar solution will pull free water out of the interstitium and into the peritoneal cavity.*

g) *Hypoalbuminemia*
  i) *Albumin loss can occur with dialysis and increases with peritonitis.*
  ii) *Plasma or colloid administration may be necessary if serum albumin drops below 1.5 g/dL.*

H. Renal biopsy

1. Indications
   a. To establish a specific diagnosis and prognosis
   b. Abnormal kidney shape
   c. Undiagnosed proteinuria or renal failure after noninvasive means of diagnosis have been exhausted
   d. To predict a probable course of the renal disease prior to undergoing expensive and prolonged therapy (e.g., peritoneal dialysis)

2. Contraindications
   a. Presence of coagulation abnormalities
   b. Renal abscesses where biopsy may contaminate the abdominal cavity

3. Procedure
   a. Fine-needle aspiration
   1) Can usually be done percutaneously, particularly in cats with suspected renal lymphoma
   2) Ultrasound-guided fine-needle aspiration is safer and assures accuracy in needle placement. Abdominal ultrasound postaspiration allows monitoring for gross complications such as hemorrhage or urine leakage.
   3) Mild sedation is recommended, although in some docile cats this may be done without sedation.
   4) Equipment for aspiration includes a 10- to 12-mL syringe and a 22-gauge (1 inch long) needle.
   5) The kidney(s) to be aspirated should be palpated and immobilized immediately under the abdominal wall closest to the kidney.
   6) The area of skin where the needle will penetrate should be clipped and scrubbed as for any sterile surgical procedure.
   7) The needle should be advanced tangentially through the renal cortex if possible.
   8) Aspiration of the syringe should be as for aspiration of any solid structure (e.g., lymph nodes, cutaneous masses).
   9) Smears of the slides should be made and submitted for cytological analysis.
   10) This technique is particularly useful when renal lymphoma is suspected.
   b. Percutaneous Tru-Cut biopsy
   1) Sedation is required for this procedure.
   2) It can usually be done percutaneously in cats and small dogs as described for fine-needle aspiration if the kidneys can be easily palpated and immobilized.
   3) Ultrasound-guided percutaneous Tru-Cut biopsy is safer and assures accuracy in placement of the biopsy needle. It also allows monitoring for complications postbiopsy.
   4) An alternative method is to make a small keyhole incision just caudal to the last rib. The kidney can then be immobilized and Tru-Cut Biopsy performed.
   5) Passage of the biopsy needle should be tangential to the renal cortex, avoiding the renal artery and vein.
   6) Specific contraindications for Tru-Cut biopsy include pyelonephritis, hydronephrosis, and extreme azotemia as well as bleeding tendencies.
   c. Surgical renal biopsy
   1) The most invasive but most productive way to obtain renal tissue for biopsy is exploratory laparotomy, and a wedge of renal tissue is obtained surgically. This allows the clinician to perform an accurate biopsy and obtain an adequate amount of tissue for histopathology.

2) Disadvantages are invasiveness and the requirement for general anesthesia.

d. Complications of renal biopsy

1) Serious complications are rare.

2) Gross or microscopic hemorrhage are rare but the most common complications.

3) Rupture of a renal abscess or leakage of bacteria-contaminated tissue from an infected kidney may cause peritonitis.

4) Uroperitoneum or retro-uroperitoneum

4. Interpretation

a. Histologic evidence of intact basement membranes and tubular regeneration warrants a good prognosis for reversal.

b. Extensive tubular necrosis, interstitial mineralization, and disruption of basement membranes suggest irreversible damage.

I. Urine protein/creatinine ratio

1. Indications

a. To determine whether substantial proteinuria is present via a "spot" test

b. To evaluate for the source of protein loss in patients with hypoproteinemia

2. Procedure

a. Urine is collected via cystocentesis, urinary catheter, or midstream free catch.

b. The sample is submitted to the clinical pathology laboratory for determination of urine protein and creatinine concentrations.

3. Interpretation

a. Substantial urinary tract hemorrhage as well as urinary tract infection, inflammation, and neoplasia will increase urine protein concentration and confuse interpretation of the test result.

b. In the dog, a ratio of <0.5 is normal, 0.5–1.0 is questionable and should be repeated at a later date, and >1.0 is significant proteinuria in the absence of the above-listed confounding factors. The magnitude of proteinuria roughly correlates with the severity of glomerular disease. Urinary tract infections usually have a P/C ration <8, while glomerulonephritis is often >20. The most significant proteinuria is usually seen with amyloidosis. The P/C ratio may be >50.

J. Fractional clearance of electrolytes

1. Fractional clearance of electrolytes can be used to evaluate tubular function.

2. It is the ratio of the clearance of the electrolyte in question to the clearance of creatinine.

3. Formula

a. Fractional clearance of electrolyte "b" = $(U_b V/P_b)/(U_{cr} V/P_{cr})$

1) U_b = urine concentration of "b", V = urine volume collected during the time period in question (usually 24 hours), P_b = plasma concentration of "b," U_{cr} = urine creatinine concentration, P_{cr} = plasma creatinine concentration

4. Values for fractional clearance of dogs and cats

a. Sodium

1) Dog: <1%

2) Cat: <1%

b. Potassium

1) Dog: 20%

2) Cat: <5%

c. Chloride

1) Dog: <1%

2) Cat: <1.3%

d. Calcium

1) Dog: 0–0.4%

2) Cat: not known

e. Phosphorus

1) Dog: <39%

2) Cat: <73%

5. A fractional excretion of sodium value is useful to help separate prerenal from renal causes of azotemia.

a. Fractional excretion of sodium = $((U_{Na}/P_{Na}) \times (P_{Cr}/U_{Cr})) \times 100$

b. Prerenal azotemia: fractional excretion of sodium <1%

c. Renal failure: fractional excretion of sodium >1%

d. The advantage of the fractional excretion of sodium versus the fractional clearance of sodium is that the former requires only a spot test, while the clearance determination requires a continuous collection of urine.

6. Fractional excretion of potassium may be increased in geriatric cats with renal insufficiency, $(U_K/P_K) \times (P_{Cr}/U_{Cr}) \times 100 > 10\%$. Oral potassium supplementation (2–4 mEq/day) can prevent muscle weakness and polymyopathy associated with chronic hypokalemia.

K. Prepubic cystostomy catheter

1. Indications

a. When urine cannot be passed through the urethra because of urethral occlusion or trauma, when all methods to relieve the urethral obstruction or to pass a urinary catheter have failed

b. For temporary stabilization of a patient with urethral obstruction while waiting for a surgeon to perform definitive treatment such as urethrotomy or perineal urethrostomy

2. Procedure

a. Procedure may need to be performed under sedation unless the patient is extremely moribund.

b. A sterile preparation of the skin of the caudal half of the abdomen should be performed as for any sterile surgical procedure.

c. A 1–2 cm incision is made in the caudal third of the abdomen. In male dogs, the skin incision is made lateral to the prepuce. The prepuce is then retracted laterally and the linea alba is incised. In cats and female dogs, the skin incision is made in the midline.

d. Once the linea alba is incised, the bladder is exteriorized and held in position with two retention sutures.

e. An absorbable purse string suture is placed through the serosa and muscular layers of the urinary bladder.

f. A stab incision is then made in the center of the pursestring circle.

g. A small Foley catheter is then placed into the urinary bladder through the incision, and the balloon is inflated with sterile saline.

h. The original retention sutures are then passed through the linea alba and tied.

i. The linea alba and skin incision are closed with simple interrupted sutures, and the Foley catheter is secured to the skin.

j. The catheter is then connected to a sterile closed urinary collection system.

k. The catheter can be removed and the bladder closed when definitive surgery can be performed, or the catheter can be deflated and removed percutaneously after 3 or more days.

3. Aftercare

a. Care should be as for any sterile urinary catheter.

b. Monitoring should be performed to be sure that urine is not leaking into the abdominal cavity.

c. Monitoring should be as for any abdominal surgical procedure.

III. MANAGEMENT OF SPECIFIC CONDITIONS

A. Acute renal failure (ARF)

1. Definition: a sudden and severe reduction in renal function

2. Causes (*Table 12-1*)

a. Hypotension from any cause: e.g., dehydration, hemorrhage, heart disease, anesthesia, surgery, trauma, renal artery occlusion, vasculitis, fluid loss from burns, heatstroke, sepsis.

b. Nephrotoxins: e.g., ethylene glycol, heavy metals, aminoglycosides, chemotherapeutic agents, nonsteroidal antiinflammatory medications, thiacetarsamide, radiocontrast agents, snake venom, certain anesthetic agents, myoglobinemia, hemoglobinemia, hypercalcemia

c. Miscellaneous: Leptospirosis, amyloidosis, pyelonephritis, neoplasia, glomerulonephritis, urinary tract obstruction, diabetes mellitus, and hypercalcemia

3. Diagnosis

a. Diagnosis is made when azotemia is accompanied with minimally concentrated urine in the absence of conditions that inhibit renal urine concentrating ability (e.g., hyperadrenocorticism, central diabetes insipidus, or diuretics.).

b. Cause may be determined by recognizing the common causes listed above combined with a thorough medical and clinical history, complete blood count, serum chemistry profile, urinalysis, imaging techniques, and appropriate blood work or tests for investigation of specific causes (e.g., leptospirosis titers, ethylene glycol concentrations, urine culture).

c. Acute versus chronic renal failure

1) Clues that renal failure is acute include a history of no previous episodes of illness, weight loss, or polyuria/polydipsia; normal or enlarged kidneys, painful/enlarged kidneys or abdominal palpation; historical evidence of a recent exposure to a nephrotoxic agent or known cause of acute renal failure; absence of anemia; and finding granular casts in the urine.

2) Acute onset of azotemia and hyperphosphatemia suggests ARF.

3) Ischemic and toxic insults usually cause oliguric or anuric renal failure. Nonoliguric ARF can occur with aminoglycosides or cisplatin.

TABLE 12.1
POTENTIAL CAUSES OF ACUTE RENAL FAILURE

Nephrotoxins

Ethylene glycol	Streptozotocin
Aminoglycosides	Mithramycin
Amphotericin B	Hypervitaminosis D (rodenticide)
Cephaloridine	Heavy metals
Sulfonamides	Hydrocarbons
Tetracyclines	Thiacetarsamide
Polymyxin B	Phosphate enemas
Colistin	Easter lily
Cisplatin	EDTA
	IV radiographic contrast agents

Ischemia/Poor Perfusion

Shock	Congestive heart failure
Hypotension	Anaphylaxis
Severe burns	Sepsis
Hypoadrenocorticism	Heat stroke
Prolonged anesthesia	

Infections

Leptospirosis	Glomerulonephritis secondary to chronic disease
Pyelonephritis	Borelliosis
Rocky Mountain spotted fever	

Miscellaneous

Myoglobinuria	Thromboembolic disease
Hemoglobinuria	Transfusion reaction
Catecholamine-induced vasoconstriction	Urinary tract obstruction
Vasculitis	Snakebite
	Trauma

---

4) Some animals can have an acute episode of renal failure on top of long-standing or chronic renal failure. Many of these animals will have signs of chronic renal failure including small irregular kidneys, weight loss, anemia, polydipsia, and polyuria.

5) The diagnosis of chronic renal failure versus acute or acute on chronic is not always clear, and a renal biopsy is sometimes necessary.

4. Treatment

  a. Treatment or removal of the underlying cause is necessary.

  b. Fluid deficits should be replaced with a balanced electrolyte solution over 4–6 hours (see fluid therapy).

    1) If the animal does not seem dehydrated, then 5% of its body weight should be infused over 4 hours to correct subclinical dehydration and encourage diuresis.

    2) Urine output should be monitored as accurately as possible as well as the amount of fluid administered. Monitoring of central venous pressure, frequent auscultation of the lungs, assessment of body weight, and measurement of packed cell volume and serum total solids will help guage the adequacy of fluid therapy and detect overhydration.

    3) Blood pressure should be monitored frequently, and a mean arterial pressure of 60–80 mm Hg should be maintained.

    4) Minimal acceptable urine output once the patient is rehydrated and minimal MAP is maintained should be 2 mL/kg/h.

  c. Electrolytes and acid–base status should be monitored closely, particularly in anuric, oliguric, or extremely polyuric patients. Electrolyte abnormalities commonly seen in acute renal failure patients include hyperkalemia, metabolic acidosis, hyperphosphatemia, hypermagnesemia, and ionized hypocalcemia. (See specific treatment for each metabolic abnormality.)

d. Treatment of oliguria/anuria

1) Oliguria is defined as an output less than 0.27 mL/kg body weight/hour. Any well-hydrated animal should have a minimum of 1–2 mL/kg/h urine output. Urine output less than this should be addressed.

a) Urinary catheter patency and adequate blood pressure should be addressed once oliguria has been recognized.

2) Diuretics

a) If blood pressure is adequate and oliguria persists, then administration of diuretics should be considered

b) Furosemide

i) 2–6 mg/kg IV every 6–8 hours.

ii) An initial IV bolus of 2 mg/kg followed by a constant rate infusion of 0.2–1 mg/kg/h combined with a dopamine infusion (see below) is considered most effective.

iii) Improved urine output should be noted within 1 hour of initiation of the furosemide. A repeat dose should be administered if no improvement in urine output is noted. If urine output is not improved after this, it is unlikely that furosemide will be effective.

c) Mannitol

i) Osmotic diuretic (may not be effective in anuric patients)

ii) Should not be used in volume-overloaded or dehydrated patients

iii) Dose: 0.5–1.0 g/kg slow bolus over 15–20 min

iv) Urine output should be improved within 1 hour of administration. If no improvement in urine output is noted within this time, a second dose may be administered, but volume overexpansion becomes more likely, and close monitoring for this possibility is necessary.

d) Hypertonic glucose (indications and contraindications similar to those for mannitol)

i) Acts as an osmotic diuretic (may not be effective in anuric patients)

ii) Dose: (10–20% concentration) Intermittent slow bolus of 25–50 mL/kg IV over 1–2 hours (BID to TID).

3) Dopamine

a) Constant rate of infusion: 1–3 μg/kg/min

b) Generally works best when combined with a furosemide infusion of 1mg/kg/h

c) Continuous ECG should be used to monitor for arrhythmias.

d) Blood pressure should be monitored.

e) Diuresis generally is noted within 1 hour of administration if the drug is going to be effective.

f) Recent evidence suggests that in cats, dopamine may be ineffective in promoting diuresis because of a lack of renal dopaminergic receptors.

g) The use of low dose dopamine to treat acute renal failure in humans is controversial because of potential side effects of tachycardia and stroke and lack of evidence of increased survival.

h) The use of dopamine in dogs is somewhat controversial because although it increases renal blood flow, it may not improve medullary blood flow. Newer agents, such as fenoldapam, may be superior to dopamine but have not been investigated in small animals.

4) Dialysis (see p. 231)

a) Should be considered when fluid and diuretic therapy has been ineffective in treating diminished urine output and uremia

b) Peritoneal dialysis is more readily available than hemodialysis but still requires personnel with the expertise and monitoring capabilities.

c) The number of veterinary hemodialysis centers is slowly increasing, and they should be considered for these patients.

B. Ethylene glycol toxicity

1. See the chapter on toxins for specific treatments for ethylene glycol toxicity.

2. The renal failure treatment is similar to that for any acute renal failure.

C. Feline urethral obstruction

1. Diagnosis

a. The typical presentation is a male cat with a history of nonproductive straining to urinate often confused with constipation by owners. Other signs commonly noted are attempting to urinate outside the litter box, hematuria, restlessness, crying as in pain, pain on palpation of the abdomen, loss of appetite, and vomiting. Physiologic status may range from stable to severe cardiovascular compromise and collapse.

b. Diagnosis is inferred with a history of nonproductive straining to urinate and palpation of an enlarged, nonexpressable urinary bladder.

　1) Corroborating signs include discoloration of the tip of the penis and the presence of a urethral plug at the tip of the penis.

　2) Absence of a palpable bladder does not rule out urethral obstruction. Rarely, the bladder can rupture, in which case the cats are generally extremely ill and uremic.

2. Treatment

a. Initial assessment and treatment should be directed toward the cardiovascular status.

　1) Critically ill cats with urethral obstruction often have decreased tissue perfusion due to hypovolemia and cardiac dysfunction secondary to metabolic derangements.

　2) An intravenous catheter should be placed, and an emergency database including PCV, TS, dipstick glucose, dipstick BUN, sodium concentration, potassium concentration, blood gas analysis, and ionized calcium values should be obtained if possible.

　3) An ECG should be obtained if a fast, slow, or irregular heart rate is noted.

　4) If poor tissue perfusion is determined on the basis of physical examination, a bolus of 30 mL/kg/h of a balanced electrolyte solution should be administered.

　5) Hyperkalemia can cause bradycardia and conduction disturbances and should be treated immediately if severe (>7.5 mEq/L). Treatment choices include

　　a) Regular insulin: 0.1–0.25 U/kg IV with a 0.25–0.5 g/kg glucose IV bolus. Add glucose to fluids to prevent hypoglycemia (2.5–5% concentration).

　　b) Calcium gluconate 10%, 0.5–1 mL/kg IV slowly over 10 minutes protects the myocardium against the effects of potassium. Monitor ECG.

　　c) Sodium bicarbonate, 1 mEq/Kg IV slowly. Caution: May decrease the ionized calcium level, resulting in clinical signs of hypocalcemia (tetany, seizures).

b. After cardiovascular status is improved, relief of the urinary obstruction should be attempted.

　1) The tip of the penis is examined, and any urethral plug present at the tip should be dislodged and the urethra catheterized with an open-end tomcat catheter (see urethral catheterization p. 227). In critically ill cats, catheterization is well tolerated without sedation. If the cat resists or struggles, sedation should be given. The most effective sedative combination is 2.5–5 mg/kg of ketamine mixed with 1–1.5 mg of Valium (per cat) and given intravenously. One half of this combination is given again if sedation is inadequate or the patient begins to wake up prior to completion of urethral catheterization. If cardiac abnormalities are present or hypertrophic cardiomyopathy is suspected, then 0.05 mg/kg of hydromorphone mixed with 1–1.5 mg of diazepam can be used in the critically ill cats that require sedation for urinary catheter placement.

　2) Sterile technique should be adhered to as closely as possible.

　3) The tip of the catheter should be lubricated with a sterile lubricant gel.

　4) The catheter should be gently fed into the tip of the penis through the external opening of the urethra. Once the catheter is seated into the opening the penis should be slipped backed into the prepuce while maintaining the catheter placement in the urethra.

　5) The prepuce is grabbed with two fingers and retracted dorsally and caudally toward the base of the tail while maintaining the position of the catheter in the penis. This motion effectively straightens the urethra, allowing easier dislodgment of the urethral plug and passage of the urinary catheter into the urinary bladder.

　6) The catheter is then advanced gently until resistance is met when the catheter meets the urethral plug.

　7) The catheter is flushed with sterile saline. If flushing is prevented because the catheter tip is obstructed by the plug, the catheter should be retracted just slightly while pressure on the flush syringe is maintained. As soon as flushing continues, retraction of the catheter should stop and the flush be allowed to continue.

　8) Catheter advancement should be attempted again. When flush resistance is felt, the catheter should be retracted as before and the flush continued. This procedure should be repeated multiple times until the plug is dislodged. The keys are patience and ample flushing.

9) Do not pass the catheter aggressively. The urethra is often very friable because of severe inflammation and can be easily perforated or ruptured.

10) If the urethral plug cannot be dislodged by the technique above, then cystocentesis (see therapeutic cystocentesis, p. 230) and drainage of the urinary bladder may relieve the back pressure on the plug and facilitate passage of the urinary catheter. Because of the high hydrostatic pressure on the urinary bladder wall, the blood supply may be compromised and the urinary bladder may be prone to rupture. Therapeutic cystocentesis should be performed only after urethral catheterization has been unsuccessful. After drainage of the urinary bladder using a stopcock and extension tubing, urethral catheterization should be attempted again.

11) If urethral catheterization is unsuccessful after cystocentesis, an emergency perineal urethrostomy will be needed or a prepubic cystostomy tube may be placed until a perineal urethrostomy can be performed.

c. Once the urethra has been successfully catheterized with a tomcat catheter, the bladder should be flushed multiple times until the amount of grit within the urine is minimized.

1) The urinary catheter should be left in place if the cat does not have a good stream of urine, the cat is uremic and sick, the bladder has detrusor atony, or the urine has large amounts of grit, hemorrhage, or blood clots likely to cause reobstruction.

2) The tomcat catheter can be sutured to the prepuce and a closed urinary collection system attached to the tomcat catheter opening.

3) Because of the stiffness of the tomcat catheter, a softer, more pliable urethral catheter is less likely to cause hemorrhage from trauma to the bladder wall. A 3.5 or 5 French red rubber feeding tube catheter is our long-term indwelling catheter of choice. The tomcat catheter should be continuously flushed as it is removed to prevent reobstruction of the urethra prior to placement of the softer catheter.

4) The catheter is left in place for 12–48 hours or longer depending upon the appearance of the urine and the stability of the patient. The catheter is generally removed when the patient is alert and stable, laboratory results are normal, and minimal grit and blood are present in the urine.

a) The catheter should be removed in the morning and the cat observed throughout the day to make sure it can urinate.

d. After catheter placement, while the cat is still sedated, an intravenous catheter can be placed in the jugular or medial saphenous vein. This will provide easy access for blood sampling and IV fluids. The cat's perfusion parameters should be monitored closely as well as urine output, PCV, TS, dipstick BUN and glucose, sodium concentration, potassium concentration, and blood gas analysis. After initial stabilization, continued fluid therapy, and return of urine flow, most metabolic abnormalities will continue to improve.

e. The most common electrolyte abnormality after stabilization is hypokalemia. Cats with postobstructive diuresis have increased losses and generally require potassium supplementation (14–20 mEq/L) to prevent hypokalemia.

f. The monitoring frequency should reflect the severity of patient compromise. Critically ill cats may require constant monitoring initially; evaluations are then extended to every 2 hours and longer as the cat improves. Very stable cats may require very little monitoring of vital signs or blood parameters.

g. Urine output should be followed closely to make sure postobstructive diuresis does not compromise the patient. Urine output can be as high as 100–120 mL/h in a cat after relief of urethral obstruction. If IV fluid rates are not increased to compensate for urinary losses, dehydration will result.

h. Rarely, urinary tract bleeding can be severe enough to require a transfusion. In these instances, coagulation profiles are warranted to rule out any coagulopathic conditions. Hemoglobinuria secondary to acute hemolysis associated with hypophosphatemia can be another cause of life-threatening anemia. Phosphate replacement may be required in rare cases (p. 331).

i. If fluid input does not match urine output, dehydration will develop. With excessive solute diuresis, cats often develop "medullary washout" and lose the ability (temporarily) to concentrate urine. In these cases, fluids must be tapered off gradually before they are discontinued. To promote dilute urine formation to dissolve crystalline and inflammatory precipitates, the cat can be given subcutaneous fluids after intravenous fluids are discontinued.

3. Prognosis
   a. Prognosis is very good even in critically ill cats if they are stabilized through the first few hours.
   b. Clients should be warned about reobstruction, and perineal urethrostomy should be considered if the problem recurs.

D. Feline lower urinary tract disease: Nonobstructed cat

1. Diagnosis, clinical signs
   a. Idiopathic stranguria, hematuria, and dysuria are common in both male and female cats.
   b. The cause is unknown, but contributing factors include stress, crystalluria, bladder inflammation (interstitial cystitis), dry diets, and alkaline or concentrated urine.
   c. Affected cats often urinate outside the litter box, have demonstrable hematuria and pollakiuria, and lick the genital area frequently.
   d. On physical examination the bladder is usually small or empty.
   e. Urine culture is usually negative unless previous catheterization has been performed.
   f. If the cat is already on a diet to promote acid urine, calcium oxalate crystalluria should be suspected. Abdominal radiographs may reveal bladder stones.
   g. Any uroliths or mucous plugs should be submitted to the University of Minnesota for stone analysis and definitive diagnosis. Cats with calcium oxalate crystalluria need a diet specifically formulated to promote alkaline urine; cats with struvite crystalluria require a diet that promotes the formation of acid urine.
   h. Male cats are at risk for developing urethral obstruction.

2. Medical management
   a. Male cats should be given subcutaneous fluids (40–60 mL/kg/day) to promote dilute urine and diuresis, and they should be watched closely for signs of obstruction.
   b. Canned diets will increase water intake and promote less-concentrated urine.
   c. Antibiotics are usually not indicated unless there is a previous history of catheterization, although many clinicians administer antibiotics to prevent infection of a severely inflamed hemorrhagic bladder.

d. Many cats improve within 5–7 days with or without therapy.
e. Recurrences are common, but episodes tend to decrease in severity and frequency as cats age.
f. Amitriptyline, 2.5–10 mg once daily in the evening, may have benefit by stabilizing mast cells, decreasing stress through mild sedation, and reducing inflammatory changes of interstitial cystitis.
g. Diazepam, 1–2 mg/cat q12–24h, may relieve stress and decrease urethral spasms, but hepatotoxicity has been reported in cats receiving oral diazepam.
h. Phenoxybenzamine, 5 mg PO q12h, can reduce urethral muscle spasms.
i. Prednisolone, 1 mg/kg PO q12–24h, may reduce inflammation and edema.

E. Ruptured urinary bladder

1. The two major causes of a ruptured urinary bladder are trauma and overdistention of the urinary bladder secondary to urethral obstruction.
2. Diagnosis
   a. Definitive diagnosis is provided by finding free urine within the abdominal cavity and contrast cystography demonstrating loss of urinary bladder integrity or direct visualization during exploratory surgery.
   b. Free fluid in the abdomen may be identified as urine by
      1) Comparison of the abdominal fluid creatinine concentration to the creatinine concentration in a simultaneously collected peripheral blood sample. If the creatinine concentration in the fluid is higher than that in the blood, then the fluid is likely urine.
      2) Finding a higher concentration of potassium in the abdominal fluid than in a simultaneously collected blood sample suggests that the fluid is likely urine.
      3) Finding a higher BUN in the abdominal fluid than in a simultaneously collected blood sample suggests that the free abdominal fluid is urine.
   c. Ureteral leakage may result in uroperitoneum if the peritoneum lining the retroperitoneal space has been ruptured.
      1) An intravenous urogram should be performed on any patient with uroperitoneum to fully assess the integrity of the urinary tract.

2) Avulsion of the ureter from the kidney can cause lumbar pain from retroperitoneal urine leakage, azotemia, and hyperkalemia.

3) Evaluation of the integrity of the ureters via exploratory surgery after trauma can often be difficult, if not impossible, in certain patients with significant retroperitoneal hematoma formation.

3. Treatment

a. Initial stabilization with intravenous fluids and perfusion support should be administered as for any critically ill patient.

b. Severe electrolyte changes and acid–base derangement should be treated to stabilize the patient.

c. Extremely uremic patients will benefit from several hours of peritoneal dialysis prior to anesthesia and surgery.

d. Once the patient is stable, surgery should be done to repair the defect.

e. Small tears in the bladder or urethra may not require surgery. A urinary catheter and closed drainage system can be left in place for 3–10 days.

4. Postoperative care

a. Treatment and monitoring should be as for any critically ill patient.

b. If the urine was infected, septic peritonitis may result and this condition should be treated if it is present (see septic peritonitis, p. 219).

F. Hematuria

1. Hematuria can range from minor to frank hemorrhage that is life threatening. The latter has been noted occasionally in cats after relief of urethral obstruction and in dogs with systemic coagulopathy.

2. Hematuria may occur because of a local problem anywhere within the urinary tract or because of a systemic coagulopathic condition.

a. Local problems include trauma, inflammation, infection, neoplasia, urinary calculi, vascular anomalies, and benign prostatic bleeding.

3. Diagnosis

a. Grossly, the urine can appear slightly red to frankly hemorrhagic.

1) Definitive diagnosis cannot be made on the basis of the gross appearance of the urine because hemoglobinuria can appear very similar to hematuria.

2) Red urine should be centrifuged.

a) *If the supernatant becomes clear then hematuria is present.*

b) *If the supernatant does not clear, pigmenturia (hemoglobinuria or myoglobinuria) is present, but hemorrhage cannot be ruled out.*

3) The presence of red blood cells on a direct smear or urinary sediment examination indicates hematuria.

a) *Blood may sometimes contaminate the urine during cystocentesis or traumatic catheterization.*

b) *A large amount of blood can sometimes contaminate the urine when a blood vessel is inadvertently punctured during cystocentesis.*

b. Urine dipsticks may be positive for blood even when only hemoglobinuria is present.

c. Diagnostic evaluation

1) Urinalysis will provide information regarding local urinary tract processes such as inflammation, infection, urinary calculi, and neoplasia.

2) Further evaluation depending upon the urinalysis may include CBC, chemistry screen, coagulation screen, platelet count, platelet function tests, urine culture, imaging procedures, and exploratory laparotomy.

d. Emergency therapy

1) Hematuria itself rarely causes any life-threatening problems.

2) Rarely, severe urinary tract bleeding can result in anemia and hypovolemia. Patients should be monitored closely for these problems when severe urinary tract hemorrhage is present.

3) Rule out any potentially life-threatening problems such as urinary tract obstruction, urinary tract rupture, or prostatic abscess.

G. Urolithiasis

1. The most immediately life-threatening problem associated with urolithiasis is urethral obstruction.

2. Urolithiasis may be an incidental finding during workup for other problems but is most often associated with lower urinary tract signs such as pollakiuria, stranguria, and hematuria.

3. Diagnosis

a. Lower urinary tract signs such as stranguria, pollakiuria, and hematuria are the most common presenting complaints.

b. Animals may present with signs consistent with the underlying disease process such as hepatoencephalopathy in patients with ammonium biurate stones due to hepatic disease.

c. Urinary tract stones may be found anywhere in the urinary tract including the renal pelvis, ureters, urinary bladder, and urethra. The most common site is the urinary bladder.

d. Radiopaque stones may be detected with plain abdominal radiography.

    1) Uroliths noted to be radiopaque include oxalates, magnesium ammonium phosphates (struvite), and calcium phosphates.

    2) Uroliths with varying density include cystine, ammonium urates and uric acid stones, mixed stones, and matrix stones.

    3) True radiolucent uroliths with properly performed radiographs are rare.

e. Uroliths may be outlined or detected by contrast radiography.

f. Abdominal ultrasonography may detect uroliths in the renal pelvis, ureters, or the urinary bladder.

4. Treatment

a. Treatment should be as for any critically ill patient.

b. The most immediately life-threatening condition associated with urolithiasis is urethral obstruction.

c. Urethral obstruction due to urolithiasis occurs most commonly in males. The uroliths usually lodge at the base of the os penis in dogs.

d. A urethral catheter should be placed as discussed above (p. 226).

e. If the urinary catheter cannot dislodge or bypass the urethral urolith, then try simultaneous flushing of the urinary catheter with sterile saline and attempts at passage of the catheter.

f. If passage of the urinary catheter is not possible at this point, then urethral hydropropulsion will be necessary (see p. 229).

    1) Another option is to place a stylet in a urinary catheter and pass it to the obstruction and gently push. Pushing too aggressively can potentially damage or rupture the already inflamed urethra. Take care to ensure that the stylet does not get outside the urinary catheter.

    2) Passage of an appropriately sized Foley catheter to the site of obstruction and slowly and gently inflating of the balloon with normal saline while the catheter is gently

pushed can sometimes free up the urolith. Again, care is needed to avoid aggressive pushing or overinflation of the balloon.

    3) Once the urinary catheter is passed, the urinary bladder should be completely emptied and the catheter should remain in place.

g. If passage of the urinary catheter is still not possible, then a urethrotomy should be performed or a prepubic cystostomy tube must be placed.

h. Further concerns

    1) Aftercare should be applied as to any critically ill patient. Give special attention to monitoring urine output and the potential for postobstructive diuresis.

    2) Analyze the urolith to provide clues to the underlying cause of its formation.

    3) Do a full evaluation to determine the underlying cause of the urolith.

H. Leptospirosis

1. Leptospirosis is caused by a spirochete that can affect the liver and the kidney and cause a systemic vasculitis.

2. Classic leptospirosis is caused by the serovars *icterohaemorrhagiae* and *canicola*. More recently, serovars *grippotyphosa*, *pomona*, and *bratislava* have been recognized in increasing frequency to cause disease.

3. Most commercial vaccines contain only antigens from serovars *icterohaemorrhagiae* and *canicola*. A new vaccine (Fort Dodge) now offers protection against *L. pomona* and *L. grippotyphosa*.

4. Outbreaks of canine leptospirosis have followed periods of heavy rainfall or flooding. It is transmitted through the urine of infected wildlife.

5. Leptospires can infect by invading mucous membranes or open skin wounds.

6. Clinical findings

    a. Fever, anorexia, vomiting, diarrhea, weight loss depression, dehydration, polydipsia, polyuria, bleeding, icterus, abdominal pain, renomegaly, myalgia, anterior uveitis, and hypovolemic shock

    b. Laboratory abnormalities include leukocytosis (primarily a neutrophilia), thrombocytopenia, increased BUN, increased creatinine, increased liver enzymes, increased total bilirubin, hypoproteinemia, hyperphosphatemia, isosthenuria, hematuria, granular urinary casts, white blood cells in urine, and glucosuria.

1) Renal abnormalities may be present without liver abnormalities, particularly with serovars *grippotyphosa* and *pomona.*

2) Laboratory abnormalities may be dynamic, depending upon the stage of disease. Serial hematologic and serum chemistry evaluations may be necessary.

7. Pathophysiology
   a. Clinical and laboratory abnormalities can be explained by the systemic spread of the organism, its replication in localized areas, and a toxin associated with the organism's outer membrane.
   b. Local replication of spirochetes in the renal tubular cells causes inflammation in the kidney and shedding of the organism in the urine.

8. Diagnosis
   a. Diagnosis is made serologically combined with consistent clinical signs.
   b. The microscopic agglutination test is the mostly widely used method for detecting antibodies against leptospires.
      1) Diagnosis of infection is definitive when at least a 4-fold increase in titers is detected 2–4 weeks apart.
      2) Usually, the serovar with the highest titer is considered to be the infecting agent.
      3) Titers may be negative during the first week of infection.
      4) A single titer >1:800 (longer than 3 months after vaccination) and compatible clinical signs are sufficient for diagnosis.
      5) Vaccine titers are serovar specific and usually are below 1:320 but can be much higher in some instances. Usually the titers drop below 1:320 3 months after vaccination.
   c. ELISA titers can distinguish between IgM and IgG antibodies and can be helpful if results of the microscopic agglutination test are confusing.
   d. Darkfield microscopy may demonstrate spirochetes in the urine (special microscope required).
   e. Spirochetes may be demonstrated on renal or hepatic biopsy specimens following silver stains.

9. Treatment
   a. Treatment should be started immediately and not be delayed for results of serology.

   b. Specific treatment for leptospirosis is antibiotics.
      1) Penicillin (20,000 to 50,000 U/kg IM or SQq12h) is effective for leptospiremia.
         a) Ampicillin and amoxicillin are also effective.
         b) Penicillins are eliminated primarily by the kidneys, and the dose should be adjusted for dogs that are in renal failure.
      2) Penicillin therapy should be continued for 2 weeks or until azotemia resolves.
      3) Either dihydrostreptomycin (10–15 mg/kg IM q12h), tetracycline (20 mg/kg PO q8h), or doxycycline (10 mg/kg PO q24h) are recommended to eliminate the leptospires from the kidney and prevent leptospire shedding. These antibiotics should be started after termination of the penicillin therapy and continued for 2 weeks.
         a) Doxycycline has fewer nephrotoxic effects than tetracycline and dihydrostreptomycin.
      4) Supportive care should be given as for any patient in acute renal failure.
      5) Disseminated intravascular coagulation may occur in patients with systemic vasculitis and should be monitored and treated as necessary (see DIC, p. 292).
      6) Leptospirosis is potentially a zoonotic disease. Animal care workers should avoid contact with urine, wear gloves when handling the animal, and wash hands after treatments.
      7) To prevent spread of leptospirosis, affected animals in the hospital should be allowed to urinate in a run with a floor drain, and the drain should be flushed with Betadine solution or other disinfectant, or the urine can be collected through urethral catheterization and closed system drainage.

10. Prognosis
    a. Acute renal failure is usually reversible.
    b. Some animals develop chronic renal failure; therefore, animals should be monitored for several months after recovery for this problem.

I. Acute on chronic renal failure

1. Chronic renal disease is common in geriatric cats and dogs. Animals with loss of 66% of nephron function lose the ability to concentrate urine and are said to have renal insufficiency.

2. As long as the glomerular filtration rate (GFR) and water intake are adequate, uremic renal failure can be avoided. Conditions that promote hypotension, such as anesthesia or dehydration, can result in acute on chronic renal failure.

3. The treatment goal is to provide fluid therapy to promote diuresis, restore hydration, and reduce the azotemia low enough to avoid the clinical signs of uremia.

4. This condition should be prevented, if possible, by avoiding nephrotoxic drugs, avoiding hypotensive agents, providing intravenous fluids during anesthesia, and avoiding dehydration in animals with known renal insufficiency.

5. Clinical signs include anorexia, vomiting, diarrhea, dehydration, polyuria, and polydipsia.

6. Nonregenerative anemia and systemic hypertension are common in animals with chronic renal failure.

7. Treatment involves supportive care and control of clinical signs of anemia.

    a. Intravenous fluid therapy is administered as for acute renal failure. To avoid hypernatremia in patients with a reduced GFR, 0.45% saline and 2.5% dextrose can be used. Polyuric patients receiving fluid diuresis often develop hypokalemia. To prevent this, 14–20 mEq/L of KCl can be added to each liter as long as hyperkalemia is not present.

    b. These animals are usually polyuric. After dehydration has been corrected, fluid input should match urine output ("ins and outs"). Animals with acute on chronic renal failure usually produce 2–5 mL/kg/h of urine.

    c. After several days of fluid therapy, serum creatinine will usually plateau and further reduction is difficult. At this time, fluid therapy can be gradually tapered off to see if the patient can maintain renal function without continued fluid diuresis. If necessary, a kidney biopsy can be done for prognostic purposes.

    d. Vomiting can be controlled with the following mediations:

        1) Ranitidine: 2–4 mg/kg IV q12h

        2) Chlorpromazine: 0.5 mg/kg IM or SQq6–12h

        3) Metoclopramide: 1–2 mg/kg/24 h added to fluids as a constant rate infusion.

        4) Sucralfate: 1 g/25 kg PO q8h

    e. If severe anemia develops, a blood transfusion can be given followed by injections of recombinant erythropoietin 50–100 U/kg SQ2–3 times per week. Approximately 30% of animals develop antibodies against erythropoietin, so this treatment is reserved for severe cases.

    f. Hypertension is common in animals with chronic renal failure and should be treated if systolic pressure exceeds 200 mm Hg or diastolic pressure exceeds 110 mm Hg. Treatments include

        1) Low-sodium diet

        2) Enalapril: 0.5 mg/kg PO q12–24h

        3) Amlodipine (cats): 0.625 mg/cat PO q24h

    g. Dietary management

        1) Phosphorus restriction or phosphorus binder

        2) Supplementation with omega-3 polyunsaturated fatty acids to reduce inflammatory precursors

        3) Protein restriction to prevent buildup of nitrogenous wastes

        4) A multiple vitamin supplement is recommended to replace water = soluble vitamins lost in the urine.

J. Glomerulonephritis

1. Pathophysiology

    a. Damage to the glomerulus can occur from immune complexes, chronic antigenic stimulation, or direct toxin injury.

    b. The hallmark of glomerular disease is proteinuria secondary to protein leakage through damaged glomerular membranes.

    c. Loss of antithrombin III predisposes these animals to thromboembolic disease.

2. Clinical signs

    a. Nonspecific signs, such as poor body condition and weight loss may be present.

    b. If albumin <1.5 g/dL, pitting edema and ascites may develop.

    c. There may be evidence of predisposing inflammatory, infectious, or neoplastic disease.

    d. Hypertension (systolic BP >160–180 mm Hg) is common.

    e. Signs of acute thromboembolism may develop, e.g., dyspnea, labored respirations, and loss of peripheral pulse.

3. Diagnosis

    a. A urine protein/creatinine ratio >1.0 is abnormal. Hematuria or urinary tract infection may elevate proteinuria (PC ratio usually less than 8) until the UTI is treated. The PC ratio may be extremely high with glomerulonephritis (usually in the range of 10–25) or amyloidosis (20–40).

b. Azotemia develops with glomerulosclerosis and a decreased GFR.

c. Nephrotic syndrome includes hypoproteinemia, proteinuria, hypercholesterolemia, and edema.

d. Normal antithrombin III activity is 80–130%. When it is <75%, a hypercoagulable state exists, and dogs are at risk for thrombus formation.

e. Ultrasound may reveal hyperechogenicity of the renal cortex and loss of the corticomedullary junction.

f. Definitive diagnosis can be made with renal biopsy.

g. The underlying condition should be sought (*Table 12-2*).

4. Treatment

   a. Recognize and treat underlying disease.

   b. Angiotensin-converting enzyme (ACE) inhibitors (enalapril 0.5 mg/kg q12–24h)

may reduce proteinuria and slow progression of disease.

c. If hypertension is still present after ACE inhibitors, additional treatment may be needed:

   1) Amlodipine 0.1 mg/kg PO q24h

   2) Prazosin 1 mg/15 kg PO q8–12h

   3) Atenolol 0.25–1.0 mg/kg q12–24h

d. Feed high quality, protein-restricted diet.

e. Aspirin 0.5 mg/kg q12–24h (dogs) or 25 mg/kg q48h (cats) may prevent thromboembolism and attenuate thromboxane induced glomerular injury.

f. Immunosuppressive therapy (prednisone, azathioprine) is used for glomerulonephritis associated with immune mediated disease.

g. H_2 blockers are used to manage gastritis

   1) Cimetidine 5 mg/kg PO or IV q6–8h

   2) Ranitidine 2 mg/kg PO or IV q8–12h

   3) Famotidine 0.5–1.0 mg/kg PO or IV q12–24h

TABLE 12.2
CONDITIONS ASSOCIATED WITH GLOMERULONEPHRITIS

Inflammatory
   Chronic dermatitis
   Pancreatitis
   Polyarthritis
   Inflammatory bowel disease
   Immune mediated diseases (SLE)

Infectious
   Bacterial endocarditis
   Borreliosis
   Pyometritis
   Babesiosis
   Hepatozoonosis
   Leishmaniasis
   Ehrlichiosis
   Dirofilariasis
   Cats—FeLV, FIV, FIP

Neoplastic
   Lymphosarcoma
   Carcinoma
   Mastocytosis
   Leukemia

Miscellaneous
   Corticosteroid excess
   Trimethoprim-sulfa
   Familial

h. Acute azotemia requires fluid therapy. If edema is present, colloids are necessary (plasma, hetastarch, or Dextran 70 at a dosage of 10–20 mL/ kg/day). Low-sodium crystalloid fluids (0.45% saline with 2.5% dextrose) are used for maintenance requirements.
i. Diuretics may be given to reduce ascites and edema.
   1) Furosemide 2 mg/kg PO q8–24h
   2) Spironolactone 1–2 mg/kg q12–24h
j. A sodium-restricted diet is recommended.
k. Prognosis is very poor for animals with uremia, hypoalbuminemia, and/or thromboembolic disease in association with glomerulonephritis.
l. Prognosis is favorable if the protein/creatinine ratio improves following treatment of the underlying disease.

K. Urethral trauma

1. Cause of trauma
  a. Blunt trauma—urethral contusion
  b. Laceration/rupture—fractures of pubis or os penis; penetrating wounds (gunshot, knife, bite); iatrogenic (traumatic catheterization)

2. Clinical signs
  a. Dysuria, hematuria, pain, swelling, ascites, discoloration of skin in perineal area.
  b. Absence of clinical signs does not rule out urethral tear. Voiding may be normal.
  c. Cellulitis, development of fistulous tracts, leukocytosis
  d. Dehydration, hypoproteinemia

3. Diagnosis
  a. Clinical suspicion
  b. Positive-contrast urethrogram (not cystogram, p. 227)

4. Treatment
  a. Correct acid–base, electrolyte, and perfusion problems.
  b. If transection is not complete, the urethra will regenerate to repair the tear if a urinary catheter is left in place for 3 weeks.
  c. If extravasation of urine has caused tissue damage, surgical exploration with drain placement may be required. The urethral tear can be sutured and a urinary catheter left in place as a stent.
  d. For complete urethral rupture, a midline symphysiotomy is performed, and the severed ends of the urethra are anastomosed by suturing them over a urinary catheter that remains

in place for 5–7 days. Sometimes a prepubic cystostomy catheter is placed to divert urine from the urethra while it heals.
  e. An Elizabethan collar is usually necessary to prevent premature removal of the urinary catheter.
  f. Closed urine drainage with periodic culture and sensitivity testing for infection is recommended.

L. Perineal hernia

1. Breakdown of muscles surrounding the rectum (coccygeus, levator ani, and external anal sphincter muscles) allows abdominal organs or tissues (urinary bladder, intestines, fat) to herniate into the perineal area.
2. Most common in older male dogs, may be secondary to prostatic hypertrophy and tenesmus
3. Predisposed breeds include the Boston Terrier, Boxer, Collie, Corgi, Pekinese, and Old English Sheepdog.
4. Clinical signs include constipation, tenesmus, and dyschezia. Stranguria occurs with bladder herniation.
5. The hernia may be unilateral or bilateral.
6. Diagnosis is made from history, clinical signs, and rectal examination.
  a. A perineal mass can be palpated and reduced with pressure.
  b. A rectal examination should be done carefully to avoid perforation. A lack of muscular support in the pelvic diaphragm makes it feel weak and "flabby."
  c. A retrograde urethro/cystogram can be done to confirm herniation of the urinary bladder.

7. The definitive treatment is surgical correction, but the animal must be stabilized prior to surgery.
  a. The surgery is not an emergency unless there is bladder herniation or intestinal obstruction.
  b. A urinary catheter should be passed to empty the bladder if it is retroflexed into the hernia.
  c. The rectum should be manually evacuated and the animal placed on stool softeners (dioctyl sodium succinate 100–200 mg PO daily) and a low-residue diet prior to surgery. Enemas and laxatives are not indicated, as liquid stool will contaminate the surgery site.
  d. Broad-spectrum antibiotics are administered pre- and postoperatively to prevent infection.

e. Immediate postsurgical complications include infection, fecal incontinence, rectal prolapse, sciatic nerve entrapment, and hernia recurrence on the same or opposite side.

f. Castration should always be performed along with hernia repair.

M. Acute prostatitis/prostatic abscess

1. Acute bacterial infection of the prostate gland can cause fever, lethargy, and signs of systemic sepsis.

2. Clinical signs include dripping of hemorrhagic or purulent fluid from the penis, stiff gait, caudal abdominal pain, and pain on rectal examination.

3. Prostatic abscessation may cause dysuria and tenesmus.

4. Ruptured prostatic abscess is a cause of acute abdomen, resulting in fever, shock, vomiting, and abdominal pain secondary to septic peritonitis.

5. Occurs most commonly in middle-aged, intact male dogs.

6. Diagnosis
   a. Urinalysis reveals pyuria and bacteruria ± hematuria.
   b. CBC—neutrophilic leukocytosis with left shift and toxic neutrophils is common. With severe sepsis, neutropenia or degenerative left shift may be present.
   c. Dogs with sepsis frequently have dehydration, hemoconcentration, hypoglycemia, elevated serum alkaline phosphatase, and increased bilirubin.
   d. Abdominal radiographs may reveal prostatomegaly and/or loss of detail in the caudal abdomen.
   e. Abdominal ultrasound may reveal focal-to-diffuse hyperechogenicity. Hypoechoic areas suggest abscessation.
   f. Prostatic wash or massage is not recommended, as acute prostatitis is very painful.
   g. Needle aspiration is not recommended because of the risk of rupturing a prostatic abscess.
   h. A Gram stain of the urine can be done. The most common bacteria is *Escherichia coli*. Others include *Staphylococcus, Proteus, Klebsiella, Pseudomonas,* and *Streptococcus/Enterococcus.*
   i. A urine sample should be submitted for culture and sensitivity testing.

7. Treatment
   a. Animals exhibiting tachycardia, painful abdomen, vomiting, weak pulses, hypo- glycemia, "muddy" mucous membrane color, and slow capillary refill time have signs of septic shock.
      1) Septic shock should be managed with appropriate supportive care (pp. 220–222).
      2) Administer intravenous bactericidal antibiotics (fluoroquinolone and β-lactam or cephalosporin).
      3) Do abdominocentesis or diagnostic peritoneal lavage (pp. 190–192) to determine if peritonitis has occurred from ruptured prostatic abscess.
      4) Surgery should be performed as soon as possible.
   b. Prostatic abscesses need to be surgically drained (Penrose drainage or marsupialization).
   c. Antibiotic therapy (based on culture and sensitivity testing) should be continued for 8 weeks for peritonitis or prostatic abscess and for 4 weeks for simple acute prostatitis. Urine should be cultured 7 days after completing therapy to prevent the occurrence of chronic prostatitis.
   d. Castration should be performed to promote shrinkage of the prostate gland and hasten resolution.
   e. Urinary catheterization with closed drainage may be required in some dogs with prostatic abscess causing dysuria and partial urethral obstruction.
   f. Therapy for chronic prostatitis requires long-term treatment (8–12 weeks) with antibiotics that have good penetration of the prostate (trimethoprim-sulfa, fluoroquinolones, or chloramphenicol).

N. Pyelonephritis

1. Bacterial infection of the upper urinary tract can result in systemic signs of anorexia, vomiting, fever, and lethargy.

2. Acute pyelonephritis can cause lumbar pain and a stiff, stilted gait.

3. Risk factors include diabetes mellitus, hyperadrenocorticism, urolithiasis, lower urinary tract infection, immunosuppression, neoplasia, and congenital or acquired anomalies of the urinary tract.

4. Most infections ascend from the lower urinary tract, but occasionally, hematogenous spread can occur from bacterial endocarditis, diskospondylitis, or periodontal disease.

5. Pyelonephritis can result in acute or chronic renal failure.

6. Diagnosis
   a. Laboratory work reveals leukocytosis ±left shift, ±mild anemia, azotemia, and hyperphosphatemia.
   b. Bacteriuria, pyuria, hematuria, ±cellular or granular casts, and low specific gravity are common findings on urinalysis.
   c. Urine should be submitted for culture and sensitivity testing. Common bacteria include *E. coli, Staphylococcus aureus, Proteus mirabilis, Streptococcus* spp., *Klebsiella pneumoniae, Pseudomonas aeruginosa,* and *Enterobacter* spp.
   d. Ultrasonography may reveal dilated renal pelvis and proximal ureter, bright renal pelvis, and changes in echogenicity of the renal parenchyma.
   e. Excretory urography may show dilation of the proximal ureter and renal pelvis, blunting of the renal diverticula, decreased uptake of contrast material, or prolonged retention of dye. These changes are not specific for acute pyelonephritis and may persist from a previous infection. A normal excretory urogram does not rule out pyelonephritis.
   f. Urine culture material can be obtained directly from the renal pelvis by ultrasound-guided aspiration or at the time of surgery if it is performed. Culture material can also be obtained from the center of uroliths.
   g. Renal biopsy may reveal pyelitis, interstitial nephritis, and leukocyte casts in tubular lumens.

7. Treatment
   a. Antibiotics should be chosen on the basis of culture and sensitivity testing. Aminoglycosides should be avoided if possible because of nephrotoxicity. Antibiotics with good renal penetration include ampicillin, amoxicillin–clavulanic acid, trimethoprim/sulfa, cephalosporins, chloramphenicol, and fluoroquinolones.
   1) Antibiotic therapy should be continued for 4–8 weeks.
   2) Urine should be cultured 5–7 days after completing antibiotic therapy.
   3) If infection is still present, continue treatment for another 6–8 weeks and reculture.
   4) Urine should be cultured q6–8 weeks until three negative cultures are obtained. Positive urine cultures require another 6- to 8-week course of therapy.

b. If casts are seen in the urine, the animal should be treated aggressively for acute renal failure (pp. 235–237) or acute on chronic renal failure (pp. 243–244).
c. Chronic recurrent infections sometimes occur.
   1) Low-dose antibiotic therapy (1/3 dose given at bedtime) may be required long term.
   2) Lightly salting food or adding bouillon to water may encourage drinking.
   3) Monitor blood pressure. Avoid salt if hypertensive. Consider a low-dose diuretic to promote diuresis.
   4) Consider dietary management.
      a) *Alkaline diets to prevent oxalate urolithiasis*
      b) *Acidic diets to prevent struvite urolithiasis*

O. Ureteral obstruction/hydronephrosis

1. Obstruction of a ureter can cause progressive distension of the renal pelvis resulting in destruction of renal parenchyma.
   a. The longer the obstruction, the less chance of reversibility.
   b. Causes of ureteral obstruction include uroliths, neoplasia, prostatic enlargement, perineal hernias, trauma, or accidental ligation during ovariohysterectomy.
2. Clinical signs may include vomiting and lumbar pain. Palpation may reveal an abdominal mass. With unilateral partial obstruction, no clinical signs may be seen and azotemia will not develop if the contralateral kidney is functional.
3. Laboratory findings include isosthenuria and progressive azotemia.
4. Diagnosis can be confirmed with ultrasound or excretory urography. Ureteral rupture may occur, causing fluid accumulation in the retroperitoneal space.
5. Treatment.
   a. Fluid and electrolyte balance should be restored. Hyperkalemia, acidosis, and dehydration must be corrected.
   b. Ultrasound or excretory urography should be done to determine the extent of damage and ensure that the contralateral kidney appears to be functioning. Intravenous contrast material should be avoided until rehydration is completed, as it may cause nephrotoxicity.

c. Unilateral nephrectomy is recommended for nonfunctional hydronephrotic kidneys, as they can become a continual source of infection if allowed to remain in situ. Bacterial infection could lead to life-threatening sepsis.

d. If the kidney is still functional, the obstruction should be removed as soon as possible. A ureteral stent may be required postoperatively.

e. Urine should be submitted for culture and sensitivity testing, and infections should be aggressively treated for 4–8 weeks.

f. If the obstruction is caused by a urolith, stone analysis should be performed so that dietary and appropriate medical therapy can be initiated.

g. If the obstruction is relieved within 1 week, renal damage is reversible; irreversible damage usually occurs after 4 weeks.

P. Urethral obstruction/urolithiasis (canine)

1. The most common uroliths in dogs are

   a. Struvite (magnesium, ammonium, phosphate) uroliths:

   1) These are often associated with a urinary tract infection with urease-producing bacteria, which cause alkaline urine, thus promoting crystal formation. Common bacteria are *Staphylococcus* and *Protease* spp.

   2) Struvite uroliths are radiopaque.

   3) Diets high in protein, magnesium, and phosphorus can supersaturate the urine, especially when it is concentrated, thereby promoting urolith formation. These diets should be avoided.

   4) Miniature Schnauzers, Shi Tzus, Lhasa Apsos, and Miniature Poodles are predisposed. Exogenous steroid administration increases the risk.

   5) Microscopic struvite crystals appear as coffin-like prisms on microscopic evaluation of urine sediment.

   6) Struvite uroliths are responsible for 50% of lower urinary tract stones and 33% of upper urinary tract stones.

   b. Calcium oxalate uroliths:

   1) These stones account for 30–35% of stones removed from the lower urinary tract and 40% from the upper urinary tract in dogs. They also have become common in cats.

   2) Predisposed breeds include the Yorkshire Terrier, Miniature Schnauzer, and Lhasa Apso. More common in male dogs.

   3) Glucocorticoids, high-calcium diets, or diets that promote acid urine predispose.

   4) These stones cannot be medically dissolved with diet.

   5) Calcium oxalate stones are radiopaque.

   c. Cystine uroliths

   1) These stones result from an inborn error of metabolism that causes cystinuria in affected animals.

   2) Seen in young to middle-aged dogs. Affected breeds include Dachshunds, English Bulldogs, Newfoundlands, Welsh Corgis, and Staffordshire Terriers.

   3) These stones are not as radiodense as struvite or oxalate, but are more radiodense than urate stones.

   d. Urate uroliths

   1) These stones are radiolucent.

   2) Dalmatians and some English Bulldogs have a breed predisposition for forming urate stones.

   3) Other breeds (especially Yorkshire Terriers) may form urate stones as a result of portosystemic shunt causing impaired metabolism of uric acid and ammonia.

   4) These stones represent 5–8% of the uroliths removed from dogs.

   e. Calcium phosphate uroliths

   1) These are uncommon and usually secondary to hypercalcemia—primary hyperparathyroidism, excessive dietary calcium, or vitamin D ingestion.

   f. Silica uroliths

   1) Seen primarily in large dogs, especially German Shepherds, Golden Retrievers, and Labrador Retrievers.

   2) A diet containing high amounts of corn gluten and soybean hulls may predispose.

2. Clinical signs of urolithiasis include stranguria, dysuria, incontinence, and hematuria.

   a. If urethral obstruction occurs, clinical signs include vomiting, depression, lethargy, abdominal pain, and abdominal distension.

3. Urethral obstruction can also be caused by strictures and tumors. The most common cause of urethral obstruction in female dogs is transitional cell carcinoma involving the bladder and urethra.

4. Treatment

   a. Urethral obstruction must be relieved.

   1) In male dogs, a common site is the level of the os penis.

2) Retrograde urohydropropulsion should be performed to try to flush the urolith(s) back into the bladder.

3) A cystocentesis using a stopcock and extension tubing may be done to empty the bladder and relieve back pressure before attempting retrograde flushing.

4) A well-lubricated urinary catheter is passed to the site of the obstruction, and gentle "bumping" and flushing is carried out. The distal urethra can be occluded at the tip of the penis around the catheter to promote urethral distension. Urethral distension can also be achieved if an assistant holds off the urethra per rectum while the urethra is filled with saline under pressure. Pressure is relieved when the assistant relieves the occlusion by lifting a finger, and the obstruction should be flushed into the bladder. This procedure may need several repetitions to clear the obstruction.

b. A urinary catheter can be left in place if excessive urine sediment remains after bladder lavage or if detrusor atony is suspected.

c. If the obstruction cannot be relieved, surgery is required.

1) A prepubic urethrotomy can be performed to remove calculi lodged near the os penis. An incision is made on the ventral midline of the prepuce through the corpus spongiosum of the penis to expose the urethral lumen. A concurrent cystotomy may be required to remove higher urethral calculi.

2) A permanent urethrostomy in which urethral mucosa is sutured to the skin is recommended for animals with recurrent urolithiasis or urethral strictures. A scrotal urethrostomy or a prepubic urethrostomy can be performed (see surgical texts).

d. Stones should always be submitted for analysis, and urine should be evaluated for culture and sensitivity testing.

e. Medical management depends on the type of urolith.

1) Struvite uroliths can be dissolved medically or removed surgically.

a) If a concurrent urinary tract infection is present, antibiotics must be administered for the entire dissolution period (usually 2–3 months).

b) Dietary therapy (e.g., Hill's S/D) should be continued for 30 days after radiographic dissolution of uroliths.

2) Calcium oxalate stones cannot be dissolved. Surgical removal is recommended unless small stones can be expelled by voiding urohydropropulsion.

a) Diets formulated for oxalate stones are available and should help prevent or slow formation of additional stones. These diets should contain citrate and should result in the formation of alkaline urine.

b) If urine remains acidic, additional potassium citrate (75 mg/kg q12h) can be given.

c) Vitamin B_6 (2–4 mg/kg q24h) may decrease oxalate excretion in the urine.

3) Urate urolithiasis

a) Diagnostic workup should be performed to rule in/out portosystemic shunt.

b) Allopurinol (15 mg/kg PO q12h) is given to Dalmatians to decrease uric acid production.

c) A low-purine diet is recommended (either Hill's U/D or homemade).

d) Potassium citrate (40–75 mg/kg PO q12h) is recommended to maintain the urine pH between 7 and 7.5.

e) Eradication of urease-producing bacteria is important if infection is present.

4) Cystine urolithiasis

a) Acid urine should be avoided (i.e., feed Hill's U/D).

b) 2-Mercaptopropionyl glycine (2-MPG) at a dosage of 15–25 mg/kg q12h in conjunction with dietary management can dissolve the stones in 1–3 months.

5) Calcium phosphate urolithiasis

a) The underlying cause of hypercalcemia should be corrected.

6) Silica urolithiasis

a) Medical dissolution cannot be accomplished.

b) Avoid diets high in plant proteins (gluten and soy).

c) Encourage water drinking to promote diuresis and avoid concentrated urine.

CHAPTER 13

NEUROLOGIC EMERGENCIES

I. CLINICAL SIGNS, DIAGNOSIS

A. Clinical signs depend on location of lesion within nervous system.

B. Cerebral lesions cause seizures, behavioral changes, pacing or circling, blindness, sensory deficits, and minimal gait abnormalities. Focal deficits are contralateral to the affected side.

C. Cerebellar disease causes ataxia, hypermetria, tremors, and possible menace deficits with normal vision and vestibular signs. Wide-based stance with normal strength and postural reactions are seen. Intention tremors are induced by purposeful movement such as reaching for food or water.

D. Brainstem lesions cause cranial nerve deficits, severe gait and postural abnormalities, and changes in mentation if the ascending reticular activating system is affected. Deficits are usually ipsilateral to the affected side when lesions are caudal to the midbrain (*Table 13-1*).

E. Spinal cord lesions cause upper motor neuron signs (e.g., exaggerated segmental reflexes, caudal to lesion) and lower motor neuron signs (depressed or absent reflexes and withdrawal at the site of the lesion) if the cervical, intumescence (C_6-T_2) or lumbosacral intumescence (L_4-S_3) are involved. Unilateral lesions cause ipsilateral signs.

F. Diseases of peripheral nerves or the neuromuscular junction cause lower motor neuron signs with or without sensory deficits.

G. Testing the specific function of each area of the nervous system allows localizing the lesion (*Table 13-2*).

II. DIAGNOSTIC AND MONITORING PROCEDURES

A. A thorough neurologic examination is the most important diagnostic tool in evaluating patients that present with neurologic signs.

B. History and general physical examination will assist in making a differential diagnosis and identifying nonneurologic disease.

C. Once neurologic disease has been identified and localized, further diagnostic steps may be indicated.

D. Radiography may aid in diagnosing intracranial disease (e.g., hydrocephalus, skull fracture) but is more helpful when assessing a patient with spinal cord signs. Spinal column fracture or luxations may be seen in trauma patients. Narrowed or wedged intervertebral disk spaces with collapsed articular facets may indicate intervertebral disk herniation. General anesthesia is often necessary for optimal positioning.

E. Myelography involves injecting positive contrast material into the spinal cord subarachnoid space to evaluate spinal cord deviation, compression, or swelling (*Table 13-3*). Myelography is indicated to help localize the surgical site or when neurologic examination findings are inconsistent with radiographic lesions, no radiographic lesions are seen, or multiple radiographic lesions are present. Seizures may be a complication of cisternal myelography but rarely occur with newer contrast agents.

F. Brain tumors and other intracranial disorders are best evaluated with magnetic resonance imaging (MRI) or computed tomography (CT). MRI is

TABLE 13.1
CRANIAL NERVES

Cranial Nerve	Function	Neurologic Examination Findings with Lesions Affecting Nerve
I, Olfactory	Smell	Crude—unable to locate food while blindfolded
II, Optic	Vision	Menace response absent; unable to navigate obstacle course or follow dropped cotton ball
III, Oculomotor	Pupil constriction, ocular movement (dorsal, medial, ventral), eyelid elevation	Pupils dilated or asymmetric; oculocephalic (doll's eye) reflex absent when head moved side to side; ventrolateral strabismus
IV, Trochlear	Eye position, innervation of superior oblique muscle	Lateral rotation of eyeball (easier to detect in cats because of vertical pupil)
V, Trigeminal	Sensory component— sensory to entire head and face	Lack of response when stimulus applied to pinna, nasal mucosa, medial canthos, or cornea (facial nerve is motor component of reflex)
	Motor component—muscles of mastication	Temporalis muscle atrophy/asymmetry; unable to chew or close mouth (if bilateral involvement)
VI, Abducens	Eye position, innervation of lateral rectus/retractor ocular muscle	Medial strabismus
VII, Facial	Facial expression	Facial muscle droop, blink reflex absent (trigeminal nerve is sensory component of reflex)
VIII, Vestibulocochlear	Eye movement/balance (vestibular portion), hearing (cochlear portion)	Nystagmus, head tilt, ataxia (vestibular component); lack of response to noise/negative brain stem auditory evoked response (cochlear)
IX, Glossopharyngeal	Sensory and motor to pharynx	Gag reflex absent; unable to swallow (dysphagia)
X, Vagus	Sensory and motor to pharynx, parasympathetic to visceral organs	Gag reflex absent; unable to swallow (dysphagia)
XI, Accessory	Motor to neck and shoulder muscles	Atrophy of neck/shoulder muscles
XII, Hypoglossal	Motor to tongue	Atrophy or asymmetry of tongue

optimal for soft tissue lesions. CT provides more sensitive evaluation of bony structure and may be optimal for detecting tumors that have invaded bone or extended through the cribriform plate. These modalities can also be used to evaluate patients with spinal cord signs in which radiography or myelography are not conclusive.

G. Cerebrospinal fluid (CSF) tap is indicated when evaluating patients with multifocal neurologic signs,

TABLE 13.2
SPINAL REFLEXES

Reflex	Peripheral Nerve Tested	Spinal Cord Segments Involved	Technique	Expected Response
Forelimb				
Biceps	Musculocutaneous	C6-8	Percuss finger placed on biceps tendon	Elbow flexion (often subtle)
Triceps	Radial	C7-T2	Percuss triceps tendon at insertion	Elbow extension
Extensor carpi radialis	Radial	C7-T2	Percuss muscle belly	Carpus extension
Withdrawal (flexor) reflex	Dorsal surface— radial Palmar surface— median, ulnar	C7-T2	Pinch toe with hemostat to create noxious stimulus	Limb flexion
Rear limb				
Patellar	Femoral	L4-6	Percuss patellar tendon	Stifle extension
Cranial tibial	Sciatic, peroneal branch	L6, 7-S1	Percuss muscle belly	Hock flexion
Gastrocnemius	Sciatic, tibial branch	L6, 7-S1	Percuss Achilles tendon	Hock extension
Withdrawal (flexion)	Medial toe—femoral Lateral toe—sciatic	L4-S1	Pinch toe with hemostat	Limb flexion
Perineal	Perineal	S2-3	Pinch perineum with hemostat	Anal sphincter constriction; tail flexion

TABLE 13.3
PROCEDURE FOR MYELOGRAPHY

1. General anesthesia is required.
2. Lateral and VD survey radiographs are obtained.
3. Use iohexol (0.25–0.45 mL/kg)
   a. Use lower dose in large or obese dogs.
   b. Use lower dose if injection is made near the suspected site of lesion.
   c. Contrast material should be warmed to body temperature.
4. Place the animal in sternal or lateral recumbency with an assistant pulling the rear legs, cranial and dorsal, to open the lumbar spaces.
5. The skin is clipped and surgically prepared.
6. The lumbar spines are palpated and a 20–22 gauge 3.5-inch spinal needle is inserted in the caudal aspect of the space between L4-L5 or L5-L6.
7. The needle is advanced carefully until bone is contacted and then it is "walked" cranially or caudally until it drops into the space.
8. The stylet is removed, and fluid is obtained by gentle aspiration.
9. Contrast material is injected slowly, and radiographs are taken.
10. Myelography may help determine which side of the spinal cord the lesion is on.
11. Extradural compression (as in disk extrusion) is evidenced by detecting loss of contrast column(s) in the area of the lesion.

> **TABLE 13.4**
> PROCEDURE FOR CISTERNAL CSF TAP
>
> 1. General anesthesia is required.
> 2. The animal is placed in lateral recumbency, keeping the spine a consistent distance from the table surface. The head is flexed ventrally and the ears pulled forward to open the atlanto-occipital space.
> 3. The dorsal cervical area is clipped and prepared.
> 4. Landmarks are the rostral wings of the atlas and the occipital protuberance on the dorsal midline. The site for needle placement is a depression between the three structures.
> 5. A spinal needle with stylet is slowly advanced through skin, subcutaneous tissue, and muscle until the dura mater and arachnoid membranes are penetrated. The stylet is withdrawn to check for fluid and replaced if the needle is advanced further.
> 6. A 3-way stopcock and manometer can be carefully attached perpendicular to the spinal needle if CSF pressure measurements are desired. The spinal needle must remain completely still. The stopcock is turned to allow fluid to flow into the manometer, and a reading is taken when the flow stops.
> 7. A syringe is fitted to the stopcock, and CSF fluid is collected by gentle aspiration.
> 8. If pressure is not increased, CSF fluid can be allowed to drip into a collection tube or it can be aspirated directly into a syringe and submitted for microscopic, chemical, and microbiologic analysis.
> 9. The spinal needle is carefully withdrawn.
> 10. Some clinicians prefer to perform this procedure with the animal in sternal recumbency with perpendicular ventroflexion of the head.

inflammatory central nervous system (CNS) signs, or unexplained pain/hyperpathia (*Table 13-4*) Contraindications include brain tumors and possibly coagulation disorders. CSF should be obtained for protein analysis, bacterial and/or fungal culture, and cytologic interpretation. Cytology should be performed immediately on a cytospin preparation to minimize cell degeneration. Cloudy CSF may indicate meningitis/encephalitis. CSF pressure may be assessed as an indicator of mass lesions (e.g., neoplasia, granuloma).

III. MANAGEMENT OF SPECIFIC CONDITIONS

A. Myasthenia gravis (MG)

1. Definition/pathology
   a. Relative or actual decrease in the number of acetylcholine receptors results in impaired neuromuscular transmission and clinical signs of weakness.
   b. Two forms exist.
      1) Acquired MG—immune response with development of antibodies (usually immunoglobulin G (IgG)) against acetylcholine (Ach) receptor on the postsynaptic membrane of the neuromuscular junction.

   2) Congenital MG—autosomal inheritance in Jack Russell Terriers, Springer Spaniels, and Smooth Fox Terriers. Clinical signs occur at 6–8 weeks of age.
      a) Acquired MG affects adult medium to large breed dogs and occurs rarely in cats, especially Abyssinian and Somali breeds.
      b) Age of onset ranges from 2 to 4 years, with a second peak in dogs over 9 years old.
      c) Thymoma is present in up to 15% of acquired cases.
      d) Megaesophagus is common.

2. Clinical signs depend on type of MG; classically see generalized muscle weakness that worsens with exercise.
   a. Focal MG—facial, pharyngeal, laryngeal, and/or esophageal dysfunction results in loss of blink reflex, gagging/dysphagia, voice change, or megaesophagus with regurgitation.
   b. Generalized MG—episodic weakness/collapse with recovery after short rest. Affected animals may stand with head and neck held low, demonstrate ataxia or stiff gait, or walk on toes. Additional signs of focal MG may or may not be seen.
   c. Acute fulminant MG—acute, rapidly progressive weakness ±recumbency that does not improve with rest. Respiratory distress due to aspiration pneumonia secondary to

megaesophagus is common. Signs of focal MG are commonly seen. Usually fatal.

3. Diagnosis
   a. Serum Ach receptor antibody titer elevated in 80–90% of cases of acquired MG.
   Send a 1- to 2-mL serum sample overnight on ice to Dr. Diane Shelton, Comparative Neuromuscular Laboratory, Basic Science Bldg, Rm 2095, University of California, San Diego La Jolla, CA 92093-0612 (e-mail: musclelab @ucsd.edu; fax: 858-534-7319).
   b. Tensilon test—IV administration of edrophonium HCl, (a short-acting acetylcholinesterase inhibitor)
      1) Dose: 1–5 mg/dog, 0.25–1 mg/cat.
      2) May result in improved muscle strength and/or return of blink reflex. Results are often equivocal, as the test is neither sensitive nor specific.
      3) Atropine, endotracheal tube, and oxygen should be readily available if signs of cholinergic crisis (bradycardia, urination, salivation, defecation, respiratory distress due to increased bronchial secretions/bronchoconstriction) develop.
      4) Effects generally last <5 minutes.
   c. Electromyography (EMG) classically shows a decremental response of compound muscle action potential (CMAP) to repetitive nerve stimulation. Single-fiber EMG is very sensitive and specific but requires specialized equipment and expertise.
   d. Muscle biopsy can be submitted (intercostals) for demonstration of Ach antibodies or decreased Ach receptors (in congenital MG).

4. Treatment
   a. Pyridostigmine bromide, 0.2–3.0 mg/kg BID–TID PO, improves skeletal muscle weakness in patients with acquired MG.
   b. Neostigmine, 0.05 mg/kg q6–8h SQ or IM, if megaesophagus precludes oral medications
   c. Prednisone, 0.5 mg/kg/day titrated upward to 2 mg/kg/day may be indicated in acquired MG if pneumonia/sepsis is not present.
      1) The use of corticosteroids in MG is controversial because of undesirable side effects and possible exacerbation of weakness.
      2) The course of disease may be shortened by reducing circulating antibody levels.
   d. Megaesophagus may require elevated feedings or placement of a gastric feeding tube to provide nutrition and administer medications.

   e. Aspiration pneumonia should be treated with bactericidal antibiotics based on culture/sensitivity of secretions by transtracheal wash, oxygen, and other supportive measures (see pneumonia, pp. 151–152). It is the most common cause of death in MG.
   f. Nursing care may be necessary for a recumbent patient and includes frequent turning, thick dry bedding, urinary bladder management, and ocular lubrication if blink reflex is absent.

B. Steroid-responsive meningoencephalitis/meningomyelitis.

1. Definition/pathology
   a. Idiopathic, probably immune-mediated, inflammation of meninges/neural tissue. Most common cause of meningitis in dogs.
   b. Repeated vaccination with modified live vaccines may sensitize pet to viral antigens resulting in immune response that cross-reacts with tissue of the CNS.
   c. Syndrome is clinically similar to infectious meningomyelitis and necrotizing vasculitis of spinal meningeal arteries.
   d. May have a genetic component (Beagle pain syndrome)

2. Clinical signs/physical examination
   a. Most often affects medium to large breed dogs 7–16 months of age. (Boxers, Beagles and Bernese Mountain Dogs are predisposed.)
   b. Signs of pain include reluctance to move, kyphotic posture, stiff gait, holding the head/neck low, and generalized or focal spinal hyperpathia.
   c. Animals resist manipulation of head/neck and react painfully to pressure along cervical or thoracolumbar spine.
   d. Focal neurologic deficits may be seen.
   e. Optic neuritis is seen occasionally.
   f. Fever is common.

3. Diagnosis
   a. Made on the basis of clinical signalment/clinical signs and exclusion of infectious causes
   b. CSF analysis reveals meningitis with nondegenerate neutrophilic/monocytic and/or eosinophilic pleocytosis and increased protein.
      1) Bacterial meningitis has a marked increase in all count(s) with degenerate neutrophils. This must be ruled out before administering steroids.

2) Neutrophils are not degenerate in steroid-responsive meningitis.

c. Viral or protozoal serologies are negative in serum or CSF.

d. CSF and blood cultures should be submitted to rule out bacterial meningitis. However, negative CSF culture does not necessarily preclude an infectious cause.

4. Treatment

a. Prednisone, 2–4 mg/kg/day for 1–2 weeks followed by gradual taper over 3–6 months to a dose of 0.5 mg/kg every other day. Relapse may occur as prednisone is tapered or discontinued. Reinstituting a higher dose for a longer period is usually effective.

b. Trimethoprim sulfa can be administered initially as 15 mg/kg BID PO pending CSF culture results. Other antibiotics with excellent CNS penetration include penicillin, enrofloxacin, metronidazole, and doxycycline.

C. Intervertebral disk (IVD) disease

1. Definition/pathology

a. Extradural spinal cord compression by IVD degeneration, protrusion, or extrusion

b. Two types are recognized.

1) Hansen type I—chondroid metaplasia of nucleus pulposus that occurs at young age, 8 months to 6 years, in chondrodystrophic breeds (Dachshunds, Lhasa Apso, Beagle, Pekingese, Cocker Spaniel, Shih-Tzu, and French Bulldogs, etc) and results in mineralization of disk nucleus and eventual extrusion through the dorsal annulus. Most common age: 3–6 years.

2) Hansen type II—fibroid degeneration of nucleus pulposus that occurs in older non-chondrodystrophic breeds (usually large dogs) and results in protrusion of fibrous mass through partially ruptured dorsal anulus. Disk calcification and extrusion is uncommon.

c. Cervical spondylomyelopathy, also called cervical vertebral instability/Wobbler's syndrome

1) Occurs in Great Danes <2 years old, Doberman pinscher 3–9 years of age, and other breeds less commonly. Causes cervical spinal cord compression due to stenosis of vertebral canal, caudal cervical vertebral instability, and hypertrophy of ligamentous structures at the floor of the vertebral canal. Disk extrusion may cause acute exacerbation of signs in affected animals.

2. Clinical signs

a. Peracute/acute onset of pain, ataxia, and paresis

1) Cervical disk disease is most commonly seen as cervical rigidity, pain on neck manipulation, muscle spasms, and reluctance to move.

2) Neurologic deficits are usually more pronounced with thoracolumbar disk disease.

b. Neurologic deficits depend on location and degree of spinal cord compression.

1) Reflexes in limbs caudal to the affected segment are spastic.

2) Lower motor neuron signs are present in the front limbs if brachial (C_6-T_2) intumescence is affected and in the rear limbs if the lumbar (L_4-S_3) intumescence is affected.

3) T3-L3 compression is most common (85%), especially T11-12, L1-2. Results in upper motor neuron signs (spastic reflexes) in pelvic limbs.

4) Animals with cervical disk disease may exhibit "root signature" (thoracic limb lameness due to compression of nerve root).

c. Mild compression causes ataxia and proprioceptive deficits. More severe compression causes loss of voluntary motor function. Severe compression results in loss of superficial and deep pain sensation of affected limbs.

d. Severe back or neck pain is common.

1) Animals with neck pain may present with anorexia and depression.

2) Cervical or T-L disk disease may be misdiagnosed as gastrointestinal disease because of abdominal muscle rigidity and splinting, thought to indicate abdominal pain.

e. Panniculus reflex is lost 1–4 dermatomes caudal to the affected spinal cord segment.

f. Neurologic deficits may be unilateral or asymmetrical.

g. The urinary bladder is often distended because of loss of voluntary control of urination and increased urethral sphincter tone.

3. Diagnosis

a. History, signalment, and neurologic examination allow presumptive diagnosis.

b. Radiographic signs of IVD disease include narrow, wedged, or collapsed disk space, collapsed articular facets, narrow or increased opacity of intervertebral foramen, and calcified disk material in the vertebral canal.

   1) General anesthesia is necessary for proper positioning.

   2) Myelography is indicated when survey films are nondiagnostic, when multiple lesions are seen on survey films, or when radiographic findings contradict results of neurologic examination.

   3) If indicated, the patient is taken directly to surgery after completion of the myelogram.

c. CT and MRI are gaining in popularity as they become more accessible and are often used in lieu of standard myelography.

d. Urinalysis with culture and sensitivity testing is recommended, as bladder infections are common.

4. Treatment

  a. Medical therapy is indicated for an initial episode of neck or back pain with minimal neurologic deficits.

   1) Cage rest or confinement to crate/carrier for 3–4 weeks followed by gradual return to normal activity is the most important aspect of conservative therapy.

    a) Antiinflammatory treatment (prednisone 0.5 mg/kg PO q24h) or analgesic therapy (butorphanol 0.2–0.4 mg/kg SQ or IM q2–6h) can be administered concurrently with strict cage rest.

    b) MEDICATION WITHOUT STRICT CAGE CONFINEMENT MAY LEAD TO WORSENING OF NEUROLOGIC SIGNS AND IS CONTRAINDICATED.

   2) Medical therapy for acute onset of severe neurologic deficits: methylprednisolone sodium succinate—30 mg/kg IV over 5–10 minutes, then 15 mg/kg 2 and 6 hours later, then 2.5 mg/kg/h for 42 hours is preferred. Prednisolone sodium succinate 10–15 mg/kg BID–TID IV can also be used. Dexamethasone preparations carry a higher risk of erosive/ulcerative gastrointestinal complications. Some clinicians question the efficacy of corticosteroids in IV disk disease altogether.

  b. Surgical decompression

   1) Indications include deterioration in neurologic status in spite of medical therapy, loss or absence of voluntary motor function, recurrent episodes of IVD disease, or pain unresponsive to medical therapy.

   2) Loss of deep pain sensation indicates severe spinal cord compression and warrants a guarded- to-poor prognosis. Surgery should be performed as soon as possible for best results.

   3) Cervical disk disease is usually treated with ventral decompression (ventral slot technique). Adjacent disk spaces may be fenestrated prophylactically to prevent extrusion in chondrodystrophic breeds.

   4) Dorsolateral hemilaminectomy is usually the procedure of choice for thoracolumbar disk disease. Adjacent disks may also be fenestrated.

D. Fibrocartilaginous embolism (FCE)

1. Definition/pathology

  a. Ischemic myelopathy resulting from presumed embolization of degenerative nucleus pulposus to vertebral vasculature. Exact mechanism by which nucleus material gains access to vasculature is not known.

  b. Young adult dogs are most commonly affected; cats rarely affected. Most common in large and giant breed dogs.

  c. There may be a history of trauma or vigorous exercise immediately prior to onset.

2. Clinical signs

  a. Acute, lateralizing, nonprogressive, nonpainful paresis or paralysis of sudden onset

  b. Upper motor neuron signs in limb(s) caudal to lesion

  c. Lower motor neuron signs if cervical, C_6-T_2, or lumbar, L4-S_3, intumescence affected

3. Diagnosis

  a. Diagnosed on the basis of history, neurologic examination findings, and **excluding** other causes of spinal cord disease

  b. Survey radiographs normal

   1) Myelography is normal or may reveal mild cord swelling.

   2) MRI may reveal spinal cord ischemia, not specific for embolization.

  c. The tendency for non-progressive lateralizing paresis, lack of back pain, and acute onset in a young large breed dog are factors that help differentiate FCE from intevertebral disk disease.

4. Treatment

   a. Glucocorticoids have been recommended, but there are no data to prove their effectiveness: prednisone, 1 mg/kg/day for 3–7 days with gradual taper over 1–3 weeks.

   b. The mainstay of therapy includes nursing and supportive care as needed based on the severity of neurologic deficits and loss of function.

   c. The prognosis for recovery is guarded to poor if no improvement is seen in 14 days or if deep pain perception is absent.

   d. Full recovery may occur over several weeks to months in animals with milder signs. Persistent deficits may remain. Owners should be warned about the committment required to care for a paretic pet.

E. Flaccid paresis

1. Definition/pathology

   Flaccid paresis is caused by diseases affecting the peripheral nerves, muscle, spinal cord, or neuromuscular junction. Five disease conditions should be considered.

   1) Polyradiculoneuritis (coonhound paralysis): idiopathic, probably immune-mediated disease, affecting motor nerves

   a) *Raccoon saliva, postvaccinal reaction, and systemic illness are sometimes associated and are thought to induce an immune reaction to peripheral nerve myelin.*

   b) *Signs begin 7–10 days after raccoon exposure and progress over 2–10 days.*

   2) Tick paralysis—A toxin secreted by a gravid female, *Dermacentor* spp. or other tick species. blocks Ach release and impairs the action potential propagation at the neuromuscular junction.

   a) *Signs begin 5–9 days after tick attachment and rapidly progress over 24–48 hours.*

   3) Botulism—Ingestion of preformed *Clostridium botulinum* toxin in spoiled food and carrion blocks Ach release at presynaptic membrane of neuromuscular junction.

   4) Spinal cord dysfunction at the level of the cervical or lumbar intumescence should be ruled out as the cause of flaccid paresis/paralysis.

   5) Severe cases of myasthenia gravis may appear to have flaccid paresis.

2. Clinical signs

   a. Ascending flaccid paresis begins in pelvic limbs and progresses to tetraparesis.

   b. Spinal reflexes are diminished or absent.

   c. Respiratory failure may occur if phrenic and/or intercostal nerves are affected.

   d. Sensation remains intact with tick paralysis, botulism, and coonhound paralysis, but the withdrawal reflex is depressed or absent.

   e. Cranial nerves may be involved, resulting in voice change, dysphagia/gagging, hypersalivation, and/or facial paralysis. Dysphagia and megaesophagus are common in botulism.

   f. Animals may retain voluntary tail movement and control of urination and defecation.

3. Diagnosis

   a. History, presence or absence of tick exposure, and neurologic examination findings are suggestive.

   b. Polyradiculoneuritis

   1) EMG suggests denervation with normal to decreased nerve conduction velocities after 7 days.

   2) CSF analysis is usually normal; increased protein may be seen on lumbar puncture.

   3) Histologic changes are more severe in the ventral (motor) nerve roots than in peripheral nerves and include infiltration with inflammatory cells and axonal degeneration.

   c. Tick paralysis

   1) EMG indicates neuromuscular blockade with fibrillation potentials appearing after 5–7 days.

   2) Rapid recovery within 1–2 days following tick removal supports diagnosis.

   d. Botulism

   1) EMG findings are similar to those in tick paralysis.

   2) Type C botulinum toxin can be assayed in serum, feces, vomitus, or affected food/carrion.

4. Treatment

   a. General

   1) Nursing care—turning q4–6h, thick dry bedding, corneal lubrication, bladder management

   2) Nutritional and hydration support if cranial nerve or esophageal dysfunction are present.

   3) Supplemental oxygen or mechanical ventilation if hypoxemia or hypoventilation, respectively, are present.

b. Specific

    1) Polyradiculoneuritis

        a) Corticosteroid use is controversial and usually avoided because of the increased potential for muscle atrophy and secondary infections.

        b) Recovery may take months.

    2) Tick paralysis

        a) Removal of tick or acaricide dip

        b) Organophosphates may exacerbate weakness and should be avoided.

        c) Check ears and interdigital spaces and clip long-haired dogs if necessary to locate and remove all ticks.

        d) Clinical improvement in 24–48 hours

    3) Botulism

        a) Polyvalent botulin antitoxin containing type C antitoxin: 10,000–15,000 units IV or IM administered twice 4 hours apart

            i) Anaphylaxis is possible. A test dose of 0.1 mL intradermally should be given 20 minutes prior to full dose.

            ii) Antitoxin inactivates circulating toxin but is ineffective once it has entered the axon.

        b) Antibiotics are probably of no benefit because the signs are due to preformed toxin and not the organism. Secondary infections should be treated, however.

        c) Recovery occurs gradually over 2–3 weeks.

F. Focal cranial nerve disorders: facial nerve paralysis

1. Definition/pathology

  a. Idiopathic inflammation of facial nerve; may be unilateral or bilateral

  b. Has been associated with hypothyroidism, hyperadrenocorticism, and lead poisoning in dogs

  c. Adult Cocker Spaniels may be predisposed.

2. Clinical signs

  a. Lip and ear droop on affected side(s)

  b. Lack of blink reflex

  c. Decreased tear production

  d. Excessive salivation

3. Diagnosis

  a. Based on clinical signs

  b. Schirmer tear test may document decreased tear production

  c. Otoscopic examination and/or radiographs of tympanic bulla should be performed to rule out otitis media.

  d. Thyroid and adrenal function tests should be done to rule out hypothyroidism and hyperadrenocorticism.

4. Treatment

  a. Spontaneous recovery may occur within 2–6 weeks, although some deficits may be permanent.

  b. Artificial tears should be administered if tear production is decreased.

  c. Nutritional support is usually not necessary unless multiple cranial nerves are involved.

  d. Thyroid hormone replacement therapy is indicated if hypothyroidism is documented.

G. Focal cranial nerve disorders: trigeminal neuropathy

1. Definition/pathology

  a. Idiopathic motor dysfunction of cranial nerve V resulting in loss of function of muscles of mastication. Sensory branches of cranial nerve V are unaffected.

  b. A seasonal increase in incidence is seen in the fall.

  c. Rule out endocrine-associated neuropathies (hypothyroidism, hyperadrenocorticism, and diabetes mellitus) and infectious causes (tick titers).

2. Clinical signs

  a. Acute onset of dropped jaw and inability to close mouth

  b. Excessive drooling, difficulty prehending food

  c. Sensory deficits and muscle atrophy are rare.

3. Treatment

  a. Nutritional support including elevated feedings

    1) Many patients have an easier time ingesting food pressed into meatballs.

    2) Placement of a feeding tube (esophagostomy/gastric) is rarely necessary.

  b. Recovery is usually complete within 2–8 weeks. Prognosis is excellent with supportive care.

H. Nervous system trauma: head trauma

1. Etiology

  a. Blunt trauma—vehicular trauma, most common, baseball bat, golf ball, etc.

b. Penetrating trauma—animal fight, gun shot

c. Cats are predisposed because of a thin calvarium and less muscle mass than dogs.

2. Pathology

a. Primary injury occurs as a direct result of trauma (skull fractures, hemorrhage, and tearing or compression of brain tissue).

b. Secondary injury occurs hours to days after trauma.

   1) Results in edema, ischemia, increased intracranial pressure (ICP) and decreased cerebral perfusion

   2) Calcium, glutamate, and other excitatory neurotransmitters and inflammatory mediators are important in secondary brain injury.

c. Treatment of head injury is aimed at controlling or reversing the secondary injury. The primary injury is not as amenable to therapy.

d. ICP elevation is the common endpoint of primary and secondary injury. The formula

$$CPP = MAP - ICP$$

where CPP is cerebral perfusion pressure and MAP is mean arterial pressure and ICP is intracranial pressure explains the relationship between factors affecting brain perfusion. Therapy is aimed at maintaining cerebral perfusion by optimizing MAP (fluid therapy) and minimizing ICP. Steps to minimize ICP may include limiting the use of crystalloids, using colloids (hetastarch) or hypertonic crystalloid (mannitol, hypertonic saline) to restore volume and provide blood pressure support, and giving corticosteroids (*very* controversial), supplemental oxygen, mechanical ventilation, and others.

3. Clinical signs

a. Location of injury and extent of damage will determine the severity of clinical signs.

   1) Cerebrum: circling, ataxia, postural deficits, blindness, altered mentation, and loss of consciousness

   2) Brainstem: coma, nonresponsive pupils, lack of physiologic nystagmus (poor prognosis)

   3) Cerebellum/vestibular system: head tilt, rolling, falling to one side, nystagmus, dysmetria, ataxia

b. Multisystem trauma may be present in animals that have been hit by a car or fallen from significant height.

c. Skull fractures cause facial or skull deformity, palpable depression in calvarium, blood

or CSF from ear or nose, and subcutaneous emphysema if sinuses involved.

d. Serious head trauma causes

   1) Stupor or coma—severe decrease in level of consciousness because of damage to the cerebral cortex or ascending reticular activating system in brainstem, resulting in minimal (stupor) to no (coma) response to noxious stimuli

   2) Pupillary abnormalities

   a) *Miotic, responsive pupils indicate cerebral injury/edema. Guarded-to-fair prognosis*

   b) *Midrange, nonresponsive pupils indicate brainstem injury and a grave prognosis.*

   c) *Progression from miotic to midrange fixed pupils indicates possible brain herniation and carries a grave prognosis.*

   d) *Asymmetric pupils are most often due to oculomotor nerve damage and compression of the nerve nucleus by herniating cerebral tissue. Direct eye injury and secondary uveitis can also cause assymmetric pupils.*

   3) Ocular position/movement abnormalities

   a) *Physiologic nystagmus indicates an intact brainstem.*

   b) *Absence of physiologic nystagmus (i.e., eye position does not change when head is moved side to side) indicates severe brainstem damage with a poor prognosis.*

   c) *Strabismus indicates damage to nuclei of cranial nerves 3, 4, 6, and/or 8 in the brainstem.*

   d) *Caloric test—instilling warm or cold water into the ear should cause nystagmus with the fast phase toward the instilled ear; lack of response indicates severe brainstem injury. Because this is an unreliable test, it is rarely done.*

   4) Respiratory pattern changes

   a) *Cheyne-Stokes respiration is a cyclic increase and decrease in the respiratory rate because of impaired responsiveness to $PaCO_2$ and indicates a severe diffuse cerebral or diencephalic lesion.*

   b) *Increased respiratory rate/hyperventilation may be due to cerebral acidosis, hypoxia, or herniation (midbrain pathology).*

   c) *Apneustic or ataxic breathing occurs as rapid inspiration with short incomplete expiration and indicates severe brainstem damage (pontine or medullary pathology).*

5) Postural changes

a) Decerebrate rigidity is characterized by opisthotonus and extensor rigidity of all four limbs and indicates severe brainstem injury and carries a grave prognosis. It may be caused by hemorrhage/infarct/ischemia, brainstem transection, or brain herniation. The animal is unresponsive and unable to detect deep pain sensation.

b) Decerebellate posture, characterized by forelimb extensor rigidity with variable extension/flexion of the rear limbs, indicates cerebellar injury or herniation. This can be differentiated from decerebrate rigidity because the animal is conscious and aware, and pupils are responsive. It carries a much more favorable prognosis than decerebrate rigidity.

c) Spinal reflexes may be normal to slightly exaggerated.

d) Serial neurologic assessment of above parameters is critical in determining progression of injury and response to treatment and should be monitored frequently during the initial 24 hours posttrauma.

4. Treatment

a. Assess and stabilize life-threatening problems as in any trauma patient.

b. IV fluids—goal is to maintain cerebral perfusion by optimizing MAP without causing increased ICP. Cerebral dehydration by fluid restriction or induction of diuresis is not currently recommended because of deleterious effects on cerebral perfusion.

1) Isotonic crystalloid solutions such as lactated Ringer's, 0.9% NaCl, or Normosol-R are usually sufficient. Volume and rate are based on hemodynamic status and parameters such as central venous pressure (CVP), blood pressure (BP), and urine production, as overhydration and hypertension should be avoided. Dextrose supplementation is generally contraindicated unless hypoglycemia is present to avoid anaerobic metabolism of glucose and increased cerebral acidosis.

2) Hypertonic crystalloids, e.g., 20% mannitol, 7.5% hypertonic saline

a) Indications—deteriorating neurologic status, signs or risk of herniation, poor neurologic assessment at presentation

b) Advantages—reduce cerebral edema, improve cerebral perfusion, lower ICP,

oxygen free radical scavenging (mannitol)

c) Disadvantages—potential exacerbation of cerebral hemorrhage/edema, transient increase in ICP, decreased cerebral perfusion due to osmotic diuresis, hyperosmolality/hypernatremia may worsen CNS signs (obtundation, etc.).

d) Dose:

i) *Mannitol 20%, 0.5 g/kg IV over 20 minutes, repeat 1–3 times q4–8h based on neurologic status/progression*

ii) *Hypertonic saline 7.5%, 4–6 mL/kg over 5–10 minutes*

3) Colloids

a) Indications

i) *Maintain plasma oncotic pressure in shock, systemic inflammatory response syndrome (SIRS)*

ii) *Some advocate use in all cases of severe brain injury.*

b) Advantages

i) *Blood volume is maintained with low fluid volume*

ii) *Decreases cerebral edema*

iii) *Increases cerebral perfusion*

iv) *Longer effect than hypertonic crystalloids*

v) *May limit vascular leak*

c) Disadvantages/contraindications

i) *Hypervolemia if overdosed*

ii) *Contraindicated with cardiac disease or oliguria*

iii) *Coagulopathy, potential for enhanced bleeding (not clinically relevant at recommended dose)*

d) Dose:

i) *Hetastarch: Dog, 5–10 mL/kg IV over 10–15 minutes for acute trauma resuscitation, total dosage 20–30 mL/kg/day; Cat, 2–5 mL/kg IV over 10–15 minutes, total dosage 10–20 mL/kg/day. Use minimal amount to maintain mean arterial blood pressure between 80 and 100 mm Hg or systolic pressure between 120 and 140 mm Hg. Avoid hypertension.*

ii) *Fresh frozen plasma: 6–10 mL/kg IV; use best reserved for patients at risk of disseminated intravascular coagulation (DIC) or other coagulopathy and/or albumin <2.0 mg/dL*

4) Corticosteroids
  a) Use is controversial.
  b) Potential advantages
    i) Decrease cerebral edema by restoring vascular integrity
    ii) Provide antiinflammatory activity through phospholipase inhibition and oxygen free radical scavenging
  c) Potential disadvantages
    i) Delay in neuronal remyelination
    ii) Potentiate neuronal damage in presence of ischemia
    iii) Gastrointestinal erosion/ulceration
    iv) Hyperglycemia (potentiates cerebral acidosis)
    v) Must be given within 4–8 hours of trauma or may not be effective
  d) Doses
    i) Methylprednisolone sodium succinate—30 mg/kg IV over 10 minutes initial dose, 15 mL/kg IV 2 and 6 hours later, then 2.5 mg/kg/h for 42 hours. This protocol has been shown experimentally to decrease ischemia and necrosis and improve neurologic outcome following spinal cord injury. In humans with brain injury, high-dose methylprednisolone neither reduced ICP nor improved long-term outcome.
    ii) Dexamethasone sodium phosphate—2 mg/kg q12h IV

5) Supplemental oxygen is indicated in all head-injured patients to limit hypoxic neuronal injury. See section for discussion of supplemental O_2 (pp. 115–117). Anemia should be identified and corrected to maximize oxygen delivery.

6) Hyperventilation
  a) Increased $PaCO_2$ results in cerebral vasodilation and increased ICP. Hyperventilation with end tidal CO_2 measurements greater than 40 should be avoided.
  b) Indications—hypoventilation, deteriorating neurologic status
  c) Precautions
    i) Excessive hyperventilation, $PaCO_2$ <25, may cause cerebral ischemia by excessive vasoconstriction
    ii) Intubation may result in increased ICP due to gag/cough. Pretreatment with lidocaine prior to intubation is recommended.
    iii) Positive pressure ventilation may increase ICP by impaired venous outflow secondary to increased intrathoracic pressure. Avoid positive end-expiratory pressure (PEEP).
  d) Goal
    i) Maintain $PaCO_2$ at 25–35 mm Hg
    ii) Lidocaine 2% (without epinephrine) should be given to prevent ICP increase during intubation. Dose: 2 mg/kg IV, (dog); 0.25 mg/kg IV, (cat).
    iii) Optimize cerebral venous outflow.
      i. Elevate head 30°—optimize gravitational drainage without compromising cerebral blood flow/perfusion.
      ii. Avoid jugular occlusion—maintain neutral head/neck position, minimal neck restraint, loose catheter bandage, etc.
      iii. Avoid PEEP if ventilatory support is necessary.

7) Nutritional support
  a) General—Severe brain injury causes a marked increase in caloric requirements above basal needs. This can be estimated by determining basal energy requirement (BER) and multiplying by an illness energy requirement (IER) factor of 2–2.5.
  b) BER (kcal/24 h) = (30 × BW (kg)) +70 for animals >2 kg, or 70 × BW (kg) 0.75 exponent for animals <2 kg
  c) Kcal to administer = BER × IER
  d) Enteral route of administration is preferred whenever possible.
  e) May require placement of gastric feeding tube, nasoesophageal or esophagostomy tube may be impractical with severe head injury.
  f) Enteral formulas (e.g., Clinicare) are used beginning at 25% of the total caloric requirement on the first day, 50% on second day, and 100% on third day. Diluting diet 1:1 with warm water on day 1 and increasing to full strength on day 3 may minimize complications such as diarrhea.
  g) Hyperglycemia should be avoided in head trauma patients. Some clinicians believe that persistent hyperglycemia in acute patients may require short term administration of a constant rate infusion of regular insulin (p. 301, Table 15-1).

8) Nursing care
   a) *Prevent decubital ulcers—thick padded bedding, turn patient q4h*
   b) *Bladder management—manually express or intermittently catheterize bladder q6–8h*
   c) *Lubricate corneas q8h if necessary*
   d) *Physical therapy—passive range of motion of limbs q6–8h; use caution if concurrent spinal injury*
   e) *Rotate recumbent animals from side to side q4–6h to prevent atelectasis.*

9) Surgery
   a) *Indications*
      i) *Depressed skull fracture*
      ii) *Subdural hematoma (rare in small animals); epidural hematomas are more common.*
      iii) *Deteriorating neurologic status despite aggressive medical management when increased ICP is suspected*
   b) *Anesthetic recommendations include rapid induction with thiopental or propofol and maintenance with inhalant anesthesia using isoflurane*

10) Additional treatments for severe brain injury
    a) *Barbiturate coma*
       i) *Advantages*
          i. *Controls seizures*
          ii. *Provides anesthesia with minimal cardiovascular depression in intubated patients*
          iii. *Decreases cerebral metabolic rate (CMRO$_2$), thereby exerting protective mechanism on marginally perfused neuronal tissue*
       ii) *Disadvantages*
          i. *Hypoventilation*
          ii. *Increases nursing and monitoring requirements*
          iii. *May lower blood pressure and cerebral blood flow if overdosed*
          iv. *Very difficult to monitor and maintain*
       iii) *Dose*
          i. *Pentobarbital—4–6 mg/kg IV bolus as needed to maintain anesthesia for 12–24 hours (longer if mechanical ventilation required)*
          ii. *Pentobarbital CRI—0.2–1 mg/kg/h*

    b) *Hypothermia*
       i) *Definition—controlled decrease in body temperature to 31–34°C. Regional cooling of head only may limit some complications of total body hypothermia. Technically challenging and not routinely done in veterinary medicine*
       ii) *Advantages*
          i. *Decreased CMRO$_2$,*
          ii. *Decreased ICP*
          iii. *Decreased production of inflammatory cytokines*
          iv. *Decreased production of excitatory neurotransmitters*
       iii) *Disadvantages*
          i. *Coagulopathy*
          ii. *Cardiac arrhythmias*
          iii. *Hypotension*
          iv. *Shivering and rewarming may increase ICP.*
    c) *Additional/experimental treatment for secondary brain injury*
       i) *Glutamate antagonist—experimental, not readily available*
       ii) *Deferoxamine mesylate (Desferal), 25–50 mg/kg IM or slowly IV, iron scavenger that limits production of oxygen-derived free radicals via Haber-Weiss reaction*
       iii) *Dimethyl sulfoxide (DMSO), 0.5–1 mg/kg IV over 30 minutes, free radical scavenger*
       iv) *21-amino steroids; not yet available in the United States*

I. Spinal cord trauma

1. Etiology
   a. External trauma—HBC, fall from height, animal fight, gunshot, etc.
   b. Internal trauma—intervertebral disk disease (see pp. 256–257).

2. Pathology
   a. Mechanical injury to spinal cord due to vertebral fracture, luxation, or subluxation resulting in compression, laceration, or vascular disruption of cord tissue
   b. Primary and secondary injury occurs as in head trauma. Severity of injury depends on degree of cord compression and diameter of spinal cord relative to the width of the vertebral column. Cervical lesions may cause less severe compression than thoracolumbar injury

because ratio of spinal cord diameter to vertebral column width is lower.

c. Myelomalacia, ascending and/or descending, may occur as mediators of inflammation responsible for secondary injury travel within central gray matter of the spinal cord, affecting segments distant from site of initial injury.

  1) Clinical signs include fever and progressive loss of pain sensation and motor function.

  2) It can lead to necrosis of the spinal cord within 24–48 hours and death from respiratory paralysis within 3–7 days. Humane euthanasia is indicated if there is an ascending or descending progressive loss of spinal cord function.

d. Spinal cord topography explains severity of neurologic deficits.

  1) Heavily myelinated fibers in the periphery of the cord mediate proprioception, hence mild compression causes proprioceptive deficits.

  2) Intermediate-sized and slightly smaller-sized fibers more centrally located within the cord mediate voluntary motor function and superficial pain sensation; hence moderate compression results in loss of these functions.

  3) Small nonmyelinated or lightly myelinated fibers deep within the spinal cord mediate deep pain sensation; therefore loss of deep pain indicates severe cord injury.

3. Clinical signs

  a. Neurologic deficits depend on location of spinal cord injury.

  1) Cervical injury, C1-C5, results in tetraparesis with upper motor neuron signs to all four limbs (stiffness, hyperextension, spastic paresis/paralysis).

  2) Respiratory failure may occur with severe caudal cervical lesions, C5-C7, because of damage to motor neurons of the phrenic nerve.

  3) Thoracolumbar (TL) injury, T3-L3, results in posterior paresis with upper motor neuron signs to rear limbs; most common location of injury.

  4) Schiff-Sherrington posture (opisthotonus and forelimb extensor rigidity) may occur with TL injury because of release of ascending inhibition from damaged border cells in

lumbar cord gray matter (indicates severe cord damage).

  5) Injury to cervical (C6-T2) or lumbar (L4-Cd5) intumescence results in lower motor neuron signs to thoracic and pelvic limbs, respectively, plus upper motor neuron signs to the pelvic limbs with injuries above L_4.

  6) Horner's syndrome can occur with injury from C5 to T2.

  a) Clinical signs include miosis, anisocoria, ptosis, enophthalmos, and protrusion of the nictitating membrane (third eyelid).

  b) Anisocoria becomes more pronounced in the dark as the normal pupil dilates.

  c) Horner's syndrome can occur with lesions in the brainstem, cervical cord, middle ear, neck, and retrobulbar area.

b. Pain is almost always present due to vertebral column injury and damage to meninges, dura, and nerve roots.

c. Findings from intracranial neurologic examination are usually normal unless head trauma has also occurred.

d. General physical examination may reveal signs of multiple trauma or shock.

e. Musculoskeletal examination may reveal fractures of long bones or pelvis. Dogs with TL vertebral injuries may have a palpable misalignment over affected vertebrae.

f. Paratetraplegia (paralysis with complete loss of voluntary movement and pain sensation) indicates possible cord transection and carries a guarded-to-poor prognosis. Spinal shock is a transient functional disruption in spinal cord function mimicking transection. Although this is uncommon in small animals, it may be difficult to assess pain sensation in a severely traumatized animal in shock. Initial lack of response should not be mistaken for permanent injury caused by spinal cord transection, and serial neurologic examinations should be performed after the animal is stabilized.

4. Diagnosis

  a. History, general physical examination, and neurologic examination often provide the diagnosis.

  b. Radiography may reveal vertebral fracture, luxation, subluxation (*Figs. 13-1* and *13-2*). Two views of the spine are optimal. In most cases, a lateral view suffices and avoids aggravating the

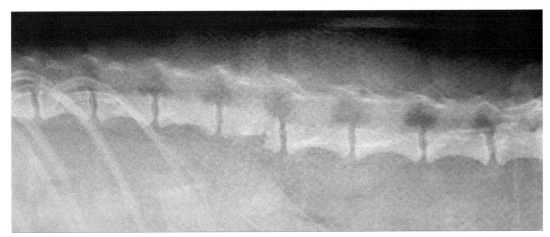

FIGURE 13.1   Right lateral view of the vertebral column in a dog after trauma reveals a compression fracture of L3. Hazy appearance is the result of a stabilizing bandage.

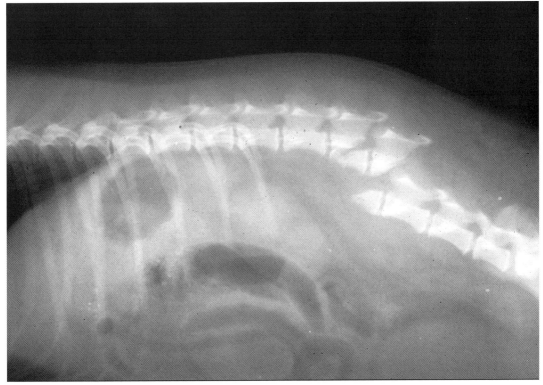

FIGURE 13.2   Lateral radiograph of a dog's spine after trauma reveals severely displaced spinal fractures. Note that one segment is almost floating.

spinal injury, which can occur with positioning for ventrodorsal projections. Normal survey radiographs may not rule out cord injury when spontaneous reduction of dynamic luxation has occurred following the initial impact.

c. Myelography is indicated in patients with severe neurologic deficits and inconclusive survey radiographs or when neurologic deficits do not coincide with radiographic findings.

5. Treatment: Always immobilize the spine when transporting the animal. Tape to a rigid board or gurney.

a. Identify and stabilize concurrent life-threatening problems as indicated by general physical examination.

b. Nonsurgical treatment of spinal cord injury

1) Corticosteroids—controversial, most effective if given within 1 hour after trauma; advantages and disadvantages similar to those for head trauma (see above).

a) Methylprednisolone sodium succinate—30 mg/kg IV over 10 minutes, 15 mg/kg IV 2 and 6 hours later, then 15 mg/kg IV q6h for 24–48 hours or begin CRI of 2.5 mg/kg/h for 42 hours

b) Prednisolone sodium succinate 10 mg/kg q8–12h IV

c) Dexamethasone sodium phosphate 2 mg/kg BID IV (not preferred because of higher incidence of erosive/ulcerative gastrointestinal complications).

d) DMSO has shown benefit in experimental studies—1 g/kg IV q24h ×3–4 days. Dilute to 20% solution in 5% dextrose in water.

2) Gastrointestinal protectants

a) H₂ blockers—cimetidine 5—10 mg/kg TID PO or IV, ranitidine 2 mg/kg TID PO or IV, dog, 2.5 mg/kg BID IV or 3.5 mg/kg BID PO, cat; famotidine 0.5 mg/kg SID or BID PO.

b) Sucralfate: 0.5–1 g TID PO, dog; 0.25 g TID PO, cat.

3) Bladder management—manual bladder expression or indwelling or intermittent urinary catheterization q6–8h is usually necessary because of impaired voluntary urination. Phenoxybenzamine and/or bethanechol may be necessary in chronic cases in which return of voluntary urination is delayed; their use is discussed in the section on urinary and fecal incontinence (pp. 276–277).

4) Confinement—critical aspect of therapy; confine to cage or crate for 4–6 weeks followed by gradual return to normal activity over 2–4 weeks.

5) External bandage/splint—various combinations of soft padded bandages, cast material, and/or aluminum rods can be used to immobilize vertebrae cranial and caudal to affected area.

6) Nursing care of paralyzed patient includes thick, dry bedding, carefully turning patient q4h, and performing passive physical therapy (without aggravating spinal instability) q8–12h.

7) Analgesics—narcotics preferred. Nonsteroidal antiinflammatory drugs should not be used in animals receiving corticosteroids, because of the increased risk of gastrointestinal ulceration. Analgesics must be used in conjunction with strict confinement to minimize risk of aggravating injury if animal feels well enough to move about.

a) Butorphanol, 0.2–0.8 mg/kg BID QID IV or SQ

b) Buprenorphine, 0.01 mg/kg TID IV or IM

c) Oxymorphone or hydromorphone, 0.1–0.2 mg/kg BID TID IV

d) Morphine, 0.5–1 mg/kg BID TID IV, SQ, IM

e) Fentanyl—transdermal patch

8) Muscle relaxants—use cautiously as enhanced muscle tone can act as a "splint" for spinal injuries

Methocarbamol, 150 mg/kg IV or 15–20 mg/kg PO q8h

c. Surgical management

1) Indications—inability to stand after spinal trauma, spinal instability with severe neurologic deficits, and/or spinal cord compression demonstrated by myelogram

2) Goal is realignment of vertebral column to provide skeletal stability and minimize spinal cord compression.

a) Decompression is usually accomplished by hemilaminectomy or dorsal laminectomy.

b) It should be done as soon as possible in animals with severe deficits.

3) Internal fixation most commonly involves combinations of bone screws, Kirschner wires, Steinmann pins, plates, and polymethylmethacrylate cement.

4) Referral to specialty surgeon is recommended.

6. Prognosis

a. Favorable if neurologic deficits and vertebral injuries are mild.

b. Poor if neurologic examination reveals loss of deep pain sensation and radiographs suggest severe vertebral injury—these are signs of possible spinal cord transection.

J. Brachial plexus avulsion

1. Definition/pathology

  a. Peripheral nerve dysfunction caused by damage to nerve roots of spinal nerves originating from C6-T2 that innervate the forelimb

  b. Most common mechanism of injury is severe traumatic abduction of forelimb. Blunt trauma to lateral or proximal shoulder is less common. Nerve roots can be stretched, torn, or contused.

  c. Histopathologic changes include degenerative necrosis, myelin fragmentation, and possible retrograde injury to ventral horn cells.

  d. Radial, median, and ulnar nerves are most commonly affected.

  e. A common cause of this injury in dogs is falling from the back of a moving pickup truck.

2. Clinical signs

  a. Total avulsion—The limb is paralyzed and flaccid. Elbow and carpus cannot extend. Sensation is lost distal to elbow. Ipsilateral Horner's syndrome and loss of panniculus reflex may occur if T1-T2 nerve roots are affected.

  b. Caudal avulsion, C8-T1—Carpus cannot extend, but proximal limb function is preserved.

  c. Cranial avulsion, C6-C7—Uncommon, caused by trauma to proximal shoulder; muscles of proximal shoulder affected and may atrophy. Limb can support weight, but elbow cannot flex. Innervation of triceps and antebrachium is preserved.

3. Diagnosis

  a. History of trauma and neurologic examination establish the diagnosis.

  b. Evaluation of cutaneous distribution of nerves can determine extent of injury.

4. Treatment

  a. Spontaneous recovery of function may occur over 1–2 weeks in partial or mild injuries, but there is no treatment for complete avulsions.

  b. Bandaging the foot may prevent injury to dorsal skin if the limb drags.

  c. Surgical techniques such as triceps tendon transposition or carpal arthrodesis can be considered in severe cases as salvage procedures.

  d. Indications for amputation include lack of return of neurologic function with discomfort, persistent skin infections caused by dragging foot, pain (rare), or persistent biting and chewing of the affected limb.

K. Seizures

1. Definition

  a. Seizures are caused by paroxysmal disturbances of electrical activity in cerebral neurons.

  b. In dogs, generalized seizures are more common than localized seizures and involve tonic–clonic activity in all limbs

  c. Partial seizures may affect one limb, one side of the body, or just the face/head.

  d. Other characteristics of seizures include loss of consciousness, involuntary urination and/or defecation, vocalization, and facial twitching.

  e. A preictal aura characterized by changes in activity or behavior and postictal mentation changes or neurologic deficits are additional characteristics of seizures.

  f. These signs aid in distinguishing seizure activity from syncope and other causes of collapse.

  g. Status epilepticus is defined as continuous seizure activity lasting longer than 5–10 minutes or multiple seizures with no interictal return of consciousness. Persistent partial seizure activity is also considered status epilepticus and should be treated accordingly.

    This represents a true emergency as prolonged seizure activity may cause permanent neuronal damage due to hypoxia, cerebral edema, hyperthermia, and lactic acidosis causing decreased cerebral tissue pH.

2. Etiology

  a. Intracranial causes of seizures include idiopathic epilepsy, head trauma, neoplasia, cerebrovascular disease, and meningoencephalitides, e.g., GME, canine distemper, feline infectious peritonitis (FIP).

  b. Extracranial causes of seizures include hypoglycemia, metabolic disease (e.g., hepatic encephalopathy and uremic encephalopathy), hypocalcemia, and toxicosis (e.g., metaldehyde, strychnine).

3. Diagnosis

  a. Perform stat blood glucose, CBC, biochemical profile and urinalysis to identify metabolic causes (or consequences) of seizures.

  b. Check for history of trauma or exposure to toxin.

  c. Age of onset of first seizure may aid in differential diagnosis.

1) <1 year of age—congenital anomaly (e.g., hydrocephalus, lissencephaly, and glycogen storage disease), head trauma, toxicity, hypoglycemia, portocaval shunt, infectious (e.g., distemper, FIP)

2) 1–5 years of age—idiopathic epilepsy, cerebral neoplasia (rare) and causes mentioned above. Epilepsy is common in large breeds and purebred dogs.

3) >5 years of age—neoplasia, hepatic encephalopathy (cirrhosis), hypoglycemia (insulinoma), acquired metabolic disorders (uremia), infectious and other causes of encephalitis

d. CSF tap—Nonspecific findings of increased protein, variable pleocytosis (mononuclear cells in granulomatous meningoencephalitis), hemorrhage or xanthochromia, and increased pressure are consistent with CNS disease.

   1) CSF tap may be contraindicated in patients with intracranial neoplasia because of risk of cerebral or cerebellar herniation.

   2) Bacterial culture, fungal culture, and/or antibody titers can be run on CSF.

e. Skull radiographs are not indicated unless trauma is suspected.

f. CT/MRI are indicated in patients with adult-onset seizures, focal or multifocal neurologic deficits that localize to the brain or brainstem of any patient in which structural lesion of CNS is suspected.

g. Cats: Consider FIP, feline leukemia virus (FeLV), toxoplasmosis, toxins, trauma, vascular accident, and metabolic disease.

4. Treatment

a. Treatment depends on condition of patient on presentation and neurologic examination findings.

   1) Stable patient that presents in stable condition after first seizure, no active seizure activity, normal neurologic examination:

   a) Perform stat blood glucose, submit CBC, biochemical profile, urinalysis to rule out metabolic causes.

   b) Instruct clients to keep log of seizure activity, date, duration, and description.

   c) No antiepileptic drug (AED) therapy necessary at this time.

   2) Stable patient that presents after one or more seizures, no active seizure activity, persistent neurologic deficits:

   a) Hospitalize for monitoring, obtain laboratory data base as above, place IV catheter.

   b) Consider CT or MRI if deficits persist >24–48 hours after last seizure.

   c) Consider maintenance AED therapy—phenobarbital 2.5 mg/kg BID PO or potassium bromide 20 mg/kg PO BID.

   3) Indications for emergency treatment—status epilepticus, single seizure lasting longer than 5 minutes, cluster seizures (more than one seizure in 24-hour period).

   a) Diazepam, 0.25–0.5 mg/kg IV, may repeat 3–4 times

   b) Phenobarbital administered simultaneously with Valium provides sustained effect.

   i) *Loading dose (mg) = desired serum level (25 μg/mL) × BW (kg) × 0.8 L/kg. (for cats, the desired serum level is 15 μg/mL).*

   ii) *This dose can be administered IV at a rate not to exceed 100 mg/min.*

   iii) *If the animal is an epileptic already receiving phenobarbital, the serum level should be checked before giving more phenobarbital. The animal should be given 1 mg/kg IV for each μg/mL of desired concentration increase. For dogs, the serum concentration should be raised in increments of 5 μg/mL up to 30 μg/mL. For cats, the serum concentration should be raised in increments of 3 μg/mL up to 25 μg/mL.*

   c) For refractory seizures, first try diazepam CRI. One of the benefits of a diazepam CRI is that it can be discontinued once the seizures subside and there is little CNS depression to complicate a neurologic examination.

   i) *Mix in 0.9% NaCl at maintenance rate (60 mL/kg/day).*

   ii) *Use 0.45% NaCl and 2.5% dextrose if animal is receiving potassium bromide, because 0.9% NaCl will lower serum bromide concentrations.*

   iii) *Begin at 0.2 mg/kg/h.*

   i. *If seizures stop, taper infusion by 50% q2h.*

   ii. *If seizures continue, (<3), increase diazepam dose to 0.5 mg/kg/h.*

iii. *If seizures continue, (>3), administer general anesthesia.*

d) *General anesthesia protocols for patients refractory to diazepam CRI:*

i) *Pentobarbital: 2 mg/kg IV slowly to effect followed by 5 mg/kg/h CRI*

ii) *Propofol: 4–8 mg/kg slow IV bolus, followed by 8–12 mg/kg/h CRI*

iii) *Inhalation anesthesia: Isoflurane is preferred because of rapid induction/smooth recovery, no hepatotoxicity, and less effect on ICP than halothane.*

iv) *Supportive care: Patients require intubation to protect airway with deflation and repositioning of tube q4–6h, frequent turning, and optimally monitoring blood pressure (direct or indirect) and oxygenation parameters (pulse oximetry).*

v) *After 23 hours, begin to taper anesthetic dosing by 25% q2–4h.*

e) *Initiate maintenance antiepileptic drug therapy.*

i) *Begin maintenance dose of phenobarbital 12 hours after loading dose.*

i. *Dogs: 2.5 mg/kg PO q12h*
ii. *Cats: 1 mg/kg PO q12h.*

ii) *For patients already on phenobarbital, use the following formula to increase the daily maintenance dose.*

i. New daily dose (mg)

$$= \frac{\text{Concentration desired}}{\text{Concentration actual}}$$
$$\times \text{Phenobarbital (mg)}$$

ii. *For dogs, desired concentration is increased by 5 μg/mL up to 30 μg/mL.*

iii. *For cats, desired concentration is increased by 3 μg/mL up to 25 μg/mL.*

b. Supportive therapy

3) IV fluids

a) *Isotonic saline at maintenance rate plus volume deficit caused by excessive seizure activity*

b) *Saline is preferred because diazepam may precipitate in other crystalloids.*

4) Glucocorticoids to treat cerebral edema

a) *Prednisolone sodium succinate, 10 mg/kg TID IV for 24 hours*

b) *Dexamethasone sodium phosphate, 0.1 mg/kg BID IV for 24 hours*

5) Dextrose, 0.5 mL/kg IV of 50% solution (diluted to 5%) if stat BG <60 mg/dL. Avoid hyperglycemia, which may potentiate cerebral acidosis due to anaerobic metabolism of glucose to lactic acid.

6) Correct the hyperthermia commonly seen with prolonged seizure activity.

a) *Administering IV fluids and controlling seizure activity is usually adequate.*

b) *Stop cooling measures when temperature reaches 102°F to avoid rebound hypothermia.*

7) Correct other metabolic derangements identified by laboratory work.

8) Provide respiratory support if hypoventilation or noncardiogenic pulmonary edema occur.

L. CNS toxins

4. General treatment guidelines

a. Few toxins have specific antidotes (see below), thus, general guidelines for managing toxicities are presented.

1) Induce emesis—apomorphine 0.02–0.04 mg/kg IV or IM, 0.08 mg/kg SQ in dog or 2–6 mg dissolved and placed in the conjunctival sac; hydrogen peroxide 3% 1–5 mL/kg PO dog or cat. Contraindicated if patient is severely depressed or exhibiting seizure activity, caustic or petroleum-based substance was ingested, or exposure/ingestion >4–6 hour prior to presentation.

2) Gastric lavage is indicated if emesis is contraindicated and is most effective within 2 hours of exposure. Activated charcoal and saline cathartic should be administered via stomach tube after lavage. (Mix 1–4 mg/kg activated charcoal powder with 250 mg/kg magnesium or sodium sulfate and dilute with 10 × volume of water).

3) Decrease further absorption—activated charcoal, pediatric suspension is most convenient and may be combined with sorbitol as cathartic.

5. Specific toxins

a. Organophosphates/carbamate

1) Mechanism: Acetylcholinesterase inhibition causes increased levels of Ach in the synaptic space of nicotinic and muscarinic receptors of somatic and parasympathetic preganglionic neurons. Sympathetic preganglionic nicotinic receptors are also affected. Result is continuous stimulation of postsynaptic nicotinic and muscarinic receptors leading primarily to increased parasympathetic activity. Increased sympathetic activity may occur along with skeletal muscle stimulation via somatic nicotinic receptors.

2) Clinical signs—salivation, lacrimation, urination, defecation, dyspnea (SLUDD), muscle tremors, miosis, occasionally seizures

3) Treatment

a) *General therapy as above*

b) *Antidote—atropine, 0.2 mg/kg $^1/_4$ dose IV, remainder SC, only if muscarinic signs are present. Atropine can be repeated q3–6h for 1–2 days if miosis, salivation, and bradycardia occur.*

c) *Pralidoxime chloride, 10–15 mg/kg BID–TID IM or SC until full recovery. Most effective within 24 hours of exposure. Not indicated in carbamate exposure because of reversible nature of acetylcholinesterase inhibition with these compounds*

d) *Diphenhydramine, 2 mg/kg IM, SQ q8h, may reverse nicotinic signs of muscular weakness caused by undetermined CNS effects. (Effectiveness is questionable.)*

e) *Supportive care on ventilator if respiratory failure occurs.*

b. Metaldehyde—snail bait, slug bait, some rat poisons.

1) Mechanism of action—unclear, proposed inhibition or reduced level of inhibitory neurotransmitter γ-aminobenzoic acid (GABA)

2) Clinical signs—hyperactivity, generalized muscle tremors, seizures, hyperthermia

3) Treatment—control seizures (see pp. 267–269)

a) *Methocarbamol, 150 mg/kg IV or 15–20 g/kg PO q8h.*

b) *Acepromazine, 0.023–0.2 mg/kg IV, SQ, IM, maximum 3 mg, effective in controlling muscle tremors. Do not administer to animals that are dehydrated, because of hypotensive vasodilatory effects.*

c) *Supportive care—IV fluids, nursing care for neurologic patients, etc.*

c. Strychnine

1) Mechanism of action—competitive inhibitor of inhibitory neurotransmitter glycine found in internuncial neurons in spinal cord. Result is uninhibited stimulation of striated muscle.

2) Clinical signs—muscle tremors progressing to tetanic seizures triggered by noise, light, and touch.

3) Treatment—control seizures (see pp. 267–269); pentobarbital often necessary

4) Maintain patient in quiet, dark environment.

5) Supportive care as above

d. Bromethalin (new rodenticide developed for warfarin-resistant rats. (Trade names, Vengeance, Assault, Trounce)

1) Mechanism of action—uncouples oxidative phosphorylation in CNS (and liver) mitochondria. Causes failure of Na–K ATPase resulting in cytotoxic edema of brain and spinal cord. Histopathology shows diffuse vacuolization of CNS white matter.

2) Clinical signs—Mild exposure causes ataxia with posterior paresis and depressed mentation. High doses can cause severe excitement, hysteria, and seizures.

3) Treatment—general therapy as above

4) Treat cerebral edema (see section)

5) Control seizures (see pp. 267–269)

e. Lead

1) Mechanism of action—inhibits essential enzymes of cellular metabolism and causes endothelial damage

2) Sources of lead include paint before 1950, lead fishing sinkers, curtain weights, storage batteries, linoleum, rug padding, decorative glazes, roofing materials, putty and caulk, solder, plumbing materials, golf balls, and improperly glazed ceramic bowls.

3) Diagnosis

a) *History of exposure, demonstrating metallic density in GI tract or metaphysis of long bones with radiographs*

b) *Nucleated red blood cells with or without basophilic stippling with only mild anemia*

c) *Whole blood level >0.35–0.6 ppm is diagnostic. Submit 2 mL of whole heparinized blood (not EDTA blood).*

4) Clinical signs

a) *GI—vomiting, diarrhea, abdominal pain, inappetence, megaesophagus*

b) *Neurologic—blindness, seizures, hysteria, dull mentation, ataxia, tremors*

5) Treatment
   a) *Remove lead from GI tract—emesis, lavage, enemas, endoscopy, laparotomy if necessary*
   b) *Chelation therapy (choose one):*
      i) *Calcium disodium versenate 100 mg/kg/day diluted to 10 mg/mL in 5% dextrose or 0.9% NaCl, given SC in divided doses q6h for 5 days. Adequate hydration is necessary to minimize risk of nephrotoxicity.*
      ii) *D-Penicillamine, 35–50 mg/kg/day PO divided q6–8h 30 minutes before feeding for 7 days. Can be repeated in one week if necessary.*
      iii) *Succimer (Chemet) is a newer chelating agent that is safe and effective when administered orally at a dosage of 10 mg/kg q8h for 10 days. It is not necessary to remove all lead from the GI tract when this method is used.*
   c) *Methocarbanol 50 mg/kg slow IV bolus, repeated to effect (not to exceed 300 mg/kg/24h) to control muscle fasiculations.*
   d) *Seizure control and supportive care (fluids, etc) as needed.*

f. Pyrethrins/pyrethroids
   1) Mechanism of action—cause repetitive nerve firing by prolonging sodium conductance in neural tissue resulting in increased afterpotentials. Readily absorbed through skin because of lipid solubility.
   2) Clinical signs
      a) *GI—hypersalivation, anorexia, vomiting*
      b) *Neurologic—ataxia, muscle tremors, seizures*
   3) Treatment
      a) *In addition to general measures to minimize absorption (discussed above), bathing animal with liquid dishwashing detergent may limit dermal absorption.*
      b) *Methocarbanol 50 mg/kg slow IV bolus, repeated to effect (not to exceed 300 mg/kg/24h) to control muscle fasiculations*
      c) *Seizure control and supportive care as indicated*

g. Tremorogenic mycotoxins—*Penicillium*
   1) Mechanism of action—mold on cream cheese, walnuts, or other spoiled food produces toxins that decrease GABA inhibitory neurotransmitters and cause cerebral vasoconstriction.
   2) Diagnosis

   a) *History of eating moldy foods*
   b) *Identification of tremorogens in stomach contents*
   3) Clinical signs
      a) *Acute onset of excitement, ataxia, tremors, opisthotonus, seizures*
      b) *Exacerbated by stress and handling*
   4) Treatment
      a) *Remove food source. Administer activated charcoal.*
      b) *Supportive care—IV fluids, quiet environment*
      c) *Full recovery is possible.*

h. Ethylene glycol
   1) CNS signs predominate in first 12 hours—ataxia, seizures, coma, stupor
   2) Diagnosis
      a) *Positive serum ethylene glycol test result*
      b) *Severe metabolic acidosis*
      c) *High serum osmolality*
      d) *±Fluorescent vomitus with Wood's lamp*
   3) Treatment—see Toxicologic Emergencies.

i. Aromatic hydrocarbons—in wood preservatives (creosote), mothballs, some disinfectants
   1) Mechanism of action—rapidly absorbed, affecting CNS, liver, and kidney
   2) Diagnosis—urine test for phenols
   3) Clinical signs—ulceration of oral mucous membranes, vomiting, ataxia, muscle fasciculation, seizures, coma
   4) Treatment
      a) *Milk/egg whites to decrease corrosive lesions orally; gastric lavage; activated charcoal*
      b) *Supportive care: IV fluids, GI protectants, seizure control*

j. Metronidazole
   1) Mechanism of action—unknown
   2) Diagnosis—history of metronidazole administration at dosages exceeding 50–60 mg/kg/day with acute onset of neurologic signs (lower doses can cause toxicity in dogs with liver disease).
   3) Clinical signs—acute onset of vestibular signs, ataxia seizures, and/or blindness
   4) Treatment—discontinuation of medication and supportive care as needed. Recovery is usually complete within 5–21 days.
   5) Treatment with diazepam (0.5 mg/kg IV as an initial bolus followed by 0.5 mg/kg PO q8h for 3 days) will result in rapid clinical

improvement with complete recovery within 3 days.

M. Acute vestibular disease

1. Overview
  a. Vestibular system is responsible for balance and coordinates movements of eyes, trunk, and limbs with respect to changes in head position.
  b. Vestibular system has both peripheral and central components.
    1) Peripheral—inner ear receptors, vestibular nerve
    2) Central—brainstem nucleus of vestibular nerve, flocculonodular lobe of cerebellum

2. Clinical signs
  a. Ataxia, head tilt, circling and nystagmus are classic neurologic signs of vestibular disease. Head tilt and circling are usually toward side of lesion.
  b. Localizing disease to peripheral or central vestibular system is important in determining differential diagnosis, diagnostic workup, and prognosis.
    1) Signs of peripheral disease
      a) Horizontal nystagmus, named by direction of fast phase, which is away from the side of the lesion
      b) Absence of long-tract signs such as proprioceptive deficits, postural changes, spinal reflex abnormalities
      c) Horner's syndrome or facial nerve deficit usually indicates a middle ear lesion.
    2) Signs of central disease
      a) Nystagmus may be vertical, horizontal, rotary, or change with head position. Vertical nystagmus is consistent with a central lesion.
      b) Long-tract signs, mentation changes, possible visual deficits with normal pupillary light and menace response (cerebellar lesion), and/or other signs of CNS involvement. Lateralizing weakness or proprioceptive deficits are often seen with central disease.

3. Peripheral vestibular diseases—common
  a. Idiopathic (old dog vestibular disease, idiopathic labyrinthitis)
    1) Acute onset of severe peripheral vestibular signs is seen most often in older dogs.
    2) Also occurs in cats
    3) Patient may roll and thrash violently; may resemble seizure but has no

tonic–clonic limb movements or loss of consciousness or pre- and postictal behavior changes.
    4) Physical examination findings including those of otoscopic examination are otherwise normal.
    5) Treatment is supportive—IV fluids at maintenance rates and nutritional support until animal can eat and drink on its own.
      a) Diphenhydramine, 2 mg/kg SC or IM, meclizine, 2 mg/kg PO q24h (cat) or 4 mg/kg PO q24h (dog), or chlorpromazine 0.25–0.5 mg/kg q6–12h SC, IM can be used to treat nausea or vomiting that is occasionally seen in these patients.
      b) Corticosteroids are of no proven benefit.
    6) Recovery is usually complete with initial rapid improvement in most cases followed by more gradual improvement within 2–4 weeks. Slight head tilt may persist permanently in a small percentage of patients. Relapse can occur.
  b. Otitis media/interna
    1) Indicated by typical findings during otoscopic examination: discharge and opaque, bulging, or ruptured tympanum. Nasopharyngeal polyp may be identified (cats).
    2) Skull radiographs or CT of the tympanic bulla may reveal fluid or osseous changes.
    3) Treatment includes systemic antibiotics, preferably based on culture/susceptibility testing of exudate obtained by myringotomy.
      a) Surgery, bulla osteotomy, lateral ear canal resection, or nasopharyngeal polyp removal, performed when indicated
      b) Identify and treat underlying cause of recurrent infection, e.g., hypothyroidism, atopy, food allergy.
  c. Trauma, neoplasia, peripheral neuropathy (hypothyroidism) and congenital disease are uncommon causes of peripheral vestibular disease.

4. Central vestibular disease
  a. Causes include inflammatory or infectious disease (viral, protozoal, GME), neoplasia, metronidazole toxicity, thiamine deficiency, and congenital cerebellar disease (hypoplasia, abiotrophy, storage disease).
  b. Clinical signs are usually progressive and may be multifocal, involving other intracranial

structures. Prognosis is more guarded than that of peripheral vestibular disease.

c. CT or MRI will demonstrate mass lesions (neoplasia, granuloma).

d. Treatment varies with diagnosis.

N. Diskospondylitis

1. Definition/pathology

a. Bacterial or fungal infection of intervertebral disk and adjacent vertebral bodies.

b. Routes of infection include hematogenous spread (e.g., urinary tract infection, bacterial endocarditis), migration of grass awn, and extension of infection from adjacent soft tissue.

c. Organisms most commonly involved include coagulase-positive staphylococci, streptococci, *Escherichia coli*, *Pasteurella multocida*, *Nocardia* spp., *Actinomyces* spp., and *Brucella canis*.

d. Predisposing factors include trauma, spinal surgery, and immunosuppression.

2. Clinical signs

a. Most commonly seen in large-breed dogs; small-breed dogs and cats are less commonly affected.

b. Back or neck pain with stiff gait with or without spinal neurologic signs. Pain may be focal over affected disk space. Multiple disk spaces may be involved or pain may be severe enough to cause generalized pain/hyperpathia. Must be differentiated from acute abdominal pain.

c. Fever, lethargy, inappetance and other signs of systemic illness may be present.

d. Neurologic deficits depend on location of lesion (s) and degree of spinal cord compression by protruding disk, bony proliferation, or vertebral luxation. Signs vary from spinal hyperpathia to paralysis or plegia.

3. Diagnosis

a. Survey spinal radiographs may reveal collapsed disk space(s) with lysis and/or proliferation and sclerosis of endplates of adjacent vertebral bodies (*Fig. 13-3*).

b. Lesions most commonly affect lumbosacral junction and caudal, cervical, and midthoracic vertebrae. Grass awn migration commonly affects attachment of diaphragmatic crura at L2-L4.

c. Sedation or general anesthesia may be necessary for optimal positioning and collimation.

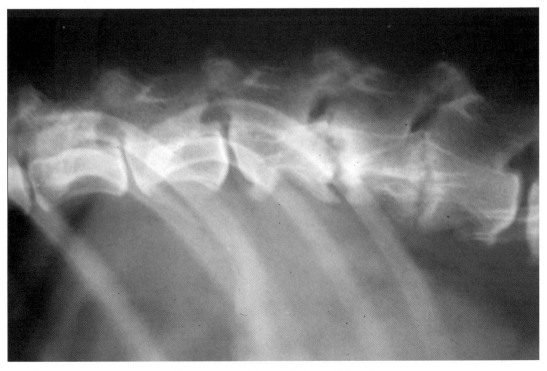

FIGURE 13.3 Lateral radiograph of spine reveals diskospondylitis at the L1-L2 intervertebral space.

d. Lesions may be mild and difficult to identify within first 2 weeks of infection; repeating radiographs may be necessary.
e. Myelography may be useful to assess spinal cord compression and identify multiple affected disk spaces if animal is a potential candidate for surgery.
f. CSF tap is usually not rewarding but is helpful in ruling out other causes of similar neurologic signs such as meningitis/encephalitis, GME.
g. CT and bone scintigraphy are very sensitive at detecting early lesions.
h. Blood and urine cultures are positive in at least 50% of patients and may yield the same organism infecting the disk space.
i. Aspirate of disk material using fluoroscopic guidance may provide material for bacterial or fungal culture and cytology.
j. Screening for *B. canis* is recommended in all cases in dogs.

4. Treatment
  a. Long term, 6–8 weeks, antibiotic therapy
  b. IV administration of cephalosporin or enrofloxacin for the first 5–7 days is a good initial choice pending culture results. Improvement is usually dramatic within 1 week of appropriate antibiotic administration.
  c. Oral therapy with the appropriate antibiotic should be continued for total of 6–8 weeks.
  d. Relapse may occur necessitating reinstitution of antibiotic therapy for up to 4–6 months.
  e. Aminoglycoside/doxycycline combination for *B. canis* infection.
    1) Minocycline 12 mg/kg PO q12h and gentamicin 2.2 mg/kg IM q8h for 14–21 days
    2) Enrofloxacin 10–15 mg/kg PO q12h for 3 weeks, then discontinue for 3 weeks; repeat 1–3 times
  f. Analgesics (butorphanol) and/or antiinflammatory agents (carprofen, aspirin, ketoprofen) may be indicated for patients with severe pain.
  g. Surgical debridement, decompression, and stabilization are occasionally necessary.

O. Tetanus

1. Etiology/pathogenesis
  a. Exotoxins tetanospasmin and tetanolysin produced by *Clostridium tetani* inhibit inhibitory neurons in brainstem and spinal cord and impair transmission, resulting in extensor rigidity and sustained contraction of striated muscles, including the facial, skeletal, and diaphragmatic muscles.
  b. Inactive spore in the environment germinates when introduced into a wound and elaborates toxin. Signs may occur 5 days to 3 weeks after infected puncture wound.

2. Clinical signs
  a. Characteristic signs include sawhorse stance with erect ears and prolapsed nictitans. Facial muscle contraction pulls lips into sustained "grin" called trismus.
  b. Severely affected animals have extensor rigidity of all four limbs with head and neck extension (opisthotonus).
  c. Animals exhibit exaggerated response to light or noise.
  d. Respiratory failure may result from laryngeal or intercostal muscle or diaphragmatic spasm.
  e. Skin wound, usually on extremities, may be present or may be difficult to identify by the time clinical signs are evident.

3. Diagnosis
  a. Purely a clinical diagnosis. Characteristic musculoskeletal and neurologic signs suffice in most cases.
  b. Presence of a wound, sometimes quite small, is supportive.

4. Treatment
  a. Intravenous penicillin, 10,000–40,000 units/kg QID IV, or ampicillin, 22 mg/kg IV TID, is treatment of choice.
  b. Tetanus antitoxin may be used early in course of disease in severely affected animals. A test dose of 0.1–0.2 mg SC is recommended, as anaphylaxis may occur. If no adverse reaction is seen within 30 minutes, daily administration of 10–100 units/kg/day IV or SC in dogs and 500 units/day in cats, divided into 3 doses for the first 2–3 days is recommended until severe signs begin to resolve.
  c. Muscle relaxants including phenothiazines such as acetyl promazine are particularly effective; diazepam or methocarbamol can also be used.
  d. Occasionally, general anesthesia with pentobarbital is necessary, especially if intubation for respiratory support is necessary.

e. Supportive care involves maintenance fluids, frequent turning, and other nursing care for recumbent patient.

f. Flush and debride any wounds.

g. Consider amputation to eliminate source of toxin production in refractory or severely affected patients.

h. Supplemental oxygen or mechanical ventilation as indicated by pulse oximetry or arterial blood gas analysis. Elevated PCO_2 levels indicate that respiratory paralysis is imminent and ventilatory support is necessary.

i. Gradual recovery occurs over 1–4 weeks.

P. Isolated peripheral nerve injury

1. Sciatic nerve

    a. Pathogenesis/etiology

    Sciatic nerve injury may be caused by lumbosacral, pelvic, or femoral fractures, lumbosacral stenosis, or iatrogenic trauma from thigh injections.

    b. Clinical signs/diagnosis

    1) Affected animal cannot flex stifle or extend hock; thus gait is stiff with leg extended and knuckling onto toes. There is loss of sensation lateral to, and below, stifle.

    2) Additional signs of trauma or vertebral abnormalities may be detected by physical examination and radiography.

    c. Treatment

    1) Identify and treat associated traumatic injuries.

    2) Surgical exploration and repair of severed nerve is indicated in severe cases.

2. Radial nerve injury

    a. Pathogenesis/etiology

    1) Traumatic injury to proximal ribs or humerus may damage or transect the radial nerve.

    2) Innervation is lost to extensors of elbow and carpus, and animal cannot bear weight on limb. If distal injury to nerve occurs, elbow extension and ability to bear weight may be preserved, though knuckling will occur.

    b. Diagnosis/clinical sign

    1) Animal stands with dropped limb and cannot bear weight. Knuckling of carpus is seen.

    2) Radiographs may reveal rib (uncommon) or humeral fracture or gunshot injury.

    3) Radial nerve injury also occurs with brachial plexus avulsion (p. 267).

    c. Treatment

    1) Identify and treat associated traumatic injuries.

    2) Bandage foot to prevent excoriation of dorsal surface through dragging the paw.

    3) Surgical exploration and repair of severed nerve is indicated in severe cases.

    4) Limb amputation may be necessary in unresponsive cases, especially if severe excoriation or self-mutilation occurs.

Q. Stupor and coma

1. Definition/pathology

    a. Altered level of consciousness caused by lesion of cerebral cortex and/or ascending reticular activating system in brainstem

    b. Stupor is a severely depressed level of consciousness from which the patient can be roused by noxious stimuli, e.g., toe pinch.

    c. Comatose patients do not respond to noxious stimuli.

2. Clinical signs and neurologic examination findings

    a. Patients are usually recumbent.

    b. Acute onset and rapid deterioration in neurologic status indicate trauma, toxicity, cerebrovascular incident, or possibly heat stroke.

    c. Gradual onset and progression indicate neoplasia, encephalitis/meningitis, thiamine deficiency (uncommon), or metabolic disease.

    d. Rule-outs for suspected metabolic disease include liver disease with hepatic encephalopathy, severe renal failure, hyperlipidemia, hypoglycemia (presentation is usually acute), hyperosmolar syndromes (hyperosmolar nonketotic diabetes mellitus, acute ethylene glycol toxicity), polycythemia, hyperviscosity syndrome (paraproteinemia), severe electrolyte or acid–base disturbance, hypoadrenocorticism, and myxedema associated with severe hypothyroidism.

    e. Signs that indicate cerebral disease include miotic responsive pupils and/or seizure history.

    f. Signs that indicate brainstem lesion include midrange unresponsive pupils and loss of physiologic nystagmus ("doll's eye") and carry grave prognosis.

    g. Spinal reflexes are usually normal or slightly increased.

    h. Changes in respiratory rate or pattern are common and are discussed under head trauma (p. 260).

i. Serial neurologic assessment is critical to assess the progression or resolution of disease and response to treatment.

j. Owners should be questioned regarding exposure to toxins and traumatic events.

3. Diagnosis

a. Complete laboratory assessment may indicate one of the metabolic rule-outs mentioned above.

b. Blood gas analysis and pulse oximetry may indicate acid–base abnormalities or the need for supplemental oxygen or ventilatory support.

c. Radiographs may reveal associated traumatic injuries, noncardiogenic pulmonary edema, or metastatic lesions.

d. Advanced imaging using CT or MRI may aid in diagnosing intracranial neoplasia.

e. Screening urine or blood may aid in diagnosing toxicity, e.g., ethylene glycol.

4. Treatment

a. Support major organ systems as indicated by thorough history and physical examination.

   1) Basic supportive measures in patients with stupor and coma include IV fluid support and possibly supplemental oxygen.

   2) Choice of fluids depends on underlying cause.

      a) Isotonic crystalloids usually suffice.

      b) Gradual reduction in serum osmolality is recommended in chronic cases to avoid cerebral edema that may occur in response to osmotic gradient created by formation of idiogenic osmoles (osmolytes).

      c) Oncotic agents such as hetastarch, or hypertonic crystalloids (e.g., mannitol, hypertonic saline) may minimize ICP elevations and may be useful when low-volume resuscitation is indicated, e.g., trauma patients with head injury.

b. Other measures to control ICP are discussed in section on head trauma and include corticosteroids (controversial), oxygen, assisted ventilation, and head elevation (see pp. 259–263).

c. Nursing care is extremely important and involves thick dry bedding and turning patient q4h to prevent decubitus and compression atelectasis, corneal lubrication, head elevation and avoiding jugular occlusion, and physiotherapy to prevent atrophy/contracture.

R. Urinary and fecal incontinence

1. Definition/etiology

a. Impaired voluntary urination or defecation resulting from damage to innervation of bladder or colon

b. Lesions of sacral or caudal spinal cord segments result in lower motor neuron signs of flaccid/atonic bladder and dilated anus. Bladder is easily expressible and overflow incontinence occurs. Rectal examination reveals loss of sphincter tone and reflex.

c. Upper motor neurons are generally inhibitory to bladder and bowel emptying. Damage to these nerves causes incomplete bladder emptying and contraction, increased sphincter tone of both urethra and anus, and difficulty expressing bladder.

d. Differential diagnosis includes spinal trauma, infection/inflammation associated with bite wounds or penetrating injury, neoplasia, congenital malformation/agenesis of sacrocaudal vertebrae or spinal cord, reflex dyssynergia, and dysautonomia Damage to the sacral cord is commonly seen in cats following trauma to the tail and damage to caudal nerve roots from stretching.

e. In trauma cases, it is important to rule out fecal and urinary incontinence with a good neurologic evaluation before owners spend a large amount of money on an animal that may no longer be a suitable pet.

2. Diagnosis

a. Clinical signs, neurologic examination, and history are important in narrowing the differential diagnosis.

b. Urinalysis and culture/susceptibility are indicated because infections are common

c. Radiography may demonstrate distended bladder, stool-filled colon, or vertebral column abnormalities.

d. Occasionally, electrodiagnostic urodynamic studies such as cystometry, urethral pressure profilometry, or simultaneous cystometry and uroflowmetry are performed to localize the lesion in cases of urinary incontinence.

3. Treatment

a. Nonpharmacologic treatment of urinary incontinence includes managing associated problems and assisting voiding by manually expressing the bladder or intermittent catheterization. An indwelling urinary catheter is not preferred because of increased risk of urinary tract infection. Bladder should be emptied a minimum of 4 times daily to prevent permanent damage to tight junctions in the detrusor muscle.

b. Digital evacuation of colon or a gentle warm water enema is used initially for fecal incontinence. After evacuation, add bulking agents, e.g., fiber, to diet.

c. Pharmacologic treatment of urinary incontinence

  1) Bethanechol hydrochloride, 5–15 mg PO q8h, dog; 1.25–2.5 mg PO q8–12h, cat; parasympathomimetic that stimulates detrusor contraction in atonic lower motor neuron bladder; cholinergic side effects such as vomiting, abdominal pain, and salivation are common.

  2) Phenoxybenzamine, 0.25 mg/kg PO q12h, dog; 0.5 mg/kg PO q12–24h, cat; α-receptor antagonist resulting in decreased urethral sphincter smooth muscle tone.

  3) Skeletal smooth muscle relaxants such as diazepam decrease tone in striated muscle of the external urethral sphincter.

  4) Combination of bethanechol and phenoxybenzamine is used commonly to treat upper motor neuron bladder and reflex dyssynergia.

  5) For older spayed female dogs with overflow incontinence

    a) *Diethylstilbestrol (DES), 0.1–1 mg PO SID for 5–7 days, then repeated weekly, increases urethral tone. Use minimum effective dose to avoid bone marrow toxicity.*

    b) *Phenylpropanolamine, 1–3 mg/kg PO q8–12h*

    c) *Pseudoephedrine, 1–2 mg/kg PO q12h*

d. Management of associated urinary tract infections may help decrease incontinence.

S. Brain and spinal cord tumors

1. Diagnosis/clinical signs

a. Tumors of the CNS cause focal neurologic deficits of gradual onset.

b. Brain tumors commonly cause seizures, behavioral changes, pacing/circling, blindness, and/or mild ataxia.

c. Spinal cord tumors cause upper motor neuron signs caudal to the lesion and lower motor neuron signs if cervical, C6-T2, or lumbar, L4-S3, intumescence involved.

d. MRI/CT is necessary to identify intracranial mass lesions.

e. Myelography may suggest cord swelling or compression with spinal cord tumors.

f. Biopsy of affected area is necessary for definitive diagnosis.

g. Results of CSF tap often are nonspecific; procedure is contraindicated if increased intracranial pressure is suspected, to avoid potential complication of herniation.

h. Chest radiographs or abdominal imaging indicated to identify metastatic lesions (or possible primary tumor with CNS metastasis).

i. Results of laboratory tests are usually nonspecific; hypercalcemia may indicate malignancy.

j. Common primary tumors in both brain and spinal cord include meningioma, astrocytoma, oligodendroglioma, and lymphosarcoma. Metastatic neoplasia is common in both locations (e.g., lymphosarcoma, hemangiosarcoma).

2. Treatment

a. These cases are generally referred to a specialist for definite diagnosis and treatment following initial stabilization.

b. Surgical debridement or decompression will reduce tumor burden and provide material for histopathology.

c. Ancillary chemotherapy or radiation therapy based on tumor type may be indicated.

d. Prednisone, 0.5–1.0 mg/kg/day, may reduce edema and improve neurologic signs as a palliative measure.

e. Phenobarbital, 2 mg/kg BID PO, may be necessary to control seizures.

T. Hydrocephalus

1. Etiology/pathogenesis/definition

a. Excessive accumulation of CSF in the ventricular system and subarachnoid spaces of the brain

b. Usually a congenital anomaly in small, toy, and brachycephalic breeds (Bulldogs, Chihuahuas, Maltese, Pomeranians, toy Poodles, Yorkshire Terriers, Lhasa Apsos, Boston Terriers, Pugs, and Pekinese)

c. May be secondary to other CNS conditions, such as neoplasia, trauma, or inflammation

2. Clinical signs

a. Seizures, dementia, visual deficits, and incoordination are commonly seen.

b. May be a cause of "fading puppy syndrome" in nursing puppies of predisposed breeds

3. Diagnosis

a. Enlarged dome-shaped calvarium with palpable open fontanelles in a young small-breed dog is highly suggestive.

b. Skull radiographs may reveal a "ground glass" appearance to the calvarium.

c. Ultrasound through an open fontanelle may reveal ventricular dilation.

d. CT, MRI, and electroencephalogram (EEG) may be useful in the diagnosis.

4. Treatment

a. Prednisone, 0.5 mg/kg q12h gradually tapered to QOD, helps decrease CSF production.

b. Acetazolamide (10 mg/kg PO q6h) is a carbonic anhydrase inhibitor that may also reduce CSF production.

c. For acute increase in intracranial pressure, osmotic diuresis with mannitol is indicated (1 g/kg IV over 20 minutes; may repeat twice over 6-hour intervals).

d. Furosemide, 1–2 mg/kg q12h IV, IM, or SC, also decreases CSF volume.

e. Phenobarbital, 2.5 mg/kg q12h, is indicated in animals with seizures.

f. Surgical placement of a shunt to transport fluid from the ventricles into the peritoneal cavity may be required in animals that do not respond to medical therapy.

CHAPTER 14

HEMATOLOGIC EMERGENCIES

I. CLINICAL SIGNS, DIAGNOSIS

A. General signs of a hematologic emergency include weakness, pallor, collapse, shock, ±evidence of trauma or blood loss, and anemia.

B. Cats and dogs with **acute** blood loss will exhibit tachypnea and weakness when the hematocrit drops to 15–20%, respectively; animals with **chronic** anemia often exhibit no clinical signs (unless they are stressed) even at very low hematocrits (e.g., 8–12%).

C. Animals with acute life-threatening anemia should be rapidly stabilized while minimizing stress.

1. Tissue hypoxia, anxiety, tachycardia, and weakness may occur because of reduced oxygen-carrying capacity of the blood when hemoglobin levels drop below 7 g/dL (PCV ~ 21%).

   a. Supplemental oxygen should be given ("flow-by" or face mask) to fully saturate available hemoglobin, but no significant improvement in oxygen delivery to tissues will occur until the hemoglobin concentration of the blood is raised, by administering either packed red blood cells, whole blood, or polymerized hemoglobin solution.

   b. The determinants of oxygen delivery are cardiac output and arterial oxygen content. The formula for arterial oxygen content is

$$1.34 \times (\text{Hb concentration})\,(\text{SpO}_2)$$
$$+\ 0.003\,(\text{PaO}_2)$$

which shows that increasing the PaO_2 without increasing hemoglobin concentration of the blood will have little effect on significantly raising the arterial oxygen content.

2. An intravenous catheter should be placed, and the hematocrit or hemoglobin concentration should be determined immediately to confirm the presence of anemia.

3. A blood smear should be made, and the hematocrit tube should be checked for evidence of hemolysis. Special attention should be exercised during the physical examination to detect evidence of blood loss or other underlying causes of anemia (melena, hematuria, icterus, petechiation).

D. In anemic animals, clinicians should attempt to characterize the anemia as regenerative or nonregenerative.

1. Nonregenerative types require a bone marrow examination and blood chemistries to differentiate intramarrow from extramarrow causes of anemia.

2. Hemorrhage and hemolysis are the causes of regenerative anemias.

E. Clinical signs may help differentiate the source of anemia.

1. External hemorrhage

   a. Laceration of artery—fractures, puncture wounds from sharp objects

   b. Parasites—fleas or hookworms may cause life-threatening anemia in young animals

   c. Epistaxis, melena, hematochezia, and hematuria may cause significant anemia. (Always do a rectal examination.)

   d. Chronic blood loss will result in a microcytic, hypochromic, nonregenerative anemia due to iron deficiency.

2. Internal hemorrhage

 a. Blunt trauma—pelvic fractures, trauma to kidney, liver, or spleen

  1) Clinical signs may include bruising and progressive distension of a body cavity. Abdominal distension may not always be noted despite substantial intraperitoneal hemorrhage. Also, retroperitoneal hemorrhage can be difficult to detect.

  2) Diagnostics

   a) Abdominal radiographs reveal loss of abdominal detail and a fluid density abdomen. Retroperitoneal hemorrhage causes increased density and streaking in the retroperitoneal space, ventral depression of the colon, and loss of kidney detail.

   b) Abdominocentesis may reveal hemorrhagic fluid. The presence of platelets on a smear may indicate acute bleeding.

   c) Compare the PCV of the fluid with systemic PCV to evaluate the severity of blood loss. Identical values can either indicate acute severe bleeding or a sample obtained by needlestick of the spleen or blood vessel. Serial PCVs should be monitored to determine whether ongoing hemorrhage is present.

   d) Diagnostic peritoneal lavage is usually not necessary with clinically significant intraabdominal hemorrhage because it is obvious. If performed, the bloody fluid will be too opaque to read through when substantial hemorrhage is present.

 b. Causes of splenic hemorrhage include hemangiosarcoma, hematoma, hemangioma, splenic torsion with vascular avulsion and gastric-dilatation volvulus.

3. Coagulation defects—clinical signs will help to differentiate clotting factor deficiencies from vascular or platelet defects.

 a. *Clotting factor deficiencies* may result in hematomas, ecchymotic hemorrhages, hemarthrosis, hemoabdomen/hemothorax, or prolonged bleeding after injury or needlestick. (*Note:* Avoid jugular venipuncture in these animals.)

  1) Congenital/inherited (*Note:* A good history is helpful here, especially questions about whether the coagulation system has ever been challenged before, as in previous surgery (spay/neuter), trauma, bleeding episodes, etc.)

   a) Specific factor deficiencies
   b) von Willebrand's disease

  2) Acquired

   a) Anticoagulant rodenticide toxicity
   b) Liver failure
   c) Vitamin K deficiency (may occur with GI malabsorption or biliary obstruction)
   d) Disseminated intravascular coagulation (DIC)

 b. *Vascular or platelet defects*—check oral mucous membranes, pinnae of ears, axillary and inguinal regions for petechial hemorrhages. Other signs include epistaxis, retinal hemorrhages, melena, hematochezia, hematuria, and prolonged bleeding after injury or needlestick.

  1) Vasculitis—additional signs often include fever, edema, and organ failure

   a) Causes include immune-mediated, infectious (e.g., feline infectious peritonitis, Rocky Mountain spotted fever, dirofilariasis, leptospirosis), drug reactions, systemic inflammatory response syndrome, and heatstroke.

  2) Platelet defects

   a) Consider tick-borne diseases in dogs with history of ticks, fever, splenomegaly, and lymphadenopathy.

   b) Immune-mediated thrombocytopenia may occur following recent vaccination or viral infection, drugs, idiopathic, other.

   c) Spontaneous bleeding usually does not occur unless the platelet count drops below 20,000–30,000.

   d) Certain drugs may impair platelet function (aspirin, phenothiazines, dextrans, cephalosporins).

   e) Inherited thrombocytopathies have been identified in Otterhounds, Great Pyrenees, Spitz, gray Collies, and American Cocker Spaniels.

4. Hemolytic anemia—differentiate intravascular from extravascular types on the basis of clinical findings. This differentiation can provide better diagnostic and prognostic information.

 a. Intravascular hemolysis

  1) Hemoglobinuria (port wine colored urine), icterus

  2) Causes include babesiosis, zinc and onion toxicity, phosphofructokinase deficiency in English Springer Spaniels, hypophosphatemia, snakebite, heatstroke, and severe forms of immune-mediated hemolytic anemia (IgM and complement fixation lead to intravascular destruction of RBCs).

b. Extravascular hemolysis

1) ±Icterus, bilirubinuria, splenomegaly

2) Most common cause is immune-mediated hemolytic anemia (IMHA)

a) *Primary IMHA is idiopathic.*

b) *Secondary IMHA may result from infections, drugs, or neoplasia.*

II. DIAGNOSTIC AND MONITORING PROCEDURES

A. A blood smear should be evaluated to characterize the anemia.

1. Regenerative anemia is characterized by

a. Anisocytosis—variation in cell size; large RBCs consistent with regenerative response

b. Polychromasia—increased basophilia of RBCs

c. Leukocytosis—neutrophilia with left shift is common when bone marrow is actively producing blood cells

d. Reticulocytosis—request a reticulocyte count from a laboratory or perform in-house

1) Mix 2 drops of fresh EDTA-treated blood with 2 drops of new methylene blue stain. Incubate 2 minutes. Make smear.

2) Count number of reticulocytes in 10 fields of 100 RBCs to determine the percentage. Absolute reticulocyte count = % reticulocytes × RBC count

3) Regenerative anemia >60,000/μL reticulocytes, >1% corrected reticulocyte count.

4) Corrected reticulocyte count =

$$\text{Reticulocyte \%} \times \frac{\text{Patient PCV}}{\text{Normal PCV}}$$

(Normal PCV = 37% cat, 45% dog)

5) RPI = reticulocyte production index =

$$\text{Reticulocyte \%} \times \text{PCV}/45 \times \frac{1}{\text{maturation time}}$$

6) The corrected reticulocyte count and the RPI help the clinician determine whether the degree of regeneration is appropriate for the severity of the anemia. A good regenerative response will have a CRC >3% and RPI >1%.

e. Macrocytosis, hypochromia: ↑MCV, ↓MCHC

MATURATION TIME	
PCV	**MT**
45	1.0
35	1.5
25	2.0
15	2.5

2. Nonregenerative anemia is characterized by

a. Normocytic, normochromic indices (MCV, MCHC normal)

b. A regenerative response requires 2–3 days following acute blood loss

c. Bone marrow evaluation is usually necessary to characterize nonregenerative anemia.

3. Specific cell types on blood smear may give a clue to the cause of anemia.

a. Spherocytes—small, dense, round RBCs lacking central pallor that strongly suggest IMHA

b. Schistocytes—fragmented RBCs seen with DIC, vasculitis, hemolysis

c. Target cells look like "bull's eye" cells—seen with liver disease

d. Nucleated RBCs—seen in increased numbers with regenerative anemia, but should be proportional to reticulocytes; also seen with hemangiosarcoma, lead poisoning, splenic contraction, hypoxia, bone marrow disease, and heatstroke

e. Howell-Jolly bodies—RBCs with small round nuclear fragments and are increased with regeneration

f. Heinz bodies—pale, spherical projections from RBC membrane; seen with oxidant exposure, toxic anemias (especially in cats)

g. Autoagglutination—To differentiate from rouleaux: Mix 2 drops of saline with 2 drops of blood. Apply cover slip. Autoagglutinating RBCs stick together like clusters of grapes and are diagnostic for IMHA. (Rouleaux forms stacks like coins and disperses in saline.)

h. Hemoparasites—chance of finding these is increased by making smear from capillary blood (e.g., ear stick)

1) *Hemobartonella* spp.—chains of cocci on RBCs; most common cause of hemolytic anemia in cats

2) *Babesia* spp.—bilobed, pyriform protozoa in canine RBCs

3) Cytauxzoon felis— "safety pin" organisms in feline RBCs
4) Ehrlichia canis morula—round basophilic inclusion body occasionally seen in cytoplasm of WBCs
5) *Hepatozoon* spp.—oblong inclusion body uncommonly seen in WBCs
i. Evaluate platelets
1) Should be at least 10–15 platelets per high power field; 1 platelet/hpf represents approximately 15,000 platelets.
2) When evaluating a blood smear for platelet estimation, the whole slide should initially be scanned at low power to check for platelet clumping. Falsely low platelet estimates are obtained when the monolayer is evaluated for platelet numbers and platelets are clumped at the feathered edge. Platelet clumping is less likely to occur when smears are made from EDTA-treated blood rather than from freshly drawn blood.
3) Giant platelets may be seen with active bone marrow response to diseases causing increased destruction of platelets.

B. Bone marrow examination is indicated for non-regenerative anemias, persistent thrombocytopenia, pancytopenia, and suspicion of intramarrow disease such as neoplasia or myelodysplasia.

1. Common sites include the iliac crest, trochanteric fossa of the femur, and craniodorsal humerus.
2. Note cellularity of sample. If poor, a core biopsy may be indicated rather than aspiration.
3. Count 3 cell lines (granulocytes, red cells, lymphoid cells). Note megakaryocyte numbers.
4. Myeloid/erythroid ratio (M:E) should be 1:1 to 2:1, with a complete and orderly maturation sequence.
5. Plasma cells and lymphoid cells should be <5% of total cells. (Increased numbers may indicate plasma cell myeloma, lymphoid leukemia, or ehrlichiosis.)
6. Hemosiderin in macrophages appears as blue-green granules. Increased iron stores are seen with anemia of chronic inflammation; iron stores may decrease with iron deficiency anemia.
7. Bone marrow hypoplasia may be due to drug toxicity, chronic ehrlichiosis, or feline leukemia virus (FeLV) infection.

C. Coagulation tests

1. In emergency practice, screening tests for bleeding disorders include the blood smear, platelet count, ACT (activated clotting time test), PIVKA (proteins induced by vitamin K absence or antagonists) test, prothrombin time, activated partial thromboplastin time, buccal mucosal bleeding time, and determination of FDPs (fibrin degradation products). All of these tests can be performed in-house.

a. Examination of blood smear, platelet estimation: If there are >5 platelets/hpf, bleeding is most likely NOT due to thrombocytopenia alone.
b. ACT (activated clotting time)

- Requires a special tube with diatomaceous earth that activates coagulation (ACT tubes, Becton Dickinson), a 37°C incubator, and a stopwatch.
- The stopwatch is started as soon as 2 mL of blood is added to tube, which is gently rocked 4–5 times.
- The tube is placed in the incubator at 37°C or placed under the arm of the investigator.
- After 60 sec, the tube is removed every 5–10 sec, gently tilted, and checked for clot formation.
- At the first sign of clot formation, the stopwatch is stopped and the time recorded.
- Normal ACT is usually 90–120 sec in dogs and is <75 sec in cats, but each hospital should establish its own normal values because of individual variations in test performance.
- The ACT measures the intrinsic and common coagulation pathways and is prolonged in DIC, anticoagulant rodenticide toxicity, liver disease, and congenital coagulopathy.
- Thrombocytopenia may cause mild prolongation of the ACT (increased by 10–20 sec).

c. Determination of FDPs

- Requires specialized tubes (Thrombo Wellco Test tubes) containing thrombin and a trypsin inhibitor
- Two dilutions are incubated with sheep anti-FDP antibodies and checked for agglutination after 2 min.
- FDPs >1:40 are commonly seen with DIC.
- FDPs >1:10 <1:40 commonly seen with liver disease, thrombosis, early DIC, and hypercoagulable states.

d. PIVKA test (Thrombotest, Accurate Chemical and Scientific Corp, Westbury, NY)

TABLE 14.1
RESULTS OF COAGULATION TESTS IN SPECIFIC DISORDERS

	PTT	PT	ACT	FDP	PLT[a]	Bleeding Time	Fibrinogen
von Willebrand's disease	N	N	N	N	N	↑	N
Vitamin K deficiency	N to ↑	↑	↑	N	N	↑	N
DIC	↑	↑	↑	↑	↓	↑	↓
Thrombocytopenia	N to SI ↑	N	SI↑	N	↓	↑	N
Platelet function defect	N	N	N	N	N	↑	N
Liver disease	↑	↑	↑	SI↑	N	↑	↓

[a] Platelet count.
N = normal, SI = slight, ↑ = increased, ↓ = decreased.

- In-house test used to diagnose anticoagulant rodenticide toxicity and monitor treatment.
- If test result is normal 48 hours after discontinuing vitamin K therapy, treatment can be stopped.
- This test is not specific for anticoagulant rodenticide intoxication, as these proteins may be increased in other diseases with prolonged clotting times.

e. Buccal mucosal bleeding time

- This test is used to evaluate platelet function in a patient with >50,000 platelets, normal coagulation test results, and a propensity to bleed.
- Requires bleeding device (Simplate II, American Diagnostics) to make a standard incision on the inner surface of the upper lip.
- A loose gauze tourniquet is used to hold the upper lip up, and filter paper is used to absorb the blood from the incision without dislodging the clot.
- Normal animals stop bleeding in about 3 min.
- This is a good screening test for von Willebrand's disease or platelet dysfunction caused by nonsteroidal antiinflammatory drugs (NSAIDS).

f. A new point-of-care coagulation analyzer is available from Synbiotics (San Diego, CA; 800-247-1725) that allows immediate in-house measurement of prothrombin time (PT), activated partial thromboplastin time (APTT), and ACT.

g. Coagulation tests commonly performed by laboratories include the PT, APTT, fibrinogen concentration, antithrombin III (AT-III) determination, and determination of FDPs. *Table 14-1* summarizes the results of coagulation testing in common bleeding disorders.

h. Concentration of AT-III, a naturally occurring anticoagulant made by the liver, may decrease in conditions such as protein-losing nephropathy, protein-losing enteropathy, subclinical DIC, vasculitis, and systemic inflammatory response syndrome (SIRS). Loss of AT-III results in a hypercoagulable state, and the animal is at risk for spontaneous thrombus formation when AT-III levels are < 50%.

D. Coombs' test—direct antiglobulin test.

1. Identifies antibody or complement on RBCs
2. Species specific—IgG, IgM, complement
3. False negatives due to
   a. Insufficient antibody on RBCs
   b. Temperature
   c. Prozone effect
   d. Previous corticosteroid therapy
4. Positive in 60–70% of cases of IMHA
5. Performed on EDTA-treated blood
6. Not necessary in patients with autoagglutination (Agglutination = end point of test).

E. Crossmatching

1. Blood typing card test (DMS Laboratories, Inc., 2 Darts Mill Road, Flemington, NJ 08822)
   a. Canine—tests for DEA 1.1 (most antigenic)
      1) "Universal donor"—DEA 1.1 negative

2) DEA 1.1 positive dogs can receive blood from DEA 1.1 positive or negative donors.

b. Feline—tests for types A, B, and AB blood

1) Most domestic short haired (DSH) cats in the United States are type A

2) Cats have preformed antibody against antigens they lack. Type B cats can have a life-threatening reaction to first-time transfusion of type A blood.

3) Cats likely to have type B blood include British breeds (Devon Rex, Cornish Rex, British Shorthair, Scottish Fold), Norwegian Forest Cat, Persian, Himalayan, Abyssinian, Birman, Sphinx, and Somali.

4) Exotic breeds/purebred cats should be typed before transfusing.

5) In cats, the card test replaces need for crossmatching.

2. Crossmatching procedure (*Table 14-2*)

a. Used primarily for dogs that have been previously transfused, even if donor is DEA 1.1 negative.

b. Major crossmatch: Donor cells are exposed to recipient plasma to see if recipient contains antibodies against any of the DEA antigens.

c. Minor crossmatch: Donor plasma exposed to recipient's cells

F. Transfusion medicine (see Table 14-3 "Uses of Blood Component Therapy," Appendix I, p. 436)

1. Sources of blood

a. Clinic blood donors

1) Dogs

a) *Ideal donors are negative for DEA 1.1, DEA 1.2, DEA 7 and have normal concentration of von Willebrand's factor.*

b) *Must weigh at least 50 lb.*

c) *Negative for heartworm disease, tick-borne diseases, brucellosis, and parasites and vaccinated, with a PCV of about 40%.*

d) *Can donate 22 mL/kg q3–4 weeks.*

e) *To prevent iron deficiency give 10 mg/kg of ferrous sulfate PO SID for frequent donors.*

2) Cats

a) *Domestic short-haired cats >8 lb*

b) *Healthy (negative for toxoplasmosis, FeLV, feline immunodeficiency virus (FIV), and Hemobartonella spp.)*

c) *Blood group A (should have access to type B cat for purebred cats that may be type B)*

d) *Iron/vitamin supplements may be needed if used frequently*

e) *Can donate up to 14 mL/kg once a month*

b. Staff/client pet donors

1) Do not use pets that have been pregnant or previously transfused. (Blood may contain alloantibodies.)

c. Commercial blood banks that will ship component therapy overnight.

1) Animal Blood Bank, Vacaville, CA 916-678-3009

2) Eastern Veterinary Blood Bank, Annapolis, MD 800-949-3822

TABLE 14.2
CROSSMATCH PROCEDURE

1. Collect blood from recipient and possible donors in EDTA tubes.

2. Centrifuge and separate plasma into labeled tubes.

3. Wash RBCs 3 times with phosphate-buffered saline and resuspend.

4. Prepare 3 tubes labeled major, minor, and recipient control for each potential donor. Add 2 drops of plasma and 1 drop of RBC suspension to each tube as follows:

Major crossmatch: recipient plasma + donor RBCs
Minor crossmatch: donor plasma + recipient RBCs
Recipient control: recipient plasma + recipient RBCs

5. Mix gently. Incubate at 37°C for 15–20 min.

6. Centrifuge. Look for hemolysis.

7. Evaluate cells for macroscopic and microscopic agglutination.

8. Any hemolysis or agglutination on the major crossmatch indicates incompatibility. Slight hemolysis or incompatibility on minor crossmatch does not preclude transfusion.

3) Hemopet, Irvine, CA 714-252-8455
4) Midwest Animal Blood Bank Services, Inc., Stockbridge, MI 517-851-8244
5) Penn Animal Blood Bank, Philadelphia, PA 215-573-7222

2. Blood collection—must be aseptic!
  a. Cats are sedated with ketamine 10 mg, diazepam 0.5 mg, and atropine 0.04 mg by IV injection.
    1) The site for venipuncture is clipped and cleaned as if for sterile surgical procedure. Blood is drawn through a 19-g butterfly catheter into 5–6 10-mL syringes, each containing 1–1.5 mL of CPD-A anticoagulant (60-mL syringe may collapse the vein).
  b. Dogs—collect blood from the jugular vein directly into a commercial plastic blood bag (Avoid vacuum glass bottles; they activate platelets and may hemolyze RBCs.)
  c. Whole blood should be administered within 6–8 hours and not be refrigerated if functional platelets and clotting factors are desired.
  d. Blood collected in CPD-A anticoagulant can be stored in a refrigerator for 1 month. Bags should be labeled with donor name, date collected, and expiration date.
  e. Clotting factors are functional in fresh frozen plasma stored for up to 1 year.
  f. Frozen plasma (for increasing colloid oncotic pressure) can be safely stored for up to 5 years, but clotting factors are not functional.

3. Blood administration
  a. Administer through blood filter (removes fibrin clots and platelet aggregates)
  b. Refrigerated blood should be prewarmed in a water bath prior to infusion. Frozen plasma can be CAREFULLY thawed in a microwave on the defrost cycle if it is mixed every 10–15 sec.
  c. It can be given by intravenous, intraosseous, or intraperitoneal routes.
  d. Blood is incompatible with lactated Ringer's (calcium can combine with citrate in anticoagulant) and D5W (hypotonicity can lyse RBCs). Only 0.9% saline can be administered in the same line.
  e. Rate of administration (see Appendix I: "Transfusion Guide," p. 436)
    1) Begin at a slow rate (0.25 mL/kg) for 10–30 min and observe for reaction before increasing the rate.
    2) Set rate so blood will be delivered within 4 hours.
    3) Most animals: 5–10 mL/kg/h
    4) Heart failure patients: 1–2 mL/kg/h
    5) The maximum recommended rate is 22 mL/kg/h (used for patients with hemorrhagic shock). However, in acute massive hemorrhage, it may need to be given as fast as possible. In severe hemorrhagic shock, blood can be administered rapidly by placing a syringe and stopcock in the line with extension tubing. Blood is drawn into the syringe and delivered rapidly by IV push.
    6) How much to give:
      a) *Rule of thumb:*
      1 mL/lb of whole blood will raise PCV by 1%
      1 mL/kg of packed RBCs will raise PCV by 1%
      b) *Blood (mL) in anticoagulant =*
      $$BW (kg) \times 90 (dog) \text{ or } 70 (cat) \times \frac{PCV (desired) - PCV (recipient)}{PCV (donor)}$$
      c) *Increase PCV to 20–30% in anemic animals or ≥20% in animals requiring anesthesia or surgery.*
    7) Always check hematocrit before and after transfusion and note any hemolysis.

4. Transfusion Reactions
  a. Most common reaction is vomiting. It usually occurs because the blood is being administered too fast. Slow the rate and monitor the animal closely.
  b. Another common reaction is fever. Stop the transfusion and rule out sepsis (discolored blood, improper collection or storage) and hemolysis. Check for urticaria and edema. Non-life-threatening immunologic reactions can occur to white blood cells and plasma proteins. The transfusion can usually be administered slowly after administering 0.25 mg/kg dexamethasone IV and 1 mg/kg diphenhydramine chloride SC, IM, or IV. Monitor.
  c. Severe acute reactions (hemolysis, DIC, shock, and renal failure) can occur in type B cats given type A blood or in previously transfused dogs that have alloantibodies. Stop the transfusion immediately and treat for anaphylaxis (Chapter 4, p. 36).
  d. Delayed hemolysis 1–2 weeks after the transfusion can occur in animals receiving mismatched blood. Blood typing and crossmatching should help avoid this complication.

e. Volume overload resulting in signs of congestive heart failure (coughing, dyspnea, tachycardia) can occur in patients with underlying heart disease or overtransfusion. Slow the rate and do not exceed a total dosage of 22 mL/kg without careful monitoring. Central venous pressure monitoring is recommended for heart failure patients receiving colloids, blood products, or large amounts of fluid.
f. Bacterial contamination of blood appears as a dark brown supernatant overlying the red cells. Such blood should be discarded. Blood products that have been opened or warmed and not used within 8 hours should also be discarded. Gram stain and culture can be used to document suspected bacterial contamination.
g. Massive transfusion can result in citrate toxicity that is manifested as signs of hypocalcemia: tetany, muscle tremors, hyperthermia, and cardiac arrhythmia. If these signs are noted, calcium gluconate (100–150 mg/kg) should be administered slowly IV. Coagulopathy may also result if too much anticoagulant is used or if the animal is autotransfused with defibrinated blood from a body cavity.

III. MANAGEMENT OF SPECIFIC CONDITIONS

A. Immune-mediated hemolytic anemia

1. May be primary (idiopathic) or secondary to drug, vaccine, erythroparasites, or neoplasia
   a. History of recent vaccination (≤30 days earlier) should prompt a recommendation against future vaccines.
   b. Drugs associated with IMHA include cephalosporins, penicillins, trimethoprim-sulfa, or NSAIDS.
   c. Examine blood smear for hemoparasites: *Babesia* spp., *Hemobartonella,* or *Ehrlichia.*

2. Antibodies are produced against the RBC membrane. Coated RBCs may be lysed via complement fixation (intravascular hemolysis) or removed by macrophages in the spleen (extravas-

---

TABLE 14.3
USES OF BLOOD COMPONENT THERAPY

Component	Indications/Comments
Fresh whole blood	1. Coagulopathy with active bleeding (ITP, DIC, warfarin toxicity) 2. Massive acute hemorrhage 3. Animals with anemia + liver disease—preoperative stabilization
Stored whole blood[a] or packed RBCs[a]	1. Nonregenerative/refractory anemia 2. Autoimmune hemolytic anemia (when PCV ~ 10%) 3. Correction of anemia before surgery 4. Acute or chronic blood loss
Fresh frozen plasma	1. Factor depletion with active bleeding: vWd, congenital factor deficiencies, warfarin toxicity, DIC 2. Acute hemorrhage replaced with PRBCs 3. Prior to surgery in hypoproteinemic animals (e.g., liver biopsy, kidney biopsy, GI surgery)
Plasma	1. Hypoproteinemia (hepatic, renal, or GI disease) when albumin <1.5 g/dL or TP <3.5 g/dL and coagulation test results are normal 2. Acute pancreatitis and other SIRS conditions (contains acute phase proteins) 3. Colostrum replacement—neonates, parvo puppies
Cryoprecipitate	Congenital factor deficiencies (vWd, hemophilia A, hypofibrinogenemia)—prior to elective surgery or to stop on-going hemorrhage
Cryopoor plasma[b]	To improve colloid oncotic pressure in hypoproteinemic patients.

[a]Not to be used in patients with liver disease.
[b]Not to be used in patients with coagulopathy.

cular hemolysis). Partial damage of cells results in spherocytes.

3. RBCs coated with antibody become "sticky" and tend to clump or autoagglutinate.

4. Common breeds include Cocker Spaniels (especially buff colored), Miniature Poodles, Irish Setters, Dobermans, and Old English Sheepdogs: Most common in young to middle-aged female dogs, especially in spring. Rare in cats.

5. Clinical signs include weakness, lethargy, collapse, pale icteric mucous membranes, tachycardia, hepatosplenomegaly, ±fever and heart murmur.

6. Abnormal laboratory findings commonly include

   a. Leukocytosis and regenerative anemia—some patients are not regenerative because condition is peracute or because antibodies are directed against RBC precursors in the bone marrow

   b. Autoagglutination, spherocytosis—diagnostic

   c. Coombs' test is positive in 60–70% of cases.

   d. Serum chemistries—↑liver enzymes; UA-bilirubinuria; hemoglobinuria with intravascular form

7. Treatment

   a. Uncomplicated case (positive Coombs' test, no autoagglutination, regenerative anemia, hepatosplenomegaly, bilirubinuria, PCV >15%)

     1) Prednisone 2.2 mg/kg PO BID

     2) Sucralfate to prevent GI bleeding

     3) Consider doxycycline if thrombocytopenia, possibility of rickettsial disease

     4) Heparin 150–250 U/kg SC q8h is recommended to prevent thrombosis in dogs with agglutination or thrombocytosis. Aspirin 0.5 mg/kg PO q12h can be given when heparin is discontinued. Heparin therapy must be tapered (not abruptly discontinued) to avoid rebound hypercoagulopathy. Decrease each dose by ½ over 48h.

     5) Continue prednisone at high dose for 1 month or until PCV >35%. Decrease to SID for 2–4 weeks and continue to taper slowly over 8–12 months.

     6) If glucocorticoid side effects become a problem, give azathioprine at 2 mg/kg PO q24h for 7–10 days, then reduce to every other day, alternating with prednisone. This allows more rapid reduction of corticosteroid dose.

   b. Complicated case (autoagglutination, intravascular hemolysis, peracute collapse,

PCV <15%, icterus); also use this protocol if there is no response to prednisone after 3 days

     1) Dexamethasone 0.3 mg/kg q12h may be initially substituted for oral prednisone if the animal is vomiting.

     2) Azathioprine 2 mg/kg PO q24h

     3) Cyclosporine 10 mg/kg/day PO or IM, 5 days on, 2 days off (inhibits cell-mediated immunity while prednisone and cyclophosphamide inhibit humoral immunity). This is a costly medication, but it has shown promise in animals with nonregenerative IMHA. Therapeutic serum concentration is 200–400 ng/mL. This test is often available at local hospital laboratories.

     4) Danazol 5 mg/kg q8–12h (dog) may inhibit extravascular hemolysis and does not suppress bone marrow. Drawbacks include high cost and potential for liver toxicity.

     5) Human IgG, 0.5–1.5 g/kg IV infused over 6–12 hours, has been effective in halting immune mediated destruction of RBCs in some dogs.

     6) Cyclophosphamide may be substituted for azathioprine or added to the protocol, depending on clinician preference. It can be given at a dosage of 50 mg/m^2 IV or PO q24h for 4 days, then skip 3 days and repeat cycle. Another protocol recommends giving IV cyclophosphamide at a dosage of 200 mg/m^2 IV once and repeating in 2 weeks if necessary. Because it may suppress bone marrow, it should not be used in dogs that do not have an active bone marrow response.

     7) Transfusion may be necessary in severely affected dogs. Transfusion increases the risk of pulmonary thromboembolism and acute renal failure. Transfusions are withheld unless the dog shows clinical signs of anemia (tachypnea, tachycardia, weakness, collapse). Transfusion is usually necessary if the PCV drops below 10%.

     8) Hemoglobin-based oxygen-carrying solutions (HBOCs) can be used instead of blood to provide tissue oxygenation in anemic animals at a dosage of 15–30 mL/kg. HBOCs provide a short-term "bridge" until the animal's bone marrow replaces RBCs and immunosuppressive therapy takes effect. At the recommended dose, HBOCs will last 24–48 hours. Precautions include elevation of central venous pressure with possible volume overload and the short half-life of these solutions compared with packed red blood cells. Low doses (7–15 mL/kg) can provide temporary benefit but must be repeated in 12–24 hours. Primary benefit is improved oxygenation of tissues without increasing the risk of thromboembolism or acute renal failure. The only way to monitor these solutions is with a hemoglobinometer. Hemoglobin levels must be kept above 3.5 g/dL.

   9) Central venous catheters should be avoided if possible because of the propensity for these animals to develop thromboemboli.

   10) Supportive care with intravenous fluids should be given to animals with nausea, vomiting, or inability to drink water. Dehydration must be avoided in animals with autoagglutination to avoid venous stasis, tissue hypoxia, local acidosis, and thrombosis.

   11) Pulmonary thromboembolism is a serious potential complication of IMHA. Clinical findings include dyspnea, tachypnea, cyanosis, and hypoxemia. Thoracic radiographs may be unremarkable (see Respiratory emergencies, pp. 153–154). Prognosis is guarded to poor.

   12) Splenectomy may be considered as a last resort in patients with extravascular hemolysis that have not responded to medical therapy. Because RBC destruction can also occur in the liver, splenectomy may not be beneficial.

B. Toxic hemolytic anemias (see also Toxicologic Emergencies, Chapter 20)

1. Oxidants can damage RBCs, leading to Heinz body anemia. Cats are particularly susceptible.

2. Oxidants include onions, onion powder in baby food or soup, zinc, acetaminophen, local anesthetics (topical benzocaine, Cetacaine spray), new methylene blue, phenazopyridine (urinary analgesic), vitamin K, propylene glycol, and phenol compounds (e.g., moth balls).

3. If there is no history of possible toxin exposure, radiograph abdomen to check for metallic density (zinc, lead).

4. Zinc toxicity can be caused by ingestion of zinc oxide ointment, pennies minted after 1983, wing nuts and bolts from pet carriers, and galvanized metallic objects (see p. 397).

5. Treatment involves removal of source of toxin and supportive care for anemia.

6. Acetaminophen causes methemoglobinemia as well as Heinz body anemia in cats. Classic signs include brown blood, "muddy" mucous membranes, facial edema, tachypnea, and weakness. Treatment includes N-acetylcystine 140 mg/kg PO or IV, followed by 70 mg/kg q6h until clinical signs resolve (usually 7 treatments). Ascorbic acid can also be administered to promote conversion of methemoglobin to oxyhemoglobin (see p. 387)

C. Increased RBC fragility

1. Hypophosphatemia may cause hemolytic anemia in animals being treated for diabetes mellitus, hepatic lipidosis, or malnutrition followed by nutritional replacement, especially with glucose-containing solutions. Other conditions that promote hypophosphatemia include polyuria, alkalosis, malabsorption, and administration of intestinal binding agents.

2. Treatment of hypophosphatemia: Recommended veterinary dosage is 0.01–0.06 mmol/kg/h phosphate added to intravenous fluids (without calcium) and given over 6 hours. Potassium phosphate solution contains 3 mmol/mL phosphate. Recommended human dose is 7.7–15 mg/kg given over 4–6 hours. Potassium phosphate solution contains 93 mg/mL phosphate and 4.3 mEq/mL potassium. Discontinue IV supplementation when serum P is ≥2.0 mg/dL. Oral supplementation: 0.5–2 mmol/kg/day (cow's milk contains .029 mmol/mL phosphate).

3. Phosphofructokinase deficiency has been reported in English Springer Spaniels and American Cocker Spaniels. Affected dogs exhibit chronic hemolytic anemia with acute hemolytic crises resulting from strenuous exercise and panting. Treatment is supportive. Diagnosis is made by genetic testing.

4. Pyruvate kinase deficiency has been reported in Beagles, Basenjis, and Abyssinian cats. It is first recognized as chronic severe hemolysis at 3–6 months of age and often ends in terminal myelofibrosis.

5. Intravenous infusion of hypotonic solutions such as 5% dextrose in water may cause hemolysis if administered rapidly in large volumes.

6. Microangiopathic hemolytic anemia occurs when RBCs are fragmented by an underlying condition such as splenic torsion, hemangiosarcoma, caval syndrome secondary to severe heartworm disease, heatstroke, vasculitis, or DIC. Schistocytes are seen on the blood smear. Treatment involves correction of the underlying disease.

D. Parasitic hemolytic anemias

1. Mycoplasma hemofelis (formerly Hemobartonella felis).

   a. Most common parasitic anemia in cats

   b. Transmitted by blood-sucking insects

   c. Mycoplasma hemocanis is uncommon in dogs unless splenectomized

   d. Risk factors—FeLV, FIV, outdoor cats (males), stress, history of cat bite abcesses.

   e. Parasites appear as small cocci on the RBC membrane surface. Transient shedding may impede definitive diagnosis. Fresh blood smears are superior to EDTA-treated blood, as parasites can be washed off cell surface by EDTA dilution.

   f. Many cats have a positive Coombs' test.

   g. Recovered cats become carriers and are at risk for recurrence of disease secondary to stress.

   h. Hemobartonella organisms were recently reclassified as mycoplasmas rather than rickettsial organisms.

   i. Another hemotropic parasite in cats has been discovered: Mycoplasma hemominutum. Infections with this smaller parasite are usually subclinical and not associated with anemia.

   j. Treatment:

- Tetracycline 22 mg/kg q8h × 14–21 days
- Prednisone 2 mg/kg q12 h for 1–2 weeks, then tapered off for cats with a positive Coombs' test
- If cats develop a drug fever associated with tetracycline, consider substituting one of the following:

   Doxycycline 5–10 mg/kg q24h for 10–14 days

   Chloramphenicol 25 mg/kg PO q12h for 10–14 days

   Thiacetarsamide sodium, 1 mL/10 lb on 2 alternate days

   Enrofloxacin 5 mg/kg PO q12h for 10–14h

- Always look for underlying disease in resistant animals.
- Cats usually become subclinical carriers and may exhibit signs of disease with stress or concurrent illness.

2. *Babesia canis* or *Babesia gibsoni*

   a. Tick-borne disease

     1) *B. canis* is common in Greyhounds.

     2) *B. gibsoni* is common in pit bull terriers.

   b. Signs may include acute intravascular hemolysis, hemoglobinuria, icterus, fever, and splenomegaly or may be chronic fever, weight loss, and anemia. Exacerbated by stress, splenectomy, or concurrent disease.

   c. Diagnosis—detection of parasitized RBCs on blood smear, IFA titer >1:40. Coombs' test may be positive, indicating secondary IMHA

     1) *B. canis*—paired piriform inclusions in RBCs

     2) *B. gibsoni*—smaller, pleomorphic, often singular

     3) IFA serology does not differentiate species. *B. gibsoni* usually results in antibody titer >1:320. PCR testing will identify the species.

   d. Treatment

     1) Imidocarb 6.6 mg/kg SC or IM, two injections 14 days apart

     2) Pretreatment with atropine (0.04 mg/kg SC) 30 min prior to imidocarb may diminish parasympathomimetic signs.

     3) Supportive care (IV fluids, blood transfusion) as needed.

     4) Doxycycline 5 mg/kg q12–24h if rickettsial disease is suspected

     5) Prednisone 2.2 mg/kg q12h is indicated if anemia is Coombs' positive. It can usually be tapered off over 3–4 weeks after parasitemia is controlled.

     6) Response to treatment is usually good for *B. canis*; *B. gibsoni* is more difficult to clear.

     7) The most effective treatment for *B. gibsoni* is atovaquone (13.5 mg/kg PO q8h given with a fatty meal) plus azithromycin (10 mg/kg PO q24h) for 10 days.

       a) *This treatment was effective in achieving negative PCR status*

       b) *Very expensive treatment*

     8) Other treatments include (variable efficacy)

       a) *Clindamycin 25 mg/kg PO divided q12h*

       b) *Metronidazole 25 mg/kg PO q12h*

       c) *Diminizene acetate: 3.5 mg/kg IM (B. canis) or 7 mg/kg IM (B. gibsoni)*

3. Cytauxzoan felis

   a. Severe, usually fatal protozoal disease of cats in endemic areas of southern United States

b. Suspected host is the bobcat. Transmitted by blood-sucking insects.

c. Forms large schizonts in spleen and bone marrow. Merozoites are released and parasitize RBCs 24–48 h prior to death.

d. Clinical signs are icterus, fever, hepatosplenomegaly, collapse, and death.

e. Treatment:

   1) Most reported animals have died.

   2) Imidocarb (5 mg/kg IM, two injections, 14 days apart) plus aggressive supportive care may be effective.

   3) Early diagnosis through bone marrow or lymph node aspirate may improve chances of survival.

E. Thrombocytopenia

1. Clinical signs include petechial hemorrhage, ecchymoses, melena, hematuria, retinal hemorrhage, and epistaxis. Dogs with infectious disease often have fever, lymphadenopathy, and splenomegaly.

2. Decreased or defective production

a. Bone marrow examination shows reduced numbers of megakaryocytes.

   1) To avoid significant bleeding, constant pressure must be applied to the bone marrow aspiration site for 5–10 minutes following the procedure.

   2) Bone marrow examination is usually not performed when the platelet count is $<2000/\mu L$.

b. Causes of decreased production include myeloproliferative disease, estrogen, chemotherapeutic agents, phenylbutazone, chloramphenicol, *Ehrlichia canis, E. platys*, FeLV, vaccines, hypothyroidism, and an immune process against megakaryocytes.

3. Increased platelet consumption and destruction

a. Bone marrow examination reveals increased numbers of megakaryocytes.

b. Causes include immune-mediated thrombocytopenia (ITP), systemic lupus erythematosus, drugs (sulfa drugs, propylthiouracil, gold salts, dextrans, heparin, cephalosporins), neoplasia, hypersplenism, gram-negative sepsis, DIC, dirofilariasis.

4. Treatment

a. Give patients with active bleeding fresh whole blood or platelet-rich plasma.

   1) Platelet-rich plasma is prepared by collecting whole blood in CPDA anticoagulant

and centrifuging at 2000 rpm for 3 minutes. The plasma is removed from the cells and kept at room temperature. It must be transfused within 28 hours of collection for platelets to be viable.

   2) Dosage of blood or plasma is 10–20 mL/kg administered over 2–4 hours.

b. If rickettsia-induced thrombocytopenia is suspected, administer doxycycline (5–10 mg/kg q12–24h) or tetracycline 22 mg/kg q8h for 2–3 weeks and submit blood for tick titer determinations.

c. ITP usually has a platelet count $<30,000$ with low mean platelet volume (MPV) if it is acute or if antibodies are directed against megakaryocytes. MPV is increased with an active bone marrow response resulting in release of immature platelets.

   1) Initial treatment is prednisone 2.2 mg/kg q12h and azathioprine 2.2 mg/kg q24h.

   2) In areas endemic for rickettsial disease, doxycycline is administered concurrently.

   3) Sucralfate at a dose of 0.5–1 g q8h PO is given for protection and treatment of GI bleeding.

   4) Refractory cases may require additional treatment.

     a) *Cyclophosphamide 200 mg/m^2 IV once may decrease antiplatelet antibody production.*

     b) *Danazol 5 mg/kg q12h may decrease immune-mediated destruction of platelets.*

     c) *Intravenous IgG infusion (0.5 g/kg over 6 hours) may modulate immune-mediated destruction of platelets.*

     d) *Vincristine 0.5 mg/m^2 IV causes megakaryocytic fragmentation and release of platelets into circulation. It may benefit animals with dangerously low platelet counts that are at risk for spontaneous hemorrhage. It should not be given unless immunosuppressive therapy has already been administered. Also, immature platelets may have decreased function, so the practice of giving vincristine to patients with ITP is controversial.*

   5) Once the platelet count reaches 200,000 cells/μL, immunosuppressive therapy is gradually tapered off (*Table 14-4*)

F. Anticoagulant rodenticide toxicity

1. Most common acquired coagulation defect

2. Pathophysiology

TABLE 14.4
TREATMENT OF ITP[a]

Month	Prednisone (mg/kg)	Azathioprine (mg/kg)
Initial	2.2 BID	2.2 SID
2	2.2 SID	2.2 QOD
3	1.1 SID	2.2 QOD
4–6	1.1 QOD	2.2 QOD
7	0.5 QOD	1.1 QOD
8	0.25 QOD	1.1 QOD
9	0.25 QOD	Stop
10	Stop	

[a]Platelet counts should be checked frequently until stable and then 1 week after each decrease in dosage. If the count begins to drop again, the dosage must be increased to the last effective dose. Some dogs must stay on 0.25 mg/kg QOD for life to prevent relapse.

a. Coumarins inhibit epoxide reductase.
b. This enzyme is necessary for activation of vitamin K.
c. Vitamin K-dependent clotting factors are II, VII, IX. and X.
d. Inactive clotting factors accumulate in the liver and are released systemically. These are called PIVKA and can be detected by the Thrombotest (Accurate Chemical and Scientific Corporation, Westbury, NY).
e. Factor VII has the shortest half-life (6 hours), so the extrinsic system (PT) will be prolonged first. The APTT will be prolonged within 24 hours after the PT.

3. Clinical signs
   a. May be delayed for 2–7 days after toxin ingestion
   b. Signs are variable and may include dyspnea, weakness, lethargy, collapse, hematomas, hemarthrosis, GI bleeding, severe bruising, bleeding into body cavity, and hemorrhage from site of trauma

4. Determine the type of rodenticide if possible, because treatment times vary.
   a. Coumarin (warfarin) types
      1) Shortest half-life, must treat for 7 days
      2) Commercial products: Coumafene, D-Con, Banarat, Rosex, Ratox, Prolin
   b. Indanediones
      1) Still first-generation compounds, but more potent with longer half-life
      2) Treatment is required for 3–4 weeks.

3) Commercial products include Chemrat, Drat, Drozol, RamiK, and Diphacin.
   c. Second-generation compounds
      1) More potent, longest half-life; must be treated for 4–6 weeks
      2) Often marketed as green or blue pellets
      3) Generic compounds include brodifacoum, bromodialone, and difethiolone.
      4) Commercial products include Talon, Demize, Rodend, Havoc, Bolt, Rapax, D-Con Mouse Prufe II, Maki, D-Cease, and Contrac.

5. Treatment
   a. If the animal is brought in within a few hours of ingestion, induce vomiting or perform gastric lavage and administer activated charcoal. Oral vitamin K is administered for 1 week and the PT checked 24–48 hours after the last dose.
   b. Severe cases with evidence of active hemorrhage should be treated with a fresh whole blood transfusion or fresh frozen plasma (10–20 mL/kg) to provide clotting factors.
   c. Vitamin K can be administered IM, SQ, or PO.
      1) IV administration is avoided because of the potential for anaphylaxis
      2) SQ administration is usually effectively absorbed within 30 minutes unless the patient is in shock, because poor perfusion can delay absorption.
      3) IM administration results in rapid absorption but may cause hematomas. Use a very small gauge needle.
      4) The initial dose is 5 mg/kg SQ of vitamin K_1 (phytonadione), followed by 1 mg/kg q12h PO with a fatty meal.
         a) Warfarin is treated for 7 days.
         b) Diphacinone and indanediones are treated for 3–4 weeks.
         c) Brodifacoum and bromodiolone are treated for 4–6 weeks.
         d) An unknown toxin is treated for 3 weeks. Two days after the last vitamin K dose, the PT is checked. If it is prolonged, therapy is continued for 2–3 more weeks.

G. von Willebrand's disease (vWD)
   1. This is the most common inherited bleeding disorder in dogs.
   2. von Willebrand's factor (vWF) is synthesized by the vascular endothelium and megakaryocytes. It is necessary for proper platelet function and adhesion.
   3. Because vWD is a platelet function defect, all coagulation tests including platelet count will be

normal except those that require functional platelets (e.g., buccal mucosal bleeding time).

4. The most common form of vWD is type I, manifested by a decrease in vWF levels. It is autosomal dominant and is common in many breeds, especially Dobermans. These dogs are usually asymptomatic but have prolonged bleeding following surgery or trauma.

5. A severe autosomal recessive form resulting in complete absence of vWF has been described in Scottish and Manchester Terriers, Shelties, Dutch Kooikers, and Chesapeake Bay Retrievers. These dogs are at risk for spontaneous mucosal bleeding and prolonged hemorrhage.

6. Clinical signs are variable and include prolonged estrual bleeding, melena, hematochezia, hematuria, hematomas, and prolonged bleeding following surgery or trauma.

7. Normal vWF activity for dogs is 70–150%; dogs with about 25% have mild-to-moderate signs and dogs below 10% have severe signs.

8. A good screening test for vWD is the buccal mucosal bleeding time. It is prolonged (>3 min) in dogs with vWD. This test should be checked before elective surgery in breeds at risk.

9. Hypothyroidism may exacerbate bleeding tendencies in dogs with vWD.

10. Treatment

a. Bleeding episodes can be terminated by administering fresh whole blood or fresh frozen plasma (10–20 mL/kg).

b. Desmopressin (DDAVP, 1 μg/kg SQ) can be administered to the donor dog 30–120 minutes prior to drawing the blood to increase vWF levels in the transfused blood.

c. Animals with vWD that require surgery should have fresh frozen plasma (10 mL/kg) or cryoprecipitate (5 mL/kg) prior to or during surgery.

H. Disseminated intravascular coagulation (DIC)

1. DIC results from diffuse and overwhelming activation of the coagulation, fibrinolytic, and antithrombotic systems. Widespread microvascular thrombi are formed resulting in multiple organ failure.

a. Platelets and clotting factors are consumed, and bleeding tendencies result.

b. Plasmin degrades fibrin and fibrinogen into FDPs, which are potent anticoagulants that also inhibit platelet function.

c. Another name for DIC is ICF (intravascular coagulation and fibrinolysis) syndrome.

2. Conditions associated with DIC include

a. Neoplasia—especially hemangiosarcoma, metastatic mammary adenocarcinoma, and leukemia

b. Infection—sepsis, leptospirosis, Rocky Mountain spotted fever, babesiosis, dirofilariasis

c. Inflammation—pancreatitis, gastric-dilatation volvulus, heatstroke, snakebite, liver disease, immune-mediated diseases, amyloidosis

3. Laboratory diagnosis of DIC

a. Prolongation of PT, APTT, ACT, and bleeding time

b. Thrombocytopenia (usually in the range of 20,000–80,000/μL)

c. Decreased fibrinogen and antithrombin III concentrations

d. Elevation of circulating FDPs (usually >40)

e. Schistocytes may be evident on blood smear.

4. Clinical signs

a. Subclinical or chronic DIC—laboratory diagnosis with absence of clinical signs: Warning signs include rapid thrombin time, low platelet count, decreased AT III, increased FDPs

b. Acute DIC—Petechial hemorrhages are common. Other signs of organ dysfunction may be evident: melena, dyspnea, hematuria, and oozing and hematoma formation at venipuncture sites.

c. Fulminant DIC—Severe bleeding tendencies are evident exhibiting petechia, hematomas, and massive bruising. These patients are very unstable.

5. Treatment

a. Basic approach

1) Correct poor perfusion, hypoxia, dehydration, and acid–base and electrolyte abnormalities to decrease conditions that predispose to thrombosis (venous stasis, ischemia, tissue acidosis, vasculitis).

2) Identify and treat the underlying cause.

3) Use a peripheral rather than a central venous catheter to avoid excessive bleeding from the jugular vein.

b. Controversial treatments—many conflicting recommendations exist concerning the treatment of DIC. These are guidelines used by the authors.

1) Subclinical or chronic DIC: Prevent coagulation cascade by decreasing platelet aggregation with low-dose aspirin therapy (0.5 mg/kg q24h, dog; or 25 mg/kg q72h, cat).

2) Acute DIC
a) Begin low-dose heparin therapy (200–250 U/kg, dog; or 75 U/kg, cat) SC q8h.
b) Try to maintain APTT at 1.5–2 times normal.
c) Heparin therapy must be tapered by gradually decreasing the administered dose. Abrupt cessation of heparin therapy causes a hypercoagulable state. It is usually tapered over 24–48 hours by progressively decreasing the administered dose.
3) Fulminant DIC
a) Animals with active bleeding must have clotting factors and antithrombin III replaced.
b) Heparin is dosed at 200–250 U/kg SC q8h. The initial dose may be given IV (500 U/kg).
c) Fresh frozen plasma or fresh whole blood is administered after incubating with 10 U/kg heparin for 30 min to activate AT III.
d) For many years, it was thought that heparin therapy must always be given concurrently with blood or plasma transfusions to avoid exacerbation of the hypercoagulable state with enhanced formation of microthrombi. In recent years, however, heparin has fallen out of favor, and some clinicians treat DIC with plasma alone.

I. Epistaxis

1. Acute epistaxis may be a sign of a primary nasal problem, evidence of a bleeding disorder, or secondary to hypertension.
  a. Nasal problems—trauma, foreign body (splinter, thorn, grass awn), bacterial rhinitis, aspergillosis, cryptococcosis, benign polyp, neoplasia (adenocarcinoma, squamous cell carcinoma, fibrosarcoma, chondrosarcoma, osteosarcoma), allergic rhinitis
  b. Bleeding disorders—multiple myeloma, ehrlichiosis, Rocky Mountain spotted fever, babesiosis, immune-mediated or other causes of thrombocytopenia, anticoagulant rodenticides, inherited coagulation defects

2. History and physical examination
  a. Look for other evidence of bleeding (e.g., bruising, petechiations, melena, hematuria). Remember that melena may result from ingested blood from nasal bleeding and does not always indicate GI bleeding.
  b. Rule out trauma.
  c. Evaluate nasal discharge.
    1) Mucopurulent, chronic, transient response to antibiotics suggests a foreign body or bacterial origin.
    2) Unilateral discharge with decreased airflow through one nostril as evidenced on glass or mirror placed near the nose suggests a nasal mass, usually neoplastic.
    3) Bilateral epistaxis suggests a coagulopathy.
    4) Look for evidence of facial swelling (fungal or neoplastic).
    5) Perform a fundic examination to check for evidence of retinal hemorrhage (hypertension, hyperviscosity, or coagulopathy) or engorged blood vessels (hyperviscosity).
    6) Cytology of the nasal swab may reveal neoplastic cells, fungal elements, or inflammation.
  d. Initial diagnostics differentiate between a primary nasal problem and a systemic coagulopathy.
    1) PCV and TS will determine if anemia is present. Elevated total protein is consistent with multiple myeloma.
    2) CBC, platelet count, and blood smear should detect the presence of thrombocytopenia or blood parasites. Reticulocytosis suggests ongoing blood loss or previous episodes of hemorrhage.
    3) Coagulation screen will rule out bleeding disorders such as anticoagulant rodenticide toxicity and DIC.
    4) Thoracic radiographs should be taken to rule out metastatic disease if neoplasia is suspected.
    5) If coagulopathy is ruled out, anesthesia will be necessary for further diagnostics (e.g., skull radiographs, computed tomography (CT) or magnetic resonance imagery (MRI), nasal flush, nasal biopsy, rhinoscopy, cytology of impression smears).
  e. Emergency management of epistaxis
    1) If coagulopathy is present, fresh frozen plasma, blood transfusion, or vitamin K may be indicated.
    2) Instillation of dilute epinephrine (1 mL added to 50 mL of saline, 1:50,000 solution) can cause peripheral vasoconstriction and may terminate bleeding. This solution is

most effective if cooled in an ice bath before instilling in the nares.

3) Active animals that are not hypotensive can be given acepromazine (0.05–0.2 mg/kg IV; maximum dosage, 2.5 mg) to calm the animal and lower blood pressure. The epistaxis often subsides with cage rest. Blood pressure should be monitored to avoid hypotension.

4) If epistaxis continues, monitor the PCV and TS closely in case a transfusion becomes necessary.

5) If epistaxis continues unabated, the animal can be anesthetized, then intubated to prevent aspiration of blood, and the nasal passages packed with epinephrine-soaked gauze.

6) Once epistaxis has been terminated and the patient stabilized, the underlying disease process should be treated.

J. Feline anemia

1. Anemia is common in cats
   a. Cats are predisposed to Heinz body anemia because feline hemoglobin has 8 sulfhydryl groups (compared with <4 in other species), which are subject to oxidative injury.
   b. Feline RBCs have a short half-life (70 days compared with 112 days for dogs).
   c. Cats have a lower blood volume than dogs (60 mL/kg vs. 90 mL/kg). Anemia is more likely to occur following hemorrhage or hemolysis because of the reduced RBC mass.
   d. Cats also have a lower hematocrit (35%) than dogs (45%) under normal conditions.

2. Causes of anemia in cats
   a. Anemia of chronic disease
      1) Nonregenerative anemia occurs secondary to sequestration of iron in bone marrow macrophages.
   b. Feline leukemia virus (FeLV)
   Anemia can result from myelodysplasia, hematopoietic neoplasia, nonregenerative macrocytic anemia, hemobartonellosis, or chronic disease.
   c. Feline immunodeficiency virus (FIV)
   Causes of anemia include bone marrow suppression, hemobartonellosis, and anemia of chronic disease.
   d. Mycoplasma hemofelis (formerly *Hemobartonella felis*)

1) Organisms appear as chains of small cocci on the RBC surface.
2) Parasitemia is intermittent and may be missed.
3) If Coomb's test is positive, empirically treat for hemobartonellosis (p. 289).

   e. *Cytauxzoon felis*
      1) Clinical signs: Depression, fever, pallor, icterus, splenomegaly, lymphadenopathy
      2) Laboratory findings: Anemia, leukopenia, thrombocytopenia, hyperbilirubinemia
      3) Aspirates of lymph nodes, spleen, or bone marrow reveal schizonts.
      4) Organisms in RBCs—bipolar "safety pins"
      5) Usually fatal within 7 days of onset of clinical signs
      6) Imidocarb 5 mg/kg IM is effective if given early in the course of disease.
   f. Heinz body anemia
   Causes include methylene blue, vitamin K, acetaminophen, lidocaine, benzocaine, *dl*-methionine, onions, zinc, propofol, propylene glycol in semimoist foods, and baby food with onion powder
   g. Hypophosphatemia (see p. 331)
      1) Hemolytic anemia has been reported in cats with diabetes mellitus following insulin therapy and in cats with prolonged anorexia after feeding is initiated.
      2) Intravascular hemolysis occurs because RBCs lack sufficient phosphorus to make ATP.
   h. Liver disease
   Anemia may be caused by coagulopathy, hypophosphatemia, or chronic disease.
   i. Chronic renal failure (CRF)
      1) Anemia results from low erythropoietin levels, GI hemorrhage, iron deficiency, Heinz body formation, myelofibrosis, and decreased RBC lifespan.
      2) Treatment of anemia associated with CRF:
         a) Ferrous sulfate 50–100 mg/cat/day
         b) Multiple vitamin supplement
         c) Correct hypertension: Amlodipine 0.625 mg PO q24h
         d) Erythropoietin 100 U/kg SQ 3 × per week; when PCV is about 30%, decrease to once weekly
   j. Neonatal isoerythrolysis
      1) Occurs in type A kittens after ingesting colostrum from type B queen.

2) Breeds with a high incidence of type B blood include Abyssinian, Birman, British Shorthair, Cornish Rex, Devon Rex, Exotic Shorthair, Himalayan, Japanese Bobtail, Persian, Scottish Fold, Somali, and Sphinx.
3) Clinical signs: Dark pigmenturia, anemia, icterus, anorexia, and sudden death within first week of life
4) Prevention: Test breeding pairs of breeds at risk to make sure they are blood-type compatible.
  k. Blood loss
    Causes: fleas, surgery, trauma

K. Ehrlichiosis

1. Most common species infecting dogs is *E. canis. E. platys* infects platelets to cause infectious cyclic thrombocytopenia.
2. Vector: *Rhipicephalus sanguineus* (brown dog tick)
3. Acute phase—nonregenerative anemia, leukopenia, thrombocytopenia, hyperglobulinemia, hypoalbuminemia, fever, pallor, lymphadenopathy, splenomegaly, bleeding tendencies (petechia, ecchymoses, epistaxis)
4. A chronic form is seen, especially in German Shepherd dogs, which is manifested by severe pancytopenia, weight loss, and organ system failure.
5. Diagnosis is usually made by serology. Rarely, morulae (inclusion bodies) can be identified in the cytoplasm of circulating mononuclear cells.
6. Treatment (choose one)
  a. Doxycycline 5–10 mg/kg PO q12h × 14–21 days
  b. Tetracycline 22 mg/kg PO q8h × 14–21 days
  c. Chloramphenicol 15–25 mg/kg q8h × 14–21 days
  d. Imidocarb 5 mg/kg IM
7. Other treatments
  a. Supportive care (IV fluids, blood transfusion)
  b. Tick control

L. Rocky Mountain spotted fever

1. RMSF is a tick-borne disease transmitted by *Dermacentor* spp.
2. The rickettsial organism replicates in the vascular endothelial cells causing vasculitis, thrombocytopenia, edema, and organ dysfunction.
3. Clinical signs include fever, lymphadenopathy, splenomegaly, petechial hemorrhages, joint and muscle pain, peripheral edema, and occasionally retinal hemorrhages.
4. Neurologic signs (ataxia, stupor, coma) may also occur.
5. Diagnosis is by demonstrating a fourfold increase in paired titers over 2–3 weeks. A very high single titer (>1:1024) is considered indicative of active infection.
6. Treatment is the same as for ehrlichiosis (see above).

M. Chronic blood loss

1. Young animals—severe flea infestation, hookworms
2. Older animals—GI ulceration (mast cell tumors, NSAID toxicity, glucocorticoids, GI neoplasia)
3. Chronic blood loss results in iron deficiency.
4. Anemia is classically nonregenerative, microcytic, and hypochromic.
5. Diagnosis is confirmed by low serum iron (N = 80–122 μg/dL), normal-to-high total iron-binding capacity (N = 280–340 μg/dL), and an absence of iron in bone marrow.
6. Treatment
  a. Ferrous sulfate, 100–300 mg/day PO (dogs) or 50–100 mg/day PO (cats)
  b. Reduce dosage by one half when PCV reaches 30%.
  c. For vomiting animals or animals with severe GI disease, use injectable iron dextran (10–20 mg/kg IM).

CHAPTER 15

ENDOCRINE AND METABOLIC EMERGENCIES

I. CLINICAL SIGNS, DIAGNOSIS

A. Clinical signs of endocrine/metabolic disease are variable but most often involve urinary, gastrointestinal (GI), neurologic, and dermatologic systems.

B. The most common urinary signs are polyuria and polydipsia (PU/PD) (e.g., diabetes mellitus, adrenal gland disorders, hyperthyroidism).

C. Signs of urinary tract infection (pollakiuria, stranguria, hematuria) are common with diabetes mellitus and hyperadrenocorticism (HAC).

D. Vomiting and diarrhea are extremely common with most endocrine diseases, especially hypoadrenocorticism, diabetic ketoacidosis, and hyperthyroidism.

E. Vomiting and diarrhea are also common with hypo- and hypercalcemic disorders.

F. Polyphagia is common with diabetes mellitus, HAC, and hyperthyroidism.

G. Neurologic signs vary from altered level of consciousness (e.g., hyperosmolar nonketotic diabetes mellitus, hyperkalemia, severe hypothyroidism, hypoadrenocorticism) to generalized seizures (e.g., hypoglycemia).

H. Muscle twitching/tetanus may be seen with severe hypocalcemia.

I. Dermatologic signs include symmetric alopecia (e.g., hypothyroidism, HAC) and calcinosis cutis (HAC).

J. Thinning of the skin is common with HAC, especially in cats.

K. Dehydration and weight loss are common.

L. Patients with hypoadrenal crisis, hypoglycemia, and diabetic ketoacidosis may present as true emergencies requiring rapid assessment and aggressive resuscitation measures.

II. DIAGNOSTIC AND MONITORING PROCEDURES

A. Low-dose dexamethasone suppression test

1. A screening test for HAC (i.e., Cushing's syndrome) used to differentiate normal animals from animals with HAC.

2. In normal animals, exogenous glucocorticoids inhibit anterior pituitary release of corticotropin (ACTH), thereby suppressing cortisol secretion from the adrenal glands; serum cortisol concentration will decrease following a low IV dose of dexamethasone.

3. With HAC, autonomous secretion of ACTH (pituitary-dependent disease) or cortisol (adrenal gland tumor) results in *lack* of suppression of serum cortisol concentration by low dosages of glucocorticoids.

4. Protocol:

    a. Obtain a baseline serum sample for cortisol determination.

    b. Administer 0.01 mg/kg IV of dexamethasone sodium phosphate.

    c. Obtain serum samples 4 and 8 hours later for cortisol determination.

5. Interpreting results:

    a. Normal: 4- and 8-hour serum cortisol concentrations are below the reference range, (<1.5 μg/dL or 40 mmol/L).

b. HAC: 8-hour serum cortisol concentration above 1.5 μg/dL or 40 mmol/L (no suppression)

c. Serum cortisol values between 1.0 and 1.5 μg/dL 8 hours after dexamethasone administration are nondiagnostic.

d. The pattern of serum cortisol concentration <1.0 μg/dL 4 hours and >1.5 μg/dL 8 hours after low-dose dexamethasone administration is diagnostic for pituitary-dependent HAC; no further discriminatory tests are necessary.

6. *Screening emergent or critical patients for HAC is not recommended because the stress of any illness may result in excess cortisol secretion leading to false-positive results (i.e., lack of suppression); screening tests should be postponed until the patient is stable.*

B. ACTH stimulation test

1. The ACTH stimulation test is used for 2 purposes:

a. Test of choice for diagnosing hypoadrenocorticism (i.e., Addison's disease)

b. Screening test for HAC (i.e., Cushing's syndrome)

2. In normal animals, exogenous ACTH stimulates the adrenal gland to secrete cortisol.

3. In animals with hypoadrenocorticism, idiopathic adrenal gland atrophy/fibrosis results in impaired secretion of cortisol in response to exogenous ACTH; serum cortisol concentration remains below the reference range.

4. In animals with HAC, either pituitary dependent or due to adrenal tumor, exogenous ACTH results in exaggerated secretion of cortisol by the adrenal glands; serum cortisol concentration is significantly above the reference range.

5. Protocol:

a. Obtain a baseline serum sample for cortisol determination.

b. Administer 0.25 mg IM or IV (dogs) or 0.125 mg IM or IV (cats) of synthetic ACTH (Cortrosyn, Organon Pharmaceuticals, West Orange, NJ). A calculated dose of 5 μg/kg synthetic ACTH can be used in either species.

c. Obtain serum sample 60 minutes (dogs) or 30 and 60 minutes (cats) after administration of synthetic ACTH for cortisol determination.

d. Natural ACTH gel preparations (porcine extracts) can be used as follows:

1) Obtain baseline serum sample for cortisol determination.

2) Administer 2.2 IU/kg IM (dogs and cats) ACTH gel.

3) Obtain serum sample after 2 hours (dogs) or 1 and 2 hours (cats) for cortisol determination.

e. Prednisone (any form) should not be administered within 24 hours of performing an ACTH stimulation test because it may cross-react with cortisol assays, leading to falsely elevated results; injectable dexamethasone should be used in the acute setting.

6. Interpreting results:

a. Normal: pre- and post-ACTH serum cortisol concentrations are within reference ranges established by the laboratory (pre: 1–4 μg/dL, or 28–110 mmol/L; post-ACTH: <20 μg/dL, or <550 mmol/L).

b. Hypoadrenocorticism: pre- and post-ACTH serum cortisol concentrations are below established reference ranges. A post-ACTH cortisol value that is within the reference range EXCLUDES hypoadrenocorticism.

c. HAC: pre-ACTH serum cortisol concentration is variable; post-ACTH serum cortisol concentration is well above established reference range (usually >22–30 μg/dL).

d. Iatrogenic HAC—results similar to those with hypoadrenocorticism

7. *Screening emergent or critical patients for HAC is not recommended (see A.6).*

C. High-dose dexamethasone suppression test, endogenous ACTH concentration

1. Tests allow discrimination between pituitary-dependent HAC and that caused by adrenal tumors.

2. They are not commonly performed in emergent or critical patients and are discussed in detail in several veterinary medicine texts.

D. Urine cortisol/creatinine ratio

1. Normal urine cortisol (nmol/L)/urine creatinine (mmol/L) ratio <13.5 (dog) or <28 (cat)

2. Low or normal ratio rules out HAC.

3. High ratio suggests HAC but may be due to stress.

E. Thyroid testing

1. Indicated for evaluation of thyroid gland disorders, primarily hypothyroidism in dogs and hyperthyroidism in cats

2. Total T$_4$
   a. Measures protein-bound and free circulating hormone concentration
   b. Preferred initial screening test for thyroid gland disorders—sensitive, inexpensive, readily available, rapid turn-around time
   c. A serum sample (1 mL) is drawn after an overnight fast for transport to laboratory; refrigeration pending assay is preferred but not essential.
   d. Methodology is evolving—radioimmunoassay (RIA) was previous "gold standard"; chemiluminescence, immunoradiometric (IRMA) are more recently developed.
   e. In-house enzyme-linked immunosorbent assay (ELISA) test kits are commercially available; results correlate fairly well with RIA values except at upper and lower limits established for the ELISA.
   f. Hemolysis and lipemia generally do not interfere with thyroid hormone analysis.
   g. Low total T$_4$ concentration is caused by
      1) Hypothyroidism—dogs (rare in cats)
      2) Nonthyroidal illness (euthyroid sick syndrome)—dogs, cats
      3) Drugs—especially phenobarbital, glucocorticoids, sulfamethoxazole
      4) Random fluctuation—total T$_4$ is below the reference range 20% of the time in normal dogs.
   h. Elevated total T$_4$ concentration is caused by
      1) Hyperthyroidism—cats (rare in dogs)
      2) Anti-T$_4$ antibodies cross-react with certain T$_4$ assays, indicate lymphocytic thyroiditis, and are seen in 25–33% of hypothyroid dogs.

3. Total T$_4$ interpretation—hypothyroidism
   a. Hypothyroidism primarily affects dogs; extremely rare in cats.
   b. A T$_4$ value within the reference range excludes hypothyroidism; no further testing is necessary.
   c. In general, a T$_4$ value below the reference range with compatible history, clinical signs, and supportive laboratory data (hypercholesterolemia, normocytic normochromic nonregenerative anemia) is diagnostic for hypothyroidism; no further testing is necessary.
   d. The diagnosis of hypothyroidism is sometimes made difficult because of overlap of total T$_4$ values between normal and hypothyroid dogs.

   e. Factors other than thyroid gland function that affect total T$_4$ values include
      1) Random fluctuation—T$_4$ values may be below normal 20% of the time in normal dogs.
      2) Nonthyroidal illness lowers T$_4$ values in an unpredictable manner (euthyroid sick syndrome).
      3) Drugs that lower T$_4$ values include phenobarbital, glucocorticoids, sulfamethoxazole and others.
      4) Circulating anti-T$_4$ antibodies (indicating lymphocytic thyroiditis) may cross-react with T$_4$ assay and falsely *elevate* values in approximately 1/4 to 1/3 of hypothyroid dogs; free T$_4$ by equilibrium dialysis is not affected by anti-T$_4$ antibodies and should be performed in dogs with signs of hypothyroidism and elevated or normal total T$_4$ values.

4. Total T$_4$ interpretation—hyperthyroidism
   a. Hyperthyroidism primarily affects cats; extremely rare in dogs
   b. A total T$_4$ value above the reference range is diagnostic for hyperthyroidism; no further testing is necessary.
   c. In older cats, >10 years of age, a T$_4$ value above 2.5–3.0 μg/dL should be considered suggestive of hyperthyroidism.
   d. Cats with hyperthyroidism *and* concurrent nonthyroidal illness may have total T$_4$ values within or below the normal range.
      1) Hyperthyroidism should be pursued if a thyroid nodule is present.
      2) Free T$_4$ by equilibrium dialysis, T$_3$ suppression test, or radionucleotide uptake scan may aid in diagnosis.

5. Total T$_3$
   a. Provides no useful information in assessing thyroid status—does not distinguish between normal animals, those with hypothyroidism, and those that are euthyroid with concurrent nonthyroidal illness
   b. T$_3$ autoantibodies occur with lymphocytic thyroiditis and may cause falsely elevated serum T$_3$ concentration; incidence low—0.3 to 4.5% of samples submitted for thyroid hormone analysis.

6. Free T$_4$ by equilibrium dialysis (free T$_4$ ED)
   a. Biologically active non-protein-bound fraction of circulating thyroid hormone that more accurately reflects thyroid gland function than serum total T$_4$ concentration

b. Potentially less affected by drugs and nonthyroidal illness than total T_4; however, phenobarbital and glucocorticoids falsely lower free T_4 ED.

c. More specific (92%) and sensitive (98%) than total T_4 in diagnosing hypothyroidism in dogs

d. May allow differentiating true hypothyroidism (low total T_4 and low free T_4 ED) from sick euthyroidism (low total T_4, normal free T_4 ED) in dogs

e. In cats, free T_4 ED may aid in diagnosing hyperthyroidism when concurrent nonthyroidal illness is present—T_4, normal or low; free T_4 ED, elevated.

7. Canine TSH

a. Should be elevated in primary hypothyroidism because of lack of negative feedback on anterior pituitary gland as the serum T_4 level falls

b. TSH level is normal in approximately 10% of hypothyroid dogs (false negatives).

c. TSH level is elevated in 10–20% of normal dogs (false positives).

d. Diagnostic accuracy may be improved when evaluated in combination with total T_4 or free T_4 ED.

e. Secondary hypothyroidism due to pituitary abnormality is rare in dogs and would be expected to cause low TSH.

f. No valid TSH assay for cats is currently available.

F. Serum insulin concentration, amended insulin/glucose ratio

1. Indicated to confirm pancreatic islet beta cell neoplasia (i.e., insulinoma) in patients with hypoglycemia

2. In normal animals, insulin secretion decreases as serum glucose concentration falls.

3. A relative (within the mid to upper normal range) or absolute increase in serum insulin concentration *in the presence of hypoglycemia* is consistent with the diagnosis of beta cell neoplasia.

4. The amended insulin/glucose ratio was designed to improve diagnostic accuracy when hypoglycemia is marginal (50–70 mg/dL) and serum insulin level is within the reference range by the following formula:

$$\frac{\text{Serum insulin} \, (\mu U/ \times 100)}{\text{Blood glucose} \, (\text{mg/dL}) \, - \, 30}, \text{Normal} < 30$$

a. The "−30" term in the denominator is derived from human medicine—in normal persons, insulin secretion is 0 when blood glucose concentration is <30.

b. If serum glucose concentration is less than 30, the number 1 is used in the denominator.

c. An elevated amended insulin/glucose ratio is not 100% specific for beta cell neoplasia; the test may offer no advantage over basal serum insulin concentration in conjunction with hypoglycemia and compatible clinical signs.

G. Parathormone (parathyroid hormone; PTH)

1. Indicated in patients with abnormal serum calcium concentration to diagnose parathyroid gland disorders

2. Preferred methodology is immunoradiometric "two-site" assay that simultaneously detects midregion/C-terminal and biologically active N-terminal amino acid sequences of *intact* PTH.

3. Assay is valid in dogs and cats.

4. A serum sample (1 mL) is collected after an overnight fast (lipemia will affect results) and kept at 4°C until assayed.

5. Hemolysis does not interfere with assay.

6. Results must be interpreted relative to serum calcium, preferably ionized calcium concentration [Cai], and serum phosphorus levels.

a. In normal animals, as [Cai] falls, PTH levels increase, and as [Cai] rises, PTH levels decrease to maintain normocalcemia.

b. Primary hyperparathyroidism—[Cai] increased, PTH mid- to high normal or elevated, low or low-normal phosphorus (unless renal function is impaired)

c. Primary hypoparathyroidism—[Cai] decreased, PTH low normal or decreased, phosphorus elevated

d. Hypercalcemia of malignancy—PTH usually low to undetectable, serum phosphorus normal to low

e. Renal secondary hyperparathyroidism—[Cai] usually decreased or normal, PTH normal to increased, high phosphorus

7. Results of history, physical examination, routine laboratory assessment, and diagnostic imaging may aid in interpreting equivocal results.

8. Serum PTH concentration may fluctuate; repeating the test is necessary in some cases.

9. A PTH-related protein is secreted by some malignant tumors (lymphosarcoma, anal sac apocrine gland adenocarcinoma) and can be measured (sampling requirements same as those for PTH) to aid in differentiating neoplasia from primary hyperparathyroidism.

III. MANAGEMENT OF SPECIFIC CONDITIONS

A. Diabetic ketoacidosis (DKA)

1. Definition: DKA is a medical emergency characterized by hyperglycemia, metabolic acidosis, ketonemia, dehydration, and loss of electrolytes.

2. Etiology

a. Absolute deficiency of insulin is accompanied by excess of stress hormones (glucagon, cortisol, epinephrine, and growth hormone).

b. Insulin is an anabolic hormone that is needed to form triglycerides and glycogen and allow glucose to enter cells.

c. Lack of insulin causes hyperglycemia because of inability of cells to use glucose.

d. Excessive stress hormone release results from some underlying condition causing stress leading to hyperglycemia through increased glycogenolysis and gluconeogenesis.

e. When hyperglycemia exceeds the renal threshold (~180 mg/dL in the dog and 290 mg/dL in the cat), osmotic diuresis results in polyuria, dehydration, and electrolyte depletion.

f. The imbalance of insulin and stress hormones results in excessive ketone body formation causing metabolic acidosis and increased anionic gap.

3. History and clinical signs

a. PU/PD polyphagia, weight loss, and sudden onset of cataracts (dogs) are signs of unregulated diabetes.

b. Vomiting, weakness, collapse, and mental dullness of recent onset are commonly seen in animals with DKA.

c. DKA most commonly occurs in older male cats (>8 years old) and middle-aged female dogs (peak age: 7–9 years).

d. Animals with concurrent pancreatitis often have a history of eating fatty foods or table scraps prior to the onset of illness.

4. Physical examination findings

a. Cats may have a plantigrade stance, rear limb weakness, and a scruffy, scaly haircoat.

b. Abdominal palpation may reveal hepatomegaly or cranial abdominal pain in animals with pancreatitis.

c. Metabolic acidosis usually causes tachypnea, but slow, deep breathing (Kussmaul respiration) can occur with severe acidosis.

d. Dehydration is manifested by loss of skin turgor, sunken eyeballs, tacky mucous membranes, slow capillary refill time, and, in severe cases, shock.

e. Stupor, coma, or obtundation can be seen in animals with severe acidosis, hyperglycemia, or hyperosmolality.

f. Cats with acromegaly have a broad, blunt face, increased interdental spaces, and respiratory stridor. Concurrent cardiomyopathy is common, as evidenced by systolic murmur, gallop rhythm, or clinical signs of congestive heart failure.

g. The breath may have a fruity or acetone odor.

5. Predisposing factors

a. Diabetic animals with underlying stress conditions are at increased risk for developing DKA.

b. Common underlying conditions include pancreatitis, pyometra, infection (wounds, urinary tract, respiratory tract), estrus, cardiac disease, renal disease, exogenous glucocorticoids, hyperadrenocortism, obesity, exogenous progestins, pregnancy, and acromegaly (cats).

c. The following breeds are at increased risk: Keeshond, Golden Retriever, Poodle, Old English Sheepdog, Labrador Retriever, Dachshund, Miniature Schnauzer, Cairn Terrier, Miniature Pinscher, Lhasa Apso, Siberian Husky, Yorkshire Terrier, and mixed breeds.

6. Diagnosis

a. Hyperglycemia, glucosuria, and ketonuria confirm the diagnosis.

b. The hematocrit and total solids are usually high secondary to dehydration.

c. The white blood cell count may be elevated or exhibit a left shift if there is underlying infection or pancreatitis.

d. Liver enzymes are usually elevated; 25–30% of cats are icteric.

e. Prerenal azotemia commonly results in elevation of BUN and creatinine.

f. Hemolysis and hypophosphatemia may occur on the second or third day of treatment.

g. Sodium concentrations are usually low to normal. Serum potassium is often low but will decrease even more with treatment because correction of acidosis and administration of insulin both shift potassium into the cell.

h. Venous blood gases often reveal acidosis: pH <7.3; HCO_3^- <15 mEq/L; TCO_2 <12 mEq/L

i. Urinalysis may show pyuria and bacteriuria consistent with urinary tract infection (UTI).

A urine sample obtained by cystocentesis should be submitted for culture.

j. Abdominal radiographs, thoracic radiographs, and abdominal ultrasound may reveal underlying conditions such as pancreatitis, hepatic lipidosis, pyometritis, urolithiasis, neoplasia, etc.

7. Treatment (*Table 15-1*).
   a. Fluid therapy

TABLE 15.1
DIABETIC KETOACIDOSIS EMERGENCY TREATMENT PROTOCOL

Initial database
   Immediate PCV, TS, Azostick, Dextrometer, Na, K, UA (dipstick and specific gravity), osmolality, blood gases, CBC, chemistry panel
   Rule out underlying infection (radiographs, urine culture, amylase/lipase, etc.)

Fluid therapy
   Place IV catheter—preferably central venous
   Calculate fluid requirements and replace 80% of deficit over 10 hours.
      Estimate percent dehydration $\times$ BW (kg) $\times$ 1000 mL/L = Fluid (mL) to rehydrate
      Estimate maintenance needs: 1 mL/lb/h
      Estimate milliliters of fluid lost with vomiting or diarrhea
   Begin with 0.9% NaCl
   Change fluids to 0.45% NaCl and 2.5% dextrose when glucose <250 mg/dL
   Add potassium to drip according to potassium replacement chart (Table 15-2)
   If pH <7.000, give $NaHCO_3$

$$0.1 \times \text{Base deficit} \times \text{BW (kg)} = \text{Fluid (mL) to add slowly over 2 hours}$$

   If serum phosphorus <1.5 mg/dL and related clinical signs (hemolysis, myopathy, respiratory paralysis, encephalopathy) are evident, give 0.01–0.03 mmol phosphate/kg/h over 6 hours and recheck phosphorus

Insulin therapy
   Use regular crystalline insulin in separate IV drip
   Dose: 2.2 U/kg/24 h (dog); 1.1 U/kg/24 h (cat)
   Add insulin to 250 mL NaCl or Ringer's solution; run 50 mL through IV tubing and discard; begin drip at 10 mL/h with infusion pump
   Slow insulin infusion rate by 25–50% according to insulin therapy chart (Table 15-3) when glucose <250 mg/dL
   Continue IV insulin infusion until ketones are negative and patient is eating
   Begin long-acting insulin (NPH, lente, or ultralente) at 0.5 U/kg SC q12–24h or regular insulin SC q6h when ketones are negative and patient is stable (Discontinue insulin CRI)

Miscellaneous
   Antibiotics if fever/systemic infection
   NPO if pancreatitis
   Monitor Dextrometer every 1–2 hours initially
      PCV, TS, Na, K, osmolality every 4 hours
      Blood gases every 6 hours
      Urine output every 2 hours

PCV, packed cell volume; TS, total solids; UA, urinalysis; CBC, complete blood cell; SC, subcutaneously; NPO, nothing per os.

TABLE 15.2 POTASSIUM REPLACEMENT		
Serum K (mEq/L)	KCl/L (mEq)	Maximum Rate (mL/kg/h)
3.6–5.0	20	24
3.1–3.5	30	16
2.6–3.0	40	11
2.1–2.5	60	8
<2.0	80	6

1) Calculate fluid requirements and replace 80% of deficit over 10 hours.

a) *BW (kg) × % dehydration × 1000 mL/L × 0.8 = mL needed to rehydrate*

b) *2.2 mL/kg/h × 10 h = maintenance*

c) *Estimate no. of mL lost from vomiting in a 10-hour period.*

Add (1) + (2) + (3) and divide by 10 to determine the hourly fluid rate for the initial 10 hours.

2) After 10 hours, reassess hydration and decrease infusion rate to 4 mL/kg/h.

3) The initial fluid of choice is 0.9% NaCl supplemented with potassium according to *Table 15-2.* If serum potassium concentration is unknown, add 20 mEq of KCl per liter until it can be measured.

4) When serum glucose levels decrease to <250 mg/dL, change fluid to 0.45% NaCl and 2.5% dextrose.

b. Fluid additives

1) Potassium supplementation is almost always required—especially after therapy has been initiated—because insulin administration and resolution of acidosis tend to drive potassium intracellularly. Serum potassium concentrations should be monitored closely during treatment and supplemented accordingly.

2) Bicarbonate supplementation is usually not required because the acidosis corrects with fluid therapy and metabolism of ketones to bicarbonate. However, if the pH is <7.000 (or total CO_2 is <12 mEq) the following formula can be used to determine the amount of bicarbonate to add to non-calcium-containing fluids and administer slowly over 2 hours:

$$NaHCO_3(mL) = 0.1 \times \text{Base deficit} \times BW \text{ (kg)}$$

or

$$NaHCO_3(mL) = 0.1 \times (18 - \text{measured venous } CO_2) \times BW \text{ (kg)}$$

This formula only replaces one third of the bicarbonate deficit, to avoid "overshoot alkalosis" when ketone bodies are metabolized.

3) Phosphorus supplementation may be required if serum P <1.5 mg/dL (dog) or <2.5 mg/dL (cat) and related clinical signs are evident (hemolysis, myopathy, respiratory paralysis, encephalopathy). Diabetic animals often have total body depletion of phosphorus that does not become evident until the second or third day of treatment.

a) *The recommended dosage for phosphorus supplementation is 0.01–0.03 mmol/kg/h administered IV for 6 hours. Serum [P] should be rechecked before continuing the infusion.*

b) *Potassium phosphate solutions contain 3 mmol/mL of phosphorus and 4.4 mEq/mL of potassium. PHOSPHORUS REQUIREMENTS SHOULD NEVER BE DOSED BY GIVING HALF THE POTASSIUM REQUIREMENT AS KPO_4. THIS CAN RESULT IN SERIOUS PHOSPHATE OVERDOSAGE!*

c) *In humans, the dosage for phosphorus supplementation is 7.7–15 mg/kg intravenously over 6–12 hours. Potassium phosphate solution contains 93 mg/mL of phosphorus.*

d) *Oversupplementation with phosphorus can cause hypocalcemia and/or metastatic calcification. Phosphate solutions should be avoided in animals with hyperphosphatemia or impaired renal function.*

4) Dextrose should be added to the fluids when the glucose drops to <250 mg/dL to prevent rapid decline in blood glucose concentration. Fifty to 100 mL of 50% dextrose solution are added per liter to make a 2.5–5% dextrose solution.

c. Insulin therapy requires regular crystalline insulin. It can be administered by the intermittent IM technique or the low-dose IV infusion technique. Subcutaneous administration is unreliable in patients with severe dehydration and hypovolemia.

1) Subcutaneous method—for patients that are not severely dehydrated or hyperosmolar *a)* Begin rehydration and delay insulin administration for 2–4 hours.

b) Then give 0.5 U/kg (large dogs) or 1.0 U/kg (small dogs) or 0.25 U/kg (cats) of regular crystalline insulin SQ q6–8h. Adjust dosage according to "mini glucose curve" over 6–8 hours. If regular insulin lasts 8 hours, consider NPH q24h once the animal is stabilized. All others should get NPH or lente insulin q12h at the same dose as regular insulin.

2) Intermittent IM technique—for sick, dehydrated patients—Initial dose, 0.2 U/kg IM; then 0.1 U/kg IM hourly until blood glucose level <250 mg/dL. Then switch to regular insulin SQ (0.5–1 U/kg) q6–8h once the patient is well hydrated.

3) Low-dose IV infusion technique—for sick, dehydrated patients with anorexia and vomiting.

a) This technique requires a syringe pump or infusion pump in a separate line.

b) The dosage is 0.05–0.1 U/kg/h. A convenient method to make the CRI is to add 2.2 U/kg (dog) or 1.1 U/kg (cat) of regular insulin to 250 mL of 0.9% saline.

c) Insulin binds to plastic tubing, so the first 50 mL of solution should be run through the tubing and discarded.

d) The initial drip rate is 10 mL/h. When serum glucose concentration drops below 250 mg/dL, the drip rate is adjusted according to Table 15-3.

e) Once the animal is stable and well hydrated, the insulin drip can be discontinued and regular insulin given SC every 6–8 hours (see above).

f) Once the animal is eating and drinking, longer-acting insulin (e.g., NPH, lente, ultralente, PZI) can be given at the same dose as the previous injection of regular insulin. Duration of effect and whether insulin is needed q24h or q12h can be determined by a 24-hour glucose curve.

8. Follow-up

a. The goal of acute management of patients with DKA is to correct the metabolic derangements so that the patient becomes a stable, uncomplicated diabetic.

b. The animal is usually discharged on longer-acting insulin (0.5–1 U/kg SQ q12–24h) and can return to the hospital in 5–7 days for "fine-tuning" of the insulin dosage by evaluating a 24-hour glucose curve.

c. If the insulin duration and time of peak effect are already known, it is not necessary to perform another 24-hour curve. Adjustments can usually be made by sampling blood at the "peak" time, when it should be >80 mg/dL and <200 mg/dL.

d. Adjustments are not indicated unless the owners complain of PU/PD, polyphagia, weight loss, and/or ketonuria. Owners can monitor the urine periodically with a urine dipstick to make sure the diabetes is not getting out of control.

e. Cats should be checked weekly, and a blood sample taken at the time of peak insulin effect. Cats may be transient diabetics that no longer require insulin once glucose levels have normalized. Continued insulin administration will result in hypoglycemia.

f. The diet should be changed to a high-fiber/low-carbohydrate prescription diet recommended for diabetic pets. High-protein,

TABLE 15.3 INSULIN THERAPY ADJUSTMENTS		
If Glucose Is . . . (mg/dL)	Fluids	Insulin (2 U/kg in 250 mL) (mL/h)
>250	0.9% NaCl	10
200–250	0.45% NaCl + 2.5% dextrose	7
150–200	0.45% NaCl + 2.5% dextrose	5
100–150	0.45% NaCl + 5% dextrose	5
<100	0.45% NaCl + 5% dextrose	Stop insulin infusion

low-carbohydrate diets are recommended for cats.

g. Cats are usually allowed to eat free choice. Animals receiving insulin q12h are fed $^1/_2$ of their daily caloric requirement with each injection. Animals receiving once-daily insulin are given a meal at the time of the injection and another meal 1–2 hours before the insulin peaks (usually 8–12 hours after the injection).

B. Hyperosmolar diabetes (HD)

1. Etiology

a. In humans, nonketotic hyperosmolar diabetes (NKHD) is characterized by the following:
  1) Glucose >600 mg/dL
  2) Osmolality >350 mOsm/kg
  3) Clinical signs of central nervous system (CNS) depression
  4) Lack of urine or serum ketones

b. In humans, NKHD occurs in mature-onset type II diabetics. Low levels of endogenous insulin prevent ketosis but not hyperglycemia. Marked dehydration results from persistent hyperglycemia and profound osmotic diuresis. Impaired renal perfusion causes rapidly rising hyperglycemia and azotemia. Human patients most at risk for NKHD are elderly diabetics with underlying cardiac or renal disease.

c. NKHD approximating the human syndrome has been reported in dogs and cats, but it is rare.

d. Significant hyperosmolality (>340 mOsm/kg) is NOT rare in diabetic pets, especially cats. Unlike humans, most small animal patients with HD are type I diabetics, and many have concurrent ketoacidosis.

e. Normal serum osmolality is 290–310 mOsm/kg. Values >340 mOsm/kg are associated with neurologic abnormalities.

2. Historical findings

a. Animals may have a history consistent with diabetes mellitus: PU/PD and weight loss despite polyphagia.

b. The animal may have underlying renal insufficiency—especially geriatric cats—that predisposes to dehydration and marked hyperglycemia.

c. Neurologic signs associated with hyperosmolality include restlessness, ataxia, confusion, nystagmus, twitching, convulsions, hyperthermia, coma, and death from respiratory failure.

d. There is often a history of vomiting or inability to drink water 12–24 hours before the onset of neurologic signs.

3. Physical findings

a. Animals are 10–12% dehydrated with decreased skin turgor, sunken eyes, tacky mucous membranes, and slow capillary refill time.

b. Cats often have a scruffy appearance due to lack of grooming. They may also exhibit the plantigrade stance that is common in feline diabetics.

c. Geriatric cats with HD are usually very thin, often because of underlying renal disease or hyperthyroidism in addition to the diabetes.

d. Animals are often obtunded or stuporous. Twitching of the extraocular muscles or limb muscles is sometimes noted. Ophthalmic examination may reveal nystagmus or slow papillary light reflex.

e. A heart murmur, gallop rhythm, or tachycardia may be noted in cats with underlying cardiac disease.

4. Laboratory tests

a. The initial database should consist of PCV, TS, glucose, BUN, Na, K, blood gases, and urinalysis.
  1) Blood glucose determination will rule out hypoglycemia as a cause of neurologic signs.
  2) Blood glucose determination and urinalysis will document presence of diabetes. Blood gases will provide assessment of acid–base status.
  3) Serum electrolyte determination will assist in choice of fluids and in calculating serum osmolality.
  4) PCV/TS will document dehydration.
  5) The BUN and urinalysis can help document azotemia and/or evidence of concurrent renal insufficiency.

b. Other tests that should be performed once diabetes has been confirmed include CBC, serum chemistries, serum osmolality, and serum T_4 (cats). Thoracic radiographs, echocardiography, and abdominal ultrasound may be indicated if underlying cardiac, renal, or pancreatic disease is suspected.

c. If serum osmolality cannot be measured directly with a freezing point depression osmometer, it can be calculated using the following formula:

Glucose BUN

Serum osmolality (mOsm/kg)

$$= 2[Na] + (Glucose/18) + (BUN/2.8)$$

5. Differential diagnosis

a. Hyperosmolar coma must be differentiated from the other diabetic emergencies that can cause similar signs: insulin overdose, hypoglycemia, and DKA.

b. Other causes of altered states of consciousness include uremia, hypoadrenocorticism, hypoxia, primary neurologic disease, hepatoencephalopathy, and toxicity.

c. Hyperosmolality can be seen with salt poisoning, ethylene glycol toxicity, or salicylate overdose.

6. Treatment (*Table 15-4*)

a. The main key to treating animals with HD is to avoid rapid fluid loading and rapid reduction of blood glucose concentration. During hyperosmolar states, the brain is protected from excessive shrinkage by the production of osmotically active substances (idiogenic osmols) within brain cells. These substances dissipate slowly. If blood glucose levels are rapidly lowered with insulin, an osmotic gradient can result, causing cerebral edema and worsening neurologic signs.

b. Treatment guidelines are identical to those listed for DKA, *except*

1) Fluid rehydration is established over 12–24 hours, (more slowly).

2) Initiation of insulin therapy is delayed until 2–4 hours after fluid therapy has been started.

3) Insulin dosage is lowered to 0.05 U/kg/h (1.1 U/kg/24 hours) for constant-rate infusion (CRI) method or 0.1 U/kg IM followed by 0.05 U/kg IM hourly until glucose approaches 250 mg/dL for the intermittent IM method.

4) The rate of decline of serum glucose should not exceed 75–100 mg/dL/h.

5) Animals with hypernatremia can be treated with 0.45% saline instead of 0.9% saline, as long as it is not administered rapidly during the rehydration process and as long as the decline in serum sodium concentration does not exceed 10–12 mEq in 24 hours (see pp. 323–326).

7. Follow-up

a. Perform serial neurologic examinations during treatment.

b. Monitor drop in blood glucose and maintain serum concentrations in the 200–250 mg/dL range by adding dextrose solution to the base solution to make a 2.5–5% concentration.

c. Monitor drop in osmolality and serum sodium. These should be within the normal range by 48 hours after initiation of therapy.

d. Avoid hypokalemia by monitoring closely and adding potassium to the fluids as directed in the DKA protocol.

e. Monitor serum [P] and watch for hemolysis or muscle weakness. Supplement if needed as directed in the DKA protocol.

TABLE 15.4
TREATMENT RECOMMENDATIONS FOR HYPEROSMOLAR DIABETES

Follow DKA protocol *except*
1. Replace fluid deficit more slowly (12–24 hours)
2. Do not begin insulin therapy until 2–4 hours after initiation of fluid therapy
3. Use lower insulin dose:

    1.1 U/kg/24 hours (CRI) or
    0.1 U/kg IM, followed by 0.05 U/kg IM hourly until glucose <250 mg/dL

4. Avoid lowering serum glucose concentration by more than 75–100 mg/dL/h

f. The goal of therapy is slow and steady restoration of normal parameters for glucose, acid–base balance, and electrolytes while correcting dehydration and azotemia. Avoid rapid fluid shifts.

C. Hypoglycemia

1. General points

   a. Euglycemia is maintained because of a dynamic balance between glucose production, storage. and release.

   b. During fasting, glucose concentration is maintained by the liver.

   1) During the first 24 hours of fasting, glucose is maintained primarily by liver glycogenolysis.

   2) After the first 24 hours, glucose is maintained primarily by liver gluconeogenesis.

   3) Gluconeogenesis and glycogenolysis are promoted by glucagon, catecholamines, and growth hormone.

   c. As hypoglycemia develops, the counterregulatory hormones—glucagon, catecholamines, cortisol, and growth hormone increase, promoting increased blood glucose concentration by inhibiting peripheral glucose use, increasing hepatic glycogenolysis and gluconeogenesis, and inhibiting insulin secretion. The early response to hypoglycemia results primarily from catecholamines and glucagon; cortisol and growth hormone are released a few hours later, yet their effects last 4–6 hours.

   d. Maintenance of normal glucose concentration depends on normal hepatic glycogen synthesis, glycogenolysis, and gluconeogenesis as well as on the availability of gluconeogenic precursors and appropriate hormone secretion. Abnormalities of any of these processes can lead to hypoglycemia.

   e. The brain is the major organ with an obligatory need for glucose, since it has minimal glycogen stores and cannot use alternative energy substrates.

2. Clinical signs of hypoglycemia

   a. The development of clinical signs depends upon the duration, degree, and rate of decline of serum glucose concentrations.

   b. Primarily manifested by cerebral dysfunction such as altered mentation, stupor, coma, seizures, behavioral changes, muscular weakness, ataxia, and collapse. Chronic hypoglycemia can cause peripheral neuropathy.

3. Diagnosis

   a. Errors of sample handling may result in erroneously low glucose concentration measurement.

   1) At room temperature, glucose in whole blood without glycolysis inhibitors is metabolized at approximately 7 mg/dL/h.

   2) Serum should be separated from red blood cells within 30 minutes of collection.

   3) Addition of 2 mg of sodium fluoride per milliliter of whole blood prevents glycolysis for up to 48 hours.

   4) Blood glucose is stable in separated serum or plasma for up to 48 hours if refrigerated.

   b. Commonly used glucometers tend to read glucose erroneously low, particularly when the hematocrit is high.

   1) This may vary from unit to unit.

   2) Glucometers tend to measure the glucose in serum or plasma more accurately than that in whole blood.

   c. Diagnosis of hypoglycemia is generally accepted as accurately measured glucose <60 mg/dL. Sudden drops in glucose to <40 mg/dL usually result in clinical signs, although clinical signs may not be evident at even extremely low concentrations (<30 mg/dL) in some animals with chronic hypoglycemia (e.g., insulinoma).

   d. In general, extremely low glucose concentrations (<40 mg/dL) are seen with insulin overdose, tumors secreting insulin or insulin-like factors, neonatal hypoglycemia, hypoadrenocorticism, and severe liver disease. Hypoglycemia due to systemic illness such as sepsis or systemic inflammatory response syndrome (SIRS) is generally in the 40–60 mg/dL range but, on rare occasions, can be extremely low (<40 mg/dL) and sometimes refractory to initial glucose intravenous boluses.

   e. Diagnostic algorithm for hypoglycemia (*Fig. 15-1*)

4. Treatment

   a. Acute symptomatic hypoglycemia requires immediate glucose supplementation because the longer the duration of hypoglycemia, the greater the potential for irreversible brain damage.

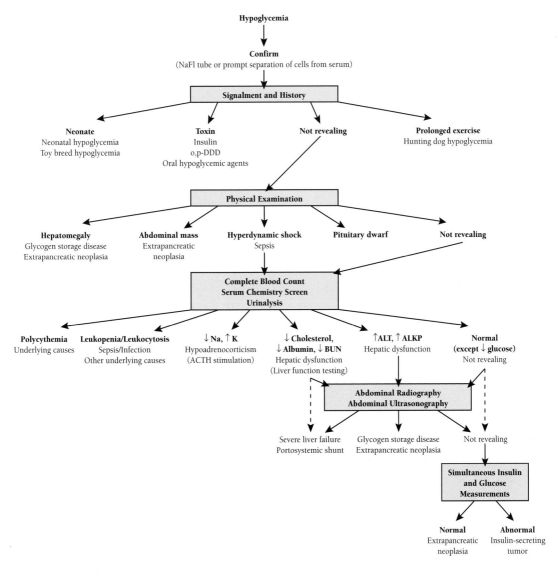

FIGURE 15.1 Diagnostic algorithm for hypoglycemia.

b. If the owner is at home and hypoglycemia is likely (e.g., a diabetic receiving insulin with clinical signs consistent with hypoglycemia), application of a glucose-containing solution (Karo syrup or pancake syrup) orally may correct hypoglycemia.

　1) There is some risk that the animal could aspirate this solution if it is severely neurologically impaired.

　2) There are no receptors for absorption of glucose on the oral mucosa, the hope is that this solution will reach the stomach where absorption can occur.

　3) Neurologic signs should improve within 1–2 minutes if adequate glucose is administered and absorbed.

　4) Owners should be warned about the potential to be bitten when working around the mouth of an animal that might be seizuring or is neurologically abnormal. Applying the glucose solution with a meat baster or bulb syringe may decrease the risk of injury to the client.

5) Whether the animal responds to home therapy or not, the owner should be advised to bring the animal immediately for evaluation.

c. At the veterinary hospital

1) Administer an intravenous bolus of 0.5 g/kg of a 25% dextrose-containing solution (1 mL/kg body weight of a 50% dextrose solution diluted in half).

a) *This dose can be repeated as necessary but should ideally be guided by serial blood glucose measurements. One cannot predict the expected glucose concentration on the basis of the dose given.*

b) *If repeated doses are necessary, a central venous catheter should be placed. Peripheral vessels can become easily irritated with resultant phlebitis if hypertonic solutions (e.g., 25% dextrose) are repeatedly or constantly infused.*

c) *Neurologic status should improve within 30 seconds to 1 minute.*

d) *Some animals may continue to seizure even after euglycemia has been achieved. Treatment with midazolam or phenobarbital may be necessary to increase the seizure threshold, and dexamethasone may be indicated to reduce cerebral edema.*

2) Once the animal has responded, then a CRI of 5% dextrose in a balanced electrolyte solution can be administered IV and the rate of infusion adjusted on the basis of serial blood glucose measurements.

3) If the animal improves substantially after intravenous infusion and is not systemically ill (e.g., insulin overdose, juvenile hypoglycemia, insulin-secreting tumor), then food should be offered.

4) Glucose infusion and monitoring of glucose should continue until the animal can eat and maintain the glucose concentration above the low end of the reference range without glucose supplementation. Monitoring: check blood glucose immediately after intravenous bolus. If normal or high, recheck in 30 minutes or if clinical signs develop. If blood glucose is not low after 30 minutes, check in another hour. If still not low, then check in 2 hours and extend rechecks to every 4–8 hours if glucose does not become low. If blood glucose is low at any interval, then readjust supplementation (e.g., increase the dextrose concentration by 50%) and repeat serial blood glucose measurements as directed above. If the glucose is extremely low and the animal has clinical signs, repeat 0.5 g/kg of 25% dextrose solution intravenously and follow assessment and adjustment steps as outlined immediately above.

5) A blood glucose concentration within the reference range is the goal of glucose supplementation. There is no advantage to producing hyperglycemia. Hyperglycemia can be deleterious to the brain, especially during hypoperfusion to the brain (excess brain lactate formation).

6) In animals with refractory or persistent hypoglycemia due to insulin overdose, glucagon administration (0.5–1 mg IM or IV once, dog or cat) may help prevent repeated or persistent hypoglycemia.

7) A CRI of glucagon in conjunction with IV glucose supplementation may help control refractory hypoglycemia that is secondary to tumors that secrete insulin or insulin-like factors.

a) *It is also indicated for iatrogenic insulin shock that is not responding to dextrose infusion.*

b) *It may help prevent the rebound hypoglycemia that occurs when animals with hyperinsulinism are treated with dextrose-containing fluids.*

c) *To make the infusion, add 1 mg of glucagon to 1 L of 0.9% NaCl to make a 1000 μg/mL solution.*

d) *Give an initial bolus of 50 ng/kg IV (for a 10-kg dog, the dose would be 0.5 mL IV) and then continue the CRI at 10–15 ng/kg/min. To maintain euglycemia, it may be necessary to increase the dosage to 40 ng/kg/min. (Note: Remember when you do your calculations, there are 1000 μg in 1 g and 1000 ng in 1 μg.)*

8) Glucocorticoids (starting at a dose of 0.5 mg/kg of prednisolone BID) in conjunction with glucose supplementation may be required to control hypoglycemia in animals with tumors that secrete insulin or insulin-like factors. The dose of glucocorticoids may be increased incrementally by 0.5 mg/kg BID if hypoglycemia is not controlled.

D. Hypoadrenocorticism

1. Primary hypoadrenocorticism (also called *Addison's disease*) results from inadequate production of mineralocorticoids and glucocorticoids by the adrenal gland.
   a. Histologically, there is bilateral adrenal atrophy.
   b. An immune-mediated process has been implicated in some cases.
   c. Other causes include iatrogenic (mitotane administration and sudden withdrawal of long-term glucocorticoid therapy), fungal infections, hemorrhagic infarctions, neoplasia, amyloidosis, and trauma.

2. Secondary hypoadrenocorticism (relatively rare)
   a. May be secondary to inflammation, neoplasia, trauma, congenital defects of the hypothalamus or pituitary gland, and exogenous glucocorticoid administration
   b. Secondary hypoadrenocorticism may result in pure glucocorticoid deficiency with normal mineralocorticoid function.

3. Hypoadrenocorticism occurs most commonly in dogs. It can occur in cats, but is quite rare in this species.

4. The clinical manifestations are a result of lack of glucocorticoids and mineralocorticoids.

5. About 70% of dogs with hypoadrenocorticism are female. The sex distribution in cats is relatively equal.

6. Usually occurs in young to middle-age dogs but can range from 4 months to 14 years

7. The most common purebreds reported in various studies include Poodles (Standard, Miniature and Toy), German Shepherd Dogs, Rottweilers, West Highland White Terriers, Great Danes, and Labrador Retrievers. Familial tendencies have been noted in Standard Poodles, Labrador Retrievers, and Portuguese Water Spaniels.

8. Diagnosis and clinical signs
   a. The reported average duration of clinical signs in most studies is 10–14 days, although waxing and waning signs may be noted as long as a year before presentation.
   b. Even patients that present in an acute crisis will have had nonspecific signs that have been present for a variable period when the owner is carefully questioned.
   c. The most common complaints are nonspecific and include the following in order of frequency (% of cases):
      1) Anorexia, lethargy, depression (~75-90%)
      2) Vomiting, (~75%)
      3) Weakness (~40%)
      4) Weight loss(~ 22%–36%)
      5) Diarrhea (22–31%)
      6) Waxing/waning course (26–40%)
      7) Shaking (27–38%)
      8) Collapse (35%)
      9) PU/PD (~25%)
      10) Sensitive abdomen (9%)
   d. Mild-to-severe mental depression secondary to poor perfusion to the brain, electrolyte disturbances, or hypoglycemia is the most common finding (~90%).
   e. Weakness secondary to electrolyte changes, poor tissue perfusion, and poor muscle tone is noted in nearly 70% of the dogs.
   f. Collapse due to hypotension and poor tissue perfusion manifested by prolonged capillary refill time and weak pulses. Some dogs with hypoadrenocorticism have an inappropriately slow heart rate (<70 beats per minute) for the degree of hypotension and poor tissue perfusion. The slow heart rate is likely due to hyperkalemia and a poor response to endogenous catecholamines resulting from the absence of glucocorticoid.
   g. Low rectal temperature secondary to poor tissue perfusion
   h. Melena or rarely massive GI hemorrhage may be present. (Glucocorticoids are necessary to maintain GI mucosal integrity.)
   i. Abdominal pain secondary to gastroenteritis may be noted in less than 10% of dogs.
   j. Initial diagnostics—as with any critically ill patient, an emergency database including PCV, TS, blood glucose, and BUN should be obtained, as well as serum sodium, chloride, potassium, ionized calcium and venous blood gas.
      1) Hyperkalemia is found in most cases except pure glucocorticoid-dependent animals in which electrolytes are relatively normal.
      2) Hyponatremia is also a common finding.
      3) Na/K ratio <27, ratios are usually <20:1 (normal ≥32:1)
      4) Mild-to-moderate azotemia is usually due to prerenal causes.
      5) Metabolic acidosis may range from mild to severe depending upon tissue perfusion.
      6) Hypercalcemia is noted in about 1/3 of cases and is generally mild; however on extremely rare occasions we have noted severe ionized hypercalcemia.
      7) Eosinophilia is noted in approximately 25% of cases.

8) Mild-to-severe hypoglycemia may occur as well, resulting in seizures in rare instances.

9) Lymphocytosis is sometimes noted

10) Mild normocytic, normochromic anemia is often noted; on rare occasions, severe anemia may be found due to GI hemorrhage.

k. Further diagnostics

1) Thoracic radiograph changes are often characteristic of hypovolemia, such as microcardia, small caudal vena cava, and pulmonary hypovascularity.

2) Electrocardiogram (ECG) can show signs consistent with hyperkalemia when this electrolyte abnormality is present, although changes can be inconsistent.

3) ACTH stimulation test shows low-to-normal baseline cortisol concentrations with no increase after ACTH administration.

4) Fecal parasite examination should always be performed in animals that have signs consistent with hypoadrenocorticism to rule out "pseudo-Addison's." This condition is attributed to GI parasite infestation (most commonly whipworm infection) and can look identical to true hypoadrenocorticism clinically but is accompanied by a normal ACTH stimulation test result.

l. Treatment

1) Initial treatment should be as for any critically ill patient.

2) Intravenous administration of 0.9% NaCl up to 80–90 mL/kg/h (40–60 mL/kg/h in cats) initially. Pulse quality, heart rate, mucous membrane color, ECG, and blood pressure should be monitored closely during resuscitation. Fluid rate should be tapered and adjusted based on frequent assessment of physical perfusion parameters (mucous membrane color, CRT, pulse quality), ECG, and blood pressure.

3) Dexamethasone sodium phosphate, 0.2–0.4 mg/kg IV, will provide glucocorticoid support. Dexamethasone sodium phosphate (a water-soluble glucocorticoid) will not cross-react with the cortisol assay used for the ACTH stimulation test.

4) 25% Dextrose, 0.25–0.5 g/kg, should be administered IV as a bolus and glucose rechecked if hypoglycemia is present. The dose should be repeated if hypoglycemia persists. Dextrose should be added to the IV

fluids to a concentration of 2.5–5% glucose (25–50 g of glucose in a liter container of fluids).

5) Hyperkalemia may cause life-threatening cardiac arrhythmias. It is rare that treatment for hyperkalemia is necessary. Intravenous fluid therapy generally promotes dilution of potassium and improves tissue perfusion. Options for treatment of hyperkalemia include

a) *50–100 mg/kg of 10% calcium gluconate IV over 2–4 minutes*

b) *0.1 U/kg of regular insulin IV followed by 1–2 g of 25% dextrose IV/unit of insulin given. Dextrose should also be added to the intravenous fluids to a concentration of 5%, as dogs with hypoadrenocorticism are particularly sensitive to the hypoglycemic effects of insulin.*

c) *Sodium bicarbonate, 1–2 mEq/kg IV, over 10–15 minutes*

6) A broad-spectrum anthelmintic should be administered empirically in case of pseudo-Addison's, as the results of the ACTH stimulation test may not be available for 1–2 days (see K.4 above).

7) Definitive therapy for hypoadrenocorticism

a) *Mineralocorticoid therapy should ideally be withheld until ACTH stimulation test is completed because of interference of these supplements with the cortisol assay.*

b) *A daily oral supplementation or injection every 3–4 weeks are two options for long-term therapy.*

i) Initial dosage of fludrocortisone is 0.02 mg/kg orally daily. The dose is adjusted on the basis of serum electrolyte concentrations, with the goal of normalizing them. The dose should be adjusted in 0.05- to 0.1-mg increments based on serum electrolyte concentrations. Electrolyte concentrations should be monitored weekly until they remain normal on consecutive assessments. Creatinine, blood urea nitrogen, sodium, and potassium concentrations should be monitored monthly for the first 3–6 months and then every 3–6 months after that, depending upon the animal's progress. Dosage requirements tend to increase initially as ongoing destruction or atrophy of the adrenal tissue continues. The median final dose in a large retrospective study was 22.6 μg/kg daily.

ii) *Desoxycorticosterone pivalate (DOCP), 2.2 mg/kg IM, may be given initially. To adjust long-term dosage, serum electrolytes should be measured 2, 3, and 4 weeks after the injection and the dose adjusted as needed. The injection must be repeated every 25–28 days.*

iii) *Maintenance glucocorticoid therapy with prednisolone (0.2 mg/kg/day divided BID, PO) will be required in dogs with secondary hypoadrenocorticism. Prednisolone may be tapered in animals with primary hypoadrenocorticism, as the glucocorticoid activity of the fludrocortisone (not DOCP) may be adequate for daily maintenance. In all dogs with hypoadrenocorticism (primary and secondary), glucocorticoid therapy should be increased 2–10 times the maintenance dose during periods of stress such as surgical procedures, general anesthesia, or boarding.*

8) Monitoring:
   a) Emergency monitoring should be as for any critically ill patient.
   b) Perfusion parameters, blood pressure, and continuous lead II ECG are warranted until the animal is cardiovascularly stable.
   c) Blood glucose should be monitored in animals that were initially hypoglycemic or when insulin has been administered for treatment of hyperkalemia.
   d) PCV and TS should be monitored if GI hemorrhage has occurred.
   e) Urine output should be monitored.
   f) Serum electrolytes (sodium and potassium) should be monitored after initial emergency fluid bolus and hourly if possible until a steady change toward normal has been noted, then intervals extended based on rate of change and clinical appearance of the animal.

9) Prognosis
   a) Prognosis is excellent with proper therapy
   b) Most animals in crisis stabilize within 12–24 hours of admission with proper fluid therapy and glucocorticoid support.

c) Long-term mineralocorticoid replacement therapy can be relatively expensive for large-breed dogs.

E. Hyperadrenocorticism

1. In dogs, functional tumors (adenomas) of the anterior pituitary gland account for 85% of cases of HAC; adrenal tumors for 15%.
   a. Pituitary macroadenomas account for 10–15% of cases of pituitary-dependent HAC and may cause intracranial neurologic signs.
   b. Iatrogenic HAC caused by chronic steroid use is clinically and biochemically indistinguishable from natural disease; the ACTH stimulation test will differentiate (see below).

2. In cats, HAC is rare and seen most commonly in conjunction with refractory diabetes mellitus.

3. Typical clinical signs of HAC include PU/PD, polyphagia, pendulous abdomen, and dermatologic changes (symmetric alopecia, thin skin over the ventrum, hyperpigmentation); these signs are rarely the cause of animals being presented as emergencies.

4. Animals with HAC most often present as emergencies due to complications of the disease or its treatment.

5. Complications of HAC include
   a. Infection—respiratory and urinary tract most commonly involved
   b. Respiratory distress—secondary to bronchopneumonia, congestive heart failure (CHF), pulmonary thromboembolism, and/or tracheal collapse
   c. Diabetes mellitus or DKA
   d. Pancreatitis (often concurrent with DKA)
   e. Neurologic abnormalities if hypertension or pituitary macroadenoma are present
   f. Glomerular disease

6. Complications of treatment with mitotane include
   a. Vomiting, diarrhea, anorexia, lethargy, weakness/ataxia
   b. Hypoadrenocorticism

7. Diagnosis
   a. Laboratory findings suggestive of HAC include elevated serum alkaline phosphatase concentration, hypercholesterolemia, mild hyperglycemia, neutrophilia, lymphopenia,

eosinopenia, erythrocytosis, and dilute urine specific gravity.

b. Laboratory findings in critical patients with HAC may include elevated amylase/lipase concentration (pancreatitis), marked hyperglycemia with metabolic acidosis (diabetes mellitus or DKA), azotemia/proteinuria (pyelonephritis or glomerular disease), leucocytosis with left shift, anemia, and/or thrombocytopenia (infection, sepsis, disseminated intravascular coagulation (DIC)).

c. Screening tests for HAC should not be performed in critical patients because stress from severe illness may cause false-positive results.

d. However, an ACTH stimulation test should be considered

   1) To rule out *hypoadrenocorticism* in patients receiving mitotane that present in shock.

   2) To rule out *iatrogenic HAC* in patients receiving long-term corticosteroids; cortisol levels do not increase after ACTH administration because of adrenal cortical atrophy secondary to long-term suppression of ACTH release from the pituitary gland.

e. Abdominal ultrasonography may suggest HAC if bilateral adrenomegaly (pituitary dependent) or unilateral adrenal mass (adrenal tumor) are detected.

f. Chest radiographs in patients with respiratory distress may reveal

   1) Bronchopneumonia—alveolar/interstitial infiltrates

   2) Pulmonary thromboembolism—blunt pulmonary arteries, hypoperfused/hyperlucent lung fields, right heart enlargement

   3) Congestive heart failure—pulmonary venous congestion/pulmonary edema or pleural effusion with left- or right-sided congestive failure, respectively.

g. Abdominal radiographs may reveal hepatomegaly, calcified adrenal mass, urinary calculi, and/or evidence of pancreatitis (loss of detail in right cranial abdomen, displaced gas-filled descending duodenum).

h. Hypertension is common in patients with HAC, especially those with renal/glomerular disease.

8. Treatment

a. The standard treatment for HAC in the dog is mitotane for pituitary-dependent disease and mitotane or adrenalectomy for adrenal tumors; in the cat, treatment options include metapyrone, adrenalectomy, or radiation for pituitary tumors.

b. Treatment for HAC is rarely *initiated* in the emergency setting; the reader is referred to veterinary medicine texts for detailed discussion of treatment for stable patients with HAC.

c. Treatment for complications of HAC or its treatment

   1) Respiratory or urinary tract infection should be treated with broad-spectrum antibiotics based on results of culture/sensitivity testing whenever possible.

   2) Patients in respiratory distress should receive cage rest, supplemental oxygen, and minimal stress pending determination of the underlying cause

   a) *Bronchopneumonia (see Chapter 9)*

   b) *Pulmonary thromboembolism (see Chapter 9)*

   c) *Congestive heart failure (see Chapter 10)*

   3) Patients with vomiting and diarrhea should receive IV fluids and nothing per os pending determination of the underlying cause.

   a) *Adverse reaction to mitotane—perform ACTH stimulation test and give prednisone, 5–10 mg/day (more if needed) until vomiting/diarrhea resolve; gradually taper the dose of prednisone; reintroduce mitotane when prednisone is discontinued, unless cortisol levels indicate hypoadrenocorticism.*

   b) *Pancreatitis (see Chapter 11, p. 202)*

   c) *DKA (see p. 300)*

   4) Patients with neurologic signs should receive supportive care and anticonvulsant therapy as needed pending blood pressure determination or CNS imaging.

   a) *Hypertension can occur in dogs with HAC. Monitor blood pressure and treat accordingly.*

   b) *Pituitary macroadenoma—treatment may include radiation therapy or surgical excision.*

   5) Patients with azotemia and proteinuria should receive IV fluids (colloids such as hetastarch may be necessary if hypoalbuminemia is severe or edema is present) and monitoring of urine production (should be at least 1.0 mg/kg/h) and blood pressure.

   6) Treatment for mitotane-induced hypoadrenocortical crisis includes

   a) *Normal saline (0.9% NaCl), 10–90 mL/kg IV, based on hydration, volume, and perfusion status b)* *Glucocorticoids—prednisone sodium succinate, 4–20 mg/kg IV over 20 minutes, repeated q2–6h prn or dexamethasone sodium phosphate, 2–4 mg/kg IV, repeat q6–8h prn*

c) *Mineralocorticoids are often not necessary because mitotane may spare the zona glomerulosa—DOCP, 2.2 mg/kg IM or SC if needed.*

d) *Discontinue mitotane until follow-up ACTH stimulation test indicates recurrence of HAC.*

e) *A small number (2–10%) of patients require lifelong treatment for hypoadrenocorticism. See pp. 310–311 for maintenance therapy for this disease.*

F. Hypercalcemia

1. General—refer to the section on hypocalcemia for an overview of calcium homeostasis (p. 315)

2. Clinical signs of hypercalcemia

a. The most important adverse effects of hypercalcemia involve the kidneys, neuromuscular system, and cardiovascular system.

b. Anorexia, lethargy, and PU/PD are the most common clinical signs.

c. Other signs include vomiting, muscle weakness, cardiac arrhythmias, seizures, and constipation.

d. Cats may be less likely to exhibit vomiting or PU/PD than dogs.

e. The presence or absence of clinical signs depends on the rate of onset, magnitude, and cause of hypercalcemia.

1) In general, most animals with total serum calcium >14–15 mg/dL show clinical signs.

2) Rapid onset of hypercalcemia (e.g., vitamin D toxicosis) may cause death; gradual onset may be less clinically apparent.

3) Animals with primary hyperparathyroidism and cats with idiopathic hypercalcemia may show no obvious clinical signs.

f. Hypercalcemia is most likely to cause mineralization of tissues when serum phosphorus levels are also high resulting in a calcium–phosphorus product >70.

g. Calcium oxalate uroliths may result from prolonged or severe hypercalcemia.

3. Causes of hypercalcemia—See *Table 15-5* for complete list.

a. In dogs, malignancy (e.g., lymphosarcoma, anal sac apocrine gland adenocarcinoma,

primary or metastatic bone tumors, multiple myeloma) is the most common cause.

b. In cats, renal failure is the most common cause.

c. Primary hyperparathyroidism is uncommon in dogs and cats but may have breed (but not sex) predilection as follows:

1) Dogs—Australian Shepherd, Dachshund, Golden Retriever, Keeshond, Labrador Retriever, Poodle, Rhodesian Ridgeback, and Siberian Husky

2) Cats—Siamese

3) Occurs in older animals, mean age 10–13 years, in dogs and cats, respectively

d. Idiopathic hypercalcemia of cats is a relatively newly recognized syndrome affecting young to middle-aged animals.

1) Both total and ionized calcium levels are increased.

2) Increases in calcium tend to be persistent, lasting months to years, but are not progressive.

3) Clinical signs are usually mild (vomiting, weight loss) or absent.

4) Azotemia, nephrocalcinosis, and calcium-containing urolithiasis may be present.

5) The cause of hypercalcemia in this disease has not been determined.

6) Increasing dietary fiber and administering prednisone may lower calcium levels in symptomatic cats or those with urinary tract abnormalities resulting from the hypercalcemia.

e. Lipemia should be ruled out, as it causes falsely high reported calcium values.

f. Hypervitaminosis D

1) Most common cause is ingestion of rodenticide containing cholecalciferol.

2) Phosphorus and serum alkaline phosphatase are usually elevated.

g. May be normal in young, growing dogs

h. Hypoadrenocorticism can present with hypercalcemia that usually resolves rapidly with fluid therapy.

i. Occasionally chronic or acute renal failure is accompanied by hypercalcemia. Since hypercalcemia can cause renal failure, sometimes it is difficult to know whether azotemia or hypercalcemia came first.

4. Diagnosis

a. In addition to documenting a repeatable increase in total serum and/or ionized calcium

---

TABLE 15.5
CAUSES OF HYPERCALCEMIA

Neoplasia
    Canine
        Lymphosarcoma
        Anal sac apocrine gland adenocarcinoma
        Multiple myeloma
        Thymoma
        Carcinoma—lung, pancreas, thyroid, mammary gland, adrenal medulla
        Myeloproliferative disease
        Leukemia
    Feline
        Lymphosarcoma—most cats with lymphosarcoma and hypercalcemia are FeLV negative
        Squamous cell carcinoma—head/neck
        Leukemia
        Multiple myeloma
        Bronchogenic carcinoma
        Sarcoma—osteosarcoma, fibrosarcoma, undifferentiated sarcoma

Renal failure—acute or chronic
Idiopathic hypercalcemia of cats
Primary hyperparathyroidism
Secondary hyperparathyroidism
    Renal
    Nutritional

Tertiary hyperparathyroidism (rare consequence of chronic renal failure)
Hypoadrenocorticism
Vitamin D toxicosis
    Iatrogenic, cholecalciferol-containing rodenticides,
    Calcipotriene (antipsoriasis cream)

Granulomatous disease
    Systemic fungal disease (e.g., blastomycosis, histoplasmosis)
    Panniculitis, injection site granuloma

Miscellaneous
    Osteomyelitis, hypertrophic osteodystrophy, thiazide diuretics, acromegaly, postrenal
        transplantation, excessive calcium supplementation

---

level, additional tests that should be considered to establish a definitive diagnosis include

1) Malignancy—imaging of chest and abdomen, lymph node aspirate, bone marrow cytology, thorough palpation of anal sacs (tumors often small), PTHrP measurement, etc.

2) Primary hyperparathyroidism—PTH measurement, ultrasonic imaging of cervical region

3) Hypoadrenocorticism—ACTH stimulation test

4) Hypervitaminosis D—thorough history, measurement of vitamin D metabolites, e.g., 25-(OH)-D_3 and 1,2-(OH)$_2$-D_3

5. Treatment

a. Identifying and correcting the underlying disease is the definitive therapy for hypercalcemia.

b. Supportive treatment is necessary in animals with severe clinical signs, rapidly rising calcium levels, calcium–phosphorus product >70, and significant acid/base disturbance or azotemia.

c. IV fluid administration using 0.9% NaCl, 100–125 mL/kg/day, increases urinary excretion of calcium.

d. Furosemide, 2–4 mg/kg q8–12h SC, IV, PO, is indicated if hypercalcemia persists *after* adequate volume expansion.

1) Cats are especially sensitive to furosemide. Taper to the lowest dose possible to prevent iatrogenic dehydration, prerenal azotemia, and hypokalemia.

2) Serial assessment of total or ionized calcium levels is indicated to obtain the optimal furosemide dose.

e. Glucocorticoids are indicated for moderate-to-severe hypercalcemia unresponsive to fluids or furosemide.

1) Prednisone, 1–2.2 mg/kg q12–24h PO, SC, IV

2) Dexamethasone (oral or short-acting injectable preparation, e.g., dexamethasone sodium phosphate), 0.1–0.22 mg/kg q12–24h PO, SC, IV

3) Like furosemide, glucocorticoids should be used at the lowest dose necessary to maintain acceptable calcium levels.

4) Important—Glucocorticoids should not be used until a definitive diagnosis is achieved. Infectious disease (e.g., fungal) may be worsened, and cytologic diagnosis of neoplasia rendered difficult with prior use of glucocorticoids.

f. Sodium bicarbonate (1–4 mEq/kg slowly IV) can rapidly lower serum ionized calcium and may be useful in a hypercalcemic crisis.

g. Calcitonin, 4–6 IU/kg q8–12h SC

1) Use as a temporary emergency treatment for severe to life-threatening hypercalcemia, (e.g., cholecalciferol rodenticide toxicity)

2) Vomiting may occur.

3) Lowers calcium levels by inhibiting osteoclastic bone resorption

h. Bisphosphonates are indicated for longer-term control of hypercalcemia.

1) Etidronate, 5–15 mg/kg q12–24h PO

2) Pamidronate, 1.3–2.0 mg/kg, give over 2 hours in 150 mL 0.9% NaCl IV; repeat in 1–3 weeks as indicated by weekly to twice-weekly serum calcium determinations.

i. Diet—high-fiber, alkalinizing diets may be useful in cats with idiopathic hypercalcemia. Low-calcium diets are only useful when hypercalcemia is caused by enhanced intestinal absorption (e.g., vitamin D toxicosis).

G. Hypocalcemia

1. General

a. Calcium is important in cardiovascular and neuromuscular function via its roles as an enzyme cofactor and a second messenger and in establishing cell membrane electrical gradients.

b. Calcium also is important in muscle contraction, skeletal support, smooth muscle tone, cell growth and division, and blood coagulation.

c. Calcium homeostasis is controlled by PTH, calcitriol (and other vitamin D metabolites), and calcitonin.

d. PTH is secreted by chief cells in the parathyroid gland in response to decreased ionized calcium levels in extracellular fluid.

1) Responsible for minute-by-minute control of [Cai].

2) Acts directly on kidney and bone and indirectly on intestine to *increase* serum [Cai].

e. Calcitriol (1,25-dihydroxycholecalciferol) is synthesized in renal proximal tubular cells. PTH increases calcitriol synthesis by activating 1-α-hydroxylase.

1) Calcitriol is responsible for day-to-day control of ionized calcium level.

2) Calcitriol acts directly on intestine and kidney and with PTH on bone to *increase* [Cai].

f. Calcitonin is secreted by C cells in the THYROID gland.

1) Calcitonin is thought mainly to limit postprandial hypercalcemia.

2) Calcitonin acts on bone to inhibit osteoclastic bone resorption and decreases [Cai].

g. Calcium exists in the body in bone (99%) and extracellular fluid (1%).

h. Extracellular calcium exists in three forms: ionized (50%), protein bound (40%), and complexed/chelated—e.g., bound to phosphate, citrate (10%).

i. Cai is the biologically active form, and its measurement is the preferred method of diagnosing disorders of calcium homeostasis.

j. Most commercial laboratories routinely measure total serum calcium concentration. Because this measurement includes protein-bound calcium, the following correction formula is used in animals with abnormal albumin levels:

Corrected calcium (mg/dL)

= Total calcium (mg/dL) − albumin (g/dL) + 3.5

(This formula may not accurately reflect ionized calcium levels and is not valid in cats.)

2. Clinical signs of hypocalcemia

   a. Muscle twitching, stiffness, ataxia, and seizures are the most common signs.

   b. Hyperthermia as a result of sustained muscle contraction is common, especially in dogs with eclampsia.

   c. Hypotension, tachyarrhythmias, and prolongation of the Q-T interval are typical cardiovascular manifestations of severe hypocalcemia.

   d. In cats, prolapse of the nictitans may be seen.

   e. Facial rubbing is a fairly typical sign, especially with primary hypoparathyroidism.

   f. Posterior lenticular cataracts may also be seen.

3. Causes of hypocalcemia

   a. Hypoproteinemia is the most common cause of decreased total calcium levels because of a low protein-bound fraction.

   1) For this reason, [Cai] should be measured if possible.

   2) There are no clinical signs when [Cai] is normal.

   b. Renal failure, eclampsia, and ethylene glycol poisoning are the most common causes of true (ionized) hypocalcemia in patients that present as emergencies.

   c. See *Table 15-6* for a complete list of differential diagnoses for hypocalcemia.

TABLE 15.6
CAUSES OF HYPOCALCEMIA

Hypoalbuminemia (total calcium low, ionized calcium *normal*)
Renal failure (acute and chronic)
Eclampsia
Pancreatitis
Ethylene glycol toxicosis
Primary hypoparathyroidism
Iatrogenic (thyroidectomy, parathyroidectomy)
Intestinal malabsorption
Phosphate-containing enema preparations (cats)
Miscellaneous
    Vitamin D deficiency
    Blood transfusion with citrate anticoagulant
    Tumor lysis syndrome
    Massive soft tissue trauma
    Rhabdomyolysis

---

4. Treatment

   a. Calcium gluconate 10%, give 0.5–1.5 mL/kg (50–150 mg/kg) IV over 5–10 minutes; (contains 9.2 mg/mL elemental calcium and is safer than 10% calcium chloride, which contains 27.2 mg/mL elemental calcium)

   1) Rapid administration may cause bradyarrhythmias; continuous ECG monitoring is recommended.

   2) Give repeated boluses as needed until neuromuscular signs resolve.

   3) Slow or discontinue administration if bradycardia, shortening of the Q-T interval, premature ventricular contractions, and/or vomiting occur.

   4) Dilute an equal volume of the amount administered IV 1:1 with saline and give SC q6-8h to prolong the duration of effect in severe cases. (Not calcium chloride—will cause tissue necrosis.)

   5) Continuous IV infusion of calcium gluconate 10%, 10–15 mL/kg/day (60–90 mg/kg/day), in 0.9% NaCl can be given for refractory hypocalcemia, e.g., primary hypoparathyroidism and postoperative thyroidectomy or parathyroidectomy patients. Avoid fluids that contain lactate, acetate, or bicarbonate to prevent formation of calcium precipitates.

   b. Administer isotonic IV fluids, 2–4 mL/kg/h, to correct hypovolemia and treat hyperthermia.

   c. Oral Vitamin D preparations enhance absorption of calcium from the GI tract and are used in long-term management of hypocalcemia. Aim for a serum calcium at the low end of the normal range (8–9.5 mg/dL) to prevent hypercalcemia.

   1) Two vitamin D_2 preparations are available:
   a) *Dihydrotachysterol, 0.03 μg/kg/day divided BID for 2–5 days (until calcium level is low normal), then 0.02 μg/kg/day divided BID for 2 days, then 0.01 mg/kg/day divided BID*
   b) *Hytakerol, 0.01–0.02 μg/kg/day for 2–5 days, then 0.01–0.02 μg/kg q24–48h.*

   2) Vitamin D_3 (calcitriol) has a shorter onset of action (1–4 days) and shorter half life (<1 day) than vitamin D_2 preparations, making it easier to titrate to the desired serum calcium level. Calcitriol, 0.02–0.03 μg/kg/day divided BID for 3–4 days, then 0.005–0.015 μg/kg/day divided BID

d. Oral calcium supplementation can be administered with vitamin D preparations for 2–4 months then gradually tapered if serum calcium levels are maintained. Enhanced absorption of dietary calcium through the action of vitamin D may make long-term supplemental calcium unnecessary.

   1) Calcium carbonate is the most commonly used oral supplement because it has a higher percentage of elemental calcium (40%) than lactate (13%) and gluconate (27%) compounds, thus making fewer pills necessary.

   2) Dose: 25–50 mg/kg/day divided BID–QID on the basis of elemental calcium content.

e. Monitor serum calcium daily while in hospital, weekly until it stabilizes in the low normal range, and then every 3 months. Watch for PU/PD that may indicate hypercalcemia.

H. Hyperkalemia

1. General points

  a. Serum potassium is determined by three major processes:

   1) Intake of potassium.(oral or parenteral)

   2) Distribution of potassium between the intracellular and extracellular space

   3) Excretion of potassium primarily through the kidneys and to a lesser extent via the colon (more important in chronic renal failure than in any acute disease process)

  b. Oral intake

   1) Oral intake rarely results in hyperkalemia by itself. Generally, increased oral intake has to be associated with decreased excretion (e.g., renal failure) or decreased intracellular translocation of potassium (see below). Oral intake of potassium is an unlikely cause of hyperkalemia in dogs and cats.

   2) IV supplementation with excessive KCl can cause iatrogenic hyperkalemia.

  c. Distribution between extracellular and intracellular spaces

   1) The Na^+/K^+ ATPase membrane pump is primarily responsible for the potassium concentration differences between the intra- and extracellular spaces.

    a) *Pumps three Na^+ out for every two K^+ in; thus is electrogenic, creating a negative potential inside relative to outside the cell.*

Intracellular potassium concentration is approximately equal to the extracellular sodium concentration.

b) *Drugs that affect the Na^+/K^+ ATPase cell membrane-associated pump:*

   i) *Inhibitors: Inhibitors of the pump may contribute to extracellular hyperkalemia by preventing translocation of potassium into the cell. Nonspecific β-blockers may contribute to hyperkalemia by inhibiting catecholamine-mediated uptake of potassium into liver and muscle cells (see below).*

   ii) *Stimulators*

    i. Catecholamines stimulate cellular potassium uptake via stimulation of the Na^+/K^+ pump.

    ii. Insulin promotes cellular uptake of potassium via the Na^+/K^+ pump; thus insulin deficiency may contribute to hyperkalemia.

2) Other effectors of cellular potassium distribution

  a) *Mineral acidosis (e.g., renal acidosis)*

   i) *Transcellular exchange of H^+ entering cell and K^+ exiting*

   ii) *Organic acidoses (e.g., lactic acidosis, ketoacidosis) are not thought to contribute to hyperkalemia because of concomitant intracellular translocation of the associated organic anion with the H^+.*

  b) *Reperfusion of ischemic tissues: e.g., acute, rapid reperfusion of hind legs of a cat with aortic thromboembolism. Serum potassium can increase rapidly and result in death if not immediately and aggressively treated.*

  c) *Acute tumor lysis syndrome: Massive cellular destruction of neoplastic cells may cause release of a large amount of potassium from the lysed cells.*

  d) *Severe crushing injuries: Massive cellular destruction can release large amounts of potassium into circulation.*

d. Decreased excretion

   1) Urethral obstruction is the most common cause of life-threatening hyperkalemia.

   2) Bilateral complete ureteral obstruction is becoming more common, particularly in cats with calcium oxalate urolithiasis.

3) Urinary bladder rupture has a generally slower onset of hyperkalemia than urethral obstruction, likely due to the greater volume of distribution available to potassium (e.g., peritoneal space).

4) Bilateral ureteral rupture

5) Anuric or oliguric renal failure

6) Hypoadrenocorticism (Addison's disease): Hyperkalemia is a strong stimulus for aldosterone release. Aldosterone promotes renal excretion of potassium.

7) Pseudo-Addison's disease: GI parasite infestation (e.g., trichuriasis)

8) Chylothorax with thoracic drainage

9) Peritoneal effusion

10) Pericardial effusion

11) Drugs

    a) Angiotensin II converting enzyme inhibitors interfere with aldosterone secretion.

    b) Prostaglandin inhibitors (NSAIDS) interfere with prostaglandin-mediated renin release.

    c) Heparin reduces aldosterone secretion.

    d) Potassium-sparing diuretics (amiloride, triamterene, spironolactone)

e. Pseudohyperkalemia

  1) Thrombocytosis

  2) Hemolysis (e.g., Akita)

f. General rules of thumb

  1) The most severe increases in potassium concentration occur with urethral obstruction and reperfusion of the hind legs in cats with aortic saddle thromboembolism.

  2) Drugs generally don't cause clinically significant increases in potassium concentration unless potassium supplementation is being provided. Even then, severe hyperkalemia is rare.

  3) Organic acidosis does not contribute to severe increases in potassium concentration. Also, inorganic acidosis does not occur in isolation and is typically associated with renal failure.

g. Physiologic consequences of hyperkalemia

  1) The most life-threatening physiologic consequence of hyperkalemia is the effect on the cardiac conduction tissue. The effects can primarily be explained by understanding the following points:

    a) Hyperkalemia results in a decrease in the potential difference across the cell membrane (less negative).

    b) Initially, the conductive tissues become hyperexcitable because of a decreased potential difference between the resting membrane potential and the threshold potential.

    c) Once resting membrane potential is equal to or less than the threshold potential, the cells cannot be repolarized, and the cells do not conduct.

    d) Initially, as the extracellular potassium concentration increases, the cell membrane becomes more permeable to potassium, and during repolarization, potassium rushes out of the cell faster, causing a narrow but peaked T-wave and shortened QT interval.

    e) Atrioventricular conduction slows as extracellular potassium concentrations become moderately high.

    f) The atrial cells are more sensitive to potassium changes than the ventricular cells. Therefore, as potassium increases to very high concentrations, the p-wave widens or even disappears. Conduction is still occurring from the sinus node to the AV node but not through the atrial tissue. Hence the term sinoventricular conduction.

    g) At the most extreme concentrations, the QRS wave becomes extremely wide and merges with the T wave, resulting in a sine wave pattern.

    h) Ventricular arrhythmias, ventricular fibrillation, and asystole may all occur as a result of hyperkalemia.

  2) ECG changes: The potassium concentration at which ECG changes occur varies among patients. The sequence of ECG changes is fairly consistent with T-wave changes occurring first, QRS changes next, P-wave changes/loss followed by sine wave form.

h. Threshold potential

  1) Threshold potential is the potential at which sodium entry exceeds potassium, resulting in sustained depolarization.

  2) Potassium concentration is not the primary determinant of the threshold potential.

  3) Calcium is the primary electrolyte that affects threshold potential.

  4) Increased calcium concentration decreases the threshold potential (makes it less negative) and increases the potential difference between resting membrane potential and the threshold potential.

5) Decreased calcium concentration increases the threshold potential (makes it more negative) and decreases the potential difference between resting membrane potential and the threshold potential.

6) Exogenous calcium protects the heart from the effects of hyperkalemia.

2. Diagnosis of hyperkalemia

  a. Potassium measurement above the reference range—rule out pseudohyperkalemia (thrombocytosis, hemolysis of blood in an Akita)

  b. Assess for underlying cause of hyperkalemia (*Table 15-7*)

   1) See above for physiologic principles.

   2) Increased supplementation

   a) *Excessive potassium concentration in intravenous fluids*

   b) *Assess for an associated potassium metabolism problem (excretion, cellular translocation).*

   3) Decreased cellular translocation or intracellular release of potassium

   a) *Diabetic?*

   b) *Associated drugs (p. 318)*

   c) *Tumor lysis syndrome?*

   d) *Reperfusion of ischemic tissue?*

   4) Decreased excretion

   a) *Renal failure(renal or postrenal)*

   b) *Hypoadrenocorticism*

   c) *Pseudo-Addison's disease*

   d) *Associated drugs*

   e) *Repeated thoracic drainage of a chylothorax*

   f) *Peritoneal effusion (cats, generally mild hyperkalemia)*

   g) *Pericardial effusion (generally mild hyperkalemia).*

   5) Life-threatening hyperkalemia is most commonly seen with decreased renal excretion and reperfusion syndrome.

3. Treatment of hyperkalemia

  a. Specific treatments of hyperkalemia are reserved for animals showing the physiologic effects of hyperkalemia (primarily ECG changes).

  b. Specific treatments of hyperkalemia include antagonizing the effects of hyperkalemia on the heart, promoting intracellular translocation of potassium, and promoting excretion of potassium.

   1) Antagonizing the effects of hyperkalemia— IV administration of 10% calcium gluconate (50–100 mg/kg IV slowly over 1–2 min) will decrease the threshold potential and increase the potential difference between resting and threshold cell membrane potentials (p. 318).

   a) *Effects should be seen within minutes of administration and last approximately 20–30 minutes.*

   b) *ECG should be monitored while administering calcium gluconate to assess for calcium-induced arrhythmias.*

   2) Promoting intracellular translocation of potassium

   a) *Insulin/dextrose administration: Administer 0.55–1.1 U/kg of regular insulin IV as a bolus followed by 1–2 g/U of insulin given of 25% dextrose IV.*

   i) *IV fluid should have glucose added to make a 5% dextrose solution to maintain glucose concentration in the normal range.*

   ii) *Hypoglycemia is possible even hours after the administration of the insulin. Therefore, blood glucose level must be monitored after insulin administration.*

   b) *Sodium bicarbonate*

   i) *Administer 1–2 mEq/kg of sodium bicarbonate IV over 15 minutes.*

   ii) *Also treats metabolic acidosis, which is often present with hyperkalemia that is associated with renal dysfunction*

   iii) *Administered cautiously in animals that are hypocalcemic, as this may lower the [Cai] resulting in tonic-clonic seizure activity.*

   3) Promoting excretion

   a) *Promoting excretion is not for immediate life-threatening hyperkalemia but is used in conjunction with the above treatments to help lower and prevent reoccurrence of hyperkalemia.*

   b) *IV fluid administration will help promote renal potassium excretion.*

   i) *Use with caution in animals with oliguric or anuric renal failure and animals with heart disease. Monitor central venous pressure (CVP) to prevent volume overload.*

   ii) *0.9% saline or any standard balanced electrolyte solution will help dilute potassium and promote diuresis.*

TABLE 15.7
CAUSES OF HYPERKALEMIA

Hypoadrenocorticism
Acute oliguric renal failure
Ruptured bladder
Urethral tear
Urethral obstruction
Severe crushing injuries
Heatstroke

Overdose of K-sparing diuretics
Overzealous KCl supplementation

Snakebite with massive tissue trauma
Tumor lysis syndrome
Overwhelming infection
Thromboembolism
"Pseudo-Addison's" (whipworms, colitis)
Chylothorax with thoracic drainage

c. Treat underlying disease: The specific treatments for hyperkalemia only temporarily stabilize the patient. Definitive therapy for the underlying disease must be provided to prevent hyperkalemia from recurring.
d. Dialysis: If all of the above fail, peritoneal or hemodialysis must be provided.

I. Hypokalemia

1. General points
a. Most common electrolyte abnormality in critically ill veterinary patients
b. Hypokalemia occurs because of one of the four reasons below or any combination of them:
1) Decreased intake/GI loss:
  a) *Anorexia*
  b) *Vomiting*
  c) *Diarrhea*
  d) *Decreased intake combined with potassium-deficient fluid*
2) Increased translocation to the intracellular space
  a) *Insulin therapy*
  b) *Catecholamines—albuterol*
  c) *Glucose administration*
  d) *Alkalemia*
  e) *Hypokalemic periodic paralysis (rare, Burmese cats)*
3) Increased loss through the kidney
  a) *Renal disease*
  b) *Diuretics (furosemide, thiazides)*
  c) *Osmotic diuresis (e.g., glucosuria, mannitol)*
  d) *Fluid diuresis with inadequate potassium supplementation or intake*

  e) *Postobstructive diuresis*
  f) *Renal tubular acidosis*
  g) *Hyperaldosteronism—may be accompanied by hypertension*
  h) *Hyperadrenocorticism*
  i) *Hypomagnesemia (most commonly seen in patients with DKA receiving insulin therapy)*
4) Drugs
  a) *Penicillins*
  b) *Other (consider any drug as a possibility and review potential complications of any drug that animal is receiving)*
c. Physiologic effects
1) Hyperpolarization of the resting cell membrane potential is the primary underlying problem for the main clinical manifestations of hypokalemia.
2) The primary clinical signs include muscle weakness, cramping, lethargy, ileus, urine retention, inability to concentrate urine, and myocardial depression.
3) Specific effects
  a) *Metabolic acidosis—Chronic hypokalemia may lead to metabolic acidosis secondary to a defect in renal tubular acidification.*
  b) *Muscle weakness*
    i) *Should be considered a possibility when potassium concentration falls below 3.0 mmol/L*
    ii) *Severe hypokalemia (<1.5 mmol/L) can lead to respiratory muscle weakness and inadequate ventilation or respiratory arrest.*
    iii) *Ventroflexion of the head (in cats) occurs due to weakness of the neck muscles.*

iv) *Smooth muscle weakness in the GI tract causes gastric atony and ileus, resulting in an inability to digest food. Feeding should not be implemented until hypokalemia is corrected.*

v) *Detrusor muscle atony can result in urine retention in hypokalemic animals.*

vi) *Animals that exercise and have hypokalemia may develop muscle ischemia and subsequent necrosis. Local potassium increase in exercising muscles results in vasodilation and preservation of blood flow to exercising muscle. Hypokalemia may lead to decreased local potassium release, resulting in ischemic necrosis.*

c) *Cardiac effects*

i) *Generally not a common clinical manifestation*

ii) *Supraventricular and ventricular arrhythmias may occur.*

iii) *Prolongation of QT and U waves may occur.*

iv) *Hypokalemia potentiates the toxic effects of digitalis.*

v) *Ventricular arrhythmias may be refractory to class I antiarrhythmics in the presence of hypokalemia.*

d) *Renal effects*

i) *Hypokalemia may result from renal disease, but hypokalemia itself can cause renal dysfunction.*

ii) *Polyuria may occur as a result of primary polydipsia and a renal-concentrating defect due to decreased responsiveness of the renal tubular cells to antidiuretic hormone (ADH).*

iii) *Hypokalemia may cause an increase in renal ammoniagenesis. Increased renal ammonia can activate complement and result in inflammation that leads to progressive renal damage. This is a greater concern with chronic disease.*

2. Diagnosis

a. Measurement of potassium below the reference range—Generally you don't see clinical manifestations until potassium is <3.0 mmol/L.

b. Assess for underlying cause of hypokalemia (see general points above).

1) In general, the most severe acute hypokalemia occurs in sick DKA patients at the start of insulin therapy.

a) *This results from a variety of causes including decreased intake (anorexia), translocation of potassium into the cell (insulin and glucose therapy), increased loss (vomiting, diarrhea, osmotic diuresis), and magnesium deficiency.*

b) *Cats with chronic polyuric renal failure and concurrent anorexia or vomiting may develop severe hypokalemia.*

c) *Cats with hyperaldosteronism may have moderate-to-severe hypokalemia.*

d) *Most other causes of hypokalemia result in mild-to-moderate hypokalemia and are from more chronic conditions.*

2) Feline hypokalemic polymyopathy

a) *First reported in 1984*

b) *Geriatric cats with muscle weakness, cervical ventroflexion, elevated creatine kinase (CPK), and severe hypokalemia*

c) *Most cats had underlying polyuric renal disease resulting in potassium losses exceeding potassium intake. Commercial diets today contain more potassium, so condition is no longer common.*

d) *Inappropriate loss of potassium can be documented by measuring fractional excretion (Fe$_x$) according to the following formula:*

$$U_k = \text{Urine K} \, (\text{mEq/L})$$

$$Fe_x = Fe_x = \frac{(U_k/S_k)}{(U_{cr}/S_{cr})} \times 100$$

where S_k = Serum K (mEq/L); U_{cr} = Urine creatinine (mg/dL); S_{cr} = Serum creatinine (mg/dL)

e) *Values above 4–6% are consistent with inappropriate potassium loss.*

f) *Cats with excessive potassium loss should receive oral supplementation at a dosage of 2–4 mEq/cat/day.*

3. Treatment

a. Stabilize as for any critically ill patient.

b. Stop giving any drugs or treatments that might be contributing to hypokalemia IF the

TABLE 15.8
POTASSIUM REPLACEMENT

Serum K (mEq/L)	KCl (mEq/L) to Add to 1L of Fluids	Max Rate (mL/kg/h)
3.6–5.0	20	24
3.1–3.5	30	16
2.6–3.0	40	11
2.1–2.5	60	8
<2.0	80	6

cessation of this therapy does not compromise the patient for other reasons, and treat underlying cause of the hypokalemia.

c. Potassium supplementation
 1) Intravenous therapy (see *Table 15–8* for dosage recommendations)
   a) *Hypokalemia can be prevented in animals receiving IV fluids who have decreased intake or excessive losses of potassium.*
    i) *IV fluids containing 14–20 mEq/L generally keep the potassium level from decreasing.*
    ii) *Animals with pancreatitis peritonitis, parvoviral enteritis, diabetes, and postobstructive diuresis usually require potassium supplementation.*
   b) *The generally accepted rule of thumb is not to exceed the rate of 0.5 mEq/kg/h for potassium supplementation. One can go as high as 1.0 mEq/kg/h in severely hypokalemic patients that are not responding to the 0.5 mEq/kg/h.*
   c) *Two primary potassium formulations are used*
    i) *Potassium chloride (2 mEq/mL)*
     i. *Also helpful for hypochloremia*
     ii. *Dilute in IV fluids. Concentrations >60 mEq/L can cause pain during infusion and injure the vessel. Ensure thorough mixing of potassium solution with fluid to prevent nonuniform potassium concentration.*
    ii) *Rapid potassium infusion—In severely hypokalemic cats a potassium "bolus" may be used to start potassium supplementation.*

   i. *Formula: Total amount of KCl for bolus = (Ideal [K$^+$] − Observed [K$^+$]) × Estimated vascular volume (L)*
   ii. *Draw up needed potassium amount and dilute in equal or two times the volume with normal saline.*
   iii. *Administer volume IV over 5–10 minutes through a central catheter to avoid pain.*
   iv. *Example: 5-kg cat with [K$^+$] = 2.0 mmol/L. Ideal [K$^+$] estimated to be 4.5 mmol/L. Estimated vascular volume is 60 mL/kg × 5 kg = 300 mL = 0.3L. Total amount of potassium = (4.5 − 2.0) × 0.3 L = 0.75 mEq of potassium as a bolus. This corresponds to 0.375 mL of the 2.0 mEq/mL KCL solution. Mix this volume with 0.75 mL of 0.9% saline to get 1.125 mL total volume of a bolus to give over 10 minutes.*
   v. *ECG should be monitored continuously when administering this bolus.*
   iii) *Potassium phosphate (KH$_2$PO$_4$) is a useful formulation in animals that have concurrent hypophosphatemia (e.g., DKA patients receiving insulin therapy).*
 2) *Subcutaneous—you can add KCl to SQ fluids, but do not exceed 30 mEq of potassium/L because of tissue irritation.*
 3) Oral potassium supplementation
   a) *Generally reserved for longer-term therapy*
   b) *Potassium gluconate—Tumil K, 1/4 teaspoon (2 mEq) per 4.5 kg body weight PO in food twice daily. Adjust dose as necessary.*
 4) Monitoring
   a) *Any animal receiving IV potassium supplementation should have potassium concentrations monitored at least initially to determine the response.*
   b) *Improvement in potassium concentration cannot be predicted from initial concentration or clinical findings of the animal. Degree of improvement can only be determined by monitoring potassium concentration after administering supplemental potassium.*

c) Special caution should be taken with animals with renal failure that are receiving IV potassium supplementation.

J. Hypernatremia

1. Important physiologic points

a. The *volume* of extracellular fluid (ECF) is determined by total body sodium content.

b. The *concentration* of extracellular sodium is determined by water balance.

c. Serum $[Na^+]$ indicates the amount of sodium in the ECF relative to the amount of water in the ECF and does not reflect total body water or total body sodium.

d. *Osmolarity* is the number of particles per liter of solution.

e. *Osmolality* is the number of particles per kilogram of solution.

    1) Osmolality is the term used most commonly regarding serum or plasma.

    2) For bodily solutions, osmolality and osmolarity are nearly equivalent.

f. Normal plasma osmolality ranges from 290 to 310 mmol/kg in dogs and slightly higher in cats (290–330 mmol/kg).

g. Sodium is the major contributor to osmolality in the normal animal.

h. Formula for calculation of osmolality:

$$2\,[Na\,(mmol/L] + [BUN\,(mg/dL]/2.8$$

$$+ \,[Glucose\,(mg/dL)]/18$$

i. Renal sodium handling

    1) Nearly 70% of the sodium in the glomerular filtrate is reabsorbed in the proximal renal tubule.

    2) 25% of sodium is reabsorbed in the thick ascending limb of the loop of Henle. Furosemide acts at this site to prevent sodium reabsorption.

    3) 5% of sodium is reabsorbed in the distal convoluted tubule and collecting duct. Thiazide diuretics act here to prevent sodium reabsorption.

    4) The remaining 3% of sodium is reabsorbed in the collecting ducts.

        a) Aldosterone is the major effector of sodium reabsorption control here.

        b) This is the primary site of regulation of sodium excretion in response to dietary variations in sodium amount.

        c) The diuretics amiloride and triamterene prevent sodium reabsorption at this site on the renal tubule.

2. Hypernatremia is defined as any sodium concentration above the high end of the reference range.

3. Hypernatremia primarily occurs by sodium gain, sodium-free water loss, or hypotonic or lower sodium-containing fluid loss. In most veterinary cases, hypernatremia is due to relatively free or lower sodium-containing water loss rather than actual sodium gain.

4. Causes of sodium-free water deficits

a. Pure water loss primarily occurs through the respiratory tract or the urinary tract.

b. Urinary loss (dilute urine)

    1) Nephrogenic diabetes insipidus

    2) Central diabetes insipidus

c. Respiratory (panting)

    1) Fever

    2) High environmental temperatures

d. Other—loss through major body cavity during surgery

e. Lack of free water intake

    1) Primary hypodipsia

    2) Neurologic disease with altered thirst mechanism

    3) Lack of access to free water

5. Causes of hypotonic fluid losses

a. Gastrointestinal

    1) Vomiting

    2) Diarrhea

b. Renal

    1) Osmotic diuresis due to diabetes mellitus, intravenous glucose supplementation, osmotic diuretics (e.g., mannitol)

    2) Chronic renal failure (polyuric)

    3) Postobstructive diuresis

c. Other—third-space losses secondary to pleural or peritoneal inflammation

6. Sodium gain

a. Ingestion of high-sodium-containing food or water (e.g., sea water, rock salt)

b. IV administration of high-sodium-containing solutions such as hypertonic saline or sodium bicarbonate

c. Sodium phosphate enema (in cats or small dogs)

d. Hyperaldosteronism or administration of excessive amounts of mineralocorticoids

7. Fluid loss in an otherwise normal animal tends to have a lower sodium concentration (hypotonic) than that of plasma and interstitium.

   a. Thus animals without pathologic losses will eventually become hypernatremic if sodium-free water is not available and imbibed.

   b. Long-term administration of normal saline solution without availability of sodium-free water for the patient

8. Diagnosis

   a. Diagnosis is based on a serum sodium measurement above the reference range.

   b. The underlying pathophysiologic cause of hypernatremia can be inferred from estimation of the volume status of the patient.

   1) If the patient is hypervolemic (distended jugular veins, high CVP, pulmonary edema), the most likely cause of hypernatremia is sodium gain.

   2) If the patient is normovolemic, hypernatremia is more likely the result of free-water loss or decreased free-water intake.

   3) If patient is hypovolemic (pale mucous membranes, weak pulse, prolonged capillary refill time, low blood pressure), the most likely cause of hypernatremia is hypotonic fluid loss.

   c. Highest concentrations of sodium tend to be associated with central diabetes insipidus.

9. Clinical signs, other than those associated with the underlying cause of the hypernatremia, most severely affect the brain.

   a. Depression, lethargy, anorexia, abnormal behavior, ataxia, obtundation, stupor, coma, or seizures

   b. Neurologic signs usually do not manifest until $[Na^+]$ exceeds 170 mmol/L, but this varies.

   c. Development of neurologic signs depends upon the rate of change of the $[Na^+]$ because of the brain's ability to produce idiogenic osmols.

   1) Slow change is associated with a higher $[Na^+]$ before neurologic signs develop.

   2) Rapid change is associated with a lower $[Na^+]$ before neurologic signs develop.

10. Treatment of hypernatremia

    a. The time period for correction of $[Na^+]$ to normal should parallel the speed with which the hypernatremia developed.

    1) For example, if the sodium concentration increased rapidly after an IV bolus of

hypertonic saline, then sodium concentration can be decreased rapidly.

2) Hypernatremia due to free water or hypotonic fluid loss generally occurs over several hours or days and should be corrected accordingly.

3) As a rule of thumb, a 0.5 mEq/L/h decrease in sodium concentration is safe.

   a) *Therefore, correction from 200 to 150 mmol/L should take approximately 100 hours or nearly 4 days!*

   b) *Practically , fine control of the rate of sodium decrease is difficult, but the rate of decline can be estimated fairly accurately by use of the formula in Table 15-9. Example: A 10-kg dog is 7% dehydrated and has a serum $[Na^+]$ of 180 mEq/L. Lactated Ringer's solution (LRS) is used to provide maintenance and rehydration over the initial 12 hours. According to the formula, each liter will decrease the serum $[Na^+]$ by 7 mEq/L:*

$$\text{Change in serum}\,[Na^+]$$
$$= \frac{\text{Infusate}\,[Na^+] - \text{Serum}\,[Na^+]}{[BW\,(kg) \times 0.6] + 1}$$
$$= \frac{130 - 180}{7} = -7$$

1 L of LRS is given over the first 12 hours for rehydration and maintenance. After 12 hours, $[Na^+]$ is 173 mEq/L. The fluid is changed to 0.45% NaCl. To determine the effect of 1 L of this solution; the formula is applied again:

$$\text{Change in serum}\,[Na^1]$$
$$= \frac{77 - 173}{7} = \frac{-96}{7} = -14$$

Each liter of 0.45% NaCl will decrease the serum $[Na^+]$ by 14 mEq/L. Because the animal is now well hydrated, the fluid rate can be reduced to 1–1.5 × maintenance (30 mL/h) so that the serum $[Na^+]$ will gradually return to normal over the next 30–40 hours. (Note: Na^+ concentration of IV fluids is found in Table 15-10.)

b. Correction of hypernatremia due to **free-water loss**:

   1) Free-water loss means that the total amount of sodium in the body is the same

---

TABLE 15.9
FORMULA FOR ESTIMATING CORRECTION OF SERUM (Na^1)

$$\text{Change in serum}[Na^+] = \frac{\text{Infusate}[Na^+] - \text{Serum}[Na^+]}{[BW(kg) \times 0.6] + 1}$$

Estimates the effect of 1 L of infusate on serum [Na1]
Rule of thumb: The rate of change should not exceed 0.5 mEq/h (~10–12 mEq/day)

---

as before the free-water loss. This point is key to understanding the calculation of free-water deficit.

2) Water moves freely between the intracellular and extracellular space. The total body water is equal to approximately 0.6 times lean body weight in kilograms.

3) The total body sodium = $[Na^+] \times$ total body water.

4) The formula to calculate free water deficit is as follows:

   a) Water deficit

   $= 0.6 \times$ lean BW (kg)

   $\times$ (Current $[Na^+]$/Desired$[Na^+]$) $- 1$

   b) *For example: A dog has [Na⁺] of 200 mmol/L and a lean body weight of 10 kg. We think that his normal [Na⁺] is 150 mmol/L. His water deficit is calculated as follows:*

   $$0.6 \times 10 \times [(200/150) - 1]$$

   $$= 2\,L\,free - water\,deficit.$$

5) Though this is appears to be an exact calculation, it should be considered only an estimate and used as a guideline for fluid therapy. One must also consider fluid maintenance requirements, ongoing hypotonic and isotonic losses, and ongoing free-water losses.

6) Once your calculation of free-water deficit has been done, you adjust the fluid rate to replace this deficit as well as replace ongoing losses and maintenance requirements. Remember that you do not want to lower $[Na^+]$ faster than 0.5 mmol/L per hour if the problem is longstanding

(>1–2 days). It is difficult to predict how fast, or sometimes even in what direction, $[Na^+]$ will change when first administering fluids. Thus $[Na^+]$ should be checked at least every 1–2 hours until a consistent change is noted. Once a consistent trend is established, the frequency of sodium checks can be adjusted accordingly.

7) Giving 5% dextrose in water is like giving pure water to the patient.

   a) *The dextrose is metabolized, leaving just water.*

   b) *Therefore, the free-water deficit can be replaced by giving 5% dextrose in water. See the formula above to estimate the change in serum [Na⁺] that will occur with each liter of 5% dextrose.*

c. Correction of hypernatremia due to **hypotonic fluid losses**

   1) Hypotonic fluid losses tend to result in greater intravascular volume losses and resultant hypovolemia than free-water losses.

   2) Patients with perfusion deficits due to hypovolemia should first be treated with fluids that will restore vascular volume. This can done using 0.9% saline or a balanced electrolyte solution (see Shock, Chapter 14). Once perfusion is adequate, treatment of the hypernatremia can be started.

   3) Lower-sodium solutions such as 0.45% saline or 1/2 strength balanced electrolyte solutions can be administered. The rate of lowering $[Na^+]$ should generally not exceed 0.5 mEq/L/h.

   4) Serial sodium measurements should be performed every 1 to 2 hours until a consistent trend is noted, then time between

TABLE 15.10
(NA⁺) OF INTRAVENOUS FLUIDS

Infusate	mEq/L
5% Dextrose in water	0
0.45% NaCl	77
Lactated Ringer's	130
Normosol-R	140
0.9% NaCl	154
3% NaCl	513
5% NaCl	855

sodium measurements can be adjusted accordingly.

d. Correction of hypernatremia due to **gain of sodium**

1) Gain of sodium tends to be associated with normovolemia or hypervolemia.

2) [Na⁺] can be corrected with 5% dextrose in water.

3) Avoid overhydration and pulmonary edema in these patients because of their existing hypervolemic or overhydrated status. CVP measurement during fluid administration may help guide fluid rates.`

4) Administration of furosemide, a loop diuretic (1–2 mg/kg IV), will help speed sodium elimination and decrease volume.

5) Rate of decrease of [Na⁺] should not exceed 0.5 mEq/L/h.

11. Maintenance of normonatremia once hypernatremia is corrected

a. Normonatremia may be obtained by continuing fluid therapy until the patient can maintain normal [Na⁺] on its own or with medical therapy for the underlying disease process.

b. Normal [Na⁺] is maintained in animals with central diabetes insipidus by administering desmopressin (DDAVP) (0.1 mg/mL). This solution is available for people as a nasal spray, but it is easier to administer to dogs by applying 1–2 drops in each eye q8–24h. One drop of the nasal spray contains 1.5–4 μg of DDAVP. The effect is reported to last for 8 to 24 hours. Therefore, dosage adjustments will depend on clinical signs of PU/PD and when they occur after drug administration.

c. Chlorpropamide (a hypoglycemic agent) potentiates the renal effects of vasopressin and thus may be useful in some patients with central diabetes insipidus (10–40 mg/kg/day orally). Side effect could be hypoglycemia.

d. Thiazide diuretics may paradoxically decrease urine volume by inducing mild dehydration. The mild dehydration will enhance proximal sodium and water reabsorption and thereby decrease distal tubule fluid delivery.

1) Chlorothiazide, 20–40 mg/kg BID.

2) Hydrochlorothiazide, 2.5–5.0 mg/kg BID.

e. Dietary sodium and protein restriction will help decrease the amount of daily obligatory solute excretion and help decrease urine volume.

K. Hyponatremia

1. General points

a. Hyponatremia may be a real finding or an artifact of measurement.

b. To determine if there is true hyponatremia, one must measure osmolality.

c. Sodium is the major contributor to osmolality in the normal animal.

d. Hyponatremia may be due to sodium loss in excess of free water, excess free-water gain over sodium, or free-water shifts from the intracellular space to the extracellular space because of the presence of other excessive or extra osmolytes (*Table 15-11*).

e. To determine if hyponatremia is real and what the underlying general cause is, one must measure osmolality. If osmolality is low, then true hyponatremia exists. If true hyponatremia is diagnosed, then physical and historical assessment of vascular volume status will help reveal the potential underlying general cause.

f. Clinically significant hyponatremia is <125 mEq/L.

g. If [Na⁺] is below 120 mmol/L, it is unlikely to be a pseudohyponatremia or a hyponatremia due to hyperglycemia or mannitol.

h. If pseudohyponatremia is occurring, then a significant lipid layer will be noted in the supernatant of a centrifuge hematocrit tube of blood; if it is due to hyperglycemia, an extremely high glucose level will be noted. Thus measurement of osmolality is not essen-

---

TABLE 15.11
CAUSES OF HYPONATREMIA

Sodium loss/depletion
   Salt-restricted diet
   Diuretics
   Hypoadrenocorticism
   GI loss—vomiting/diarrhea
   Burns, large wounds
   Uroperitoneum
   Peritoneal dialysis
   Chylothorax

Excess water gain
   Water replacement of electrolyte
     losses
   Iatrogenic-hypotonic IV fluids
   Congestive heart failure
   Nephrotic syndrome
   Severe liver disease
   Psychogenic polydypsia
   Syndrome of inappropriate ADH
     secretion
   Hyperglycemia
   Mannitol

Pseudohyponatremia
   Hyperlipidemia
   Hyperproteinemia

---

tial to make a diagnosis of true hyponatremia. It can be inferred by ruling out the conditions mentioned above.

2. Diagnosis:
   a. Clinical signs specific for hyponatremia:
      1) Clinical signs include weakness, hypotension, and shock.
      2) Cerebral edema can result in neurologic signs including depression, seizures, and focal or diffuse deficits.
      3) GI signs may include vomiting, anorexia, abdominal cramping, and ileus.
      4) Clinical signs depend upon how rapidly the true hyponatremia (hypoosmolality) developed.
         a) Faster onset—more likely to manifest clinical signs. In people this is a rate faster than 0.5 mEq/L/h and to a level below 120 mmol/L. Anecdotally, the authors feel that similar levels are applicable to dogs and cats.

b) Clinical signs can range from a normal appearing animal to mild lethargy, weakness, vomiting, seizures or coma.

b. A diagnosis of hyponatremia is first indicated by [Na$^+$] below the reference range.

c. If hyponatremia is indicated by [Na$^+$] measurement, then measurement of osmolality is indicated.
   1) Normal plasma osmolality
      a) Dogs: 290–310 mOsm/kg
      b) Cats: 290–330 mOsm/kg

d. If measured plasma osmolality is normal, pseudohyponatremia exists.
   1) This suggests a large amount of lipid or protein in the plasma. The false measurement occurs when the laboratory evaluating [Na$^+$] uses a flame photometer, which measures the number of sodium ions in a specific volume of plasma. Therefore, [Na$^+$] is calculated by the measured number of sodium molecules divided by the total volume of plasma evaluated. Sodium does not dissolve in the lipid or protein phase of plasma. Therefore, if lipid or protein content is high, there will be less aqueous phase of the plasma and therefore fewer sodium molecules in the total volume of plasma (including the nonaqueous phase). [Na$^+$] will be measured as low, but if measured by the volume of the aqueous phase, [Na$^+$] will be normal.
   2) A 1-mg/dL increase in lipid decreases [Na$^+$] by 0.002 mEq/L.
   3) Each g/dL increase in total protein above 8g/dL decreases [Na$^+$] by 0.25 mEq/L.
   4) One can see that extreme or even moderate decreases in [Na$^+$] are not likely to be due to pseudohyponatremia.
   5) If pseudohyponatremia is diagnosed, no further specific therapy for hyponatremia is necessary.

e. If measured plasma osmolality is high, then hyperglycemia or an unmeasured osmolyte (e.g., mannitol) is present.
   1) Each 100-mg/dL increase in glucose decreases [Na$^+$] by 1.6 mEq/L. This decrease is due to free-water translocation from the intracellular fluid to the extracellular fluid.
   2) Treatment for high plasma osmolality and low [Na$^+$] is usually treatment of the underlying cause (e.g., treat diabetes mellitus

if present or allow mannitol to be metabolized or excreted).

f. If measured plasma osmolality is low

    1) This indicates true hyponatremia.

    2) True hyponatremia can result from sodium loss, low-sodium water gain, or a combination. Therefore, the next step is a physical examination and assessment of volume/perfusion status and fluid retention or loss.

       a) Determine from history about fluid loss (e.g., vomiting, polyuria, etc..)

       b) Assess physical perfusion/hydration status (pulse quality, mucous membrane color, capillary refill time, heart rate, jugular pulses, etc..)

       c) Assess for fluid retention such as peripheral edema, ascites, pleural effusion.

    3) If physical examination shows hyponatremia with evidence of fluid loss, consider fluid loss through renal or extrarenal sites

       a) Extrarenal fluid loss

         i) Gastrointestinal (vomiting, diarrhea)

         ii) Third space (peritoneal or pleural)

       b) Renal losses

         i) Hypoadrenocorticism—can be confirmed by a lack of response to ACTH and a Na/K ratio <25:1.

         ii) Diuretic administration (particularly furosemide)

    4) If physical examination shows hyponatremia with evidence of fluid excess or retention, three major considerations are heart failure (including pericardial effusion), nephrotic syndrome, and severe liver disease. These three diseases all have in common decreased effective circulating volume. This results in decreased renal perfusion and concomitant nonosmotic (hypotension induced) ADH release that results in water retention.

    5) No change in volume or fluid status with hyponatremia—consider

       a) Psychogenic polydipsia

       b) Syndrome of inappropriate ADH secretion (SIADH)

         i) Very rare condition in dogs and cats

         ii) Reported to be associated with dirofilariasis, hypothalamic tumor, and pure glucocorticoid deficiency

       c) Drugs may potentiate the effects of ADH or stimulate its release.

         i) Release—cholinergic drugs, β-adrenergic drugs, narcotics, nitrous oxide, barbiturates, tricyclic antidepressants, vincristine

         ii) Potentiation—chlorpropamide, NSAIDS

3. Treatment

    a. Nearly all severe hyponatremia in dogs and cats developed for more than 48 hours. Therefore, in most patients, $[Na^+]$ should be raised slowly rather than rapidly, unless the condition developed over <48 hours). If in doubt, raise it slowly.

    b. Treat the underlying cause of the hyponatremia.

    c. Hypertonic saline is rarely if ever required in treating a hyponatremic patient.

    d. Use 0.9% saline intravenously.

    e. Aim to correct hyponatremia NO FASTER than 0.5 mEq/L/h. Err on the side of caution. If sodium is corrected too quickly, brain dehydration, brain shrinkage due to fluid loss, and osmotic demyelination may occur. Also, cerebral hemorrhage may occur as the brain shrinks and tears subarachnoid blood vessels. Clinical signs (neurologic dysfunction signs) may not occur until several days after the overzealous correction of hyponatremia.

    f. Volume and perfusion deficits should be corrected with balanced electrolyte solutions or 0.9% saline.

    g. In patients with normal volume, restrict water so that water intake is less than urine output.

    h. Discontinue any drugs that might stimulate the release, or enhance the effects, of ADH.

    i. The best treatment for patients with hyponatremia due to heart failure should be aimed at improving cardiac output by treating the heart failure with appropriate cardiac drugs (see heart failure) and decreasing the dosage of loop diuretics.

    j. Serial sodium measurements should be performed at least every 1 to 2 hours initially to establish the trend of sodium change. It is very difficult to predict the rate of sodium change when initially starting therapy, but the same formula used for correction of hypernatremia can be used to estimate the effect of various fluids on $[Na^+]$.

L. Hypothyroidism (myxedema coma)

1. Myxedema coma is a rare, but life-threatening, complication of prolonged hypothyroidism.

   a. Myxedema refers to accumulation of hyaluronic acid and mucopolysaccharide in the dermis, which causes water retention and non-pitting edema.

   b. Doberman Pinschers may be predisposed.

   c. Precipitating causes include respiratory depression from disease or drugs, exposure to cold temperatures, heart failure, and hypovolemia.

3. Clinical signs

   a. Severely altered mentation—depression, stupor, coma

   b. Hypothermia without shivering (hypometabolism prevents normal shivering response to cold)

   c. Nonpitting edema of head and face. Thickening and folding of skin may cause "tragic expression."

   d. Hypotension

   e. Hypoventilation

   f. Typical dermatologic manifestations of hypothyroidism—e.g., alopecia, dry skin, pyoderma

C. Laboratory findings

   a. Arterial blood gas abnormalities—hypoxemia, hypercarbia, metabolic and respiratory acidosis

   b. Hypoglycemia.

   c. Low-to-undetectable thyroid hormone concentration

   d. Typical abnormalities associated with hypothyroidism—hypercholesterolemia, nonregenerative anemia, hyponatremia

   e. Prolonged clotting times and/or evidence of DIC may occur

4. Electrocardiographic abnormalities

   a. Bradyarrhythmias—sinus bradycardia, slow atrial fibrillation, idioventricular rhythm. These arrhythmias are normally NOT responsive to atropine and resolve spontaneously as normal body temperature and euthyroidism are restored.

   b. Low-voltage complexes

5. Treatment

   a. Assess respiratory status and provide supplemental oxygen via face mask, nasal cannula, or endotracheal tube as indicated.

   b. Place peripheral and central intravenous catheters.

     1) All medication must be given IV to ensure adequate drug delivery.

     2) Absorption from oral, subcutaneous, and intramuscular routes is impaired because of poor perfusion and hypometabolism.

     3) Omit central IV catheter if coagulopathy is present.

   c. Administer warmed isotonic crystalloids such as 0.9% NaCl or Normosol

     1) Give an initial bolus of 5–10 mL/kg IV and subsequent volume to maintain CVP between 3 and 10 cm H_2O, urine output >1 mL/kg/h, adequate pulse strength, and normal capillary refill time.

     2) If possible, avoid fluids that contain lactate, because impaired hepatic metabolism may cause lactate accumulation that might exacerbate myocardial dysfunction and acidosis.

     3) Supplement fluids with dextrose, 2.5–5.0%, if hypoglycemia is present.

     4) Fluids must be administered cautiously and CVP monitored carefully in dogs with severe bradycardia or reduced contractility.

   d. Levothyroxine, 1–5 ng/kg IV q12h

     1) Start at the low end of the dose range and gradually increase in animals with myocardial disease.

     2) Monitor serum T_4 levels daily.

     3) Begin oral levothyroxine, 22 μg/kg q12h, when serum T_4 is normal and appetite has resumed.

   e. For anemia or coagulation abnormalities, administer packed RBCs or fresh frozen plasma (6–10 mL/kg IV) as indicated.

M. Magnesium

1. General

   a. Magnesium is the second most abundant intracellular cation (calcium is most abundant).

   b. Magnesium exists in three forms: protein bound, complexed with divalent anions (e.g., sulfate, phosphate), and ionized.

   c. The biologically active form is the ionized form.

   d. Magnesium is distributed in the body as follows: bone 80%, skeletal muscle 19%, remainder in heart, liver, and other tissue.

e. Some 99% of Mg^{2+} is intracellular; only 1% is found in serum.

f. Serum Mg^{2+}, therefore, may not accurately reflect total body concentration.

g. Magnesium functions as a cofactor in all reactions involving ATP and is important in maintaining cell membrane electrical gradients in nervous, musculoskeletal, and cardiovascular systems.

2. Hypomagnesemia

   a. Common in critically ill dogs and cats

   b. Associated with increased morbidity and mortality in hospitalized dogs and cats

   c. Commonly occurs with hypokalemia, hyponatremia, and hypocalcemia

   d. Clinical signs

   1) Neuromuscular and cardiovascular systems are most severely affected.

   2) Neuromuscular signs include muscle weakness, ataxia, twitching, hyperreflexia, seizure, and coma.

   3) Cardiovascular signs include tachyarrhythmias (ventricular and supraventricular) and hypertension.

   4) Signs may be exacerbated by

   a) *Refractory hypokalemia*

   b) *Hypocalcemia (hypomagnesemia impairs PTH secretion, resulting in secondary hypoparathyroidism in dogs)*

   e. Causes of hypomagnesemia

   1) Common causes include administration of fluids deficient in magnesium, diarrhea, and renal loss.

   2) See *Table 15-12* for complete list.

   f. Treatment

   1) Administer magnesium (as either magnesium chloride or magnesium sulfate) in 5% dextrose solution at 0.75–1.0 mEq/kg/day IV for 24–48 hours.

   2) For critical patients with life-threatening cardiac arrhythmias give 0.15–0.3 mEq/kg IV over 5–15 minutes. If hypomagnesemia is the underlying cause of arrhythmia, rapid improvement will follow the IV bolus.

   3) Correct the underlying disease.

3. Hypermagnesemia

   a. Uncommon.

   b. Clinical signs

   1) Neuromuscular signs include weakness, flaccid paresis, and respiratory depression.

TABLE 15.12
CAUSES OF HYPOMAGNESEMIA

Decreased intake
  Prolonged anorexia

Gastrointestinal loss
  Diarrhea

Urinary loss
  Primary renal disease
  Diabetic ketoacidosis
  Diuretics

Altered distribution
  Trauma
  Sepsis
  Pancreatitis
  Insulin therapy

Iatrogenic
  Mg deficient IV fluids
  Diuretics
  TPN (refeeding syndrome)

Drugs
  Aminoglycosides
  Ticarcillin

Miscellaneous
  Hyperthyroidism

---

   2) Cardiovascular signs include bradycardia, atrioventricular conduction block, and hypotension resulting from peripheral vasodilation.

   c. Causes of hypermagnesemia

   1) Acute renal failure is the most common cause.

   2) Iatrogenic causes include the use of cathartics that contain magnesium and overdosage of $MgCl_2$ or $MgSO_4$ used to correct hypomagnesemia.

   3) In cats, hypermagnesemia may occur with thoracic neoplasia and other causes of pleural effusion, probably resulting in part from impaired renal excretion.

   4) Rarely, endocrine disease (hypoadrenocorticism, hyperthyroidism, hypothyroidism) may cause hypomagnesemia.

   d. Treatment

   1) Discontinue exogenous magnesium administration.

   2) Diurese using 0.9% NaCl, lactated Ringer's at 2–4 mL/kg/h IV.

3) Furosemide, 1–2 mg/kg q12h PO, SQ, IV, to enhance diuresis; use caution not to cause dehydration, which might impair magnesium excretion.

4) Calcium gluconate may directly antagonize the effect of magnesium on neuromuscular and cardiac function.

a) Dose: 0.5–1.5 mL/kg IV over 5–10 minutes

b) Slow or discontinue injection if arrhythmia worsens or vomiting occurs.

N. Disorders of Phosphorus

1. General concerns
a. Phosphorus is primarily located within cells.
1) 80% is in bone.
2) 20% is in soft tissue (i.e., muscle).
b. Phosphorus is important for energy production (cofactor for glycolysis, needed to form ATP) and cell membrane maintenance (component of phospholipid membrane).

c. Serum phosphorus concentration is maintained in a narrow range by dietary phosphorus intake, factors that promote transcellular influx (insulin, alkalosis, carbohydrates) or efflux (glucagon, acidosis, proteins), renal excretion, vitamin D, and PTH.

3. Hypophosphatemia (see *Table 15-13*)
a. Defined as serum phosphorus <2.5 mg/dL.
b. Mild hypophosphatemia (2.0–2.5 mg/dL) is common and often transient.
c. Clinical sequelae of significant hypophosphatemia include hemolysis, skeletal muscle weakness, leukocyte dysfunction, poor oxygenation of tissue due to decreased 2,3 DPG levels, rhabdomyolysis, ileus, decreased cardiac contractility, and death.
d. "Refeeding syndrome," or "nutritional recovery syndrome," was first recognized in humans when prisoners of war were fed aggressively after prolonged malnutrition.
1) Severe hypophosphatemia can also develop in veterinary patients receiving

TABLE 15.13
CONDITIONS ASSOCIATED WITH HYPOPHOSPHATEMIA

Factors promoting intracellular translocation
 Glucose
 Insulin
 Amino acids
 Steroids
 Alkalosis—respiratory, metabolic
 Sodium bicarbonate
 Diuretics
 Postprandial (alkaline tide & insulin)
 Nutritional recovery syndrome

Diabetes mellitus
Eclampsia
Hyperparathyroidism (primary/pseudo)
Starvation
Intestinal binding agents (sucralfate; aluminum, magnesium, or calcium hydroxide)
Malabsorption
Hypovitaminosis D
Renal tubular loss
Dialysis
Severe hypothermia
Hyperalimentation
Laboratory error

enteral or IV nutrition following a period of malnutrition.

2) Carbohydrate metabolism causes insulin secretion with transcellular movement of phosphorus and consumption of enzymes and energy stores.

3) Hypophosphatemia can be prevented in at-risk patients by gradually increasing feeding to attain caloric requirements over several days and avoiding overfeeding with high-carbohydrate diets.

4) General recommendations for beginning nutrition in a malnourished patient

　　a) *Determine caloric requirement using the formula*

$$30 \times BW(kg) + 70$$

$$= Resting\ energy\ requirement.$$

　　b) *Feed 1/3 the first day, 2/3 the second day, and the full amount on day 3.*

　　c) *Avoid high-carbohydrate diets—use peripheral parenteral nutrition (PPN) instead of total parenteral nutrition (TPN) to avoid high concentrations of glucose in at-risk patients.*

e. Another cause of hypophosphatemia in veterinary patients is DKA.

1) The problem usually occurs several days after beginning treatment with insulin and fluids.

2) Serum phosphorus concentration may drop precipitously with insulin therapy, resulting in acute lethargy, weakness, and hemolysis.

3) Rhabdomyolysis can mask hypophosphatemia and maintain the serum concentration in the normal range. CPK is usually very high in these animals. IV phosphate replacement should still be considered even if serum phosphorus levels are low normal in at-risk patients with high CPK values.

f. Intravenous phosphate replacement.

1) Potassium phosphate solution contains 3 mmol/mL (93 mg/mL) phosphate and 4.3 mEq/mL potassium.

2) The recommended dose is 0.01–0.03 mmol/kg as a CRI over 6 hours. Phosphorus levels should be checked and the solution continued for another 6 hours if serum levels remain low.

3) Complications associated with IV phosphorus replacement include hyperphosphatemia, hypocalcemia, tetanic seizures, soft tissue mineralization, and hypotension. These complications can be avoided by slow infusion and close monitoring of serum P levels.

4) The recommended dose in humans is 7.7 mg/kg IV over 4 hours.

5) Potassium phosphate must be administered in calcium-free fluids (e.g., 0.9% NaCl instead of lactated Ringer's solution).

6) Some texts recommend giving half of the potassium requirement as potassium phosphate, but this practice has resulted in hyperphosphatemia and tetany in some cases and is not recommended.

TABLE 15.14 **CONDITIONS ASSOCIATED WITH HYPERPHOSPHATEMIA**	
Lipemia (spurious reading)	Metabolic acidosis
Young growing animal (normal)	Ingestion of radiator fluid
Acute or chronic renal failure	Vitamin D intoxication
Postrenal obstruction	Hypoparathyroidism
Uroperitoneum	Phosphate enema
Hyperthyroidism (cats)	Phosphate-supplemented fluids
Massive cellular destruction	Acromegaly
Hemolysis	Laboratory error
Rhabdomyolysis	
Tumor lysis syndrome	
Snakebite	
Massive tissue trauma/necrosis	

g. Oral phosphorus replacement can be administered at a dosage of 0.5–2 mmol/kg/day. Cow's milk contains 0.029 mmol/mL of phosphorus.

2. Hyperphosphatemia (see *Table 15-14*)
   a. Defined as serum phosphorus concentration >6.0 mg/dL
   b. Most common cause is renal failure. Decreased glomerular filtration rate (GFR) causes phosphorus retention.
   c. Other causes include massive cellular damage (tumor lysis syndrome, rhabdomyolysis, snakebite, thromboembolism), hyperparathyroidism, and poisoning from hypertonic phosphate enemas or vitamin D-containing rodenticides.
   d. Mild elevation in phosphorus level is normal in young growing dogs (6.0–9.0 mg/dL).
   e. Clinical findings associated with hyperphosphatemia include diarrhea, hypocalcemia, tetany, hyperosmolality, hypernatremia, and metastatic soft tissue calcification when the Ca × P product exceeds 70.
   f. Hyperphosphatemia contributes to the progression of renal disease by stimulating renal secondary hyperparathyroidism. Animals with renal failure should have a low-phosphorus diet and intestinal phosphate binders.
   g. Treatment of hyperphosphatemia
      1) IV fluids—correct acidosis, promote phosphorus excretion through diuresis
      2) Consider dextrose-containing fluids to move phosphorus intracellularly.
      3) Correct underlying cause—urethral obstruction, ruptured bladder.
      4) Administer intestinal phosphate binders:
         a) *Aluminum or calcium hydroxide, 30–180 mg/kg/day with meals*
         b) *Sucralfate, 0.5–1 g/25 kg q6–12h, is also an effective intestinal binding agent.*

CHAPTER 16

REPRODUCTIVE EMERGENCIES

I. CLINICAL SIGNS, DIAGNOSIS

Consider the possibility of an underlying reproductive disorder in all intact animals presenting for emergency care.

A. Physical examination/history

1. Female
   a. Determine date of last estrus, parturition, breeding history.
   b. Check for vaginal discharge—do cytology if present.
   c. Evaluate mammary glands, gently squeeze to express milk. Evaluate gross appearance and cytology.
   d. Palpate abdomen, *gently* if suspect pyometra. Uterus may be friable or very distended. Aggressive palpation could cause uterine rupture and peritonitis.
   e. Do not attempt cystocentesis if you suspect pyometra.
   f. Always rule out pyometra in sick intact females (abdominal radiographs, ultrasound, complete blood count (CBC)).
   g. Best time to palpate for pregnancy is 21–28 days in cats, 25–36 days in dogs.

2. Male
   a. Palpate abdomen for masses, painful caudal abdomen.
   b. Painful, soft, or hard testicles; epididymitis—suspect brucellosis
   c. Ask owner if dysuria, tenesmus (prostatic disease)
   d. Ruptured prostatic abscess can cause peritonitis and shock.
   e. Male feminizing syndrome—scrotal edema, hair loss, gynecomastia—can be seen with testicular tumors.
   f. Testicular tumors may cause life-threatening anemia and/or thrombocytopenia from estrogenic bone marrow suppression. Check for petechial hemorrhages on mucous membranes or low hematocrit.
   g. Cryptorchid testicles are prone to torsion and neoplasia.
   h. Prostatitis can cause fever, stiff gait, tenesmus, lethargy and depression. Painful rectal examination.

B. Abdominal radiographs

1. Fetal skeletons are visible after 45 days.
2. Signs of fetal death (6–48 h post) include overlapping skull bones, spinal collapse, and intrafetal gas patterns.
3. Free gas, fluid density abdomen may indicate peritonitis secondary to uterine rupture or tear or prostatic abscess leakage.
4. Examine the radiograph for homogeneous tubular densities in the caudal abdomen as seen with pyometritis.
5. Check fetal position and number for dystocia cases (count skulls and spines).
6. Check for sublumbar lymphadenopathy and metastasis to pelvic bones that can be seen with prostatic neoplasia.

C. Abdominal ultrasound

1. Best method to assess fetal viability after 24 days (check for fetal heartbeats).
2. Can also be used to detect abdominal masses—cryptorchid testicle, neoplasia. Definitive

diagnosis may require aspiration cytology or biopsy.

3. Ultrasound ±guided aspirate can be used to differentiate prostatic hyperplasia from cystic prostate, abscess, or neoplasia.

4. Ultrasound can easily identify a fluid-filled uterus.

II. DIAGNOSTIC AND MONITORING PROCEDURES

A. Vaginal cytology

1. Moisten swab with saline. Introduce at dorsal commissure of vulva and direct dorsally through the vestibule.

2. Roll swab on slide; air dry; stain.

3. For high vaginal culture, use sterile vaginal speculum or guarded swab.

4. Interpretation

   a. Anestrus—Noncornified epithelial cells, occasional nondegenerate PMN

   b. Proestrus—Numerous RBCs, noncornified epithelial cells, occasional WBC

   c. Estrus—Cornified epithelial cells; disappearance of RBCs and WBCs, no bacteria or debris

   d. Diestrus—Noncornified cells, leukocytes

   e. Infection—Masses of degenerate leukocytes and bacteria, foul odor

   f. Common pathogens include *Escherichia coli*, *Staphylococcus* spp., *Streptococcus* spp., *Klebsiella* spp., *Proteus* spp., *Mycoplasma* spp.

B. *Brucella* testing

1. Indicated for spontaneous abortion, infertility, orchitis, diskospondylitis

2. Rapid slide agglutination test—Good screening test; negative result rules out disease; positive result should be followed up with alternate testing (blood culture, agar gel immunodiffusion (AGID) test).

3. Tube agglutination test still has false positives. Follow up with AGID test (send 2 mL of serum to Diagnostic Lab CVM, Upper Tower Road, Cornell University, Ithaca, NY 14853. Phone: 607-253-3900) or submit blood culture to microbiology lab.

C. Plasma progesterone enzyme-linked immunosorbent assay (ELISA) (Icagen TARGET Canine Ovulation Timing Test, International Canine Genetics, Inc., Malvern, PA; EstruCHEK, Synbiotics, Kansas City, MO)

1. In pregnant animals >5 ng/mL

2. Decreases to <2 ng/mL 12–24 hours prior to parturition

3. Increases >2 ng/mL at time of ovulation/ estrus

4. Can be used to verify pregnancy, determine time of parturition, or choose best breeding time

D. Prostatic wash

1. Not performed frequently in emergency room because of prostatic pain. Urine culture usually suffices.

2. Indications—culture and sensitivity testing for chronic (nonpainful) prostatitis; cytologic evaluation for neoplasia, infection

3. Bladder is emptied and male urinary catheter is passed into bladder. Preprostatic sample is obtained with saline rinse of bladder. Catheter is withdrawn to just distal to prostate. Prostate is massaged per rectum for 1 minute. Urethral orifice is occluded, and 5 mL of saline is infused and then aspirated for cytology and culture.

E. Blind perineal prostatic aspirate

1. Can be a useful technique to identify prostatic neoplasia; may be dangerous with large prostatic abscesses, because perforation may result in ruptured abscess and bacterial contamination of caudal abdomen or surrounding tissue

2. Use spinal needle, 2–3$^1/_2$ inches long

3. Palpate prostate rectally and stabilize with index finger. (Assistant may need to push prostate over the brim of the pelvis with caudal abdominal palpation).

4. Clip and prepare perirectal area.

5. Guide needle into prostate. Stabilize needle, remove stylet, and have assistant aspirate for cytology and culture.

F. Ultrasound-guided aspirate/biopsy

1. May be required for definitive diagnosis

2. Avoid biopsy if you suspect prostatic infection, abscess.

3. May result in peritonitis if abscess ruptures

III. MANAGEMENT OF SPECIFIC CONDITIONS

A. Dystocia

1. Rule out pseudocyesis and failure to conceive with physical examination, history, abdominal radiographs, plasma progesterone test, and/or ultrasound.

2. Rule out abnormalities in fetal size, fetal positioning, maternal conformation (pelvic canal, vagina, vestibule) through sterile vaginal examination, radiographs.

3. Abdominal ultrasound is the most useful technique for detecting fetal viability.

4. Reasons to seek veterinary assistance:

    a. Crying/biting at vulva area

    b. No sign of labor 24–36 hours after temperature drops below 100°F.

    c. Abnormal vaginal discharge: foul odor, profuse hemorrhage, green without production of offspring

    d. More than 1 week overdue

    e. No fetus produced 4 hours after onset of labor

    f. Strong contractions for more than 50–60 minutes without birth

    g. Fetal membranes in vulva for longer than 15 minutes

    h. Toxemia of bitch

    i. More than 3 hours between births; failure to deliver all offspring within 18–24 hours

5. Manual assistance is indicated when offspring caught in pelvic canal.

    a. Apply diluted lubricant around offspring with soft catheter and syringe.

    b. Use sterile gloves. Grasp fetus and gently rock. Push up on abdomen and pull fetus caudoventrally.

    c. Avoid obstetrical instruments if possible—may perforate/traumatize bitch.

6. Medical stimulation of uterus

    a. Indicated if cervix is dilated, normal fetal presentation, birth canal not obstructed, weak or absent contractions

    b. Oxytocin: 1–2 mg/kg, not to exceed 20 U IM q30 min ×3 or as IV drip (10 U/L) to effect

    c. If no improvement, 10% calcium gluconate: 1–3 mL in cat or 3–5 mL in dog slow IV bolus (monitor ECG)

    d. 0.5 g/kg 10% dextrose IV if no response

7. Cesarean section

    a. Indications: narrow pelvis, uterine torsion, oversized fetus, no response to above medical therapy

    b. Ovariohysterectomy indicated if dead/necrotic fetuses, uterine rupture, unwanted future pregnancies

    c. Anesthetic considerations

        1) Supportive care with IV fluids and supplemental oxygen should be administered prior to anesthesia if the dam is dehydrated or toxic.

        2) Premedications

            a) *Glycopyrrolate—does not readily cross placenta*

            b) *Metoclopramide—enhances gastric emptying, reduces nausea*

            c) *Ranitidine—helps prevent esophagitis, aspiration pneumonia from gastric reflux*

        3) Induction/maintenance protocols

            a) *Dog—butorphanol (0.45 mg/kg IM) and diazepam (0.45 mg/kg IM) + mask induction with isoflurane*

            b) *Cat—Midazolam (0.25 mg/kg IV) and ketamine (5 mg/kg IV) for induction; isoflurane for maintenance or local block.*

            c) *Midazolam (0.2 mg/kg IV or 0.5 mg/kg IM) followed by etomidate (1.0–3.0 mg/kg IV). Etomidate can be repeated at low doses if needed.*

            d) *Propofol 6 mg/kg IV for induction, followed by 0.3–0.5 mg/kg/min IV infusion.*

            e) *Epidural in lumbosacral space (peaks at 20 min, lasts 60–90 min)*

                i) *Drug (choose one):*

                    0.5% bupivacaine (1 mL/kg)

                    Morphine (without preservatives) 0.1 mL/kg

                    2% lidocaine without epinephrine 1 mL/3.5–4.5 kg

                ii) *The needle is placed at the indentation between the 7th lumbar vertebra and the sacrum. The dorsal process of L_7 can be palpated just caudal to an imaginary line drawn from the cranial aspect of the wings of the ilium.*

                iii) *Epidural analgesia produces minimal depression of the newborn.*

                iv) *Some bitches may need additional sedation to prohibit movement of the front legs and head.*

8. Resuscitation of neonates

    a. Remove placental membranes from oropharynx; gently suction with bulb syringe or red rubber catheter on syringe.

    b. Carefully wrap in towel to support neck and gently swing neonate with head down to expel fluids if you cannot clear the oropharynx with suction.

c. Stimulate respiration with rough towel drying.

d. Reverse anesthetic agents by applying 1–2 drops of naloxone or flumazenil on tongue or in umbilical vein.

e. Doxapram (1–2 drops on tongue or in umbilical vein) can be used to stimulate respiration.

f. Provide mask oxygen until puppy can nurse. In the case of respiratory arrest, the puppy can be intubated with a small feeding tube and ventilated with 100% O_2.

g. If unable to nurse, rub 50% dextrose on oral mucous membranes or give 2–4 mL/kg 5% dextrose SQ or by the intraosseous route (IO).

h. For bradycardia

Epinephrine 0.1 mL/kg IV or IO (1:10,000)
Atropine 0.03 mg/kg IM, IV, IO

i. Keep warm and dry.

B. Mastitis

1. Common bacteria—*E. coli*, *Staphylococcus aureus*, β-hemolytic streptococci

2. Cytology of milk reveals degenerate neutrophils, intracellular bacteria, and macrophages.

3. Antibiotics with good penetration of mammary tissue include trimethoprim sulfa, erythromycin, lincomycin, clindamycin, ampicillin, cephalosporins, and chloramphenicol. Avoid aminoglycosides.

4. For galactostasis (red, swollen, hard, painful glands—no abscessation or necrosis), apply hot compresses and allow offspring to nurse to encourage drainage. Observe offspring carefully for signs of dehydration or toxicity.

5. Remove offspring immediately if bitch is febrile or persistent crying of offspring is noted.

6. To promote drying of secretions, wean offspring, reduce caloric intake, and give furosemide (0.5 mg/kg q12h) for two to three doses. This approach is usually best when offspring are at least 3 weeks old.

7. Abscessed, necrotic, or gangrenous mammary glands require surgical debridement, drainage, and flushing. Remove offspring from bitch.

8. Give supportive care with IV fluids until stable; systemic antibiotics for 10–21 days.

C. Pyometritis

1. Middle-aged intact female dogs and cats during diestrus (4 weeks–4 months postestrus)

2. May be open cervix (purulent vaginal discharge present) or closed cervix (more prone to endotoxemia and sepsis)

3. Clinical signs—anorexia, depression, lethargy, vomiting, polyuria, polydypsia, ±shock

4. Laboratory values—leukocytosis ±left shift, elevated BUN and creatinine, low urine specific gravity despite dehydration, proteinuria, pyuria

5. Renal impairment may be reversible. Prerenal azotemia, impaired concentration secondary to *E. coli* endotoxins, and immune-mediated glomerulonephritis are potentially reversible causes of azotemia that may be corrected with aggressive fluid therapy and surgical removal of the infected uterus.

6. Abdominal radiographs and ultrasound reveal homogeneous enlargement of both uterine horns.

7. Stabilize the patient for ovariohysterectomy with IV fluids, bacteriocidal antibiotics, and correction of acid–base and electrolyte abnormalities.

8. Prostaglandins (PGs) can be used in valuable breeding animals when surgery is not an option.

a. Dogs: 0.25 mg/kg $PGF_{2\alpha}$ (Lutalyse, Upjohn) SQ SID for 5 days. Repeat in 2 weeks if vaginal discharge is still present.

b. Cats—0.1 mg/kg SQ SID for 3–5 days

c. Broad-spectrum antibiotics should be administered concurrently and continued for 3–4 weeks.

d. Breed on next estrus.

e. Side effects (vomiting, nausea, anxiety, tachycardia) are common but usually not serious.

f. Avoid synthetic prostaglandins (too potent).

D. Eclampsia

1. Usually occurs in small-breed dogs, rarely in cats within first 21 days after whelping.

2. Hypocalcemia results when calcium loss through lactation exceeds calcium absorption from bones and the gastrointestinal (GI) tract.

3. Early signs include restlessness, panting, pacing, salivation, tremors, whining, and stiffness.

4. Later signs include tonic–clonic muscle spasms, miosis, fever, tachycardia, seizures, coma, and death.

5. Treatment is based on clinical signs:

a. Give calcium gluconate slowly IV to effect (3–20 mL of 10% solution until patient "licks its lips").

1) Muscle tremors will subside and patient will become more alert.

2) Monitor ECG—Stop injection if arrhythmias or bradycardia occur.

b. Administer IV fluids to correct dehydration and/or hypoglycemia.

c. Repeat same dosage of *calcium gluconate* diluted 50:50 with saline by subcutaneous injection.

d. Administer oral calcium (50 mg/kg q8h) during lactation until offspring are weaned.

e. Wean offspring early. Hand raise if problem reoccurs.

f. Avoid calcium supplementation during gestation—reduces GI absorption and inhibits parahormone secretion for maintaining calcium homeostasis.

g. Never give *calcium chloride* SQ or IM— causes tissue necrosis and skin sloughs.

E. Acute metritis

1. This is a bacterial infection of the uterus that occurs 1–7 days after parturition.

2. May be secondary to dystocia, obstetrical manipulation, retained fetuses or placental membranes, poor sanitation

3. Clinical signs include fever, vomiting, dehydration, foul-smelling vaginal discharge, decreased lactation, and turgid uterus.

4. Vaginal cytology reveals degenerate neutrophils and bacteria.

5. Treatment—supportive care with IV fluids and bacteriocidal antibiotics followed by ovariohysterectomy

6. Alternate therapy—$PGF_{2\alpha}$ (0.25 mg/kg SQ SID for 2–5 days) to promote uterine evacuation; systemic antibiotics for 21 days

7. Remove offspring and hand raise.

F. Uterine prolapse

1. More common in cats than dogs

2. Occurs following parturition or spontaneous abortion

3. Attempt external reduction.

a. Anesthetize animal.

b. Lubricate liberally with sterile lubricant.

c. Flush sterile saline into uterine horn under pressure.

d. Administer 5–10 U of oxytocin IM after replacing uterus.

e. Cervix should close 24 hours after parturition, preventing further prolapses.

4. Internal reduction can be accomplished if necessary with a ventral abdominal incision and laparotomy

5. Ovariohysterectomy is recommended if the tissue is damaged or necrotic.

6. If reduction is impossible because of extreme engorgement, the external segment can be amputated followed by ovariohysterectomy.

7. A ruptured uterine or ovarian artery may cause hemorrhagic shock—a serious complication.

G. Uterine torsion

1. This is an uncommon condition of the gravid uterus involving one or both horns or the entire uterus.

2. Clinical signs of dystocia, abdominal pain, and shock

3. Abdominal radiographs reveal a fluid-filled uterus, fetal skeletons, and intrauterine gas.

4. Treatment—ovariohysterectomy and supportive care for shock

H. Postpartum hemorrhage

1. Excessive bleeding may indicate uterine tear, vessel rupture, coagulation defect, or subinvolution of placental sites (SIPS).

a. Possible coagulation defects include von Willebrand's disease, anticoagulant rodenticide toxicity, thrombocytopenia, and disseminated intravascular coagulation (DIC).

2. Diagnosis/treatment

a. Obtain baseline hematocrit and coagulation tests.

1) von Willebrand's disease—all coagulation test results normal except buccal bleeding time

2) Anticoagulant toxicity—prolongation of prothrombin time (PT), elevated proteins involved in vitamin K antagonism (PIVKA)

3) Thrombocytopenia—decreased platelet count

4) DIC—prolongation of PT, partial thromboplastin time (PTT), activated clotting time (ACT); decreased platelets; decreased fibrinogen; increased fibrin degradation products

b. Administer 5–20 U of oxytocin IM to cause involution of uterus.

c. Monitor for continued hemorrhage and shock.

d. Administer transfusion if hemorrhage continues ±exploratory laparotomy and ovariohysterectomy to identify and correct source of bleeding.

  e. Subinvolution of placental sites
  1) Occurs in healthy bitches (most commonly first-time breeders) with serosanguinous vaginal discharge >3 weeks post-whelping.
  2) Negative for brucellosis, coagulopathy, or infection
  3) Ergonovine maleate (0.002–0.05 mg/kg IM) may stop hemorrhage by causing vasoconstriction of uterine vessels.
  4) Definitive treatment is ovariohysterectomy.

I. Spontaneous abortion

1. If possible examine offspring for fetal abnormalities.
2. Culture fetal lung and liver for *Brucella* sp., *Campylobacter* sp., *Mycoplasma* sp., staphylococci, streptococci, and coliforms.
3. Submit serologic tests for brucellosis, toxoplasmosis, canine herpesvirus (dog) and feline leukemia virus, feline infectious peritonitis, feline immunodeficiency virus, feline herpes virus, and toxoplasmosis (cats).
4. Assess viability of remaining fetuses with ultrasound (may continue to term).
5. If no viable fetus is present, promote uterine evacuation with $PGF_{2\alpha}$ (0.25 mg/kg SQ) or consider ovariohysterectomy.

J. Pregnancy termination

1. Avoid estradiol or diethylstilbestrol because of side effects (bone marrow suppression, aplastic anemia, endometritis, pyometritis, prolonged estrus).
2. Consider ovariohysterectomy if future offspring are not wanted.
3. Pregnancy termination can be confirmed after forced abortion with abdominal ultrasound or by measuring plasma progesterone levels <1 ng/mL for 2 consecutive days.
4. $PGF_{2\alpha}$ (Lutalyse, Upjohn)
  a. Administer 0.25 mg/kg SQ q12h for 4–9 days.
  1) Side effects—salivation, panting, emesis, trembling, whining (not life threatening)
  2) Side effects are reduced if dam is walked for 20–30 minutes after injection. Severity usually decreases as treatment progresses.
  3) Progesterone levels must be <2 ng/mL for 2–3 days for abortion to occur.
  b. Discontinue prostaglandin injections when abdominal ultrasound indicates complete uterine evacuation.

  c. Prostaglandin treatment is recommended for midgestation abortion. It is given approximately 30 days after breeding.
  d. Prostaglandin may also be effective for early pregnancy termination if administered at the same dose on days 5–10 of diestrus. Treatment can be repeated on day 30 if pregnancy is still viable.

5. $PGF_{2\alpha}$ plus intravaginal misoprostol
  a. Misoprostol (1–3 μg/kg SID intravaginally) promotes cervical dilation, causes more rapid abortion, allows reduced PG dose.
  b. $PGF_{2\alpha}$—Give 0.1 mg/kg SC q8h for 2 days, then 0.2 mg/kg SC q8h to effect. Abortion usually occurs after 5 days.

6. Synthetic PGs can be used, but are much more potent and must be diluted carefully according to the following protocol:
  a. Cloprostenol (Estrumate, Mallinckrodt; 250 μg/mL) should be diluted 1:10 in saline (9 mL saline + 1 mL Estrumate). The dose is 1 mL/10 kg (2.5 μg/kg) or 1 mL/25 kg (1 μg/kg). The diluted solution should not be reused.
  b. Dose: 1–2.5 μg/kg SC q24–48h for 5 days (25–30 days after breeding)

7. Side effects can be reduced by combining dopamine agonists with low-dose PGs.
  a. Bromocriptine, 10 μg/kg q8h PO
  b. $PGF_{2\alpha}$, 100 μg/kg SC q8h
  c. Discontinue bromocriptine when abortion begins.
  d. Continue $PGF_{2\alpha}$ for 2 days longer.

8. A highly effective drug, the progesterone antagonist (aglepristone—RU534), is available for veterinary use in some European countries. Two injections (10 mg/kg SC 24 hours apart) will terminate pregnancy between days 1 and 45 of gestation with no side effects.

K. Acute bacterial prostatitis

1. Clinical signs—fever, anorexia, lethargy, hemorrhagic or purulent urethral discharge, stiff gait, painful prostate, $\pm$dysuria, $\pm$tenesmus
2. Inflammatory urinalysis (pyuria, hematuria, bacteriuria)
  a. Culture urine by cystocentesis.
  b. Perform Gram stain to aid antibiotic selection.
  c. Common bacteria—*E. coli*, staphylococci, streptococci, *Mycoplasma* spp.

3. Abdominal radiographs, ultrasound
   a. Metastasis to pelvic bones, sublumbar lymphadenopathy, prostatomegaly seen with neoplasia
   b. Prostatic cysts, abscesses may need surgical drainage. Septic shock and peritonitis can result from a ruptured prostatic abscess.
4. Recommended antibiotics include trimethoprim sulfa, enrofloxacin, clavulanic acid–amoxicillin, and chloramphenicol for 3–4 weeks.
5. Supportive care includes IV fluids, stool softeners, and castration.
6. Urine culture, prostatic wash should be performed 1 week after completion of antibiotic therapy to rule out persistent chronic infection.

L. Testicular torsion

1. Occurs most often in cryptorchid dogs—Intraabdominal testicle more prone to torsion and neoplasia.
2. Clinical signs—acute abdominal pain; palpable abdominal mass; slow stiff gait; vomiting, shock
3. Treatment—castration through abdominal approach and supportive care

M. Paraphimosis

1. Inability to retract penis into prepuce
2. Clinical signs: engorged penis; excessive licking; drying or necrosis of exposed penis; stranguria, hematuria, anuria
3. Preputial hair may cause penile strangulation. Other causes include trauma, infection, and neoplasia.
4. Initiated/aggravated by sexual excitement

5. Treatment
   a. Sedate or anesthetize dog.
   b. Clean exposed penis. Gently remove hair; debride if necessary. Apply liberal amount of lubrication and attempt replacement in prepuce.
   c. Hyperosmotic solutions or preputial incision may aid replacement.
   d. If necessary, the preputial opening can be surgically enlarged on the dorsocranial aspect.
   e. The prepuce can be flushed daily with diluted Nolvasan, and the penis extruded to prevent adhesions from forming.
   f. If stranguria is present, a urethral catheter should be placed and the bladder emptied.
   g. In rare instances (thrombosis, necrosis, anuria), penile amputation, castration, and scrotal urethrostomy may be necessary.

N. Testicular tumors

1. Occur in older dogs (9–11 years old)
2. May cause signs of feminization—bilateral symmetrical alopecia, gynecomastia, hyperpigmentation of inguinal skin, and attraction of male dogs
3. May cause prostatic enlargement
4. Tumor types—Sertoli cell, seminoma, interstitial cell
5. Estrogen-producing tumors cause bone marrow suppression—thrombocytopenia, aplastic anemia, leukopenia.
6. May need fresh whole blood transfusion for anemia and thrombocytopenia before surgery.
7. Orchiectomy is the definitive treatment.
8. Prognosis for dogs with bone marrow suppression is guarded to grave.

CHAPTER 17

PEDIATRIC EMERGENCIES

I. RESUSCITATION OF NEONATES (BIRTH TO 2 WEEKS)

A. Clinical signs of sick neonate

1. Constant crying—unusual for neonate to cry longer than 20 minutes
2. Poor muscle tone/listlessness—unable to nurse or remain with bitch/queen/littermates
3. Mucous membranes pale, gray, or cyanotic
4. Flexor dominance—abnormal after 3 days of age
5. Diarrhea
6. Absent/diminished bowel sounds
7. Weight loss or failure to gain weight: Healthy puppies should gain 1–1.5 g/day for each pound of expected adult weight. A gram scale is necessary to allow proper dosing of drugs, nutrition, and fluid therapy.

B. Procedures used in neonates

1. Intraosseous fluids: An 18- to 20-gauge needle inserted through the trochanteric fossa of the proximal femur provides a route for administering fluids, drugs, and blood products when venous access is difficult (*Fig. 17-1*).
    a. Other sites for intraosseous administration include tibial tuberosity, greater tubercle of humerus, and wing of the ilium.
    b. Using a spinal needle with a stylet or a commercially marketed intraosseous needle (Cook) avoids the complication of needle impaction with cortical bone.
2. Subcutaneous fluids: Isotonic crystalloids can be given subcutaneously at 1 mL/25 g body weight (BW) q4–6h prn; 2.5% dextrose in 0.45% NaCl

can be given subcutaneously to correct mild dehydration and prevent hypoglycemia.
3. Intraperitoneal fluids—least preferred route
    a. Neonate is held in dorsal recumbency with hind limbs retracted caudally as 25- to 22-gauge needle is inserted in inguinal region and advanced craniad.
    b. Isotonic crystalloid solutions are absorbed rapidly.
    c. Blood absorbed more slowly; 70% of red blood cells are absorbed within 48–72 hours.
    d. Warmed isotonic fluids can be given to correct hypothermia.

4. Orogastric tube feeding
    a. Necessary when neonate fails to nurse, must be separated from bitch/queen, or is orphaned
    b. Soft red rubber feeding tube is preferred.
    c. Proper tube measurement is critical—measure from nose to last rib and mark tube with tape or indelible ink.
    d. Desired amount of warmed milk replacement formula is drawn into syringe with feeding tube attached (to avoid introducing air into the stomach).
    e. Neonate should be aroused, held in sternal recumbency, and allowed to swallow the tube to avoid intratracheal placement.
    f. After administering the formula, the tube is kinked and quickly withdrawn to prevent aspiration.
    g. The caloric requirement for basal energy can be calculated using the formula $70 \times BW (kg)^{0.75}$ for both kittens and puppies, or the amount fed can be determined on the basis of

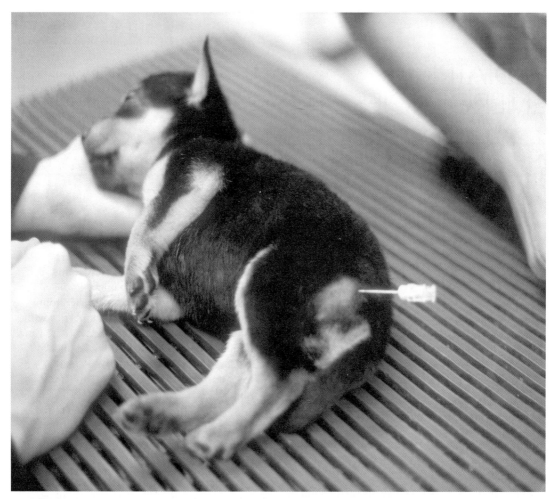

FIGURE 17.1   Correct placement of intraosseous needle in the femur of a neonatal puppy.

weight according to the label of the milk replacer. The total amount should be divided into six feedings and fed every 4 hours.

h. The neonatal stomach capacity of 50 mL/kg should not be exceeded in one feeding.

C. General approach to sick neonate

1. Correct hypothermia

a. Clinical signs of hypothermia include isolation from littermates, crying, and, if severe, weakness, ileus, hypoventilation, bradycardia, and depression/coma.

b. Normal body temperature of neonate is 95–99°F (35–37°C).

c. Gradual rewarming to an ambient temperature of 90–95°F (55–65% humidity) using

neonatal incubator is preferred because it provides internal (warm inspired air) and external heating.

d. Circulating warm water blankets, warm water bottles, and heating pads can be used but should be covered to avoid burns due to direct exposure; neonate should be able to move away from heat source.

e. In critical neonates, internal rewarming can be accomplished by administering warmed fluids via intravenous, intraosseous, or intraperitoneal routes or as an enema.

f. Frequent monitoring of body temperature is necessary to avoid overheating.

g. Feeding should be delayed until temperature is normal and borborygmus sounds are present; digestion will not occur with hypothermia.

2. Correct dehydration

   a. Fluid requirements of neonates exceed those of adults because of their higher surface area/body weight ratio, larger percentage of total body water, and increased losses through immature kidneys and skin.

   b. Estimating dehydration is difficult—skin turgor is not reliable because of their higher water and fat content.

   c. Mucous membranes should be moist and not tacky.

   d. Pale mucous membranes and slow capillary refill time in the absence of anemia indicate severe, 12–15%, dehydration.

   e. Fluids can be administered by intravenous, intraosseous, subcutaneous, or intraperitoneal routes, in order of decreasing preference.

   f. Isotonic crystalloid solutions containing 2.5% dextrose are preferred. (0.45% NaCl with 2.5% dextrose)

   g. Intravenous access is most easily achieved via jugular vein; through the needle catheter cut short, over the needle catheter, or a butterfly catheter can be used.

   h. Before administration, fluids should be warmed to body temperature of the *neonate* (95–99°F).

   i. Fluid rate of 1 mL/30 g over 5–10 minutes can be used initially and repeated at 30-minute intervals until the patient is stable.

   j. Maintenance fluid rate for neonate is 60–180 mL/kg/day.

3. Correct hypoglycemia

   a. Hypoglycemia is *extremely* common in sick neonates because of their limited glycogen stores, immature hepatic function, limited fat to provide free fatty acid substrate, and increased glucose requirement (2–4 times that of adult).

   b. Glucose can be given orally, 1–2 mL of 5–15% dextrose, if hydration and body temperature are normal.

   c. Hypoglycemic neonates with neurologic dysfunction, shock, or severe dehydration should receive 0.25 mL/25 g of 20% dextrose IV or IO.

   d. Nutrition and/or maintenance fluids with 2.5–5% dextrose can be given to maintain normal blood glucose concentration once the neonate has been stabilized.

   e. Avoid giving hypertonic dextrose-containing solutions subcutaneously.

4. Provide nutrition.

   a. Healthy neonates should receive all nutritional requirements from nursing for the first 3–4 weeks of life.

   b. Excessive crying, inactivity, and failure to gain weight indicate the need for nutritional support.

   c. Oral milk replacement formulas are used; Esbilac (Pet Ag, Inc; Elgin, IL) for puppies, KMR (same) for kittens.

   d. Stomach capacity of neonate is approximately 50 mL/kg.

   e. Daily caloric requirements for puppies and kittens of nursing age is approximately 100 Kcal/day.

   f. Initially, puppies are fed 10 mL q4–6h, and kittens are fed 5 mL q4–6h of warmed milk replacement formula.

   g. Feeding volume is increased 1 mL/feeding (dog) or 1 mL/day (cat) until requirements are met.

   h. The perineum or ventral abdomen is rubbed gently with cotton soaked in warm water after each feeding to stimulate urination and defecation.

   i. If diarrhea occurs, the formula should be diluted 1:2 with an oral balanced electrolyte solution (e.g., Pedialyte) until diarrhea resolves; gradually switch back to full-strength formula. (Normal stool is yellow to brown with paste consistency. Puppies with diarrhea have liquid stool with red, edematous anus).

D. Management of specific conditions

1. Neonatal dermatitis (acute moist dermatitis of neonates)

   a. Characterized by superficial yellow pustules on head, neck, ventral abdomen, or inguinal fold that appear between 4 and 10 days of age

   b. Lesions may crust or scab.

   c. Poor sanitation may be a predisposing factor.

   d. Treatment involves bactericidal shampoo and, in severe cases, systemic antibiotics. (amoxicillin–clavulanate, 10–20 mg/kg BID PO; cephalexin, 20 mg/kg BID PO).

   e. The neonate's environment should be thoroughly disinfected.

   f. Spontaneous resolution usually occurs after 4 months of age.

2. Umbilical infection

   a. Usually occurs during first 4 days of life.

b. Clinical signs include redness, swelling, or purulent discharge from umbilicus, anorexia, lethargy, and abdominal distention.

c. Infection is most commonly due to *Streptococcus* spp., though other organisms may be involved.

d. Treatment involves systemic antibiotics (amoxicillin or cephalexin), topical therapy with dilute Betadine or Nolvasan solution, and establishing drainage when necessary.

e. Prevention involves proper sanitation and disinfecting umbilicus at birth.

3. Neonatal conjunctivitis (ophthalmia neonatorum)

　　a. Characterized by swelling and purulent discharge from beneath eyelids prior to lid separation at 10–16 days of age

　　b. Usually bilateral

　　c. May be associated with herpesvirus infection in kittens

　　d. Treatment involves warm compress followed by gentle separation of eyelids, flushing with sterile saline or eyewash solution to remove discharge, topical antibiotic ointment, and cleaning periocular tissues.

　　e. Prognosis for vision is usually excellent; corneal scarring or deep corneal ulceration with globe rupture rarely occurs.

4. Neonatal septicemia

　　a. Clinical signs include persistent crying, abdominal distention, tachypnea, and, in severe cases, weakness, coma, and death.

　　b. Signs may spread from single neonate to littermates within 24 hours.

　　c. Predisposing factors include failure to receive colostrum, dissemination of umbilical or skin infection, nursing from bitch/queen with mastitis or metritis, and/or environmental problems such as poor sanitation, poor ventilation, and excess humidity.

　　d. Causative organisms include *Escherichia coli*, *Streptococcus* spp., *Staphylococcus* spp., *Pseudomonas* spp., and *Proteus* spp.

　　e. Necropsy abnormalities include serosal petechiation and gas-filled intestines.

　　f. Treatment involves isolating affected neonates and administering fluids, antibiotics, and supportive care *(Table 17-1)*.

5. Canine herpesvirus.

　　a. Infection usually occurs from 1 to 3 weeks of age; in utero infection is possible.

b. Clinical signs include acute onset of lethargy, crying, anorexia, hypothermia, bloating, and death within 18 hours.

c. The entire litter may be affected; subsequent litters are often completely normal.

d. Diagnosis may be made on the basis of clinical signs or necropsy findings of hemorrhagic lesions and intranuclear inclusions within kidneys, liver, and lungs.

e. Treatment involves increasing ambient temperature to 100°F for several hours then 90–95°F (inhibits viral replication, which occurs at lower temperatures), administering fluids, and providing nutrition (Table 17-1).

f. Prognosis is poor.

6. Toxic milk syndrome

　　a. Clinical signs include crying, abdominal distention, green diarrhea, edematous rectum, and discomfort in puppies 3–14 days of age.

　　b. May be caused by incompatibility to, or toxins (bacterial, other) in, milk.

　　c. Bitch may have mastitis, metritis, or uterine subinvolution.

　　d. Treatment involves removing puppies from bitch, supplementing dextrose, and maintaining hydration until abdominal distention resolves, then feeding milk replacement formula.

　　e. Neonate may be reintroduced to bitch if infection (mastitis/metritis) is eliminated.

7. Fading puppy/kitten syndrome

　　a. Characterized by a healthy puppy/kitten at birth that fails to thrive and dies within the first 3–4 weeks of life.

　　b. Affected neonates may be normal to below normal body weight at birth but develop anorexia, weakness, and weight loss proceeding to emaciation within 3–4 weeks.

　　c. Many causes are implicated including congenital abnormalities, teratogenic effects, trauma during or shortly after birth, possibly low birth weight, toxins, environmental factors, infection, neonatal isoerythrolysis, thymus dysfunction, feline leukemia virus (FeLV), feline immunodeficiency virus (FIV), feline infectious peritonitis (FIP) and canine herpesvirus.

　　d. In most cases, no cause is identified.

　　e. Treatment involves correcting any underlying cause if known and providing supportive care

---

TABLE 17.1
MANAGEMENT OF A SEPTICEMIC PUPPY OR KITTEN

I. Place IV or intraosseous catheter. Obtain blood for PCV, TS, blood glucose.

II. Parenteral fluid therapy
   A. Weigh neonate on gram scale to get accurate weight.
   B. Estimate percent dehydration. Puppies or kittens in shock will be 10–12% dehydrated.
   C. For initial resuscitation, calculate amount of fluid needed to restore deficit and divide into 4 parts [(% Dehydration ×BW (kg) = Fluid (mL) needed]. Administer by slow IV or intraosseous bolus every 15 minutes until color, CRT, and pulse quality improve.
   D. Fluids should be warmed before administration. Use a balanced electrolyte solution supplemented with 5% dextrose.
   E. After initial resuscitation, decrease fluid rate to 90–180 mL/kg/day. Add KCl (20 mEq/L) to prevent hypokalemia.
   F. If anemia or hypoproteinemia is present; blood, plasma, or hetastarch may be indicated. A total dose of 20 mL/kg can be given over 4 hours, and the crystalloid infusion temporarily discontinued before being started again at a reduced rate of 40–60 mL/kg/day.

III. Glucose replacement
   A. Animals with seizures, profound depression, or known hypoglycemia should receive 1 mL/kg of 50% dextrose diluted to a 5–10% solution to restore normoglycemia immediately.
   B. Blood glucose concentration should be monitored q4–6h and maintained in the range of 80–250 mg/dL.

IV. Antimicrobial therapy
   A. Collect culture samples (blood, urine, exudate, feces).
      1. For blood culture, collect 1 mL aseptically and inoculate directly into 5–10 mL of enriched broth. Examine for bacterial growth in 6–18 hours.
      2. Collect urine by cystocentesis.
   B. Begin empirical treatment by IV or IO route.
      1. Cefoxitin: 15–30 mg/kg IV q6–8h
      2. Timentin: 40–50 mg/kg IV q6–8h

V. External warming
   A. Use circulating hot water blanket, rice bags, or hot water bottles or place in environment with warm inspired air or heat lamp.
   B. Do not place animal directly on heating pad, and make sure it is able to move away from the heat source.
   C. Record rectal temperature hourly and turn animal.

VI. Provide oxygen and nutrition
   A. Administer oxygen by mask, nasal catheter, or neonatal incubator to prevent tissue ischemia.
   B. Begin enteral nutrition after hypothermia, hypoglycemia, and dehydration are corrected.

VII. Monitor
   A. Watch for signs of overhydration—serous nasal discharge, tachypnea, labored breathing, pulmonary crackles.
   B. Assess hydration—mucous membrane color, CRT, urine output.
   C. Weigh 3–4 times daily.
   D. Observe for improved demeanor and mentation.

(fluids, nutrition, proper environmental conditions).

   f. Prognosis is poor.

8. Neonatal isoerythrolysis

   a. Hemolytic disease that occurs in type A (or AB) kittens that receive colostral anti-A antibody from queens that are blood type B.

   b. Kittens are normal at birth; signs appear hours to days after nursing and receiving colostrum.

c. In severe cases, peracute death occurs.

d. In milder cases, kittens develop pallor, icterus, hemoglobinuria, weakness, tachypnea, and tachycardia typical of hemolytic anemia.

e. Unusual presentations include tail tip necrosis (a form of cold agglutinin disease) or subclinical Coombs'-positive anemia.

f. Treatment involves immediate removal of affected kittens from the queen, bottle or tube feeding milk replacement formula, and, if anemia is severe, blood transfusion.

g. Blood for transfusion must be compatible with the *queen's* type B blood, since her anti-A antibody is the only antibody circulating in the neonatal kitten.
  1) Ideal donor is the queen.
  2) Washed type B blood can be used.
  3) Blood can be administered at 20 mL/kg over 2 hours IV or IO.
  4) Oxyglobin (20 mL/kg IV over 4 hours) can be given in lieu of blood.

h. Subsequent transfusions after 5 days, if necessary, should be of washed type A blood, since kitten forms its own anti-B antibodies soon after birth.

i. Kittens may be allowed to nurse again, 24 hours after birth, because colostral antibodies will no longer be absorbed.

9. Trauma

a. Traumatic injuries may occur during difficult birth (obstetrical instruments, manipulation) or after birth (stepped/laid on, falls, bite wounds, etc.).

b. Clinical signs depend on cause and extent of traumatic injury.

c. Treatment is similar to that for adult trauma, with added emphasis on maintaining normothermia and normoglycemia and providing nutrition.

d. Prognosis is favorable even with severe trauma because of the resilient nature of the neonate.

II. DISEASES OF INFANT ANIMALS (2-6 WEEKS)

A. Parasites

1. Internal

a. Neonates may have heavy burdens of roundworms (*Toxocara canis/Toxascaris leonina*) and/or hookworms (*Ancylostoma*) at 2–4 weeks of age.

b. *Toxacara* sp. may be transmitted across the placenta; *Ancylostoma* may be ingested through dam's milk.

c. Protozoal parasites affecting neonates include *Giardia* and coccidia.

d. Clinical signs of intestinal parasites include diarrhea, anorexia, lethargy, and poor weight gain.

e. Treatment for roundworms and hookworms includes pyrantel pamoate (5–10 mg/kg PO) repeated every 3 weeks until 12 weeks of age.

f. Giardiasis is treated with metronidazole (60 mg/kg PO q24h for 5 days) or fenbendazole (50 mg/kg PO q24h for 3–5 days).

g. Coccidiosis is treated with sulfadimethoxine 50 mg/kg on the first day, followed by 25 mg/kg/day for 10 days or until signs resolve.

h. Hookworms may cause life-threatening anemia in neonates, requiring transfusion of whole blood, packed red blood cells, or Oxyglobin at 20 mL/kg given over 2 hours through a Millepora filter.

i. Ferrous sulfate (50–100 mg PO q24h) or iron dextran injections (10–20 mg/kg SC) should be given with blood loss anemias.

j. Proper deworming of bitch/queen prior to pregnancy and good husbandry should prevent severe infestation.

2. External

a. Severe flea infestation may cause life-threatening anemia and should be treated by flea removal and transfusion if necessary (see Section 1.h above for transfusion protocol).

b. Most flea and tick products are not safe for use on nursing animals; some pyrethrins contain appropriate label instructions. Advantage (Bayer) or Capstar can also be used safely in neonates.

c. For safe removal of fleas, spray a towel with pyrethrin insecticide and wrap neonate leaving head exposed; dead fleas can be combed or rinsed away using *warm* water (to avoid hypothermia).

d. The bitch/queen should be treated, but nipples should be avoided or rinsed.

e. Blankets and bedding should be cleaned or discarded.

B. Hypoglycemia

1. Juvenile

a. Caused by the same factors that result in hypoglycemia in neonates (see p. 343).

b. Clinical signs include weakness, tremors, facial muscle twitching, seizures, and coma.

c. Emergency treatment is similar to that described above for neonates (p. 343).

d. Fluids containing 2.5–10% dextrose are administered intravenously or intraosseously with frequent (q4–6h) blood glucose monitoring until the juvenile is eating and maintaining normoglycemia.

e. Dextrose concentrations above 5% should be given only through the jugular vein or intraosseously to avoid hyperosmolar phlebitis.

f. Juvenile hypoglycemia resolves spontaneously as puppy/kitten develops mature glycogen stores.

2. Fatty liver syndrome (hepatic steatosis)

   a. Occurs almost exclusively in toy breeds 4–16 weeks of age.

   b. Often preceded by a period of anorexia after a stressful event.

   c. Clinical signs include acute-onset anorexia, depression, persistent crying, and diarrhea in addition to typical signs of hypoglycemia.

   d. Death occurs within 1–6 days in spite of aggressive attempts at resuscitation and supportive care.

3. Glycogen storage disease

   a. Glycogen storage diseases are hereditary deficiencies of glycogenolytic enzymes that inhibit the production of glucose from glycogen, resulting in an inability to maintain normal glucose homeostasis.

   b. Breeds predisposed include toy breeds, Maltese, and German Shepherds.

   c. Enzyme deficiencies result in glycogen accumulation in liver, hepatomegaly, and hypoglycemia.

   d. Clinical signs are due to hypoglycemia.

   e. Diagnosis is suggested by persistent or recurrent hypoglycemia with hepatomegaly and is confirmed by liver biopsy (glycogen accumulation) and glycogenolytic enzyme assays performed on frozen liver tissue.

   f. Treatment involves frequent glucose feeding between meals and uncooked cornstarch at night (to sustain glucose levels overnight). Prognosis is poor; this is a fatal congenital inborn error of metabolism.

C. Diarrhea

1. Common causes of diarrhea in infants include infection, endoparasites, and dietary factors (overeating, toxic milk syndrome, dietary indiscretion).

2. Dehydration and hypoglycemia are common.

3. Treatment involves removing the underlying cause and maintaining hydration.

4. Milk replacement formula diluted 1:2 with a balanced electrolyte solution or dextrose (5–10%) can be given to maintain hydration and prevent hypoglycemia in mild cases that resolve within 24 hours.

5. More aggressive fluid therapy may be necessary in severe or prolonged cases.

6. Hypokalemia should be anticipated; supplement fluids with KCl (20–40 mEq/L) as necessary.

D. Congenital problems

1. Regurgitation/megaesophagus

   a. Causes include idiopathic megaesophagus, vascular ring anomaly (e.g., persistent right aortic arch), and myasthenia gravis (MG).

   b. Breeds predisposed to congenital idiopathic megaesophagus include Great Dane, German Shepherd, Irish Setter, Labrador Retriever, Sharpei dogs, and Siamese cats.

   c. Breeds predisposed to vascular ring anomalies include Irish Setter, Boston Terrier, German Shepherd; less common in cats, no breed predisposition

   d. Breeds predisposed to congenital MG include the Jack Russell Terrier, Springer Spaniel, and Smooth Fox Terrier.

   e. Clinical signs often develop at weaning with the introduction of solid food.

   f. Diagnosis is based on regurgitation of undigested food, often in tubular shape, and radiographic evidence of dilated esophagus.

     1) Generalized dilation is seen with idiopathic megaesophagus and MG.

     2) Focal dilation of the esophagus cranial to the heart is seen with vascular ring anomalies.

   g. MG in juveniles may be congenital (deficiency of acetylcholine receptors) or acquired (autoimmune response against receptors).

     1) Diagnosis of congenital MG requires assay of fresh frozen intercostal muscle to determine receptor concentration.

     2) Diagnosis of acquired MG is made by demonstrating increased serum anti-acetylcholine receptor antibody concentration.

   h. Aspiration pneumonia is a potentially life-threatening complication of megaesophagus of any cause.

i. Treatment includes broad-spectrum antibiotics if aspiration pneumonia is present and upright feeding.

j. MG can be treated with pyridostigmine bromide, 0.5–3 mg/kg BID–TID PO.

k. Surgery is indicated for vascular ring anomaly.

l. Prognosis is guarded to poor with idiopathic megaesophagus and MG.

n. Early surgical intervention prior to permanent dilation of the esophagus may cure juveniles with vascular ring anomalies.

2. Cleft palate

a. Caused by failure of primary (lip/premaxilla) and/or secondary (hard/soft) palate closure.

b. Clinical signs include poor growth, drainage of milk from nares during nursing, nasal discharge, sneezing, and respiratory distress if aspiration pneumonia is present.

c. Diagnosis is made by identifying the defect during examination of the oral cavity.

d. Treatment involves surgical correction of the palate defect and antibiotics for secondary bacterial rhinitis and/or aspiration pneumonia.

3. Hydrocephalus

a. Hydrocephalus is defined as excessive accumulation of cerebrospinal fluid (CSF) within (internal hydrocephalus) or outside (external hydrocephalus) the ventricular system of the brain.

b. Internal hydrocephalus is by far the most common congenital form and is due to structural defects that prevent CSF outflow or absorption.

c. Dog breeds predisposed include small and toy breeds such as Yorkshire Terriers, Chihuahua, and Maltese; uncommon in cats.

d. Clinical signs vary from mild to severe and include depression, ventrolateral strabismus ("sunset sign"), circling, head pressing, blindness, and seizures.

e. Physical examination reveals a dome-shaped calvarium and often an open fontanelle.

f. Skull radiographs may reveal open suture lines and "ground glass" appearance due to lack of cerebral gyri.

g. Ultrasonography through an open fontanelle reveals dilated ventricles.

h. Progression of neurologic signs is variable.

i. Treatment is not necessary for mildly affected dogs with nonprogressive signs.

j. Oral dexamethasone, 0.1 mg/kg every other day, may improve mild neurologic signs; it is less effective in puppies younger than 8–12 weeks of age.

k. Surgical placement of ventriculovenous or ventriculoperitoneal shunt can be considered in severe cases.

l. Prognosis is poor for infants that exhibit severe or progressive neurologic signs due to permanent compressive/ischemic damage to cerebrum.

4. Spinal cord diseases (spinal dysraphism)

a. Spinal dysraphism is defined as failure of neural tube closure leading to congenital abnormalities of the spinal cord, vertebral column, or skin.

b. Spina bifida (failure of vertebral arch closure) is the most common vertebral column abnormality; meninges (meningocele) or meninges with nerve roots (meningomyelocele) protrude through vertebral defect.

c. Sacrocaudal vertebral dysgenesis occurs as an inherited (autosomal dominant) defect in Manx cats.

d. Other vertebral abnormalities include hemivertebra and vertebral stenosis.

e. Lesions affecting the spinal cord include cystic spaces within the parenchyma (syringomyelia), spinal clefts (myeloschisis), and dilated central canal (hydromyelia).

f. Breeds predisposed include brachycephalic dogs and Manx cats.

g. Clinical signs include hind limb paresis/plegia and urinary–fecal incontinence.

h. Diagnosis is based on clinical signs and radiography.

i. With the exception of surgical excision of meningoceles, there is no treatment for most congenital spinal lesions.

5. Heart murmurs

a. Heart murmurs in infants are usually functional or due to congenital heart defects.

b. Functional murmurs are soft early systolic murmurs heard best at the left heart base and are due to increased velocity of blood (fever, excitement) or decreased viscosity of blood (anemia); most resolve by 16 weeks of age.

c. Murmurs associated with congenital heart disease vary with type of disease and persist beyond 16 weeks of age.

d. In dogs, the most common congenital heart defects are patent ductus arteriosus (PDA), aortic stenosis, pulmonic stenosis, and tetralogy of Fallot.

e. In cats, mitral valve malformation, ventricular septal defect, and endocardial elastosis are common.

f. Clinical signs vary, depending on type and severity of defect.

g. Diagnosis is based on results of physical examination, electrocardiography, chest radiographs and echocardiography with Doppler flow analysis.

h. Treatment involves medical management of left- or right-sided congestive heart failure as for adult animals.

i. Surgical correction is possible with PDA, pulmonic stenosis, and possibly tetralogy of Fallot.

III. DISEASES OF JUVENILE ANIMALS (6-12 WEEKS)

A. General considerations

1. At 6–8 weeks of age, renal function, liver function, laboratory parameters (including coagulation parameters), and immunologic status is similar to that of adults.

2. Maintenance fluid requirements (120–180 mL/kg/d) and caloric requirements (180 Kcal/kg/day) still exceed those of adults.

3. Due to loss of maternal antibody during this period, susceptibility to infectious disease increases.

4. Some congenital disorders (e.g., cardiac anomalies) are diagnosed at this age because it is often when puppies/kittens are first examined by a veterinarian.

5. As puppies/kittens become more mobile and curious, the risk of gastrointestinal foreign body, electric cord injury, and trauma increases.

B. Infectious diseases

1. Feline leukemia virus

a. Type C oncornavirus of retrovirus group.

b. Vertical and horizontal transmission places juveniles at risk of exposure and infection.

c. Saliva is the most important route of horizontal transmission.

d. Susceptibility to persistent infection after exposure is highest in neonates (70–80%), decreases to 30–50% in cats older than 8 weeks of age, and is less than 30% in adolescent/adult cats.

e. Virus-induced thymic atrophy may cause fading kitten syndrome.

f. May predispose to infection by other viruses, e.g.., panleukopenia, FIV, feline herpesvirus, FIP

g. Clinical signs in juveniles are due to immunosuppressive effects of virus and include low birth weight and infections of respiratory, urinary, and gastrointestinal tracts.

h. FeLV testing is valid at any age; a positive ELISA for viral p27 antigen is diagnostic for viremia. Test results can revert from positive to negative with latent or cleared infections. The test should be repeated in 1–3 months to confirm persistent infection.

i. False-negative results with the ELISA method may be seen with severe leukopenia and/or thrombocytopenia.

j. A positive IFA test result indicates that infection has progressed through all stages, including bone marrow, and indicates persistent infection.

k. Treatment is supportive and aimed at controlling secondary infections; infected cats should be isolated.

2. Feline immunodeficiency virus

a. Lymphotrophic lentivirus of retrovirus group

b. Juveniles are most commonly exposed by horizontal transmission through oral inoculation or nursing acutely infected queens.

c. Some strains of FIV may cross the placenta and infect kittens before birth.

d. Vertical transmission is less common than with FeLV and occurs most often in queens acutely infected during the first trimester of pregnancy or chronically infected, with a $CD4^+$ count below 200 cells/μL.

e. Clinical signs are indistinguishable from those described above in FeLV-infected juveniles.

f. Diagnosis is made by demonstrating circulating antibodies in serum, plasma, or whole blood.

g. Maternal colostral antibodies may cause false-positive results; therefore, testing kittens less than 4–6 months of age is not recommended.

h. Treatment when the disease is suspected in juveniles is similar to that described above for FeLV-infected kittens.

3. Feline panleukopenia (feline distemper)

a. A member of the parvovirus family—closely related to canine, mink, and raccoon parvovirus

b. The virus is restricted to replicating in rapidly dividing cells (e.g., thymus, bone marrow, intestinal crypt cells).

c. Transmission is by direct contact or exposure to contaminated environment (virus may persist in environment from months to years).

d. Clinical signs include acute onset of fever, lethargy, anorexia followed in 1–2 days by severe vomiting, diarrhea, and dehydration.

e. A peracute form exists with depression, hypothermia, and death within 24 hours.

f. In utero exposure via an infected queen may result in cerebellar hypoplasia due to viral destruction of rapidly dividing cells of the cerebellum.

g. Diagnosis is made by clinical signs, moderate-to-severe neutropenia/lymphopenia (and thrombocytopenia in severe cases), and (in the acute stage) positive results on the CITE test for *canine* parvovirus antigen.

h. Treatment is supportive and consists of intravenous fluids supplemented with potassium, dextrose, and B vitamins and broad-spectrum antibiotics.

i. Affected kittens should be isolated, and the environment thoroughly disinfected.

j. In severe cases, blood transfusion (to transiently increase white cell count, reverse anemia, and replace plasma proteins lost through damaged intestinal mucosa) and nutritional support may be necessary.

k. Recovery in all but the most critical cases is usually complete within 7–14 days and results in protective immunity.

l. Prevention is by vaccination and good husbandry.

m. The final vaccination in the kitten series should be given after 12 weeks of age to avoid interference by maternal immunity.

4. Feline upper respiratory disease complex

   a. The most common etiologic agents are rhinotracheitis (i.e., feline herpesvirus type 1) and calicivirus.

   b. Less common causative agents include *Bordetella, Chlamydia,* and *Mycoplasma* spp.

   c. Clinical signs in most affected kittens include sneezing, oculonasal discharge, conjunctivitis, fever, lethargy, and anorexia.

   d. Rhinotracheitis may also cause ulcerative keratitis and panophthalmitis.

   e. Calicivirus may also cause ulcerative stomatitis, pneumonia, and arthritis.

   f. The disease complex is highly contagious and may affect all cats in household or cattery.

   g. The diagnosis is made by history and clinical signs.

   h. Viral isolation or serologic testing may be useful in cattery situations.

   i. Treatment for mild infections consists of outpatient antibiotics (amoxicillin, 20 mg/kg BID PO, or amoxicillin/clavulanate, 12.5–25 mg/kg BID PO), topical antibiotic ointment if conjunctivitis is present (tetracycline or chloramphenicol ointment), and nursing care (remove discharge from eyes/nares, heat food and/or add tuna/clam juice to encourage appetite).

   j. Treatment for anorectic, dehydrated, or debilitated cats includes hospitalization for intravenous fluids, intravenous antibiotics, and nutritional support.

   k. Hospitalized patients MUST be isolated due to the highly contagious nature of the disease.

   l. Prolonged hospitalization (days to weeks) is necessary in the most severe cases, but outcome is usually good.

   m. Sequelae of upper respiratory disease include nasopharyngeal polyp, pneumonia, scarring of the nasolacrimal duct leading to persistent ocular discharge, chronic rhinitis due to viral destruction of nasal mucosa, and recurrent infections during periods of stress (rhinotracheitis).

5. Canine distemper

   a. A member of the Morbillivirus genus of the Paramyxovirus family

   b. Highly contagious viral disease spread by aerosol or infective droplets from body secretions

   c. Most commonly affects dogs from 2 to 6 months of age

   d. The virus replicates in lymphoid tissue, epithelial cells of the respiratory and gastrointestinal tracts, and the nervous system.

   e. Clinical signs of acute distemper include fever, oculonasal discharge, conjunctivitis, rhinitis, vomiting, diarrhea, coughing, anorexia, and dehydration.

   f. Neurologic signs include myoclonus (involuntary muscle twitching), focal facial or "chewing gum" seizures, circling, ataxia, and generalized seizures.

   g. Physical examination may reveal enamel hypoplasia (most obvious in canine teeth) due to direct viral injury to ameloblastic layer during dental development.

h. Hyperkeratosis of footpads ("hard pad" disease) may be present.

i. Chorioretinitis may be detected during retinal examination.

j. Diagnosis is made by history and the combination of respiratory, gastrointestinal, and neurologic signs in an incompletely vaccinated or unvaccinated puppy.

k. Lymphopenia is a common laboratory abnormality that supports the diagnosis of distemper.

l. Viral inclusion bodies composed of nuclear capsid are occasionally seen in circulating red blood cells, neutrophils, or lymphocytes.

m. A definitive diagnosis can be made by polymerase chain reaction (PCR) testing for viral RNA on whole blood, virus isolation, or identifying viral inclusions in conjunctival epithelium or blood cells by direct immunofluorescence.

n. Serologic tests may be unreliable in acute distemper because of failure of infected puppies to respond immunologically; a positive IgM titer or rapidly increasing IgG titer may be supportive.

o. Treatment for acute distemper involves supportive measures such as intravenous fluids supplemented with potassium and B vitamins, antibiotics to prevent secondary bacterial infections, and nutritional support.

p. There is no effective treatment for neurologic signs caused by distemper virus.

q. Dogs that survive may develop neurologic sequelae months to years after acute infection.

r. Prevention is by vaccination and good husbandry; the virus is inactivated by routine disinfectants.

6. Canine parvovirus

   a. Canine parvovirus type 1 is found in normal dogs and is pathogenic only in neonates.

   b. Canine parvovirus type 2 emerged as an important pathogen in 1978.

   c. Transmission of this highly contagious disease is by the fecal–oral route as the virus is shed in feces of infected dogs.

   d. The virus replicates in mitotically active cells—primarily intestinal crypt cells, bone marrow, and lymphoid tissue.

   e. Breeds predisposed to severe disease include the Rottweiler, Doberman Pinscher, and Staffordshire Terrier.

   f. Infection is most common in puppies from 6 to 20 weeks of age.

g. Clinical signs include fever, anorexia, lethargy, dehydration, vomiting, and severe bloody diarrhea.

h. Diagnosis is based on clinical signs and positive fecal ELISA results for parvoviral antigen.

i. Vaccination with modified live parvovirus vaccine may cause a weak positive reaction on the fecal ELISA from 5 to 15 days postvaccine; false negative results can occur in acute cases and testing should be repeated if suggestive clinical signs are present.

j. The complete blood count (CBC) typically reveals lymphopenia (direct lymphocytolysis during viremic phase) and neutropenia (peripheral consumption and destruction of white blood cell precursors in the bone marrow).

k. In severe cases, abnormalities in the biochemical profile may include panhypoproteinemia, elevated liver enzymes, and azotemia.

l. Treatment includes intravenous fluids; rate and volume to be administered is dictated by severity of clinical signs and varies from shock doses to 1–2 times maintenance rate.

m. Colloids, hetastarch (20 mL/kg/day) or plasma (10–20 mL/kg) are necessary if serum albumin concentration is less than 1.5 g/dL or total protein is less than 3.5 g/dL.

n. Intravenous broad-spectrum antibiotics, ampicillin (20 mg/kg TID IV) or cefazolin (20 mg/kg TID IV), with the addition of amikacin (20–30 mg/kg SID IV) in severe cases if renal function and hydration are normal or enrofloxacin (5 mg/kg IV BID).

o. Antiemetic therapy with metoclopramide (0.2–0.5 mg/kg IV or IM TID or 1–2 mg/kg/day by constant infusion) or chlorpromazine (0.5 mg/kg IM or SC) can be given if vomiting is severe.

p. For severe neutropenia, granulocyte colony-stimulating factor can be given at 5 μg/kg q24h SC, though cost and questionable efficacy limit its use.

q. Serum from recovered dogs (2–4 mL/kg IV) or plasma (5–10 mL/kg IV) can provide passive immunity and may shorten the duration of illness and limit severity when given in conjunction with standard treatment.

r. Nutritional support may be necessary in prolonged cases. Early enteral nutrition dripped in slowly through a nasoesophageal tube can shorten the hospitalization time and repair damaged enterocytes.

s. Strict isolation procedures are indicated because of the extremely contagious nature of this disease.

t. Prevention is by vaccination and good husbandry.

u. Parvovirus is extremely resistant and can survive in the environment for months to years; bleach is the only effective disinfectant.

C. Electric cord bite

1. The curiosity of puppies and kittens predisposes them to electric cord injury.

2. Common injuries include burns of the tongue, oral mucous membranes, and commissures of the lips.

3. A potential life-threatening complication of electric shock is noncardiogenic pulmonary edema resulting in severe respiratory distress.

4. Treatment for juveniles with mild thermal injury consists of wound debridement and broad-spectrum antibiotics.

5. Treatment for respiratory distress includes supplemental oxygen, cage rest, bronchodilator administration, aminophylline (5–10 mg/kg IV or IM BID (kittens) or TID (puppies)), furosemide (1–2 mg/kg IV q6–12h), and one injection of a short-acting corticosteroid, prednisolone sodium succinate (15–30 mg/kg IV) to stabilize lysosomal membranes (efficacy not proven).

6. Sequelae in severe cases may include cardiac arrhythmias, seizures, and secondary bacterial pneumonia.

7. Outcome is generally favorable if affected juveniles survive the initial 48 hours after injury.

D. Juvenile cellulitis (puppy strangles, juvenile pyoderma) is discussed in the section on dermatologic emergencies (see p. 376).

CHAPTER 18

OCULAR EMERGENCIES

I. CLINICAL SIGNS, DIAGNOSIS

A. Red eye is the most common owner complaint for ocular emergencies.

1. Focal redness is most often caused by hemorrhage or mass lesions.
2. Prolapse of the gland of the third eyelid may be reported as a red eye by clients.
3. Generalized external redness is caused by lesions involving conjunctiva, cornea, and or sclera.
4. One must differentiate between superficial (conjunctival) and deep (scleral or episcleral) redness.

    a. Superficial redness due to conjunctivitis is not likely to threaten vision and is characterized by vessels that readily blanch when topical epinephrine or phenylephrine is applied and are freely movable.
    b. Deep or scleral vessel involvement indicates intraocular disease and is more likely to threaten vision; involved vessels do not blanch, are not freely movable, and may radiate in short straight lines from the limbus.

5. Uveitis and glaucoma are the most common rule-outs for scleral or episcleral vascular engorgement.
6. Intraocular hemorrhage indicates blood in the anterior chamber (hyphema) or vitreous and is seen with coagulopathy (thrombocytopenia, vasculitis associated with rickettsial disease, anticoagulant rodenticide toxicity), trauma, uveitis, hypertension, retinal detachment, and neoplasia.

B. Other reasons animals are brought in as ocular emergencies include loss of vision, ocular discharge, and ocular pain.

1. Loss of vision can occur with
    a. Severe corneal pigmentation, keratoconjunctivitis sicca, or corneal edema
    b. Cataracts, lens luxation
    c. Anterior uveitis, intraocular hemorrhage, neoplasia
    d. Posterior segment disease—retinal dysplasia, retinal detachment, retinal degeneration, optic neuritis, chorioretinitis, Collie eye anomaly
2. Ocular discharge can occur with diseases of the eyelids (e.g., entropion), conjunctiva, nasolacrimal system, cornea, and globe.
3. Conditions that cause **ocular pain** include trauma, foreign body, eyelid disease (entropion, distichiasis), glaucoma, uveitis, corneal erosions/ulcers/lacerations, and retrobulbar masses including orbital cellulitis and neoplasia.

II. DIAGNOSTIC AND MONITORING PROCEDURES

A. Schirmer tear test (STT)

1. Measures aqueous tear production in millimeters/minute of wetness
2. Normal values in dogs >15 mm/min.
3. Normal values in cats can be quite variable.
4. Test procedure involves bending test strip at notch and inserting into conjunctival fornix at junction of middle and lateral third of lower eyelid margin (*Fig. 18-1*).
5. Test should be performed before manipulating ocular structures or administering topical

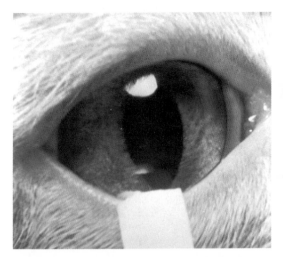

FIGURE 18.1   To estimate aqueous tear formation, the Schirmer tear test paper strip is inserted into the lower conjunctival fornix of the cat. (From Gelatt KN, ed. Veterinary Ophthalmology. 3rd ed. Baltimore: Lippincott Williams & Wilkins, 1999:457.)

medications that could influence tear production, especially topical anesthetic or saline eye rinse.
6. Excessive handling or improper storage of strips may lead to erroneously high results.

B. Fluorescein dye test

1. Used primarily to diagnose corneal ulcers/erosions
2. Should be performed as part of every ocular examination
3. Fluorescein penetrates corneal defects, enters stroma, and stains intercellular spaces bright green.
4. A cobalt blue filter on the end of a Finnoff transilluminator or ultraviolet light (e.g., Wood's lamp) causes dye to fluoresce and makes detecting small defects easier.
5. Test can also be used to assess patency of nasolacrimal duct.
   a. Dye is applied to both eyes and should reach the external nares within 5 minutes in normal animals.
   b. If none is seen within 5 minutes, a Wood's lamp should be shined in the mouth to detect dye that was either licked from external nares (cats) or entered nasopharynx through ducts that drain into internal nares (brachycephalic breeds).

C. Tonometry

1. Used to measure intraocular pressure (IOP)

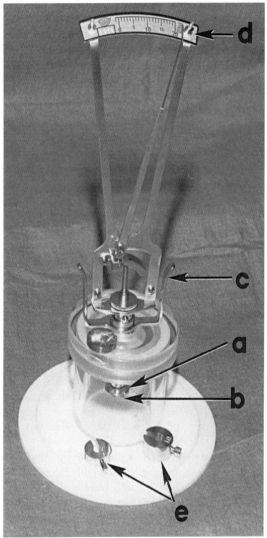

FIGURE 18.2   The Schiötz tonometer. Note the corneal foot plate (A), plunger (B), holding bracket (C), recording scale (D), and 7.5- and 10.0-g weights (E). (From Gelatt KN, ed. Veterinary Ophthalmology. 3rd ed. Baltimore: Lippincott Williams & Wilkins, 1999:457.)

2. Normal IOP in dogs and cats is 15–25 mm Hg with <5 mm Hg difference between eyes.
3. Schiötz tonometer.
   a. Degree to which instrument indents cornea reflects IOP.
   b. Test is performed by applying topical anesthetic and placing foot of instrument on center of upturned cornea (*Figs. 18-2* and *18-3*).

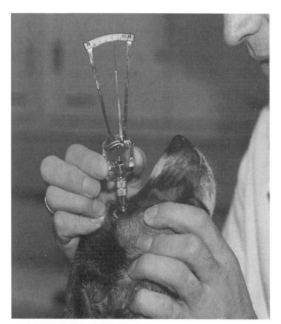

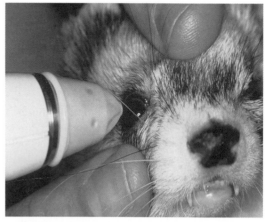

FIGURE 18.4   Tonopen applanation tonometry in a ferret. (From Gelatt KN, ed. Veterinary Ophthalmology. 3rd ed. Baltimore: Lippincott Williams & Wilkins, 1999:461.)

FIGURE 18.3   For Schiötz tonometry in the dog, the instrument is held vertically and placed on the center of the cornea. (From Gelatt KN, ed. Veterinary Ophthalmology. 3rd ed. Baltimore: Lippincott Williams & Wilkins, 1999:450.)

c. IOP is determined by measuring the deflection of the needle on the instrument's scale and using a conversion table to arrive at IOP in mm Hg: the average value of three to five measurements is used if agreement is good. *Note:* When assessing Schiötz tonometry readings, the scale reading should be ±2 from the weight on the tonometer. For example, for a 5.5-g weight, the scale reading should be between 3.5 and 7.5 if the pressure in the eye is within the reference range. If the reading is <3.5 or >7.5, then the IOP is outside the reference range.

d. Small or minimal deflections of instrument needle correspond to minimal indentation of the cornea, low numbers on the instrument scale (mm), and high IOP on the conversion table.

e. Large deflections reflect a soft eye and are read as large numbers on the Schiötz scale (mm) and low IOP on the conversion chart.

4. Tonopen (Oculab, Glendale, CA)
   a. Handheld device slightly larger than a penlight that is applied to anesthetized cornea and gives accurate digital readout of IOP in dogs and cats *(Fig. 18-4)*.
   b. Advantages:

1) Easier to use than Schiötz (less cumbersome, animal looks straight ahead, digital readout of IOP does not require using a conversion chart).
2) Accuracy
   c. Disadvantages:
   1) Expense
   2) Sensitivity—Pressure on eyelids or jugular vein during restraint may increase pressure reading; one may detect transient changes in IOP caused by excitement/fear.

5. Digital tonometry is a crude indicator of IOP; all emergency clinics should have instrumentation to determine IOP accurately.

D. Cytology is sometimes performed in animals with conjunctivitis, ocular discharge, retrobulbar disease, or ocular masses.

E. Conjunctival scrapings are made using topical anesthetic and a small, flat spatula to check for canine distemper, chlamydia, mycoplasma, bacterial infections, or eosinophilic inflammation. Intracytoplasmic inclusion bodies can be found on slides stained with Dif-quick or modified Wright's stain.

F. Fluorescent antibody tests can be performed on conjunctival scrapings for canine distemper, feline herpesvirus, and chlamydia. There is also a polymerase chain reaction (PCR) test for feline herpesvirus.

III. MANAGEMENT OF SPECIFIC CONDITIONS

A. Corneal laceration

1. Most common causes are trauma or foreign body
2. Superficial lacerations often appear as linear defects or flaps.
3. Iridal tissue prolapse or anterior chamber collapse may be seen with deep or full-thickness lacerations *(Fig. 18-5)*.
4. Injuries caused by cat claws should be evaluated carefully for anterior lens capsule damage, which may result in severe lens leakage uveitis. Lens leakage uveitis (phacoclastic uveitis) can cause a severe panophthalmitis that results in loss of vision.
5. Diagnosis is usually straightforward, though severe corneal edema, deflation of the anterior chamber, iris prolapse, and hyphema may make full assessment of intraocular structures difficult. Topical anesthetic facilitates the examination.
6. Consensual pupillary light reflexes and dazzle response are positive clinical signs, but they do not ensure that the posterior segment is normal.
7. Ocular ultrasound can be performed to assess damage of deeper ocular structures, but do not allow the coupling gel to enter the eye. The animal should be anesthetized or heavily sedated during this procedure to prevent further injury of the globe.
8. Treatment depends on depth of laceration.
9. Superficial or small wounds are treated as superficial corneal ulcers (see p. 365) and usually heal within 5–7 days.

10. Surgery is recommended for full-thickness lacerations, those deeper than 1/2 thickness of the cornea, and those with gaping edges.
   a. General anesthesia is recommended prior to manipulating the globe to avoid further prolapse of iridal tissue or globe rupture.
   b. Wound edges are *not* debrided, to preserve as much corneal tissue as possible.
   c. Prolapsed iridal tissue is gently replaced if wound is <6–8 hours old or is resected in older or contaminated wounds. Excision can be done with electrocautery (Accu-Temp Surgical Cautery Concept, Inc, Clearwater, FL).
   d. Before suturing severe wounds, the anterior chamber should be flushed with sterile saline to remove blood and fibrin clots; an iris spatula or intraocular forceps are used if necessary to free up the iris from the lacerated cornea edges
   e. Simple interrupted sutures of 7-0 to 10-0 absorbable material (e.g., Vicryl-Ehticon, Somerfield, NJ, spaced 1–1 1/2 mm apart are used to close the wound.
   f. Sutures are partial thickness and should not enter the anterior chamber.
   g. After sutures are placed, the anterior chamber should be filled with sterile saline and a small air bubble to prevent the iris from adhering to cornea.
   h. Postoperative treatment consists of topical antibiotics and atropine, systemic antibiotics, analgesics if necessary, and placement of an Elizabethan collar.

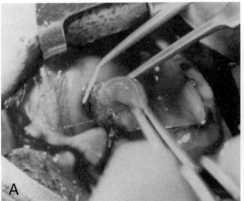 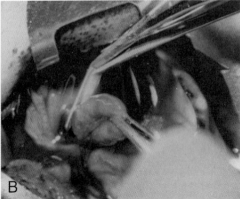

FIGURE 18.5   Corneal laceration with iris prolapse in a 1-year-old male Doberman Pinscher. (From Gelatt KN, ed. Veterinary Ophthalmology. 3rd ed. Baltimore: Lippincott Williams & Wilkins, 1999:655.)

TABLE 18.1
CAUSES OF ANTERIOR UVEITIS

Ocular causes
    Disruption of lens capsule
    Ocular trauma
    Ocular neoplasia

Systemic infectious disease
    Fungal (blastomycosis, histoplasmosis, cryptococcosis, coccidioidomycosis, candidiasis)
    Rickettsial (RMSF, ehrlichiosis)
    Protozoal (toxoplasmosis, neosporosis, leishmaniasis)
    Bacterial (sepsis, brucellosis, leptospirosis, Lyme borelliosis, bartonellosis)
    Viral (canine adenovirus, herpesvirus, FIP, FeLV, FIV)
    Protothecosis
    Parasitic—aberrant larval migration (toxocariasis, dirofilariasis, ancylostomiasis, *Cuterebra* spp.)

Immune-mediated
    Panuveitis with depigmentation skin lesions in Arctic circle breeds (Malamute, Husky, Akita, Chow Chow, Samoyed)

Other
    Systemic hypertension
    Hyperviscosity syndrome
    Idiopathic

---

    i. Prognosis depends on depth of laceration and extent of intraocular inflammation.

B. Anterior uveitis

  1. Defined as inflammation of iris and ciliary body

  2. Causes include blunt trauma/penetrating injury, infection, nonseptic inflammation, neoplasia, autoimmune disease, or metabolic disease (*Table 18-1*).

  3. Unless trauma is evident, a search for an underlying systemic disorder is always warranted; however, many cases remain idiopathic.

  4. Ocular signs include iris congestion/swelling/hyperemia, miosis, and aqueous flare.

  5. Tonometry reveals low IOP.

  6. Additional signs include blepharospasm, epiphora, corneal edema, conjunctival hyperemia, perilimbal scleral injection, photophobia, aqueous flare, and miosis.

  7. Chronic cases may reveal keratic precipitates, anterior or posterior synechiae, iris bombe, secondary glaucoma, secondary cataract, corneal neovascularization, and blindness.

  8. Determining the underlying cause should include routine laboratory investigation as for any systemic illness.

  9. Additional diagnostic tests to consider in selected cases might include fungal, protozoal, or retroviral (cats) serology, radiography, and coagulation assessment.

    a. Cats: Rule out toxoplasmosis, cryptococcosis, bartonellosis, feline immunodeficiency virus (FIV), feline leukemia virus (FeLV), and feline infectious peritonitis (FIP).

    b. Dogs: Rule out fungal disease, rickettsial disease, brucellosis, and leptospirosis.

  10. Cytology or serology can be performed on aqueous fluid aspirated with a 30-gauge needle at limbus.

  11. Treatment

    a. Treat underlying disorder if identified.

    b. Topical and systemic glucocorticoids are mainstays of treatment.

    c. Topical preparations include dexamethasone or 1% prednisolone acetate (Econopred, Alcon) and are administered 4–6 times daily (solution) or 3–4 times per day (ointment). Do not use if a corneal ulcer is present.

    d. Oral prednisone is given at 0.5–1.1 mg/kg PO q24h for 7 days followed by gradual taper to the lowest effective alternate-day dose if infectious disease has been ruled out and topical steroids are ineffective.

e. Oral prednisone can be used in presence of corneal ulcer but should be discontinued if ocular or systemic signs worsen.

f. Subconjunctival injection of corticosteroids can be considered in severe cases unless there is corneal infection, ulceration, or fungal uveitis.

    1) Triamcinolone, 4–8 mg

    2) Methylprednisolone acetate, 4–8 mg

g. Topical nonsteroidal antiinflammatory drugs (NSAIDs) including flurbiprofen 0.03%, suprofen 0.1%, and diclofenac 0.1% can be administered 2–4 times daily and can be used if corneal ulceration is present.

    1) May exacerbate intraocular hemorrhage

    2) Best used in conjunction with topical steroids in severe cases; rarely effective as monotherapy

    3) Can still delay corneal healing.

h. Atropine 1% should be applied 1–2 times daily to minimize synechia formation, alleviate pain, and stabilize the blood-aqueous barrier to minimize inflammation.

    1) For refractory miosis, atropine can be applied 3–6 times daily or topical 2.5% phenylephrine can be added.

    2) If secondary glaucoma or dry eye is a concern, tropicamide 1% can be used because the duration is short (1–4 hours).

i. Topical antibiotics, chloramphenicol, or tetracycline, are given for 10–14 days to prevent bacterial keratitis.

j. Systemic antibiotics are given as prophylaxis against more widespread ocular infection.

k. Drugs that cross the blood-aqueous barrier include amoxicillin, cephalosporins, trimethoprim/sulfadiazine, and especially chloramphenicol. Doxycycline is recommended for suspected tick-borne diseases while awaiting titers.

l. Enucleation is recommended if there is blindness, severe pain, secondary glaucoma, or no response to therapy or to remove a potential nidus of infection.

C. Glaucoma

1. Increased IOP that results in impaired vision due to damaged retinal ganglion cells and optic nerve

2. Primary glaucoma is caused by an inherited defect in trabecular meshwork (open angle) or iridocorneal angle (closed angle), resulting in impaired outflow of aqueous humor.

3. Angle-closure glaucoma is the most common cause of primary glaucoma in dogs.

4. Breeds predisposed to angle-closure glaucoma include Shar-peis, Cocker Spaniels, Basset Hounds, Akitas, Springer Spaniels, Samoyeds, Golden Retrievers, and Flat-Coated Retrievers.

5. Breeds predisposed to open-angle glaucoma include Beagles, Great Danes, Keeshonden, Miniature and Toy Poodles, Samoyeds, and Siberian Huskies.

6. Primary glaucoma is most often bilateral, with both eyes affected within 6–12 months of onset, although the eyes usually do not manifest signs at the same time.

7. Secondary glaucoma is caused by obstruction of aqueous outflow by inflammatory debris, fibrin, lens luxation, or neoplasia and is the most common cause of glaucoma in cats.

8. Ocular signs include pain, dilated pupil, corneal edema, scleral injection, buphthalmus, and loss of vision. Lens luxation may result from tearing of zonular fibers

9. Initially, fundic examination is normal except for papillary edema; later changes include attenuation of retinal vessels, tapetal hyperreflectivity, and cupping of the optic disc.

10. Diagnosis is confirmed by tonometry with IOP >35–40 mm Hg.

11. Treatment must be initiated early to preserve vision.

12. Treatment for acute glaucoma:

    a. Mannitol 20%, 1–2 g/kg IV over 20 minutes; repeat in 4–6 hours if necessary based on serial tonometry.

        1) Mannitol should be warmed to dissolve crystals and given through blood administration set or other in line filter.

        2) Contraindicated in animals with congestive heart failure or dehydration.

    b. Water should be withheld for 2–4 hours to maintain intraocular dehydration. Use caution in animals with preexisting renal disease, as dehydration or hypovolemia secondary to mannitol diuresis may further compromise the kidneys.

    c. Oral 50% glycerol, 1–2 mg/kg PO repeated in 8 hours can be used but is less effective and has more side effects (hyperglycemia, vomiting) than mannitol. Contraindicated in animals with diabetes or congestive heart failure.

    d. Latanoprost (Xalatan) is a synthetic prostaglandin analogue that can result in a dramatic drop in IOP within 20–40 minutes. Place 1 drop in the affected eye.

e. Oral carbonic anhydrase inhibitors (CAIs) are indicated in most cases but can cause metabolic acidosis or electrolyte abnormalities. If excessive panting, vomiting or diarrhea develops, the dose should be decreased or the drug discontinued.

    1) Dichlorphenamide (Daranide, Merck) 2–4 mg/kg q8–12h (dog), 1–2 mg/kg q8–12h (cat).

    2) Methazolamide (Neptazane, Lederle) 2–4 mg/kg q8–12h.

    3) Acetazolamide (Diamox, Lederle) 4–8 mg/kg q8–12h. Side effects are most common with acetazolamide and include vomiting, anorexia, polyuria/polydipsia (PU/PD), and lethargy.

f. Topical CAIs are safer than the oral drugs because they lack side effects.

    1) Dorzolamide (Trusopt), 1 drop to affected eye q8–12h

    2) Brinzolamide (Azopt), 1 drop to affected eye q8–12h

g. Pilocarpine (to constrict the iris and open the drainage angle) 2% topically q6–12h, 4% gel q24h. Contraindicated with anterior uveitis or anterior lens luxation. It causes severe miosis and can potentiate an existing uveitis. It is no longer used or recommended

h. If these measures successfully normalize IOP, then therapy is maintained with topical medications ±oral CAIs. Timolol maleate is a topical nonselective β-blocker (1 drop q12h) that can be used with latanoprost (1 drop q12–24h) for maintenance therapy.

i. Prophylactic medication of the unaffected eye is recommended to delay onset of disease.

    1) Timolol 0.5%, 1 drop q12h

    2) Demecarium bromide 0.125% (available from compounding pharmacies), 1 drop q12h

    3) Ideal pressure for visual eyes is 15–20 mm Hg.

j. Surgery is indicated if medical management is ineffective at maintaining IOP <30 mm Hg and in almost all cases of primary glaucoma.

k. Surgical procedures include cryosurgery or laser surgery to destroy the ciliary body and decrease aqueous production and/or gonio implants (Ahmed valve) that shunt aqueous fluid from the anterior chamber to sub tenon capsule area where it is absorbed.

13. Prognosis for vision is guarded to poor in most cases of severe acute glaucoma or if corneal edema, scleral injection, or buphthalmus are present.

D. Proptosis

1. Proptosis is a forward displacement of the globe outside the orbital socket.

2. Brachycephalic breeds are predisposed because of a shallow orbit. Minor trauma or only retracting eyelids during restraint may cause proptosis.

3. In nonbrachycephalic dog breeds and cats, major trauma is required, and fractures of orbit, sinuses, or oral cavity may coexist.

4. Blunt trauma (hit by car) and bite wounds are the most common causes.

5. Diagnosis is readily made by clinical signs.

6. Favorable signs for vision include miotic pupil, consensual light reflex in contralateral eye, positive menace response, short duration of proptosis, and minimal damage to extraocular muscles and soft tissue.

7. Treatment

a. Emergency surgery is indicated in all cases to optimize the chances for preservation of vision.

b. Surgery can be delayed if optic nerve is severed or globe is ruptured, as vision is hopelessly lost in either case.

c. Cornea is lubricated with artificial tears or sterile ophthalmic antibiotic ointment to prevent drying.

d. Surgery is performed under general anesthesia; therefore, assessment and stabilization of concurrent traumatic injuries is important.

e. Surgical procedure

    1) Globe and conjunctival sac are flushed with sterile irrigating solution to remove debris.

    2) Globe is replaced using forceps or preplaced sutures on margins of upper and lower eyelids while pushing on the globe with the flat surface of a scalpel handle or digital pressure.

    3) Lateral canthotomy may be necessary if swelling prohibits replacement.

    4) Sutures can be used to pull lid margins over globe while assistant applies gentle pressure on cornea with lubricated scalpel handle.

5) Once globe is replaced, the globe/conjunctiva are thoroughly irrigated to remove remaining debris.

6) Eyelids are sutured together with horizontal mattress sutures using stents, or button, IV tubing, or red rubber catheter to evenly distribute tension.

a) *Sutures must be placed carefully so they do not rub on the cornea or cause inversion of the eyelids.*

b) *Sutures should go directly into the orifices of the meibomian glands.*

7) Medial canthus is left partially open to administer topical medication.

8) Permanent lateral and/or medial canthorrhaphy may be indicated to prevent recurrence in brachycephalic breeds.

f. Topical antibiotic ointment and atropine ointment are administered q6–8h.

g. Systemic antibiotics are given for 7–10 days or until orbital swelling resolves.

h. Prednisone, 1–2 mg/kg PO q24h for 3–7 days then tapered over 1–2 weeks, is recommended to treat optic neuritis and associated uveitis.

i. An Elizabethan collar is worn until suture removal in 10–14 days.

j. Pain can be managed with butorphanol, 1 mg/4.54 kg PO q12h.

8. Potential sequelae include blindness, exposure keratitis, endophthalmitis, strabismus, keratoconjunctivitis sicca, secondary glaucoma, and phthisis bulbi.

9. Enucleation is indicated with globe rupture or optic nerve transection, persistent infection, or persistent discomfort.

E. Hyphema

1. Hyphema is blood in the anterior chamber, usually originating from iridal vessels. Blood may be clotted or unclotted.

2. Causes include head trauma, uveitis, coagulopathy, hypertension, neoplasia (primary ocular or metastatic), hyperviscosity syndrome, and glaucoma.

3. Hemorrhage in the anterior chamber may cause secondary glaucoma because of obstruction of aqueous outflow by fibrin.

4. If there is no history of trauma or systemic disease and ocular examination is otherwise normal, assess coagulation (prothrombin time (PT), partial thromboplastin time (PTT), platelet

count, buccal mucosal bleeding time, von Willebrand disease (VWD) factor assay) and blood pressure.

5. Consider serology for infectious diseases that cause vasculitis and thrombocytopenia (ehrlichiosis, RMSF, borelliosis).

6. Ocular ultrasonography is indicated with spontaneous hyphema to detect neoplasia, lens luxation, vitreal hemorrhage (carries guarded prognosis for vision) and retinal detachment.

7. Treatment

a. Treat underlying disease whenever possible.

b. Topical corticosteroids are applied 3–6 times daily until resolution for potential underlying anterior uveitis.

1) Prednisolone acetate 1%

2) Dexamethasone 0.1%

c. Atropine ointment q8–12h is indicated, though IOP should be monitored to detect any rise in IOP due to potential obstruction of aqueous outflow.

d. Pilocarpine, 2% solution q6–12h or 4% gel q24h, may facilitate removal of blood or aqueous humor by promoting vasoconstriction and mydriasis, although posterior synechia formation is a potential complication with this therapy.

e. Fibrin clots may occlude drainage angle and can be removed by irrigating the anterior chamber with saline.

f. Fibrin clots can be dissolved with tissue plasminogen activator (0.1–0.3 mL intracameral injection of a 250 μg/mL solution—Activase (Genentech, South San Francisco, CA))

1) Most effective within 48 hours of clot formation

2) Primary risk is rebleeding.

g. Monitor for secondary glaucoma.

h. Treat any associated traumatic injuries, coagulopathy, hypertension, or other ocular pathology as indicated.

i. Prognosis for return of vision is variable.

F. Ocular foreign body

1. Ocular foreign bodies may be found in conjunctival sac, in cornea, or within the globe.

2. Conjunctival foreign bodies include grass awns, seeds, glass, wood, and insects.

a. Clinical signs include conjunctivitis, blepharospasm, ocular discharge, and/or corneal edema.

b. A foreign body may be difficult to find if in conjunctival fornix or on bulbar surface of nictitans.

c. Corneal erosion/ulcer is a common sequela.

d. Sedation and topical anesthesia is required for effective exploration of the eye and foreign body removal.

e. Forceps and/or irrigating solution can be used to gently remove some foreign bodies.

f. Topical antibiotics may be necessary for 5–7 days or longer if severe conjunctival injury is present.

g. Fluorescein staining is indicated to identify corneal erosion/ulcer.

h. An Elizabethan collar may be necessary if the animal is causing self-trauma to the eye.

3. Corneal foreign body

   a. Superficial foreign bodies (e.g., plant material, metal flakes, wood, or paint chips) are removed by irrigation, moistened cotton-tipped applicator, or ophthalmic forceps.

   b. Fluorescein staining is indicated to detect corneal erosion/ulcer.

   c. A corneal ulcer should be treated if secondary corneal ulcer or abrasion is present.

   d. An Elizabethan collar is worn if the animal is causing self-trauma to the eye.

   e. Foreign bodies embedded in the cornea are removed by incising cornea with no. 65 Beaver blade or razor blade and gently lifting from the corneal stroma.

   f. Topical therapy is as that for superficial foreign body; sutures are not necessary.

4. Penetrating foreign bodies

   a. "In-and-out"–type injuries may seal spontaneously and cause minimal damage.

   b. Damage to anterior lens capsule may cause lens leakage uveitis in some cases, which can be severe enough to ultimately result in loss of the eye.

   c. Treat penetrating injuries as for anterior uveitis and corneal ulcer, avoiding topical corticosteroids until corneal epithelium has healed (see p. 357).

   d. Significant penetration may cause iridal or uveal prolapse and should be treated as anterior uveitis and corneal ulcer without topical steroids (see p. 357).

   e. Resection of prolapsed tissue and corneal suturing is discussed under corneal laceration (see p. 356).

   f. Foreign bodies in anterior chamber, lens, or posterior chamber are uncommon and are treated as uveitis pending referral to an ophthalmologist for removal or enucleation (see p. 357).

G. Chemical injury

1. Topical shampoos/dips, bleaches, other household cleaners, and fire smoke exposure commonly cause corneal and/or conjunctival inflammation.

2. Ocular signs include blepharospasm, ocular discharge, conjunctival hyperemia, and possibly corneal edema.

3. Owners can be advised to immediately rinse the eye with contact lens solution or water if contact lens solution is not available.

4. Copious irrigation followed by topical antibiotic/steroid ointment (assuming no corneal defect) usually suffices.

5. Alkali exposure causes severe corneal damage (deep ulceration/melting stromal ulcers) and possibly uveitis. Treatment includes copious irrigation, topical collagenase inhibitor (see corneal ulcer treatment, p. 365), and topical antibiotic and atropine ointments.

6. A conjunctival flap (see corneal ulcer treatment, p. 365) may be necessary in severe cases.

7. Systemic antibiotics are indicated (amoxicillin, 22 mg/kg q12 h).

H. Lens luxation/subluxation

1. Lens luxation occurs when all zonular attachments are disrupted, allowing the lens to lodge in anterior chamber, posterior chamber, or vitreous.

2. With subluxation, the partially detached lens remains in the pupil but out of its normal position, resulting in "aphakic crescent" (*Fig. 18-6*).

3. The most common causes are trauma, glaucoma, and congenital zonular defects.

   a. Inherited luxations usually manifest between 3 and 7 years of age.

   b. Predisposed breeds include terriers, Border Collies, and German Shepherd Dogs.

4. Clinical signs include blepharospasm, epiphora, corneal edema, episcleral injection, and acute blindness.

5. Ocular examination findings include

   a. Aphakic crescent in which the margin of the lens is clearly visible within the pupil and highlighted by the tapetal reflection

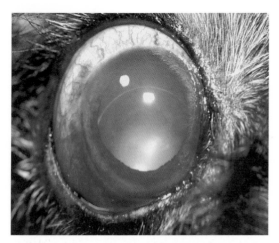

FIGURE 18.6 Focal lens subluxation associated with advanced lens fiber resorption with a hypermature cataract. Note the dorsal, irregularly shaped aphakic crescent. (From Gelatt KN, ed. Veterinary Ophthalmology. 3rd ed. Baltimore: Lippincott Williams & Wilkins, 1999:821.)

b. Shallow anterior chamber with anterior luxation

c. Deep anterior chamber with posterior movement of iris

d. Iridodonesis or fluttering of the iris when eye is moved

e. Signs of glaucoma or polytrauma may be seen.

6. Tonometry is recommended to rule out glaucoma or uveitis, either of which may cause or be caused by lens luxation.

a. IOP may be quite high (50–90 mm Hg).

b. Damage or degeneration of lens may cause leakage of nascent proteins and lead to uveitis.

7. Emergency treatment is directed at normalizing IOP if high and controlling associated ocular or traumatic injuries.

a. Anterior lens luxations require emergency treatment.

b. Posterior lens luxations are not considered an emergency.

8. Temporary reduction of anterior lens luxation can be attempted by first dilating the pupil with tropicamide, tipping the nose upward to "flip" the lens into the posterior chamber, then constricting the pupil with pilocarpine. This is sometimes done under general anesthesia after the animal has been given mannitol to soften the eye. Then the animal is placed in dorsal recumbency and the cornea is pushed so that the lens moves back behind the iris and then the iris is constricted.

9. The risk of secondary glaucoma is greatest with anterior luxation, therefore surgery is recommended as soon as feasible.

10. Surgery involves intracapsular lens extraction or enucleation for uncontrolled glaucoma and blindness.

11. Treatment for subluxation or posterior luxation is controversial.

a. IOP should be monitored for development of secondary glaucoma.

b. Surgery may not be necessary unless glaucoma develops.

I. Acute blindness

1. Confirm blindness

a. Menace response, dazzle response, obstacle course (dim and bright light), following dropped cotton balls

b. Perform complete physical examination. Rule out hearing loss, vestibular disease, seizures, and neurologic disorders.

2. Ophthalmic examination

a. Corneal disease or cataracts may result in vision loss.

b. A clear anterior segment is seen with diseases of the posterior segment or cerebral cortex.

c. Normal fundus—sudden acquired retinal degeneration (SARD)

1) Middle-aged to older dogs

2) Most common cause of acute blindness in dogs with clear eyes.

3) Vision loss may be preceded by transient polyphagia, polyuria, and polydipsia.

4) The electroretinogram (ERG) is flat.

5) Vision loss is permanent.

6) Dachshunds and Miniature Schnauzers are predisposed, but it may occur in any breed.

d. Abnormal fundus

1) Optic neuritis—Optic disc appears swollen with indistinct margins ±chorioretinitis *(Fig. 18-7).*

a) *Causes include systemic mycoses, viruses, rickettsial diseases, protozoal diseases, prototheosis, neoplasia, trauma, toxicity (lead, ivermectin), and idiopathic.*

b) *Evaluate for signs of systemic disease: fever, lymphadenopathy, joint swelling, hemorrhage, and neurologic, cardiac, or pulmonary abnormalities.*

c) *Treatment*

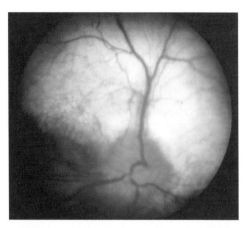

FIGURE 18.7   Optic neuritis caused by reticulosis appears as a swollen, hyperemic disc with indistinct margins. There is no apparent physiologic cup. (From Gelatt KN, ed. Veterinary Ophthalmology. 3rd ed. Baltimore: Lippincott Williams & Wilkins, 1999:989.)

     i) *Oral prednisone: 0.5–1 mg/kg q12h for 14 days, then taper*
     ii) *Treat underlying disease if possible.*
  2) Progressive retinal atrophy (PRA)
    a) *Begins with night blindness with progressive loss of vision over a period of years but may seem sudden to owners*
    b) *Congenital photoreceptor dysplasia results in early onset and rapid progression in Alaskan Malamutes, Belgian Shepherds, Collies, Greyhounds, Irish Setters, Miniature Schnauzers, and Norwegian Elkhounds.*
    c) *Late-onset PRA results from abnormal photoreceptor development that occurs early but progresses slowly. Affected breeds include Akita, English Cocker Spaniel, Labrador Retriever, Miniature Long-Haired Dachshund, Miniature Poodle, Samoyed, Swiss Hound, and Tibetan Terrier.*
  3) Chorioretinitis
    a) *Dull gray raised foci with indistinct margins indicate active inflammation.*
    b) *Look for systemic disease and treat underlying cause.*
  4) Retinal detachment
    a) *Rule out systemic hypertension, coagulopathies, hyperviscosity syndromes, systemic disease*
    b) *Treat underlying problem.*

J. Conjunctivitis

  1. Inflammation of conjunctiva is extremely common in dogs and cats.
  2. In dogs, noninfectious causes such as allergies, systemic disease, or eyelid/eyelash abnormalities are most common.
  3. In cats, infectious causes are most common and include bacteria, mycoplasma, chlamydophila (chlamydia), calicivirus, and herpesvirus.
  4. Ocular irritants and foreign bodies commonly affect both species.
  5. Clinical signs include blepharospasm, hyperemia of conjunctival vessels, chemosis (conjunctival edema), and ocular discharge.
  6. Corneal ulcers may be present with foreign bodies and in cats with herpesvirus-1 infection.
  7. Chemosis may be extensive in cats with chlamydial infections.
  8. Diagnosis is made by clinical signs.
  9. History should be thorough to rule out exposure to irritants or other animals.
  10. Examination should include a thorough search for a foreign body, especially behind the nictitating membrane (e.g., grass awn/seed), and fluorescein staining.
  11. Conjunctival scraping or swab is indicated in refractory cases to obtain material for cytology, bacterial culture, or PCR testing (herpesvirus).
  12. In dogs, initial treatment involves topical antibiotic preparation such as BNP (bacitracin-neomycin-polymyxin), Terramycin, or chloramphenicol.
  13. Topical corticosteroids applied 3–6 times daily or 0.2% cyclosporine ointment BID can be added if follicular or lymphoplasmacytic conjunctivitis is present in dogs.
  14. In cats, initial treatment is directed against chlamydophilial (chlamydial) infection using tetracycline, erythromycin, or chloramphenicol-containing products.
  15. Topical antiviral medications, idoxuridine or vidarabine, can be used if no response is seen to the antibiotic.
  16. These antiviral medications can be irritating and are expensive and often ineffective.
  17. Oral L-lysine, 500 mg q–24h, may decrease clinical signs and prevent recurrence in cats with herpesvirus but efficacy is unproved.
  18. Topical corticosteroids are rarely indicated in treating feline conjunctivitis because of the infectious etiology of most cases.

19. Refractory cases should prompt a diligent search for foreign body, distichia/ectopic cilia, keratoconjunctivitis sicca, etc.

20. If cytology reveals eosinophils or lymphocytic/plasmocytic inflammation, treatment involves topical corticosteroids ±systemic steroids or azathioprine.

K. Keratoconjunctivitis sicca (KCS)

1. Decreased production of aqueous, and to lesser extent mucous, tear layer, resulting in inflammation of, and possible injury to, cornea and conjunctiva

    a. Primary KCS results from failure of aqueous tear production.

    b. Secondary KCS results from obstruction of the lacrimal ducts.

2. Causes include heredity, infection/inflammation/immune-mediated inflammation of lacrimal tissue, trauma, drugs (sulfonamides), systemic diseases, radiation therapy, and removal of prolapsed nictitans.

    a. Most cases are idiopathic and probably immune mediated.

    b. KCS is uncommon in cats.

3. Ocular signs include thick mucoid or mucopurulent discharge, conjunctivitis, blepharospasm, and a dull corneal surface. Corneal opacification, hyperpigmentation, and neovascularization are common.

4. Diagnosis is confirmed by documenting decreased tear production with the STT.

    a. Values <5 mm/min indicate severe KCS; 6–14 mm/min indicates early, subclinical, or mild disease.

    b. The STT is less reliable in cats; normal values are probably similar to those in dogs.

    c. Fluorescein staining is indicated because corneal erosion/ulceration are common.

    d. A thorough history of recent medication or prior illness is important to identify potential underlying etiologies.

5. Treatment of choice is cyclosporine (.2–2%) applied topically 2–3 times daily for 4 weeks.

    a. Increased tear production is seen in 80% of animals with initial STT ≥2 mm/min.

    b. Response decreases to about 50% if initial STT is 0–1 mm/min.

    c. If improvement in tear production is noted, once-daily maintenance administration can be continued indefinitely (usually lifelong).

    d. Cyclosporine can be safely administered in presence of corneal ulcers.

    e. In severe cases, (i.e., severe corneal changes without ulceration, excessive discharge), concurrent oral antibiotics and corticosteroids, topical antibiotic/ steroid ointment, and artificial tears should be given.

    f. Administer artificial tears 4–6 times daily while awaiting a response to cyclosporine.

6. If tear production does not improve within 4–8 weeks, a trial with oral pilocarpine can be tried, or parotid duct transposition is indicated.

    a. For oral pilocarpine trial, 1–2 drops/10 lb is administered q12h in food. (It is very bitter.)

    b. Side effects include increased salivation, lacrimation, urination, and defecation. If these occur, drug use should be discontinued until GI side effects resolve and then restarted at a lower dose.

7. Topical atropine for the treatment of concurrent corneal ulceration with ciliary spasm should not be used because it may lead to decreased tear production.

L. Retinal detachment

1. Rarely a cause of emergency presentation unless detachment is bilateral and results in blindness

2. Congenital retinal detachment is seen in Collies as part of the Collie eye anomaly syndrome and in other breeds predisposed to retinal dysplasia.

3. Acquired retinal detachment may be secondary to systemic hypertension, trauma, neoplasia, or exudate caused by infectious/inflammatory disease.

4. A common clinical scenario is an older cat with hypertension secondary to hyperthyroidism and/or chronic renal disease.

5. Ocular examination reveals dilated pupils.

6. Pupillary responsiveness correlates inversely with degree of detachment.

7. Fundic examination reveals billowing of the retina with vessels that appear raised and out of focus.

    a. Raised area may be partial or complete.

    b. A veil or film can be seen attached to the optic disc.

    c. Retinal hemorrhage may be present.

    d. Exudate beneath the detached portion may cause the retina to appear dull, gray, or red in cases of hemorrhage.

8. Diagnosis is made by ocular examination.

9. Additional testing to detect underlying disease might include routine laboratory work as for any systemic medical problem, blood pressure measurement, thyroid hormone assay, and/or coagulation assessment.

10. Serologic assays for systemic fungal disease, toxoplasmosis, coronavirus (FIP), or rickettsial agents should be considered where appropriate.

11. Treatment is aimed at underlying disease if identified.

   a. Amlodipine (0.5 mg/kg PO q24h in dogs, 0.625–1.25 mg PO q24h in cats) is used for initial therapy of hypertension.

   b. Immune-mediated or inflammatory detachments can be treated with 2.2 mg/kg prednisone PO q24h. Reattachment and regain of function is possible.

   c. Retinal tears can sometimes be repaired surgically (laser photocoagulation, transscleral cryopexy, vitrectomy).

M. Corneal ulceration

1. Causes include trauma, foreign body, keratoconjunctivitis, sicca, exophthalmus, and abnormalities of eyelids or lashes.

2. Ocular signs include blepharospasm, ocular discharge, epiphora, and miosis.

   a. If the ulcer extends to the stroma, there is a mucopurulent discharge, aqueous flare, and a visible defect.

   b. If the ulcer extends to Descemet's membrane, there is a smooth, clear area that does not retain fluorescein dye.

   c. If the ulcer perforates the cornea, there will be intense blepharospasm and fibrin or iris prolapsing from the ulcer.

3. Diagnosis is confirmed by demonstrating fluorescein dye uptake; using a Wood's lamp is useful to detect small ulcers.

4. Treatment of superficial ulcers includes topical antibiotic ointment q6–8h and atropine ointment q8–12h for 7 days.

   a. An Elizabethan collar is placed to prevent self-trauma.

   b. Healing is often complete within 7 days.

5. Deep corneal ulcers (i.e., >50% depth of stroma) require aggressive therapy to prevent globe rupture and preserve vision (see descemetocele, p. 372).

6. Bacterial culture of specimen obtained by corneal swab will determine definitive topical antibiotic therapy; triple antibiotic ointment q 8 hr is used initially.

7. Options for surgical therapy include the following (*Table 18-2*):

   a. Third eyelid flap

   1) Useful for ulcers due to exposure keratitis or KCS

   2) Contraindicated for rapidly progressive ulcers because of inability to monitor progression

   3) A mattress pattern is used to suture the third eyelid to the upper lid or superior bulbar conjunctiva.

   b. Conjunctival flap

   1) Indicated for descemetoceles or deep stromal ulcers. A thin flap of conjunctiva is dissected from the limbus with tenotomy scissors as a pedicle or bridge and sutured over the ulcer with 6-0 or 8-0 suture.

   c. Primary closure

   1) Can be used to close small perforations

   2) Use 7-0 or 8-0 suture, and re-form anterior chamber as needed.

   d. Corneoscleral transposition, corneal lamellar graft—used for large defects with adjacent healthy cornea. A partial-thickness corneal graft attached to a conjunctival pedicle flap is sutured over the defect with 7-0 or 8-0 absorbable suture.

8. Soft contact lenses can be used for superficial nonhealing erosions.

9. Atropine is applied as for superficial ulcers.

10. Melting ulcers are deep progressive lesions caused by excessive production of collagenase and/or proteases by inflammatory cells or bacteria, especially *Pseudomonas* spp.

   a. May be a complication of any corneal ulcer

   b. Often seen when topical corticosteroids are used on eyes in which subtle corneal defect was not detected on initial examination

11. Topical collagenase inhibition using acetylcystine (Mucomyst, Bristol Meyers-Squibb) diluted to 5–10% solution with artificial tears applied q1–2h for 24–48 hours may be successful, though efficacy is questionable.

12. Autologous serum (1 drop q2–4h) can also inhibit collagenase.

13. Topical fluoroquinolones (ocufloxacin, levofloxacin) or gentamicin is used because of efficacy against *Pseudomonas* spp. Culture and sensitivity testing should be performed to determine the most effective antibiotics for rapidly progressive ulcers.

TABLE 18.2
EMERGENCY SURGICAL PROCEDURES FOR CORNEAL DEFECTS

Procedure for third eyelid flap *(Figs. 18-9 and 18-10)*
- Horizontal mattress sutures are placed through horizontal cartilage of nictitans approximately 3 mm from free margin using 2-0 to 3-0 nylon suture material.
- Sutures exit upper eyelid after penetrating palpebral conjunctiva at fornix.
- Stents using red rubber feeding tube or IV tubing or buttons can be used to secure flap and evenly distribute tension on sutures

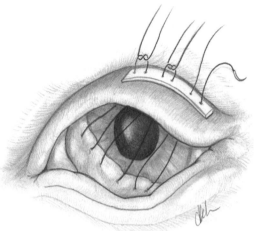

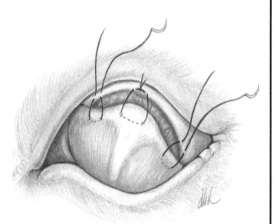

FIGURE 18.9   NM-to-superior-lid flap. Two to three horizontal mattress sutures of 3-0 monofilament non-absorbable material are placed between the free edge of the NM and the lateral aspect of the superior lid. The lid sutures should be placed well within the superior cul-de-sac, and the NM sutures should be approximately 2 mm from the free edge, incorporating cartilage into the center suture. Alternatively, a single mattress suture can be placed between the superior lid and the midpoint of the cartilage shaft. (Reprinted with permission from University of Tennessee College of Veterinary Medicine, 1997.)

FIGURE 18.10   NM-to-episclera flap. Suturing the free edge of the NM to the superotemporal episclera allows the cornea and flap to move in concert, thus minimizing corneal trauma. (Reprinted with permission from University of Tennessee College of Veterinary Medicine, 1997.)

Procedure for conjunctival flap *(Figs. 18-11 to 18-13)*
- Advantages over third eyelid flap include better blood supply and enhanced delivery of fibroblasts, immunoglobulins, systemically administered antibiotics, and anticollagenase enzyme effects of serum.
- The bulbar conjunctiva is incised near the fornix with tenotomy scissors, and a thin layer is under-mined toward the limbus.
- Care is taken to dissect just conjunctiva and not deeper tenon capsule.
- Similarly, a thin layer of conjunctiva is incised and undermined around the complete circumference of the limbus.
- The flap is pulled ventrally over the cornea and sutured with 7-0 nylon suture material.
- The flap is anchored to sclera at limbus to prevent retraction.
- Systemic antibiotics are administered for 2 weeks.
- The flap is removed by transecting it at the limbus after 2 weeks.

TABLE 18.2
(continued)

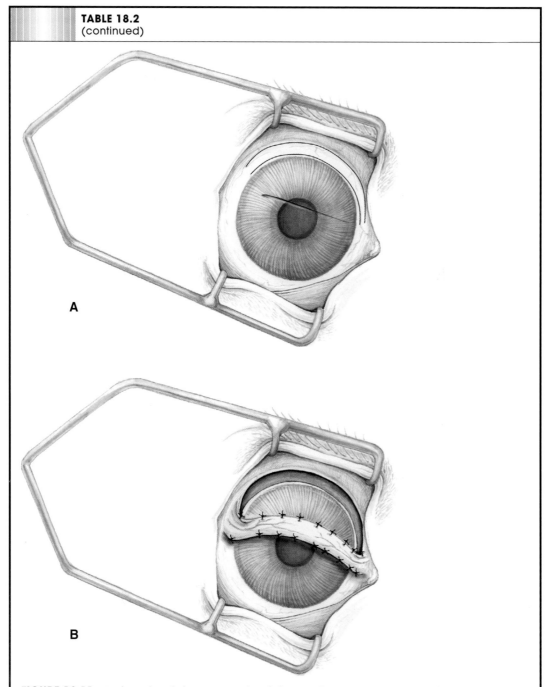

A

B

FIGURE 18.11 Bridge or bipedicle conjunctival graft/flap. **A.** The conjunctiva is excised from the limbus for approximately 180° both adjacent and parallel to the linear corneal lesion. This area is extensively undermined, and the underlying fibrous tissue is removed. A second conjunctival incision is made 5–8 mm peripheral and parallel to the original conjunctival incision, thus creating a "bridge" of conjunctiva. **B.** and **C.** The bridge is advanced over the lesion and then sutured, using simple interrupted sutures into the cornea around the lesion. **D.** The original graft-harvesting site is closed by opposing the remaining conjunctiva with a simple continuous suture. From Gelatt KN, ed. Veterinary Ophthalmology, 3rd Ed. Baltimore: Lippincott Williams & Wilkins, 1999:682.

TABLE 18.2
EMERGENCY SURGICAL PROCEDURES FOR CORNEAL DEFECTS (continued)

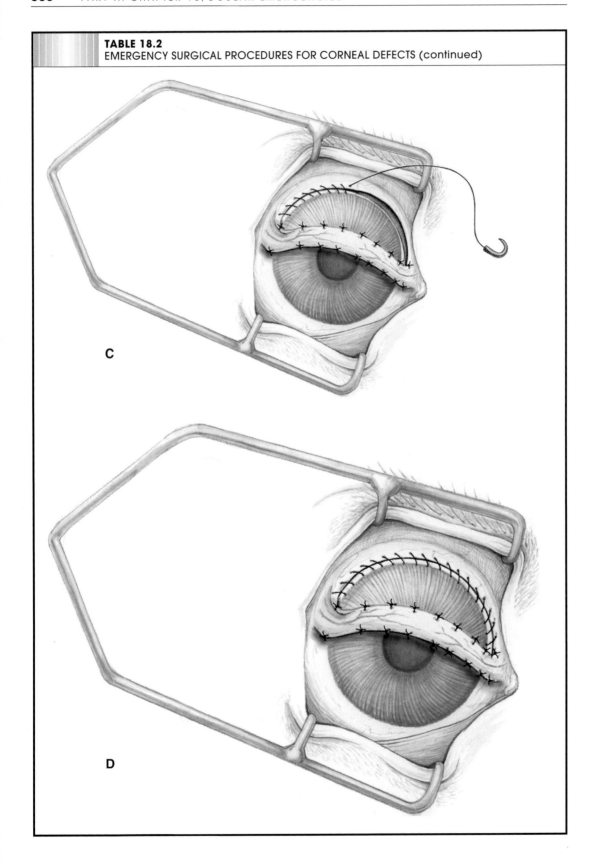

C

D

TABLE 18.2
(continued)

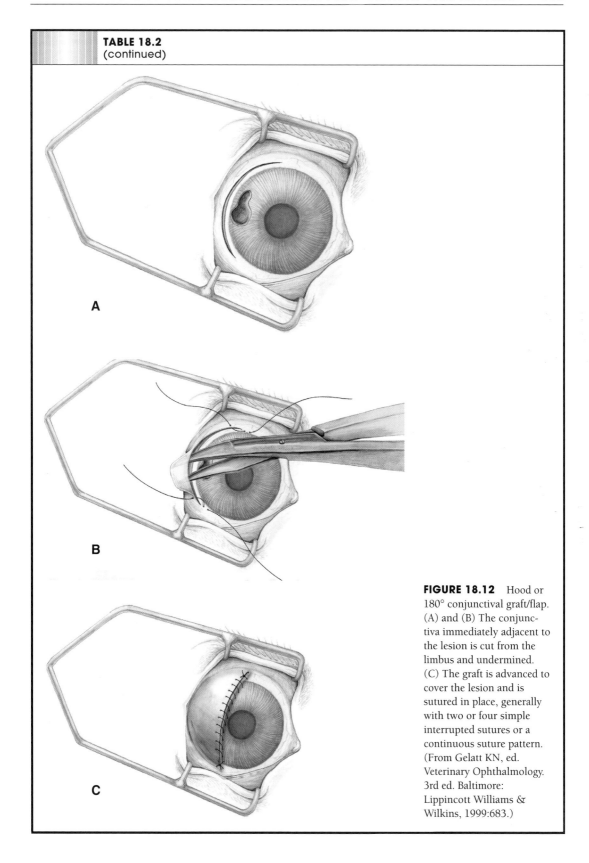

A

B

C

FIGURE 18.12 Hood or 180° conjunctival graft/flap. (A) and (B) The conjunctiva immediately adjacent to the lesion is cut from the limbus and undermined. (C) The graft is advanced to cover the lesion and is sutured in place, generally with two or four simple interrupted sutures or a continuous suture pattern. (From Gelatt KN, ed. Veterinary Ophthalmology. 3rd ed. Baltimore: Lippincott Williams & Wilkins, 1999:683.)

TABLE 18.2
EMERGENCY SURGICAL PROCEDURES FOR CORNEAL DEFECTS (continued)

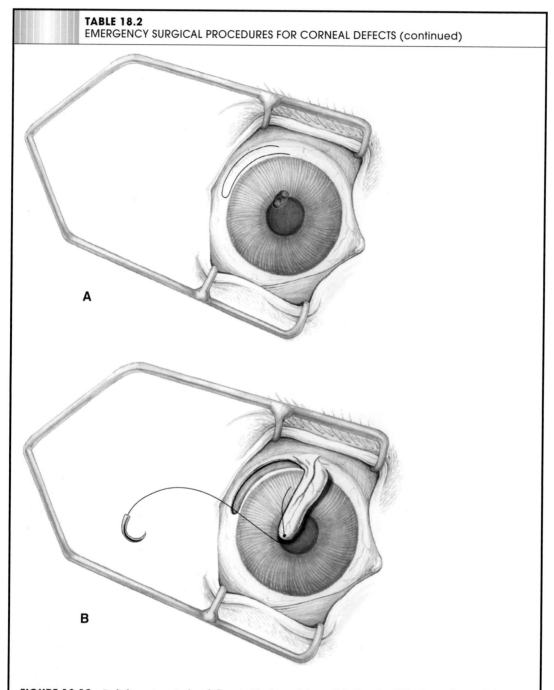

FIGURE 18.13 Pedicle conjunctival graft/flap. **A.** The base of the pedicle flap should be directed toward the area of the limbus nearest to the lesion. Once the location of the base is determined, a site 1.0–1.5 cm temporal to the base is located, at which the flap will be initiated. Through a small slit in the conjunctiva, the entire conjunctival flap site is undermined using blunt dissection. Two parallel cuts are then made to create a strip of conjunctiva. **B.** The strip of conjunctiva is rotated to cover the corneal lesion. The flap is sutured to the cornea with simple interrupted sutures of 7-0 to 9-0 polyglactin 910 or nylon. **C.** The sutures are placed first at the distal end of the flap and then 1.0–1.5 mm apart. (From Gelatt KN, ed. Veterinary Ophthalmology. 3rd ed. Baltimore: Lippincott Williams & Wilkins, 1999:684.)

TABLE 18.2
(continued)

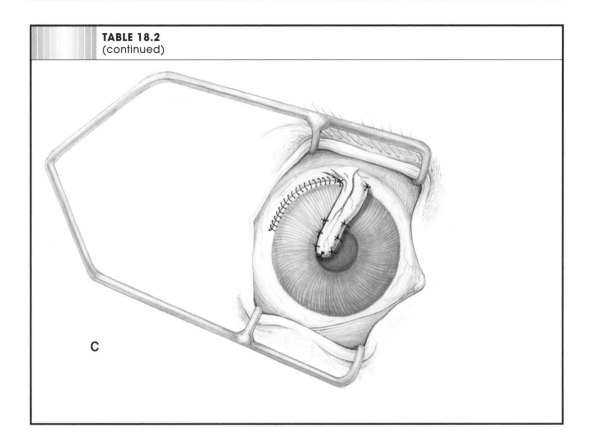

C

14. Prognosis is guarded, and globe rupture may occur.

N. Descemetocele

1. Defined as deep corneal ulcer with exposure of Descemet's membrane
2. Appears as a corneal ulcer with dark center that is negative for fluorescein uptake surrounded by fluorescein-positive rim of cornea (*Fig. 18-8*).
3. Emergency surgery is required to prevent globe rupture.
4. Small, 2- to 3-mm ulcers can be closed with simple interrupted sutures of 7-0 Vicryl placed to a depth of 50–70% of cornea.
5. Larger lesions require placement of conjunctival flap prior to referral for corneoscleral transposition, keratoplasty, or corneal transplant.
6. Topical antibiotics and atropine are given as for deep corneal ulcer.
7. Systemic antibiotics are indicated when the cornea is perforated.
8. An Elizabethan collar is placed.

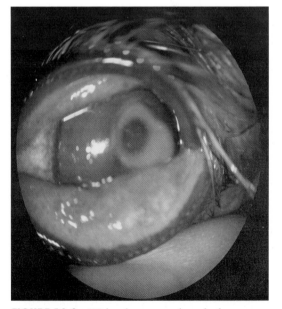

FIGURE 18.8 With a descemetocele, only the surrounding edge of the exposed corneal stroma retains topical fluorescein dye. From Gelatt KN, ed. (From Gelatt KN, ed. Veterinary Ophthalmology. 3rd ed. Baltimore: Lippincott Williams & Wilkins, 1999:647.)

O. Eyelid laceration

1. Most often caused by fight wounds or sharp object
2. Surgical closure is recommended in almost all cases, especially if lid margin is involved.
3. Prior to closure, minimal clipping and copious lavage with sterile saline are performed.
4. Only minimal debridement is recommended to "freshen" wound edges while preserving as much tissue as possible to avoid lid deformity.
5. A two-layer closure is recommend:
   a. Conjunctiva is sutured with 4-0 to 6-0 absorbable material.
   b. Skin is closed using 5-0 to 7-0 nonabsorbable material.
6. The lid margin should be perfectly realigned to preserve cosmetic appearance and lid function.
7. Topical and systemic antibiotics (amoxicillin or cephalosporin) are administered for 7–10 days with contaminated wounds.
8. Lacerations involving the medial canthus may affect lacrimal puncta or nasolacrimal duct and should be repaired by an ophthalmologist.

P. Prolapsed gland of the nictitans (cherry eye)

1. Caused by weak connective tissue attachment between gland and orbit.
2. Breed predisposition in Boston Terrier, Sharpei, Lhasa Apso, St. Bernard, Bassett Hound, Beagle, English Bulldog, American Cocker Spaniel, and others.
3. Exposed gland becomes hypertrophied and causes epiphora, conjunctivitis, ocular discharge, and corneal erosion/ulcer.
4. Gland appears as smooth, red, rounded subconjunctival mass ("cherry eye").
5. Topical lubricating ointment or triple antibiotic ointment is applied q6–8h pending surgical replacement of the prolapsed gland.
6. Removal of the prolapsed gland may predispose to KCS and is strictly contraindicated.
7. To perform pocket imbrication
   a. Pull the third eyelid forward, exposing the bulbar surface.
   b. Make parallel incisions on either side of the prolapsed gland.
   c. Close the far edges of the two incisions with 6-0 absorbable suture in a continuous pattern, causing the prolapsed gland to be tucked into the pocket as the suture line is closed.

CHAPTER 19

DERMATOLOGIC EMERGENCIES

I. CLINICAL SIGNS AND DIAGNOSIS

A. Pruritus is defined as a sensation that causes scratching.

1. Seasonal pruritus is most often due to flea allergy dermatitis or atopic dermatitis.
2. Nonseasonal pruritus can be caused by mite infestation (scabies, demodecosis, cheyletiellosis), food allergy, acral lick granuloma, and pyoderma.
3. Less common causes of pruritic skin disease include contact dermatitis, drug eruptions, chiggers, psychogenic pruritus, and others.
4. Pruritus causes self-trauma, which may obscure the inciting lesion making diagnosis difficult.
5. Self-trauma also may perpetuate the scratch-itch cycle, worsening signs.

B. Alopecia is another very common dermatologic complaint.

1. Alopecia may be generalized or partial and focal or diffuse.
2. The most common cause of alopecia in both dogs and cats is self-trauma due to pruritus.
3. Localized alopecia may be caused by mites, dermatophytes, injection reaction, and others.
4. Diffuse, patchy alopecia may be caused by mites, dermatophytes, pyoderma, follicular dysplasia, and others.
5. Symmetrical alopecia that is nonpruritic is usually caused by hypothyroidism or hyperadrenocorticism.
6. Generalized alopecia may be caused by endocrinopathy, seasonal alopecia, pattern baldness, epidermotropic lymphoma, and others.

C. Erosions (basement membrane intact) and ulcerations may be seen with infectious, metabolic, neoplastic, physical/chemical, and immune-mediated disorders.

1. Immune-mediated skin disease is commonly associated with erosions/ulcerations (resulting from disruption of vesicles). However, immune-mediated or autoimmune disease is uncommon to rare.
2. Skin biopsy is often necessary to diagnose the cause of erosions/ulcerations.

D. Scaling and crusting are nonspecific signs of dermatologic disease associated with parasites, bacterial infections, allergic disorders, dermatophytosis, keratinization defects (e.g., zinc deficiency), autoimmune disease, and neoplasia.

E. Papules and pustules are most commonly caused by bacterial skin infection.

1. A papule is a raised skin lesion caused by infiltration of inflammatory cells.
2. A pustule is a raised pus-filled epidermal lesion.
3. Because pyoderma is rare in cats, papules and pustules are also rare in this species.

F. General considerations

1. Many diseases present with similar dermatologic signs, making diagnosis using the history and physical examination alone difficult.
2. The basic workup for most dermatologic patients should include skin scraping for parasites, fungal culture for dermatophytes, and appropriate laboratory tests as indicated by historical and

physical examination findings (e.g., CBC, biochemical profile, urinalysis).

3. Most skin disorders are not life threatening, although patient discomfort may be significant.

4. Extensive loss of the barrier function of the skin, as occurs with generalized ulcerative dermatoses, burns, or trauma (bites wounds, degloving injuries), may predispose to sepsis.

II. DIAGNOSTIC PROCEDURES

A. Wood's lamp

1. Indicated when evaluating patient for dermatophytes (ringworm).

2. Emits ultraviolet light causing fluorescence of tryptophan metabolites in 50% of *Microsporum canis* strains.

3. Lamp should be warmed up for 5–10 minutes to reach ideal wavelength and directed at lesion(s) for 5 minutes in a completely dark room to optimize results.

4. True fluorescence is seen as apple-green color and usually involves hairs or broken hair shafts at periphery of lesion.

5. False-positive fluorescence is white or blue and may be caused by scales, topical medications, or bacteria.

6. Negative results are seen with 50% of *M. canis* strains and all *Trichophyton spp.* Thus, Wood's lamp examination is an insensitive test for diagnosis of dermatophytosis.

B. Fungal culture

1. Used to confirm diagnosis of dermatophytosis.

2. Procedure:
a. Clip hair if necessary to height of 1 cm.
b. Disinfect lightly with 70% alcohol.
c. Use sterile hemostat to collect hair and scales from periphery of lesion
d. Use a sterile toothbrush over entire hair coat in animals that are being tested as possible carriers or to document response to therapy.
e. Collected material is pressed into dermatophyte test medium (DTM), kept in the dark at room temperature with humidity >30%, and checked daily for 14 days.
f. A sample should also be placed on Sabouraud's medium to permit macroscopic and microscopic identification of isolates.

3. Positive result—pathogenic dermatophytes produce alkaline metabolites that turn DTM pH indicator red at the time that mycelia develop. DTMs older than 14 days may turn red when contaminated by saprophytic fungi.

4. Confirm positive results by microscopic examination and fungal culture.

C. Skin scraping

1. Indicated in all cases with alopecia and scaling to rule out ectoparasites.

2. Procedure:
a. Prepare lesion by clipping hair with scissors if necessary and cleaning with mild disinfectant (e.g., chlorhexidine solution).
b. Scrape area using No. 20 scalpel blade held at 45–90°.
  1) *Demodex*—squeeze skin to extrude mites from follicles and scrape deep enough to cause capillary bleeding.
  2) *Sarcoptes*—scrape a large area (20 cm²) and collect as many crusts as possible; capillary bleeding is not necessary.
c. Multiple scrapings from new lesions should be taken.
d. Use mineral oil to coat scalpel blade, skin surface, and microscope slide to improve adherence of collected material.
e. Applying a cover slip may aid microscopic examination by compressing crusts and spreading material evenly over slide.
f. Examine the entire slide at 4X and 10X magnification for mites, ova, and feces.

3. Sensitivity varies with parasite—high with *Demodex* and *Notoedres;* low with *Sarcoptes.*

D. Skin biopsy

1. Indications include vesicular skin disease, suspected neoplasia, nonresponsive dermatosis, persistent ulcerations, and/or unusual or severe lesions.

2. Biopsy should be performed during the initial examination when above findings are present or within 3 weeks of therapy in unresponsive cases.

3. Procedure:
a. Site selection is important—multiple samples of primary lesions (vesicles, papules, bullae, etc.) and secondary lesions (crusts, scales, etc.) are recommended.
b. Preparation of site should be minimal to avoid distorting histology and should be limited to gentle clipping of hair coat and alcohol disinfection. NEVER SCRUB a skin biopsy site.

c. Punch biopsy using local anesthesia is adequate for most lesions.

d. Excisional biopsy is recommended for vesicles or deep lesions.

e. Samples should be handled gently, blotted to remove blood, and immediately placed in formalin and possibly Michel's medium if immune-mediated disease is suspected.

f. When appropriate, a sample should be submitted for culture and susceptibility testing (contact laboratory for preferred sample submission).

g. Suture biopsy site(s) with simple interrupted or cruciate pattern.

4. Prior to biopsy, corticosteroids should be discontinued for 2–3 weeks, and secondary pyoderma should be treated with systemic antibiotics.

E. Bacterial culture

1. If possible, locate an intact pustule.

2. Prick the top of the pustule with a 25 g needle and touch with culture swab.

3. If crusts are present, they can be peeled back so that a culture can be taken from the fluid beneath the crust.

4. Cultures can also be taken from skin biopsies placed directly in the culture medium.

5. Cytology can be performed to identify inflammatory cells, neoplastic cells, or acantholytic cells (pemphigus complex).

III. MANAGEMENT OF SPECIFIC CONDITIONS

A. Bite wound abscess

1. Overview

a. More common in cats than dogs.

b. Most common in intact males due to roaming and aggression.

c. Bite introduces microorganisms from the oral cavity under the skin resulting in infection 2–7 days later.

d. In cats, small wounds often seal over and are not visible when presented for examination.

2. Diagnosis

a. History of exposure to the outdoors, other animals, or witnessed fight.

b. Physical examination may reveal fever, bite wound(s), firm swelling, fluctuant subcutaneous swelling, or purulent discharge, as well as nonspecific signs of lethargy and anorexia.

c. Clipping hair may aid in detecting small wounds and determining extent of involved tissue. Note: The presence of two adjacent punctures suggests a bite injury, whereas a single wound more likely indicates another cause of penetrating injury.

d. Common locations for bite wound abscesses include face and neck, tail base, shoulder, and distal limb.

e. The absence of pus does not exclude bite wounds; cellulitis occurs prior to abscess formation.

3. Treatment

a. Prior to drainage, the area should be liberally clipped and surgically prepared.

b. Using light sedation or general anesthesia, depending on extent and severity of wound, the abscess is lanced using a No. 12 or 15 blade at the ventral most aspect and flushed with copious volumes of sterile saline.

c. The subcutaneous space should be probed to fully assess the amount of dead space. This is often much larger than the area indicated by physical examination.

d. Any necrotic tissue should be debrided.

e. Penrose drain placement is indicated with large wounds. Often, more than one drain is necessary (e.g., for wounds that extend across the dorsal midline of the neck or tail base/lumbar area).

f. The importance of establishing adequate ventral drainage cannot be overstated. The most common cause of recurrent abscessation is incomplete treatment of the initial wound.

g. Bite wounds should never be completely sutured. Large wounds can be partially closed with nonabsorbable monofilament suture material leaving an opening for the Penrose drain.

h. An Elizabethan collar should be placed to prevent the animal from removing any drains and causing self-trauma.

i. Subcutaneous or intravenous fluids should be administered in patients that are febrile, anorectic, or that undergo prolonged anesthesia for wound treatment.

j. Broad spectrum antibiotics effective against oral microflora (e.g., *Pasteurella, Streptococcus, Bacteroides*) are administered for 7–10 days.

   1) Amoxicillin—22 mg/kg q12 h PO

   2) Amoxicillin/clavulanate—12.5–22.5 mg/kg q12h PO

k. Intact males should be neutered to minimize recurrence by reducing aggression and roaming.

l. Refractory or recurrent infections are caused by resistant or unusual pathogens, immunosuppression (e.g., retroviral disease in cats), foreign bodies, and most often inadequate debridement or drainage.

B. Acute moist dermatitis (pyotraumatic dermatitis, "hot spot")

1. Overview

  a. Lesions are self-induced in response to pruritus or pain.

  b. Allergic skin disease (flea bite hypersensitivity, atopy), grooming complications, otitis, and pyoderma are common underlying etiologies.

  c. Breed predisposition includes Golden and Labrador retriever, German Shepherd, Collie, St. Bernard, and others.

2. History and clinical signs

  a. Acute development of a moist, erythematous, circumscribed lesion that is intensely pruritic and variably painful.

  b. Lesions range in size from 1–2 cm to over 10–15 cm.

  c. The full size of the lesion is often not apparent until hair is clipped.

  d. Common locations of lesions are side of face, tail base, caudal thigh, and groin.

3. Diagnosis is straightforward based on typical history and clinical signs.

4. Treatment

  a. The hair coat is clipped liberally until healthy skin is revealed around the entire circumference of the wound.

  b. The wound is then cleaned with dilute chlorhexidine or Betadine solution or antimicrobial shampoo containing benzyl peroxide.

  c. Sedation is recommended for large and/or painful wounds to permit thorough clipping and cleaning.

  d. Systemic antibiotics with activity against Staphylococcus intermedius are given for at least 14 days.

    1) Cephalexin—22 mg/kg q8–12h PO

    2) Amoxicillin/clavulanate—12.5–22.5 mg/kg q12h PO

    3) Enrofloxacin 5 mg/kg q12–24h PO

    4) An antibiotic injection can be given to more rapidly attain therapeutic concentration.

  e. Corticosteroids are given to relieve pruritus and break the scratch-itch cycle.

    1) Prednisone—1 mg/kg q24h for 3–5 days, 0.5 mg/kg q24h for 3–5 days, then 0.5 mg/kg every other day for 3–5 treatments.

    2) A single injection of a short-acting corticosteroid can be given initially to hasten effect.

  f. The wound should be kept dry using topical astringents such as Dermacool (Virbac) or Domboro solution.

  g. An Elizabethan collar is placed to prevent further self-trauma.

  h. The underlying disease should be identified and treated.

C. Juvenile cellulitis (puppy strangles)

1. Overview

  a. Defined as steroid-responsive granulomatous pustular skin disease affecting the face, pinnae, and submandibular lymph nodes of puppies between 3 weeks and 4 months of age.

  b. Etiology is unknown but steroid responsiveness suggests an immune disorder.

  c. Breed disposition includes Golden retriever, Dachshund, and Gordon setter and is also suggested that heredity may be involved.

2. Clinical signs and diagnosis

  a. Affected puppies have severe swelling of face, ears, eyelids, and submandibular lymph nodes.

  b. Skin lesions begin as papules and pustules, which eventually break open and become crusted.

  c. Systemic signs are seen in approximately 25% of cases and include fever, lethargy, anorexia, and joint pain.

3. Treatment

  a. Prednisone—2.2 mg/kg q24h then gradually taper the dose over the next 1–2 weeks.

  b. Cephalexin—22 mg/kg q8–12h for 10–14 days.

4. Prognosis

  a. Recovery is usually complete and relapses are rare.

D. Otitis externa/aural hematoma

1. Overview

  a. Causes of otitis externa include atopy, food hypersensitivity, endocrine disease (e.g., hypothyroidism), seborrhea, ear mites, and foreign body (e.g., foxtail).

b. Other predisposing factors include abnormal conformation, polyps, or neoplasia, which permit growth of microorganisms in the external ear canal by allowing moisture and debris to accumulate.

c. Infection with bacteria or yeast is almost always secondary to the above problems.

d. Aural hematomas may occur with or without concurrent infection; an immune-mediated etiology has been suggested but not proven.

2. Clinical signs include head shaking, scratching, foul odor, and discharge.

a. If unilateral, causes such as foreign body, conformation, polyp, or neoplasia are more likely.

b. Bilateral involvement is more typical with endocrine disease, allergy, seborrhea, and other generalized conditions.

c. With middle ear involvement ipsilateral Horner's syndrome and/or peripheral vestibular (head tilt, horizontal nystagmus) may be seen.

d. With aural hematoma, affected ears have fluctuant nonpainful swelling of the pinnae. Hematomas are most often unilateral, although both ears are occasionally affected.

3. Diagnosis

a. Thorough history and physical examination confirm the presence of infection or hematoma formation.

b. The character of the discharge provides diagnostic clues:

1) Black, crusty discharge in young animal—ear mites.

2) Moist, brown discharge—staphylococci or yeast.

3) Purulent, cream colored—Gram-negative infection.

c. Otoscopic examination

1) Indicated in all cases to identify foreign object or mass lesion, examine the tympanic membrane for evidence of rupture or otitis media, and to characterize discharge and changes (redness, thickening, obstruction) of the external ear canal.

2) The unaffected ear is examined first if unilateral disease is present. This prevents spread of pathogens to the normal ear and avoids sensitizing the animal to pain thereby optimizing success in evaluating the affected ear.

3) Sedation should be considered if pain is severe (or temperament dictates) to allow thorough evaluation, minimize patient discomfort, prevent iatrogenic trauma to ear structures, and allow for thorough flushing and cleaning of the external ear canal.

d. Radiographs of the osseous bullae are indicated in chronic cases or when signs of middle/inner ear involvement are present.

4. Treatment

a. The most important aspect of treatment is thorough flushing of the external ear canal to remove ALL discharge and debris.

1) Tympanic membrane rupture is the exception.

2) Material should be collected for cytologic evaluation and culture/susceptibility testing prior to flushing.

3) Sedation is necessary to permit thorough flushing.

4) Room-temperature water, dilute chlorhexidine, or ear cleansing/ceruminolytic agents can be used.

5) A bulb syringe or 6–12 mL syringe without a needle attached is used to perform copious low pressure lavage. This minimizes complications such as tympanic membrane rupture or acute vestibular disease.

6) Cotton applicator swabs are then used to remove remaining discharge and thoroughly dry the ear canal. A red rubber catheter can be passed into the ear canal to suction out remaining fluid after thoroughly rinsing with saline.

b. Foreign bodies are retrieved under direct visualization using alligator forceps passed through an appropriate sized otoscope cone.

c. An ear loop can be passed through an otoscope cone under direct visualization to remove debris deep within the external canal or on the surface of the tympanic membrane.

d. A rare complication of ear flushing is the development of acute peripheral vestibular disease due to irritation/inflammation of the 8th cranial nerve. Owners should be informed of this potential complication.

e. Myringotomy

1) Indicated with otitis media when the tympanic membrane is intact in order to obtain samples for cytology and culture and allow for flushing and drainage of the middle ear.

2) The tympanic membrane can be punctured in the caudoventral quadrant using a spinal needle attached to a syringe and gently aspirating or using a small sterile culture swab (Calgiswab Type I, Hardwood Products Company, LP, Guilford).

3) All debris should be removed and the ear canal thoroughly cleaned before attempting myringotomy.

f. Topical treatment:

1) Bacterial otitis—antibiotic or antibiotic-glucocorticoid containing preparations are given for 10–14 days.

> **a)** *Mix 2 mL injectable enrofloxacin in 1 bottle of Synotic for* Pseudomonas *otitis externa.*
>
> **b)** *Antibacterial agents should be chosen based on cytology and culture/sensitivity testing.*

2) Yeast otitis—miconazole or clotrimazole alone or in combination with glucocorticoids for 14–21 days.

3) Ear mites—thiabendazole (Tesaderm, MSD, AgVet) is used in breeds sensitive to systemic ivermectin (e.g., collies).

4) Topical steroid-containing solutions are contraindicated in middle ear infections with tympanic membrane rupture to avoid brain abscessation due to spread of infection along the 8th cranial nerve. In most other cases, glucocorticoids are recommended to reduce inflammation, epithelial proliferation, fibroplasia, and sebum production.

f. Systemic treatment:

1) Bacterial otitis—cephalexin, 22 mg/kg q8–12h PO for 14–21 days

2) Recurrent Pseudomonas infection—enrofloxacin (Baytril), 15–20 mg/kg q24h PO. (Caution using high dose enrofloxacin (Baytril) in cats due to potential to cause blindness.)

3) Ear mites—ivermectin, 300 μg/kg SQ every 10 days for 3 treatments.

4) Prednisone, 1 mg/kg q24h for 5–7 days, then taper, when severe inflammation or swelling is present.

5. Aural hematoma surgery

a. Performed under general anesthesia.

b. Clip medial and lateral surfaces of affected pinna.

c. Place cotton balls in external ear canal to keep dry during prep and procedure.

d. Perform standard surgical scrub of both surfaces of pinnae.

e. Excise a vertical 3–4 mm strip of skin over extent of swelling from medial surface of pinna.

f. Thoroughly flush the pinna to remove all blood and fibrin.

g. Place through and through sutures in two rows of simple interrupted pattern on either side of the space left after excision parallel to the long axis of the pinna. The skin edges are NOT opposed before suture placement and a 3–4 mm gap in the skin of the medial pinna should remain. Use monofilament nonabsorbable suture material on a cutting needle and avoid blood vessels while penetrating the ear. Sutures should be placed no more than 5 mm apart. Make sure that all dead space has been opposed to avoid recurrence.

h. Place an Elizabethan collar.

i. Note: There are several acceptable alternative techniques to the procedure described here. The goal of all techniques is to drain the hematoma and oppose dead space to avoid recurrence and maintain acceptable cosmetic appearance. Drainage alone usually resolves pain, but recurrence is highly likely unless the dead space is opposed.

6. Refractory cases require investigation for primary and/or predisposing conditions mentioned above, radiographs/CT/MRI of osseous structures, and possible surgery (e.g., lateral ear canal resection or total ear canal ablation).

E. Sarcoptic mange

1. Overview

a. Etiologic agent is *Sarcoptes scabei var. canis,* which causes an intensely pruritic, nonseasonal, transferable skin disease.

b. The same mite infests both dogs and cats though feline scabies is caused by *Notoedres cati.*

c. Mite is transmissible to humans with pruritic papules/pustules developing primarily on trunk and arms within 24 hours of exposure.

d. Pruritus is due to a hypersensitivity reaction to parasitic cuticular or fecal antigens.

2. Clinical signs

a. Intense pruritus leading to self-excoriation.

b. Skin lesions appear as red papules that break open forming crusts with yellowish exudate.

c. Lesions are distributed on ears, lateral elbows, chest, legs, and ventral abdomen.

d. Hyperpigmentation, lymphadenopathy, hyperkeratosis, and secondary bacterial skin infection may occur with chronic or severe cases.

3. Diagnosis

a. Confirmed by microscopic identification of mite, ova, or feces obtained by skin scraping.

1) Skin scraping may be positive in only 20% of cases.

2) Maximize yield by obtaining multiple scraping of nonexcoriated areas with crusted papules on ears, elbows, and hocks.

3) Diagnosis is often inferred by eliminating other causes of nonseasonal pruritus and a positive response to therapy for scabies.

b. Pinnal reflex—a scratch response elicited by rubbing the ear is present in 75–100% of cases but is not specific for scabies.

c. Typical signs in young animals and pruritus that does not respond to antiinflammatory dosages of corticosteroids are supportive findings.

4. Treatment

a. Ivermectin, 300 μg/kg SQ or PO every 2 weeks until signs resolve. (Must be heartworm negative.)

b. In collies and other breeds sensitive to ivermectin, milbemycin oxime, 2 mg/kg PO on day 0, 7, and 14.

c. Acaricidal dips

1) Lime sulfur, 2–3%, weekly until 2 weeks after signs resolve.

2) Amitraz, 250 ppm, every 2 weeks for 1–3 treatments.

d. All household pets should be treated.

e. Prednisone, 1.1 mg/kg q24h PO for 3–5 then tapered may relieve pruritus.

f. Keratolytic shampoos may provide symptomatic relief.

F. Burns

1. Overview

a. Causes of thermal injury include fire, heating pads, chemical burns, electric hair dryers, and scalds.

b. Burns are classified as:

1) Partial thickness—superficial (epidermis only), deep (extend to dermis)

2) Full thickness—entire dermis with destruction of adnexa (nerves and vessels); may destroy subcutaneous tissue including muscle and bone.

c. Superficial partial thickness wounds in which basal layer of epidermis is preserved may heal completely with minimal scarring or hair loss.

d. Deep partial thickness wounds and full thickness wounds require extensive wound management followed by surgical closure or grafting and may result in significant scarring and permanent hair loss.

e. Burns involving more than 40–50% of body surface area have a high mortality rate due to systemic complications such as sepsis and multiple organ failure. Survival is rare when greater than 80% body surface area is involved (humans).

2. Clinical signs

a. Erythema and blister formation indicate partial thickness burns.

b. Deep partial wounds and full thickness wounds appear dry or leathery, are not painful due to destruction of sensory nerves, and do not bleed due to destruction of blood vessels.

c. Scar tissue (eschar) may cause a wound to appear dry but often covers an area of abscessation.

d. Chemical burns are ulcerative and necrotic.

e. Singed facial hairs and whiskers and corneal lesions indicate possible smoke inhalation necessitating careful monitoring of respiratory status.

f. Note: The full extent of injury may be obscured by hair coat and may not be apparent for 24–48 h. Thus, liberal clipping and careful monitoring are necessary during the initial management of burn patients.

3. Treatment

a. Cool water should be applied to wounds immediately if possible to minimize extent of injury.

b. Superficial partial thickness wounds

1) Clip hair from wounds and lavage with saline to remove surface heat, debris, and chemicals.

2) Apply silver sulfadiazine ointment to keep the wound moist and prevent colonization of the wound by skin flora.

3) Cover with sterile occlusive dressing.

c. Deep, partial thickness or full thickness wounds

1) Resuscitate patient as indicated by extent of injury—supplemental oxygen, intravenous fluids, etc.

2) Sedation or anesthesia is required for adequate wound management.

3) Aggressive lavage and debridement is necessary to remove debris and necrotic, nonviable tissue.

4) Apply silver sulfadiazine ointment and cover the wound with sterile occlusive dressing.

5) Daily debridement is indicated until wound healing begins.

6) Sterile technique is critical to prevent infection.

7) Splints should be used when necessary to prevent excessive movement during healing.

8) Ultimately, surgical closure or skin grafts are necessary.

d. Systemic antibiotics are not indicated in most cases and may predispose to infection with resistant organisms.

1) With severe or refractory wounds antibiotics should be chosen based on culture of full thickness biopsy of the wound.

e. Once healed, skin that remains scarred or hairless should be protected from sun exposure by applying zinc oxide cream.

G. Degloving injury

1. Overview

a. Degloving injuries or shear wounds are traumatic injuries causing avulsion of skin and exposure of deep soft tissue structures and bone.

b. These injuries most often occur on distal extremities when limbs are compressed between an automobile tire and pavement.

2. Clinical signs

a. Loss of skin to varying degrees usually affecting the medial aspect of distal limbs.

b. Bleeding is usually minimal due to traumatic injury to blood vessels.

c. Extensive damage to ligament and bone resulting in exposed unstable joints is common with severe injury.

d. Wounds are often contaminated with dirt, hair, and other debris.

e. Signs of other traumatic injuries are often present (e.g., shock, fractures of long bones/pelvis, respiratory distress).

3. Treatment

a. Life-threatening traumatic injuries are stabilized following basic principles of trauma management.

b. Initial wound care in unstable critical patients should include clipping and flushing the wound and placing a protective stabilizing splint/bandage while more serious injuries are addressed.

c. Once the patient is stabilized, more aggressive wound management is performed.

1) Severe injuries are treated as open wounds with daily debridement, copious flushing, and use of sterile wet-to-dry bandages until surgical closure.

2) Sedation or anesthesia is necessary.

3) Flush with large volumes of sterile saline to remove debris.

4) Debride the wound of all necrotic tissue.

5) Remove bone fragments that are not connected to tissue or blood vessels.

6) Tendons, ligaments, or bone with soft tissue attachments are left in place. Tag transected tendons with nonabsorbable suture to make locating them easier when anastomosis is performed.

7) Evaluate muscle for viability using the "four C system"—consistency (firm not friable), color (pink/red not gray/brown), contractility (should contract when pricked), and circulation (should bleed when cut).

8) Preserve as much skin as possible to facilitate wound closure.

9) Initially, wound edges should be partially opposed using nonabsorbable suture to permit drainage, minimize exposure of deep tissues, and provide some stability.

10) Temporarily stabilize orthopedic injuries with splints or external fixators until soft tissues have healed.

d. Systemic antibiotics

1) Cephalexin, 22–44 mg/kg q6–8h IV for 1–3 days, then 22 mg/kg q8–12h PO for 10–21 days depending on severity of injury.

2) For refractory infection wound tissue should be cultured to determine appropriate therapy.

e. Pain management

1) Analgesic support using injectable or transdermal narcotics and/or nonsteroidal anti-inflammatory drugs is necessary as in most trauma patients.

H. Immune-mediated skin disease

1. Overview

a. As the diagnosis of immune-mediated skin disease requires biopsy in most cases, the role of the emergency clinician in evaluation such patients is to know when to suspect immune-mediated disease, obtain skin biopsies if intact vesicles/bullae/pustules are present, and treat severe pruritus and/or secondary infection.

b. Immune-mediated skin disease should be suspected when animals are presented with vesiculobullous, pustular, crusting, or depigmented lesions involving the face, ears, feet/toenails/footpads, and/or mucocutaneous junctions.

c. The pemphigus complex of diseases shares the histologic feature of acantholysis or loss of intercellular adhesion between keratinocytes in the epidermis.

d. Pemphigus foliaceous is the most common immune-mediated skin disease.

2. Clinical signs

a. Pemphigus foliaceous—pustular, crusting lesions (not vesicular) on face, ears, feet/foot pads, toenails, or nipples (cats). Mucocutaneous junctions are NOT involved.

b. Pemphigus erythematosus is a more benign form of P. foliaceous.

c. Pemphigus vulgaris—vesiculobullous lesions involving mucocutaneous junctions primarily of the oral cavity.

d. Bullous pemphigoid is distinguished from the pemphigus complex by involvement of the epidermal basement membrane leading to subepidermal clefts/bullae, not acantholysis.

e. Both c and d are rare.

f. Discoid lupus—lesions begin as depigmentation of nasal planum followed by ulcer and crust formation involving bridge of nose, pinnae, palate, or tongue. ANA titer is negative.

g. Systemic lupus erythematosus—skin lesions similar to discoid lupus with multisystemic signs such as polyarthritis, glomerulonephropathy, anemia, and thrombocytopenia. ANA titer is positive in 90% of cases.

3. Diagnosis

a. Skin biopsy of intact vesicle/bullae is diagnostic method of choice.

b. When intact vesicles/bullae are absent multiple punch biopsies of representative lesions are recommended.

c. Tissue can be submitted in buffered formalin for routine histopathology and demonstration of autoantibody (IgG) via immunoperoxidase testing.

d. Tissue must be submitted in Michel's fixative if direct immunofluorescence testing is desired.

e. Whenever possible biopsy should be performed before glucocorticoid administration or after 2–3 weeks of discontinuing prior treatment.

4. Treatment

a. Prednisone, 2.2 mg/kg q12–24h PO until active lesions resolve than gradual taper.

b. Azathioprine, 2.2 mg/kg q24h PO tapered to every other day, or chlorambucil, 0.1–0.2 mg/kg q24–48h (q48 h in cats) can be added to prednisone therapy if response to prednisone is inadequate or side effects are severe.

c. Aurothioglucose, 1 mg/kg weekly IM until remission is achieved, can be used in refractory cases; response is variable.

d. Cephalexin, 22 mg/kg q8–12h PO, for secondary pyoderma.

I. Drug Eruption

1. Overview

a. Two categories

1) Nonimmunologic or predictable—dose dependent reaction due to pharmacologic properties of the drug.

2) Immunologic or unpredictable—idiosyncratic, dose independent reactions caused by a variety of host and drug factors.

b. Reactions may occur with topical, systemic, or injectable medications as well as preservatives or dyes.

c. Antibiotics, especially trimethoprim-sulfonamide, cephalosporin, or penicillins, cause most drug eruptions in small animals (*Table 19-1*).

d. Genetic factors may be involved, as Doberman pinchers appear to be susceptible to sulfonamide reactions.

2. Clinical signs

a. Vary from mild injection site reactions, pruritus, or urticaria-angioedema to severe vesiculobullous, maculopapular, or ulcerative lesions with systemic signs.

b. Mucocutaneous junctions may be affected.

c. Lesions may take weeks to months to resolve.

TABLE 19-1
DRUGS ASSOCIATED WITH ALLERGIC REACTIONS IN ANIMALS

Sulfonamides
Penicillins
Cephalosporins
Propylthiouracil
Levamisole
Gold salts
L-asparaginase
Doxorubicin
Tetracyclines
Streptokinase
Antivenom
Vitamin K
Vaccines

3. Diagnosis

a. A history of skin lesions that appear within days to weeks of beginning medication (or vaccination) and then resolve when the medication is discontinued supports the diagnosis.

b. Skin biopsy is important in ruling out other dermatoses.

4. Treatment

a. Discontinue suspected offending medication or any unnecessary medications the animal might be receiving.

b. Antihistamine and glucocorticoids can be given to provide symptomatic relief if pruritus is present.

c. Systemic antibiotics are indicated when secondary pyoderma or erosive/ulcerative lesions are present.

J. Urticaria-angioedema

1. Overview

a. Most commonly caused by type I IgE-mediated hypersensitivity reaction to insect bite or envenomation.

b. Other causes include drugs, vaccine components, blood products, food, and inhaled allergens.

2. Clinical signs

a. Characteristic signs include pruritus, erythema, and swelling usually involving muzzle and eyelids.

b. Urticaria (hives) may be generalized involving trunk and ventrum and be obscured by hair coat.

c. In short haired breeds raised urticarial plaques (wheals) cause overlying hair to be raised making identifying lesions easier.

d. Systemic signs are rare and may include respiratory distress due to laryngeal or pulmonary edema, vomiting, diarrhea or circulatory collapse.

3. Treatment

a. Glucocorticoids (choose one)

1) Dexamethasone sodium phosphate, 0.1–0.2 mg/kg SC, IM, or IV

2) Prednisone sodium succinate, 0.5–1.0 mg/kg IV

3) Prednisone aqueous suspension, 0.5–1.0 mg/kg IV

4) Prednisone, 0.5–1.0 mg/kg q24h PO for 3 days then tapered.

b. Antihistamine

1) Diphenhydramine, 2 mg/kg SQ

2) Oral forms can be given by the owner in early stages of recurrence to minimize severity of signs.

i) Diphenhydramine, 2–4 mg/kg q8h PO

ii) Chlorpheniramine, 4–8 mg/dog q8–12h, 2–4 mg/cat q12h.

iii) Hydroxyzine, 0.5–2.0 mg/kg q6–8h.

K. Hepatocutaneous syndrome (superficial necrolytic dermatitis)

1. Overview

a. Ulcerative, crusting skin disease, seen with liver disease, diabetes mellitus, or glucagon-secreting pancreatic neoplasia.

b. Pathogenesis unknown but thought to be related to nutritional deficiency and excess circulating glucagon.

2. Clinical signs

a. Skin lesions range from alopecia and erythema to crusting plaques, erosions, or ulcers.

b. Distribution includes mucocutaneous junctions, face, ears, feet and ventrum.

3. Diagnosis

a. Diagnosis is based on finding skin lesions described above in a patient with clinical signs of concurrent metabolic disease, elevated liver enzymes, hyperglycemia (usually), and hypoalbuminemia.

b. Hepatic abnormalities

1) Ultrasonography—characteristic "swiss-cheese" like pattern of hyperechoic areas surrounding hypoechoic lesions.

2) Histopathology—vacuolar hepatopathy, parenchymal collapse, and nodular regeneration.

4. Treatment

a. Treat underlying liver disease, diabetes, and any other metabolic problems.

b. Diet—good quality protein supplemented with zinc, omega 3 fatty acids, and niacin.

c. Skin lesions—benzyl peroxide-containing shampoo, systemic antibiotics, and clipping hair from affected areas as indicated.

5. Prognosis

a. Severity of lesions is correlated with severity of underlying disease and prognosis is poor.

L. Fleas

1. Animals with flea allergy can present as emergencies because of open wounds from self-mutilation, excoriation, and severe pruritus. For treatment, see Acute Moist Dermatitis (p. 376).

2. In very young animals (i.e., nursing puppies and kittens) severe flea infestation can cause life-threatening anemia. Options for removing fleas from young animals include:

a. Use a flea comb to remove adults and eggs (not 100% effective, but safe).

b. Bathe with a pyrethrin based shampoo. Dry neonate thoroughly to prevent chilling. Use low heat on hand held dryer to avoid burns and over heating. No residual activity.

c. Spray towel with pyrethrin spray and wrap neonate in towel with head exposed. Use flea comb to remove dying fleas. This has weak residual activity.

d. Give oral nitenpyram (Capstar). Kills adult fleas within 30 minutes, but the residual effect only lasts 24–48 hours. It has low toxicity.

e. Imidacloprid (Advantage). Apply between shoulder blades as spot-on preparation. It has a long residual effect. This is safe for neonates. Maximum effectiveness is after 12 hours.

f. Fipronil (Frontline) spray or topical can be used. It has long residual effect with maximum efficacy after 24 hours.

g. Selamectin (Revolution) topical spot-on has low toxicity (concentrates in sebaceous glands) and long residual activity, but does not achieve maximal efficacy until after 36 hours.

CHAPTER 20

TOXICOLOGIC EMERGENCIES

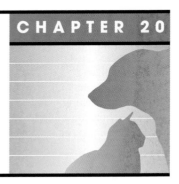

I. DIAGNOSIS, CLINICAL SIGNS

A. Telephone triage

1. The immediate aims of the initial telephone triage are to determine if the patient needs to be examined and what the owner can do for the pet.
2. Animals with respiratory distress, neurologic abnormalities, protracted vomiting, slow or rapid heart rate, bleeding from body orifices, weakness, or pale mucous membranes should be evaluated as soon as possible.
3. If there is any question about poisoning, the animal should be evaluated.
4. The owner should be instructed to bring any packages or material that the pet might have access to, as well as any material the patient might have vomited. The material should be placed in a clear plastic bag or glass container for potential evaluation.

B. Home management

1. Animals that have had a topical exposure should be bathed immediately with a mild pet shampoo (if liquid exposure). If powder has been applied to the coat then vacuuming the coat prior to bathing will be more effective. The owners should wear protective clothing such as gloves and aprons while bathing the animal.
2. All owners should be warned that pets may develop an aggressive nature while intoxicated and to take precautions when handling their pets.
3. The eye should be flushed with copious amounts of water if ocular exposure has occurred.
4. Emesis may be induced at home (see Emesis, p. 385).

5. In most instances, it is more efficient and safer to have the patient brought into the clinic rather than managed at home by the owner.

C. Initial assessment of the poisoned patient involves applying the basic principles of assessment of the emergency patient (see Approach to the Emergency Patient).

D. Diagnosis of toxicity

    a. The working diagnosis is based on a history of witnessed exposure; characteristic, suggestive, or suspicious signs and symptoms; and chemical analysis.
    b. In veterinary medicine, diagnosis is most commonly made from a history of possible exposure and consistent clinical signs.
    c. Remember that many common diseases mimic toxins and toxins mimic common diseases.
    d. It is common for owners to think that their pets have been poisoned whenever they become sick. Pointed questions to an owner regarding the basis of this thought will often validate or discount it.
    e. Clinically, a toxin should be suspected when there is a sudden onset of neurologic signs or sudden organ failure in an otherwise healthy patient or in a situation in which all other common diseases that could explain the clinical signs have been ruled out.

II. INITIAL APPROACH TO THE POISONED PATIENT

A. Poison control resource information

1. National Animal Poison Control Center: 1-900-680-0000 or 1-800-548-2423 (charge per case, credit cards only)
2. Arizona Poison Drug Information Center (University of Arizona) 1-800-363-0101
3. National Pesticides Telecommunication Network, Texas Tech University: 1-800-858-7378
4. Oklahoma City Poison Control Center (snakebites): 405-271-5454

B. General treatment of the poisoned patient
1. Elimination of further absorption
   a. Skin
      1) Bathe the pet with a mild pet shampoo or a mild liquid dishwashing detergent. Patients with powder exposures should have their haircoats vacuumed to remove the bulk of the toxin prior to shampooing. Shampooing should be continued until contamination is reduced as much as possible or eliminated. The handler should take care to protect against self-exposure to the toxin.
      2) Decontamination of the gastrointestinal (GI) tract involves induction of emesis, gastric lavage, and administration of adsorbents and cathartics as well as high enemas.
   b. Emesis
      1) Emesis should be considered if the toxin has been ingested within the last 3 hours. Beyond this time it is likely that the toxin has been absorbed or moved farther down the GI tract. Some exceptions exist (e.g., a massive dose of aspirin may ball up in the stomach and remain there for several hours).
      2) Contraindications to induced emesis:
         a) *Respiratory distress*
         b) *Ingestion of a caustic material (petroleum distillates, acids, alkalis)*
         c) *Decreased gag reflex*
         d) *Seizures*
         e) *Extreme weakness*
         f) *Neurologic impairment, central nervous system (CNS) depression, unconsciousness*
         g) *Laryngeal paralysis*
         h) *Bradycardia—ingestion of tranquilizers*
      3) Syrup of ipecac (1.0–2.5 mL/kg in the dog; 3.3 mL/kg in the cat)
         a) *Induces emesis by local GI irritation and central activation of the chemoreceptor trigger zone*
         b) *Emesis may be delayed as long as 20 minutes after administration.*
         c) *Reported side effects generally result from chronic administration or are associated with the fluid extract and include cardiotoxicity, hemorrhagic diarrhea, and skeletal muscle weakness. These side effects are rarely associated with a single administration of syrup of ipecac. If side effects are noted, activated charcoal binds well with syrup of ipecac.*
         d) *Syrup of ipecac should be diluted 50:50 with water to increase acceptability by cats.*
      4) 3% hydrogen peroxide (1.0–2.0 mL/kg orally in dogs or cats)
         a) *Induces emesis by local gastric irritation*
         b) *Induction of emesis is inconsistent.*
         c) *A second dose should be administered if emesis has not occurred within 10 minutes after the initial dose.*
      5) Table salt has been recommended as a pharyngeal stimulant to induce vomiting, but if swallowed, it can result in sodium toxicity and death. For this reason, table salt is not recommended for use as an emetic.
      6) Liquid dishwashing detergent
         a) *Mix with 8 parts water and give 10 mL/kg PO.*
         b) *Do not use laundry detergent or automatic dishwasher detergent—these are too irritating.*
      7) Apomorphine (Anthony Products Co., Arcadia, CA) is the most reliable emetic in dogs. The dose is 0.03 mg/kg IV, 0.04 mg/kg IM, or 0.08 mg/kg SC. The topical conjunctival dose is 0.3 mg/kg, or a tablet can be placed in the conjunctival sac and rinsed out with saline after vomiting has been accomplished. Cats have a much higher threshold for apomorphine-induced emesis and therefore it is not recommended for use in cats.
         a) *Side effects include mild sedation and mild conjunctivitis from topical application.*
         b) *Advantage of the conjunctival route is dose titration. When vomitus has clear stomach contents, the drug can be flushed from the conjunctiva to terminate the effects.*
      8) Xylazine
         a) *Mechanism of emesis is central.*
         b) α_2 *agonist*

c) Induces emesis in cats (0.44 mg/kg IM), usually within 3–5 minutes of administration

d) Side effects include sedation, overall decrease in cardiac output (may be as much as 30%) and prolonged hypotension. For these reasons we don't recommend the use of this drug as an emetic. Yohimbine HCl can be used to reverse the effects of xylazine (0.1 mg/kg IV in dogs, 0.5 mg/kg IV in cats).

9) Patients that ingest toxins often vomit. Despite a history of this, induction of vomiting is still recommended because the amount of vomitus or ingested toxin is often unknown.

c. Gastric lavage

1) The main indications for gastric lavage are when emesis is contraindicated or when induced emesis was ineffective.

2) Technique

a) Light anesthesia, but deep enough to allow intubation with endotracheal tube cuff inflation

b) Intubate and inflate endotracheal tube cuff to protect airway from aspiration of gastric contents or lavage fluid. The tube should extend several inches beyond the mouth or be attached to anesthetic tubing to avoid aspiration of gastric contents during the lavage procedure.

c) Premeasure a large-bore stomach tube (similar to endotracheal tube in diameter) from the tip of the nose to the last rib.

d) The tube should be lubricated with sterile KY gel and then gently passed down the esophagus into the stomach.

e) Ten to 20 mL/kg body weight of tepid water (45°C) (not hot or cold) should then be administered through the stomach tube. The free end of the tube is then rapidly lowered below the level of the stomach and placed into a bucket to allow drainage by gravity. Aspiration may be facilitated by an aspiration bulb, 60-mL syringe, or stomach pump. The procedure should be repeated until the fluid that is returned to the bucket is clear.

f) Gentle compression of the stomach often helps drainage of the fluid from the stomach.

g) Lavage should be repeated with the animal in different positions to ensure complete evacuation of stomach contents.

h) Mixing the lavage fluid with activated charcoal may enhance the effectiveness of gastric lavage.

i) The stomach tube should be kinked when removed, to prevent any drainage of residual fluid into the esophagus, oropharynx, or mouth.

j) The esophagus, oropharynx, and mouth should be suctioned to prevent aspiration of any remaining fluid that may be present.

k) Take care to avoid injury to the esophagus or stomach during this procedure.

l) Close monitoring of anesthetic recovery is recommended in these patients.

d. Activated charcoal

1) Effective absorbent for many organic compounds, but ineffective for heavy metals

2) Standard dose 1–4 g/kg of body weight mixed in 50–200 mL of water (6–12 mL/kg PO)

3) May be given orally or via a stomach tube after gastric lavage

4) Capsules containing activated charcoal may be used in cats and some small dogs.

5) Give activated charcoal with a cathartic (see below) every 4–6 hours for toxins that undergo enterohepatic circulation.

6) Side effects reported with activated charcoal are minimal; the most common complaint is constipation.

7) Warn the owner that the stool may be black for a few days.

8) Activated charcoal can be very messy. The veterinarian and technical staff should take adequate precautions, including protective clothing and covering surfaces that may stain.

e. Cathartics

1) Assist in hastening the elimination of the ingested toxins and toxin-bound activated charcoal

2) Sodium sulfate

a) Dose is 250–500 mg/kg body weight mixed in 5–10 times as much water.

b) Dose may be administered orally or via stomach tube.

3) Magnesium sulfate

a) Dose is 250–500 mg/kg body weight mixed in 5–10 times as much water.

b) Dose may be administered orally or via stomach tube.

4) Magnesium citrate: 2–4 mL/kg orally

5) Sorbitol (70%): 1–3 mL/kg PO

6) Use caution with the above cathartics in very old or young patients and patients with preexisting renal disease or ingestion of nephrotoxic substances, corrosive ingestions, recent intestinal surgery, hypertension, or congestive heart failure.

2. Eliminating absorbed toxin

a. Fluid diuresis may be used to speed elimination of some toxins that are excreted through the kidneys. Each toxin should be evaluated for this possibility.

b. Other options for speeding the elimination of toxins include urine ion trapping by administration of sodium bicarbonate, hemodialysis, peritoneal dialysis, hemoperfusion, and the use of drug antibodies. Most of these options are not routinely available in veterinary medicine, and each toxin should be evaluated individually concerning whether the technique would be useful or not.

3. Corrosive intoxication

a. Occurs rarely in veterinary medicine

b. Acids

1) Produce coagulative necrosis and rarely penetrate the entire mucosal thickness

2) In general, tend not to be as severe as alkalis

c. Alkalis produce liquefactive necrosis, potentially yielding deeper and more penetrating burns than acids.

d. Clinical signs

1) Range from mild mucosal irritation and pain to life-threatening hypovolemic shock

2) Initial signs are usually due to local irritation and corrosion of the mucosal surfaces and may include vocalization, panting, depression, difficulty swallowing, hematemesis, abdominal pain, hypersalivation, polydipsia, and/or respiratory distress.

3) Esophageal or intestinal perforation may result in hypovolemic or septic shock.

4) Absence of oral lesions does not rule out ingestion of a corrosive chemical.

5) Esophageal strictures may develop 2 weeks after ingestion of a corrosive chemical.

e. Treatment

1) Basic emergency principles should be applied to any critically ill patient that has ingested a corrosive chemical.

2) Do NOT induce vomiting.

3) Attempt immediate dilution with milk or water.

4) Exposed eyes or skin should be flushed extensively with water.

5) Chemical neutralization is not recommended because the exothermic reaction may cause further mucosal damage.

6) Activated charcoal and gastric lavage are not effective.

7) Antibiotics are controversial; they may be useful with GI ulceration and are definitely indicated in the presence of confirmed infection.

8) Administer sucralfate for gastric ulceration or esophagitis.

9) Other gastric protectants such as antacids and synthetic prostaglandins may provide protection against further ulceration.

10) Antiinflammatory doses of corticosteroids within the first 24–48 hours may prevent stricture formation.

11) Analgesics may be necessary in patients with pain.

III. MANAGEMENT OF SPECIFIC TOXICITIES

A. Acetaminophen

1. Aspirin-free pain relievers often contain acetaminophen.

2. Phenacetin is metabolized to acetaminophen.

3. Acetaminophen can be rapidly absorbed from the stomach (often <60 minutes after ingestion:

4. Susceptibility to intoxication varies from species to species; cats are the most sensitive.

5. Mechanism of action

a. Acetaminophen is initially metabolized by the cytochrome P-450 system in the liver to a reactive metabolite. The metabolite is then rapidly glucuronidated or sulfated to a relatively inert compound. The reactive metabolite will (if not glucuronidated or sulfated) bind to cell macromolecules, resulting in cell death. Glutathione is consumed rapidly when an overwhelming amount of metabolite is formed, especially in species that lack glucuronyl transferase (cats).

b. Hepatic damage occurs as a result of the metabolite binding to the liver cells.

c. Methemoglobinemia results from oxidation of heme iron. This is reversible. Methemoglobin cannot carry oxygen, resulting in tissue hypoxia.

d. Heinz body formation occurs as a result of oxidative denaturation of hemoglobin. This results in decreased red blood cell survival and anemia. Heinz body formation is not reversible.

6. Clinical signs

   a. Dogs

   1) Usually no signs until dose exceeds 100 mg/kg.

   2) Methemoglobinemia is rare but has been seen with doses >200 mg/kg.

   3) Hepatic necrosis is the most common lesion manifesting as anorexia, vomiting, and painful abdomen. These signs may not develop until 24–48 hours after ingestion.

   b. Cats

   1) Cats may develop signs with doses of 40 mg/kg, and susceptible cats at even lower doses.

   2) Methemoglobinemia (dark brown blood, cyanotic or dark brown mucous membranes) is the most common and serious problem. Cats exhibit open-mouthed breathing, anxiety, and respiratory distress.

   3) Other signs include depression, weakness, anorexia, vomiting, facial and front paw edema, and tachypnea.

   4) Hepatic lesions do occur in cats but are often overshadowed by the methemoglobinemia.

   c. Treatment

   1) If recently ingested (<3 hours), apply basic principles of treatment of oral ingestion of toxins.

   2) N-Acetylcysteine acts as a glutathione precursor, supplies sulfhydryl groups, and directly binds acetaminophen metabolites. It is considered a specific antidote for acetaminophen toxicity. Give 140 mg/kg (PO or IV) initially, then 70 mg/kg PO QID for a total of 6 doses after the loading dose. (For IV administration, mix the solution to a 5% concentration and give slowly over 15 minutes).

   3) Ascorbic acid (30 mg/kg, PO or SQ QID for 7 treatments) helps convert methemoglobin back to oxyhemoglobin.

   4) Cimetidine (5 mg/kg IV QID) inhibits cytochrome P-450 and may decrease formation of the toxic intermediate. This treatment has not been clinically evaluated in dogs and cats.

   5) Supportive care as for any critically ill animal

   6) Generally, if a cat makes it past the first 48 hours it will survive.

B. Salicylates

1. Two types of toxicity occur:

   a. Toxicity similar to that of other nonsteroidal antiinflammatory medications (NSAIDs) (i.e., renal disease, gastric ulceration, hepatotoxicity, and inhibited platelet aggregation)

   b. Acute severe toxicity

   1) Very high doses of aspirin may uncouple oxidative phosphorylation and result in hyperglycemia or hypoglycemia.

   2) Acidosis may occur due to salicylates themselves, lactic acidosis, and decreased renal excretion of acids.

   3) Stimulation of the respiratory center

   4) Pulmonary edema may occur.

   5) Salicylates are highly protein bound and are eliminated as conjugates of glycine and glucuronic acid (cats and neonates have limited glucuronyl transferase and are therefore predisposed to toxicity).

   6) Signs include tachypnea, fever, vomiting, depression/stupor, seizures, and death.

   c. Toxic dosage—dogs, 50 mg/kg/day; cats: 25 mg/kg/day

   d. Treatment

   1) Initial treatment as for any ingested toxin (see above)

   2) Occasionally, aspirin forms insoluble accumulations within the stomach that prolong absorption.

   3) Sodium bicarbonate to treat the acidosis: 50 mg/kg PO q8–12h or measure blood gases and calculate amount needed, $0.3 \times$ BW (kg) $\times$ (desired HCO_3 – measured HCO_3). Give $1/4$–$1/2$ of the calculated amount slowly IV.

   4) Hypoglycemia should be treated with intravenous glucose.

5) See NSAID toxicity for treatment of gastric ulceration and renal failure (p. 390).

C. Methylxanthines

1. Major methylxanthines encountered in veterinary medicine include theophylline, caffeine, and theobromine (chocolate). Sources include diet pills, fatigue reduction pills, tea leaves, coffee products, colas, and chocolate.

2. Milk chocolate contains 44 mg/oz of theobromine, semisweet contains 140 mg/oz, and unsweetened baking chocolate contains 390–450 mg/oz. The toxic dose for dogs is 100–150 mg/kg.

3. Methylxanthines are eliminated primarily by liver metabolism.

4. The LD_{50} of caffeine is 110–175 mg/kg in dogs and 80–150 mg/kg in cats.

5. The LD_{50} of theobromine in dogs ranges from 250 to 500 mg/kg.

6. Mechanism of action
 a. Antagonism of cellular adenosine receptors
 b. Inhibition of phosphodiesterase, causing accumulation of intracellular cyclic adenosine monophosphate (AMP)
 c. Interference with uptake and storage of intracellular calcium in striated muscle, causing contraction
 d. Smooth muscle relaxation
 e. CNS stimulation.
 f. Increased concentration of circulating catecholamines
 g. Increased gastric secretion, causing mucosal irritation
 h. Diuresis

7. Clinical signs—vomiting, hyperactivity, restlessness, tachycardia, tachypnea, ataxia, tremors, convulsions, cardiac arrhythmias, and death

8. Treatment
 a. General principles of orally ingested toxins should be followed—induce vomiting, +/− gastric lavage, activated charcoal and cathartic. (See pp. 384–387).
 b. There is no specific antidote for methylxanthines.
 c. Apply general principles for support of any critically ill patient.
 d. Monitor continuous ECG.
  1) Ventricular tachycardia should be treated with lidocaine boluses (2–4 mg/kg) followed by continuous-rate infusion (CRI) (25–80 μg/kg/min) if the boluses were effective.

2) Supraventricular arrhythmias may be treated with esmolol (10–100 μg/kg/min CRI), propranolol (0.05–0.3 mg/kg slow IV q8–12h), or metoprolol (0.5–1 mg/kg PO q8h).

e. Blood pressure should be closely monitored.

f. Tremors and seizures
 1) Diazepam or midazolam boluses (0.2–1 mg/kg IV)
 2) Phenobarbital (4 mg/kg IV BID to QID)
 3) If patient is refractory to anticonvulsants, induce general anesthesia with pentobarbital.

g. Administration of activated charcoal with a saline cathartic q3h for 72 hours will hasten elimination.

h. Gastric lavage or emesis may be effective even several hours after chocolate ingestion, because of its slow absorption.

i. Catheterize the urinary bladder to keep it empty and prevent reabsorption of methylxanthines and their metabolites.

j. Intravenous fluid diuresis (2–3 times maintenance rate) can speed renal elimination.

k. Gastric protectants (ranitidine or famotidine and Amphojel) may decrease GI irritation.

D. Cholecalciferol

1. In very potent rodenticides, skin preparations

2. Toxic doses
 a. In dogs, clinical signs can occur with 0.5–3 mg/kg, 10–20 mg/kg is fatal.
 b. Cats are more sensitive; lethal doses are 5–10 mg/kg.

3. Mechanism of action
 a. Cholecalciferol is eventually converted to vitamin D_3, increasing the ionized calcium concentration.
 b. Increased calcium concentration affects four major organ systems—neurologic, cardiovascular, GI, and renal.

4. Clinical signs
 a. Generally develop within 12–36 hours and worsen over the ensuing 24 hours
 b. Lethargy, weakness, anorexia, hematemesis, bloody diarrhea, depression, vomiting, polyuria, polydipsia, pulmonary hemorrhage, muscle twitching, seizures, bradycardia, cardiac arrhythmias, shock, stupor, and death
 c. Result from ionized hypercalcemia and calcification of tissues

d. Acute renal failure may result from renal arterial vasospasm and renal tubular calcification.

e. Blood work may reveal hyperphosphatemia, hypercalcemia, and azotemia.

f. Radiographs may reveal dystrophic calcification of bronchi and other soft tissues.

g. The prognosis is guarded to poor, with death usually occurring within 2–5 days after onset of signs.

5. Treatment

a. Administer general treatment as for any orally ingested toxin.

b. Specific measures to reduce calcium concentration:

   1) Normal saline diuresis (4–6 mL/kg/h or above)

   2) Furosemide (2–5 mg/kg IV q8–12h)

   3) Prednisolone (0.5 mg/kg PO, SQ, IM q12h)

   4) Salmon calcitonin (4–6 IU/kg SQ q2–3h). *Note:* This is a foreign protein, and anaphylaxis may occur. Preevaluation with an intradermal skin test is recommended.

c. After calcium level is stabilized in the normal range, long-term therapy will be required (sometimes several weeks) because cholecalciferol is fat soluble.

   1) Furosemide (2–4 mg/kg PO q8–12h)

   2) Oral prednisolone (0.25 mg/kg q12h).

   3) Low-calcium diet (no milk or dairy products)

   4) Continued salmon calcitonin may be helpful, although tachyphylaxis can occur.

E. Cocaine

1. A rare intoxication in veterinary medicine, likely because of minimal exposure opportunity and reluctance of owners to admit to the possibility

2. There are reports of dogs who have been force-fed balloons filled with cocaine for smuggling. These must be surgically removed if obstruction occurs.

3. Cocaine is rapidly absorbed through the mucous membranes.

4. Mechanism of action: CNS stimulation through sympathetic discharge, also resulting in vasoconstriction, tachycardia, cardiac arrhythmias, hypertension, dilated pupils, and seizures

5. Clinical signs: CNS changes ranging from depression, stupor/coma to hyperactivity or seizures. Panting, vomiting, hypersalivation, tachycardia, arrhythmias, hyperthermia, and pulmonary edema have also been reported.

6. Treatment

a. General treatment as for any orally ingested toxin (see pp. 384–387)

b. Control seizures with midazolam (0.5–1 mg/kg IV), phenobarbital (2–4 mg/kg IV), or pentobarbital (2–30 mg/kg slowly IV to effect).

c. Propranolol may help control cardiac arrhythmias (0.04–0.06 mg/kg slowly IV)

d. Control hyperthermia and hypoglycemia if present.

e. Apply basic emergency and critical care principles as for any critically ill patient.

f. The prognosis is fair to guarded.

F. Hypertonic sodium phosphate enema

1. Toxicity most commonly seen in cats

2. Mechanism of action—The high sodium and phosphate content results in serum hypernatremia, hyperosmolality, hyperphosphatemia, and hypocalcemia. The rapid electrolyte changes result in CNS dehydration and dysfunction as well as tetany from hypocalcemia.

3. Clinical signs

a. Depression, ataxia, vomiting, diarrhea (sometimes bloody), stupor/coma, miosis, tetany

b. Signs occur within 30–60 minutes postenema.

4. Treatment

a. Primarily supportive with low-sodium-containing fluids. Sodium concentration may be rapidly decreased in this situation because the increase is rapid and of short duration. Fluid diuresis will also lower phosphorus concentration. If treatment is delayed by several hours, isotonic fluids should be used to lower the sodium more slowly and avoid cerebral edema.

b. Extreme hypocalcemia may be treated with 10% calcium gluconate (50–100 mg/kg slow IV).

G. NSAIDs

1. Examples include aspirin, indomethacin, ibuprofen, naproxen, flunixin meglumine, phenylbutazone, piroxicam, and carprofen.

a. Carprofen has been associated with idiosyncratic hepatic toxicosis, primarily in Labrador Retrievers. Liver failure occurs 5–30 days after initiating therapy and is 50% fatal.

b. Ibuprofen and indomethacin are very toxic and should not be given to small animals.

2. Mechanism of action

a. Primarily due to inhibition of prostaglandin production.

b. Inhibition of prostaglandin production can cause gastric irritation and ulceration.

c. Decreased renal perfusion may occur in hypotensive patients due to inhibition of vasodilatory prostaglandin production.

d. Platelet dysfunction may occur.

e. Blood dyscrasias and hepatic damage have been reported with some NSAIDs.

f. Gastric irritation is the most common problem encountered.

3. Clinical signs

a. Anorexia, vomiting (sometimes bloody), and abdominal pain

b. Hypovolemia due to dehydration, blood loss, or peritonitis from GI perforation

c. The most severe GI signs and ulceration often occur in animals that have been given a combination of NSAIDs and corticosteroids.

d. Animals appear to vary on an individual basis in their ability to tolerate NSAIDs.

4. Treatment

a. General treatment as for any ingested oral toxin (pp. 384–387)

b. Emesis and lavage may be effective several hours after ingestion with massive doses of aspirin because of formation of concretions.

c. For acute, severe gastric hemorrhage, gastric lavage with ice water may curtail blood loss.

d. Activated charcoal with a cathartic may be necessary every 4–6 hours for some NSAIDs that undergo enterohepatic circulation.

e. If renal failure is suspected or diagnosed, dopamine (2–3 μg/kg/min CRI) combined with a bolus of furosemide (1mg/kg IV) can be given, followed by a CRI of 1 mg/kg/h. These methods should be used in conjunction with adequate fluid administration and blood pressure support. (Renal failure associated with NSAIDs is usually reversible.)

f. Gastric irritation may be treated with sucralfate (1 g/30 kg BW PO QID), misoprostol (2–5 μg/kg q8h PO), ranitidine (0.5–2 mg/kg q8h) or famotidine (0.5–1 mg/kg IV q12h), and omeprazole (0.7 mg/kg PO SID).

g. Control vomiting with antiemetics: metoclopramide (0.2 mg/kg SC or IM or 1 mg/kg/day CRI), chlorpromazine (0.05–0.1 mg/kg IV q4–6h), or prochlorperazine (0.25–0.5 mg/kg SC or IM q6–8h).

h. Blood transfusions may be necessary with severely affected patients. This is most commonly found in animals that have received a combination of NSAIDs and corticosteroids.

i. Perforating ulcers can cause shock and life-threatening peritonitis. Surgical gastrectomy and copious lavage is indicated.

H. Lead

1. Sources of lead include old paints (usually paints prior to 1950) but may still be present in newer paints, batteries, linoleum, plumbing material, grease, golf balls, caulking materials, toys, lead pipes, fishing and window weights, drapery weights, shotgun pellets and bullets. Lead projectiles that are present in muscle or subcutaneous tissues generally are walled off and inert, but if they are ingested, the acid content of the stomach allows absorption.

2. Lead is more readily absorbed (from the GI tract) and more readily crosses the blood/brain barrier in animals less than 6 months old.

3. Most commonly absorbed through the GI tract, but absorption through the lungs may occur with inhalation of lead particles.

4. Lead can cross the placenta.

5. Lead is excreted in the bile.

6. Mechanism of action

a. Primarily affects the GI and central nervous systems.

b. Interferes with thiol-containing enzymes and may replace zinc in some enzymes.

c. May lower γ-aminobenzoic acid (GABA) concentrations in inhibitory interneuron junctions in the CNS

d. May increase red cell fragility, resulting in anemia as well as interfering with red blood cell production in the bone marrow. Can cause increased number of nucleated red blood cells in the circulation as well as basophilic stippling

7. Clinical signs

a. GI system and CNS are most commonly involved, alone or in combinations.

b. Neurologic signs

1) Seizures, hysteria (barking, biting, crying, restlessness), behavioral changes, ataxia, tremors, blindness, and jaw clamping

2) Gastrointestinal

a) Anorexia, vomiting, abdominal pain, diarrhea

b) Regurgitation may be present, as megaesophagus has been rarely reported with lead intoxication.

8. Diagnosis

    a. Large numbers of nucleated red blood cells in the face of mild or no anemia may suggest lead toxicity in combination with clinical signs.

    b. Basophilic stippling is difficult to recognize and cannot be detected reliably.

    c. Abdominal radiographs may reveal a metallic foreign body in the GI tract but more commonly show diffuse radiopaque densities with paint ingestions. These cannot be differentiated from other causes of opacities but should prompt the clinician to consider lead intoxication with compatible clinical signs.

    d. Blood lead levels are the definitive diagnosis (>0.6 ppm is diagnostic). Lead is carried on the red blood cells, so whole blood must be submitted. Consult your laboratory for the appropriate amount of blood and container that it should be sent in. Do not collect in EDTA tube (chelates lead). Submit heparinized sample.

    e. Analysis of liver lead level is the best post-mortem method of diagnosis.

9. Treatment

    a. Remove large lead objects from the GI tract.

    b. Small paint chips and diffusely distributed pieces in the GI tract may be removed via enemas, inducing emesis, and cathartics such as magnesium sulfate (Epsom salt) or sodium sulfate. These cathartics precipitate lead as lead sulfate and also speed transit through the GI tract. The intestines should be cleared of any residual lead source prior to administration of chelating agents. Chelating agents may enhance absorption of any lead that remains in the GI tract.

    c. Chelating agents

    1) Calcium EDTA—25 mg/kg SC q4h for 2–5 days; dilute to 10 mg/mL with 5% dextrose

      a) *Do not exceed 2 g/day.*

      b) *All lead must be removed from GI tract prior to chelation therapy.*

    2) Penicillamine

      a) *33–55 mg/kg divided QID for 7 days, off 1 week, then repeat*

    3) Succimer (Chemet)

      a) *10 mg/kg PO q8h for 10 days*

      b) *Less toxic, effective, does not require GI tract to be free of lead*

      c) *Expensive*

    d. Repeat blood lead assay after 10–14 days. Continue chelation therapy if lead concentration is ≥0.4 ppm.

    e. Supportive care

    1) IV fluids

    2) Seizure control—Consider mannitol, furosemide, and corticosteroids to decrease cerebral edema.

I. Amitraz

1. Amitraz is used as a pesticide to control ticks, mites, and other insects on cattle and to control demodectic mange in dogs.

2. Amitraz is used primarily in collars and dips for dogs and cats. Toxicity occurs when the animals ingest the collars or dipping solution.

3. The amitraz collars weigh 27.5 g with a 9% concentration of amitraz. Therefore each collar has approximately 2500 mg of amitraz. The LD_{50} for dogs is reported to be 100 mg/kg but may actually be higher.

4. Clinical intoxication may be seen at a dose as low as 10 mg/kg.

5. Mechanism of action:

    a. The toxic effects may be primarily attributed to α_2-receptor agonism.

    b. α_2-Receptor agonism results in CNS depression, vomiting, ileus, bradycardia, hypotension (more common) or acute hypertension, mydriasis, hyperglycemia, and hypothermia.

6. Clinical signs

    a. (In order of frequency)—Depression, ataxia, pale mucous membranes, bradycardia, vomiting, hyperthermia, hypothermia, gastric dilatation, mydriasis, diarrhea, hypersalivation, dyspnea, anorexia, ileus, shock, tachycardia, urinary incontinence, disorientation, miosis, tremors, and coma

    b. Clinical signs may be observed as early as 30 minutes after exposure.

7. Treatment

    a. As for any ingested toxin (pp. 384–387)

    b. Endoscopy or surgery may be necessary to remove the ingested collar if emesis is ineffective.

    c. Administer activated charcoal with a cathartic every 8 hours while the collar is still in the GI tract.

    d. Xylazine is contraindicated as an anesthetic if surgery or endoscopy is required because it is also an α_2-receptor agonist.

e. Atropine is not indicated in the treatment of amitraz-induced bradycardia because it potentiates the pressor effects, resulting in hypertension and cardiac arrhythmias. Atropine also decreases intestinal motility, which is already compromised with this toxicity.

f. Yohimbine (0.1 mg/kg, IV) is the antidote of choice. It competitively displaces amitraz from the α_2-adrenoreceptors and reverses the bradycardia, hypotension, sedation, and GI ileus.

g. Antipamezole (Antisedan®) can also be used as an antidote at a dose of 50 μg/kg IM in the dog, repeated q3–4h as needed.

h. Basic principles of critical care should be applied as for any critically ill patient.

J. Metaldehyde (snail bait)

1. It is a polymer of acetaldehyde.

2. Mechanism of action
   a. Not clearly known
   b. Acidosis occurs in some animals, which may be due to metabolism of acetaldehyde or from lactic acidosis from muscle tremors.

3. Clinical signs
   a. Occur within 1–4 hours
   b. Tachypnea, hyperpnea, tachycardia, restlessness, hypersalivation, vomiting, cyanosis, diarrhea, and hyperthermia
   c. Neurologic signs include ataxia, nystagmus, muscle tremors, hyperesthesia, convulsions, stiff legs/gait, cortical blindness, depression, and stupor/coma (later stages).
   d. Delayed-onset (2–3 days) liver failure
   e. Most predominant sign is muscle tremors.
   f. Severe hyperthermia of 108°F may occur.

4. Diagnosis
   a. Metaldehyde in the material ingested can be measured.
   b. Metaldehyde may be analyzed from the liver, urine, or plasma.

5. Treatment
   a. General management principles should be applied as for any orally ingested toxin (pp. 384–387).
   b. Diazepam or midazolam is the drug of choice for control of convulsions or muscle tremors (0.5–1 mg/kg IV or 1–4 mg/kg per rectum).
   c. Barbiturates such as phenobarbital or pentobarbital may be used if benzodiazepines do not control the seizures. These should be used as a

last resort, because they compete with an enzyme that degrades acetaldehyde.
   d. Methocarbamol (150 mg/kg IV) is a muscle relaxant that may decrease muscle tremors as needed.
   e. Basic supportive care as for any critical patient

K. Cholinesterase inhibitors (organophosphates and carbamates)

1. Seen most frequently in the warm seasons when fleas proliferate

2. Most commonly due to ectoparasite control products

3. Cats and younger animals seem to be the most frequently affected.

4. Mechanism of action
   a. Inhibition of acetylcholinesterase enzymes, thus allowing an increase in acetylcholine.
   b. Acetylcholine acts as a neurotransmitter at several sites including autonomic ganglia of both sympathetic and parasympathetic nervous systems; between postganglionic parasympathetic nerve fibers and cardiac muscle, smooth muscle, and exocrine glands; at neuromuscular junctions of the somatic nervous system; and at cholinergic synapses in the CNS. The increased acetylcholine at these sites accounts for all the clinical signs.
   c. Binding of the acetylcholinesterase enzyme is irreversible with organophosphate (may be time related, i.e., the longer binding is allowed, the more irreversible the binding is) and reversible with carbamates.

5. Clinical signs
   a. Onset occurs within minutes to hours after exposure. Cats that are dipped or sprayed show signs within minutes to 1 hour, although onset may vary depending upon formulation of the insecticide, rate of metabolism and elimination, and concurrent drug administration or medical problems. Clinical signs may be delayed several days in some cats exposed to chlorpyrifos.
   b. Acetylcholine receptors may be classified as muscarinic or nicotinic. Clinical signs differ among organophosphates, depending on which receptors are maximally stimulated.
   c. Nicotinic signs (primarily striated muscle related)—skeletal muscle stiffness, fasciculations, tremors, weakness, and paralysis, as well as diaphragm and intercostal muscle dysfunction

d. Muscarinic signs (primarily smooth muscle and secretory glands related)—hypersalivation, lacrimation, urination, defecation, increased respiratory sounds, respiratory distress (increased respiratory secretions and bronchoconstriction), bradycardia, and miosis

e. Clinical signs may vary depending upon the balance of acetylcholine at the various sites mentioned above in the mechanism of action. For example, ganglionic stimulation may predominate in some cases resulting in tachycardia, mydriasis etc. or CNS effects may predominate causing restlessness, anxiety, hyperactivity, seizures, or depression.

f. Death may occur, usually resulting from respiratory paralysis (particularly in cats).

6. Diagnosis

a. Cholinesterase activity may be measured in blood, plasma, or serum. These measurements are not consistently reliable. A decrease in cholinesterase activity of 50% or more is suggestive, combined with compatible history and clinical signs.

b. Samples that can be saved and frozen for insecticide determination include vomitus, exposed hair, stomach contents, liver, body fat, and skin with subcutaneous tissue. The source of the poison can be analyzed as well.

c. If 0.02 mg/kg of atropine IV does not cause anticholinergic effects (mydriasis and tachycardia), then cholinesterase inhibition is possible.

7. Treatment

a. As for any orally ingested or topically applied toxin (pp. 384–387)

b. Atropine (0.1–0.2 mg/kg, $\frac{1}{4}$ dose IV, $\frac{3}{4}$ dose IM or SQ). Overatropinization should be avoided. Goal is to relieve the CNS signs and the respiratory signs. The amount and frequency of the dose should be tapered to the individual patient. Atropine primarily relieves the muscarinic and CNS signs and minimally affects the nicotinic signs

   1) Atropine can be repeated as needed q3–6h if salivation recurs.

   2) Glycopyrrolate does not cross the blood/brain barrier as does atropine and so is not effective in the treatment of the CNS signs.

c. Nicotinic signs may be symptomatically treated with midazolam 0.5–1 mg/kg IV and diphenhydramine 1–4 mg/kg SC or IM q8h.

d. For known organophosphate intoxication, pralidoxime chloride (Protopam chloride, 2-PAM) should be administered in addition to atropine (10 mg/kg q12h IV). 2-PAM frees the acetylcholinesterase enzyme and binds the organophosphate. This complex is then excreted in the urine.

   1) The longer the organophosphate is bound to the acetylcholinesterase enzyme, the more difficult it is for 2-PAM to reverse this binding, thus 2-PAM should be given as soon as possible. No matter how long after the toxin exposure, 2-PAM should still be administered. If improvement is not seen within 24–36 hours, then administration of 2-PAM should be discontinued. If improvement is noticed, then administration of 2-PAM should be continued until the patient is asymptomatic.

   2) Carbamate binding of acetylcholinesterase is rapidly reversible, so 2-PAM is not necessary with that toxicity.

e. Diphenhydramine (1–4 mg/kg orally q6–8h) has been recommended for treatment of nicotinic effects of organophosphate intoxication in the dog, but this treatment is no substitute for proper atropine and 2-PAM therapy.

f. Apply treatment principles as for any critical patient.

L. Petroleum distillate

1. Some examples of petroleum distillates include benzene, gasoline, kerosene, fuel oil, lubricating oil, grease, paint thinners, charcoal lighter fluids, and engine cleaners.

2. Mechanism of action

a. Pathogenesis is not completely defined. The pulmonary system is the major system affected and is primarily characterized by aspiration pneumonia. It is thought that the less viscous petroleum distillates cause the worst pulmonary compromise. One mechanism of action proposed is an alteration of pulmonary surfactant function.

b. They are fat solvents that can disrupt pulmonary, CNS, liver, and kidney function.

c. CNS signs may develop including excitability, depression, shivering, incoordination, head tremors, and convulsions. Seizures can occur in animals that have had massive dermal exposure to lubricating oil.

d. Dissolution of skin lipids and cell membrane damage are thought to cause the skin lesions.

3. Clinical signs

   a. CNS signs—hyperactivity, coma, seizures, tremors

   b. Respiratory system signs may range from coughing and mild tachypnea to life-threatening respiratory distress, depending upon the severity of the intoxication.

   c. Vomiting and diarrhea may be noted with ingested petroleum distillates.

   d. Skin irritation may range from mild dermatitis to skin necrosis.

   e. Corneal irritation may occur with ocular exposure.

   f. Lead in some petroleum distillates may cause lead toxicity.

4. Diagnosis

   a. History and clinical signs are usually the basis of diagnosis.

   b. The inhaled/ingested/topical material can be analyzed.

5. Treatment

   a. Oil can be removed from the haircoat with repeated washing using a liquid dishwashing detergent. Tar material may be removed by bathing the animal in highly lipid-soluble compounds such as butter, lard, vegetable oils, or peanut butter.

   b. Supportive care of the respiratory system may be necessary, and treatment as for any inflammatory condition of the lung should be applied. Corticosteroids are not indicated.

   c. Avoid inducing emesis, because of the potential of aspiration of vomited petroleum distillates.

   d. Irrigation of the eyes with an eye flush is indicated with ocular exposure.

M. Pyrethrins

1. Flea control products are the primary source of toxicity in dogs and cats.

2. Young female cats are most commonly affected.

3. Mechanism of action

   a. Slowed closing of the sodium activation gate on the cell membrane results in repetitive discharges or membrane depolarization.

   b. GABA-dependent chloride flux within the brain is inhibited.

4. Clinical signs—hypersalivation, vomiting, diarrhea, hyperexcitability, ataxia, muscle fasciculations, depression, disorientation, seizures, and dyspnea

5. Diagnosis—Clinical signs and history of exposure are the primary factors in arriving at a diagnosis.

6. Treatment

   a. General treatment is as for any topical exposure or oral ingestion of an organic toxin. Enterohepatic recirculation may occur with some pyrethrins, and activated charcoal administered 4 times per day may be necessary in animals with persistent clinical signs.

   b. Seizures should be controlled with diazepam (0.2–2.0 mg/kg IV).

   c. Phenobarbital (6 mg/kg IV) or pentobarbital (4–20 mg/kg IV) may be given. The onset of effects of phenobarbital may take as long as 20 minutes; pentobarbital is faster and effects should be seen within 2–3 minutes.

   d. Methocarbamol (50–150 mg/kg IV, not exceeding 300 mg/kg/day) may be used to control muscle tremors. It is not effective for seizures.

N. Toad poisoning

1. Two types are poisonous: *Bufo marinus* (Florida and Hawaii, most toxic) and *Bufo alvarius* (desert southwest USA).

2. Toxins contained in toad parotid glands include catecholamines and cardiac glycosides.

3. Clinical signs include profuse salivation, pawing at mouth and vocalizing, brick-red mucous membranes, cardiac arrhythmias, seizures, and hyperthermia.

4. Treatment

   a. Instruct owners to flush mouth copiously with water before transport if they call first.

   b. Treat hyperthermia (p. 399).

   c. Flush mouth

   d. Stop seizures

      1) Midazolam, 0.5–1 mg/kg IV or per rectum

      2) Phenobarbital, 2–4 mg/kg

      3) Pentobarbital, 2–30 mg/kg slowly IV

   e. An antiinflammatory dose of steroids may reduce oral irritation (dexamethasone, 0.1 mg/kg IV).

   f. Atropine may reduce salivation and treat bradycardia (0.02–0.04 mg/kg IV).

   g. Monitor ECG for arrhythmias.

O. Tricyclic antidepressants

1. Main source for animals is human antidepressant medication.

2. Small animal poisoning is increasing.

3. Used as small animal behavior modification drugs (canine separation anxiety, inappropriate urination, aggression).

4. Mechanism of action

a. The most life-threatening action is quinidine-like and atropine-like effects on the heart, characterized by bradycardia, tachycardia, prolonged QRS duration, and ventricular tachyarrhythmias.

b. Inhibit biogenic amine uptake within the CNS, causing generalized CNS stimulation (seizures, cyclic comas)

c. Competitive antagonism of histamine receptors

d. Anticholinergic effects

e. Very lipophilic, highly protein bound, and may go through enterohepatic circulation

5. Clinical signs

a. Lethargy, ataxia, behavioral changes, mydriasis, tremor, seizure, vocalizing, and crying

b. Vomiting

c. Death, tachycardia, dyspnea, bradycardia, arrhythmias

1) Death is usually attributed to cardiac arrhythmias

2) Animals ingesting 15 mg/kg or more should be considered in danger.

6. Diagnosis—Compatible clinical signs and history of exposure or witnessed ingestion are adequate for a clinical diagnosis.

7. Treatment

a. As for any orally ingested toxin (pp. 384–387. Emetics should not be administered unless the ingestion was observed within the last 15 minutes and the animal is asymptomatic. The potential for seizures is very high, and use of an emetic is dangerous under those conditions. Gastric lavage is recommended over an emetic

1) Magnesium sulfate is not recommended as a cathartic because the anticholinergically induced decrease in GI motility may prolong elimination of this cathartic, resulting in hypermagnesemia.

2) Activated charcoal should be given every 3–4 hours for 24–48 hours because of enterohepatic circulation of the drug.

b. Sodium bicarbonate should be used to treat acidosis.

1) Increased pH is thought to increase lipid solubility of the toxin, increase protein binding, and increase cardiac automaticity.

Recommendation is to maintain blood pH at approximately 7.5.

2) Alkalinization increases urinary excretion of the drug.

3) Give 1–3 mEq/kg IV slowly over 20 minutes. Repeat as needed until the pH is 7.45–7.55.

c. Intravenous fluid therapy should be used with caution to avoid pulmonary edema.

d. ECG should be monitored for 5 days. Arrhythmias can be treated with lidocaine or propranolol.

e. Severe arrhythmias, convulsions, or coma may respond to treatment with physostigmine (dogs: 0.5–1 mg; cats: 0.25–0.5 mg, slowly IV or IM).

f. Avoid dopamine, isoproterenol, quinidine, procainamide, or disopyramide; they are contraindicated.

g. Control seizures and provide supportive care.

P. Marijuana

1. All parts of the plant may be toxic. Fresh plants are not considered as poisonous as dry or smoked plants.

2. Mechanism of action—primarily a CNS depressant

3. Clinical signs

a. Ataxia, vomiting, depression, mydriasis, and disorientation are the most common signs.

b. Bradycardia or tachycardia may occur.

c. Depression can last as long as 36 hours.

d. Most typically, dogs act sleepy.

4. Diagnosis—history of exposure and compatible clinical signs. Owners often hesitate to provide exposure potential. Owners must be reassured that the primary interest is for the health of the pet.

5. Treatment

a. As for any orally ingested organic toxin (pp. 384–387)

b. Closely monitor for respiratory depression in the most severely affected patients.

c. Monitoring and nursing should be as for any CNS compromised patient.

d. The prognosis is usually fair to good with supportive care.

Q. Strychnine

1. Used in pesticides for control of small mammals

2. May be used to poison coyotes

3. Restricted in some states

4. Mechanism of action—Reversible, competitive inhibition of glycine at the postsynaptic neuronal sites in the spinal cord and medulla. Glycine is an inhibitory neurotransmitter that opens the chloride channels in the neuronal membrane, causing hyperpolarization and decreasing the chances for depolarization. Inhibition of glycine results in unchecked muscular stimulation.

5. Clinical signs

  a. Stiffness, sawhorse stance, rigid extension of all four limbs; respiratory muscle stiffness/rigidity may result in apnea and death.

  b. Tetanic seizures are often brought on by external stimuli but may be spontaneous. Stimulus-induced tetanic seizures is considered a diagnostic feature of strychnine poisoning but should be avoided as the tetanic seizures may result in death.

6. Diagnosis

  a. Analysis may be performed on the substance ingested, stomach contents, frozen liver, frozen urine (may not be accurate if death occurred rapidly after ingestion).

  b. Clinical signs and history of exposure/ingestion

7. Treatment

  a. As for any ingested organic toxin (pp. 384–387)

  b. Pentobarbital may be used for relaxation.

  c. Methocarbamol (150 mg/kg IV, repeat 90 mg/kg IV PRN) if pentobarbital is not used

  d. Diuresis may hasten elimination of the toxin in the urine.

  e. Acidifying the urine may hasten elimination, but clinically this is difficult to achieve.

  f. Keep the patient in a quiet and dark room to avoid stimulation-induced tetany.

R. Chlorinated hydrocarbons

1. Lindane toxicoses in dogs and cats are the most common. Lindane is used as a shampoo/dip for fleas, ticks, and sarcoptic mange.

2. Insecticides such as DDT are no longer available in many areas.

3. Mechanism of action—competitive inhibitor of GABA (inhibitory neurotransmitter within the brain); CNS stimulation

4. Clinical signs

  a. Salivation and vomiting may occur within minutes to days of exposure.

  b. Excitation, depression, ataxia, tremors, seizures

  c. Muscle twitching may begin in the face and neck and move posteriorly.

  d. Hyperthermia is common.

5. Diagnosis—compatible clinical signs after known exposure to the toxin

6. Treatment

  a. Bathe as for any topical toxin exposure. Gloves and protective clothing should be worn to protect the handler.

  b. If oral exposure, use treatment as for any orally ingested toxin (pp. 384–387).

  c. Treat seizures with diazepam. If ineffective, use pentobarbital short term, and for longer-term management (if necessary) use phenobarbital. Avoid phenothiazines.

  d. Promote urinary excretion with fluid diuresis.

S. Zinc toxicity

1. Common sources of zinc are zinc oxide-containing skin preparations, metallic hardware items, pennies produced since 1982/83, and galvanized metal objects.

2. Mechanism of action

  a. Poorly characterized but increased numbers of Heinz bodies have been noted in dogs suffering from zinc-induced hemolytic anemia.

  b. Zinc is an emetic and can cause vomiting in patients that ingest it.

3. Clinical signs

  a. Depression, vomiting, diarrhea, weakness, pigmenturia (hemoglobinuria), hemolytic anemia, and icterus

  b. Renal failure has been reported in dogs.

4. Diagnosis

  a. Findings of hemolytic anemia and ingestion of zinc-containing objects or detection of metallic densities in the GI tract is highly suggestive.

  b. Measurement of zinc concentration in serum, plasma, urine, or tissue specimens. Samples should be collected in tubes specifically made for trace metal evaluation, as the commonly used tubes have zinc in them (toxicity, $>0.7 \ \mu g/mL$)

  c. Radiography may demonstrate metallic objects in animals with hemolytic anemia.

5. Treatment

a. Supportive therapy with blood transfusions, critical care therapy, and removal of the source of zinc. Hemolysis generally resolves within about 48 hours after removal of the zinc.
b. Chelation therapy with calcium EDTA may be necessary in severe cases (25 mg/kg SC q6h for 2–5 days).
c. In severe cases, chelation can be continued with oral penicillamine 35 mg/kg PO divided QID for 7–14 days.

T. Boric acid

1. Found in ant and roach baits, flea products, herbicides, and cleaning compounds.
2. Cytotoxic irritant—concentrates in the kidneys, causing renal damage
3. Clinical signs include ptyalism, vomiting, abdominal pain, tremors, seizures, oliguria, coma, and death.
4. Laboratory work reveals metabolic acidosis, elevated BUN and creatinine, and casts/renal tubular epithelial cells in the urine.
5. Treatment
  a. Induce vomiting or perform gastric lavage.
  b. Administer activated charcoal. Avoid cathartic use if diarrhea is present.
  c. Treat acute renal failure.
  d. Correct metabolic acidosis $(0.3 \times BW/kg) \times$ (desired HCO_3 − measured HCO_3) = mEq of HCO_3. Give up to $1/2$ of this slowly IV, and add the rest to fluids.

U. Bromethalin

1. Rodenticide neurotoxin
2. CNS signs include extensor rigidity, hyperexcitability, anisocoria, miosis, seizures, tremors, and death.
3. Treatment
  a. Decontamination: Induce vomiting, activated charcoal, cathartic, whole bowel irrigation
  b. Treat cerebral edema.
    1) Mannitol, 0.5 g/kg IV over 20 minutes
    2) Furosemide, 1 mg/kg IV
    3) Use colloids to avoid excessive amounts of crystalloid fluids.

V. Ivermectin

1. Antiparasitic agent
2. Idiosyncratic toxicity occurs in Collies, Australian Shepherds, Old English Sheepdogs, Shelties, and their crosses at doses as low as 100 μg/kg.
3. Clinical signs—mydriasis, apparent blindness, ataxia, aggression, bradycardia, cyanosis, disorientation, dyspnea, seizures, coma, and death.
4. Treatment
  a. Avoid benzodiazepine tranquilizers for seizure control.
  b. Induce vomiting, gastric lavage, activated charcoal, cathartic
  c. Physostigmine (0.06 mg/kg IV q12h) may relieve signs.
  d. IV fluids, supportive care.

W. Mushroom toxicosis

1. Toxicity varies with species of mushrooms.
  a. Some cause CNS signs and hallucinations.
  b. Some affect the autonomic nervous system (primarily muscarinic receptors).
  c. Some are hepatotoxic.
  d. Some are extremely toxic resulting in cellular damage to heart, liver and kidney and death.
2. Clinical signs can include ataxia, coma, depression, seizures, vomiting, diarrhea, shock, disseminated intravascular coagulation (DIC), acute liver failure, acute renal failure, and death.
3. Treatment
  a. Control seizures.
  b. Correct hypoglycemia, hyperthermia.
  c. Give activated charcoal and repeat q4–6h.
  d. Give cathartic.
  e. IV fluids for supportive care and diuresis.

X. Ethylene Glycol

1. A relatively common poisoning in dogs and cats likely due to its widespread presence in antifreeze and its sweet taste.
2. Ethylene glycol toxicity is most commonly seen in spring and fall when people change their antifreeze solutions in their cars. We have seen it in the winter as well when it particularly cold and the only liquid that is not frozen is antifreeze that has leaked onto the ground.
3. The most common source of ethylene glycol is antifreeze in automobiles though some color film-processing solutions may also contain it.
4. The minimum lethal dose of undiluted ethylene glycol in the dog is 4.2–6.2 mg/kg and 1.5 mg/kg for the cat.

5. Once ingested, ethylene glycol is rapidly absorbed from the gastrointestinal tract reaching peak concentrations within 1–3 hours of ingestion.
6. The metabolites of ethylene glycol are primarily responsible for the severe acidosis and renal injury.

Ethylene Glycol

↓

Glycoaldehyde

↓

Glycolic Acid

↓

Glyoxylic Acid

↓

Oxalic Acid

7. The first step (ethylene glycol to glycolaldehyde) is catalyzed by alcohol dehydrogenase, which is the focus of the specific therapy in the initial treatment.
8. Clinical signs
  a. The initial clinical signs are a result of ethylene glycol and its metabolism to its toxic metabolites.
  b. After absorption from the gastrointestinal tract, serum osmolality increases due to ethylene glycol and its metabolites.
  c. Serum osmolality often exceeds 400 mOsm/kg (normal is approximately 300 mOsm/kg).
  d. Increased osmolality stimulates thirst and also results in an osmotic diuresis. Therefore, polydipsia and polyuria are often the initial clinical signs that are often missed by the owner.
  e. Vomiting may also occur as a result of gastric irritation and possible stimulation of the emetic center.
  f. The unmetabolized ethylene glycol has about the same toxicity as ethanol causing similar CNS dysfunction. Therefore, initially the animal may appear intoxicated as from an alcoholic beverage, be stuporous or even comatose or just have an ataxic gait. This is the first stage of ethylene glycol and it lasts from $^{1}/_{2}$–12 hours.
  g. As ethylene glycol is metabolized, more serious effects occur. Glycoaldehyde is thought to contribute to the CNS disturbance but is quickly metabolized to glycolate that causes

severe metabolic acidosis. This stimulates respiratory compensation and the animal may become tachypneic and tachycardic.
  h. Glycolate (glycolic acid) is metabolized to glyoxalic acid, which is the most toxic metabolite on a per weight basis because it inhibits cellular energy metabolism by citric acid cycle enzyme inhibition and substrate level phosphorylation inhibition.
  i. Renal damage results from calcium oxalate precipitation within the renal tubules as well as damage from oxalate and glycolate.
  j. Stage 2 signs include cardiopulmonary signs such as tachypnea, tachycardia, as well as pulmonary edema and heart failure. (Usually occurs between 12 and 24 hours after ingestion.)
  k. Stage 3, the final stage, is characterized by renal failure and its associated clinical signs. The kidneys maybe painful because of necrosis as well as swelling and edema. This stage usually occurs 24–72 hours after ingestion in dogs and 12–24 hours after ingestion in cats.
It is important to note that many of these clinical signs and stages overlap and in the clinical situation it may be hard to recognize what stage the patient may be in. We generally see patients in Stage 1 when they are neurologic and have very high serum osmolality or they present in acute renal failure. Therefore, ethylene glycol should be considered in any patient presenting with depressed or abnormal mentation of acute onset and in patients with evidence of acute renal failure. Many patients may be neurologic, recover, and then develop renal failure.

9. Diagnosis
  a. The diagnosis is made on history, physical examination findings, clinicopathology, renal biopsy, and/or measurement of ethylene glycol within the blood or urine. It should be remembered that serum and urine concentrations of ethylene glycol are usually undetectable 76 hours after ingestion.
  b. Since ethylene glycol contributes to osmolality, calculating the osmolar gap in an animal that is suspicious of having ingested ethylene glycol may be helpful in arriving at the diagnosis. Determining the osmolar gap requires that one can measure the osmolality
    1) Determining the osmolar gap:
      a) Measure osmolality with an osmometer.

b) Calculate the osmolality using the following formula:

2 (Na$^+$) + (glucose/18) + (BUN/2.8) = calculated osmolality.

(Sodium is in mmol/L; glucose and BUN are in mg/dL.)

c) Calculate osmolar gap: Measure osmolality—calculated osmolality.

i) Normal osmolar gap is between 10–15. Values substantially greater than this indicate an unmeasured osmol is present. Some authors suggest that multiplying the osmolar gap by 6.2 gives an estimate of the ethylene glycol present in mg/dL.

c. Blood gas analysis may show a severe metabolic acidosis that is usually associated with a large anion gap. The anion gap is calculated with the following formula: Anion gap = (Na$^+$ + K$^+$) − (HCO$_3$ + Cl). The normal gap is approximately 10<en>15 mEq/L. An increased anion gap indicates that an unmeasured anion is present such as ethylene glycol.

d. Ionized calcium is often low when severe metabolic acidosis associated with ethylene glycol is present.

e. Calcium oxalate crystalluria is classically associated with ethylene glycol intoxication. These crystals may be seen in the urine of normal dogs and cats but should definitely raise suspicion in any patient that has these. The most common shapes of these crystals are six-sided prisms identical to hippuric acid crystals. Less common forms include dumbbell shapes and envelope shapes. These crystals may be seen as early as 5 hours after ingestion in the dog and three hours in cats. It should be emphasized that it's not unusual for a patient to have ingested toxic amounts of ethylene glycol and crystals cannot be seen during examination of the urine.

f. Actual measurements of ethylene glycol may be performed in certain commercial clinical laboratories. Very often this is not available when we need it most, which is immediately. A qualitative test is available commercially (PRN Pharmacal, Inc., Pensacola, FL 32504). However, some authors report that some drugs that have preservatives in them (such as diazepam) can cross-react and give false positive reactions.

10. Treatment

a. As with any recently ingested toxin, general treatments to decrease absorption including induction of emesis and application of activated charcoal and a cathartic is warranted.

b. Because ethylene glycol's metabolites are so toxic, aggressive measures should be employed to eliminate the absorbed ethylene glycol via aggressive intravenous fluid diuresis and peritoneal/hemo dialysis. Prevention of the metabolism of the ethylene glycol may be achieved by using ethanol to compete with the alcohol dehydrogenase enzyme. Another competitive inhibitor of alcohol dehydrogenase is 4-methylpyrazole. This is now our treatment of choice over ethanol.

c. The formation of calcium oxalate crystals may be minimized with the use of pyridoxine and thiamine. These are co-factors for alternate pathways in the metabolism of ethylene glycol.

d. The following is a step-wise approach to the patient with ethylene glycol intoxication:

1) Place intravenous catheter. Collect blood for a CBC, chemistry profile, blood gas analysis, ethylene glycol analysis, and osmolality. Immediate PCV, TS, dipstick BUN, blood glucose, and ionized calcium tests should be performed. Urine for analysis should be obtained as well.

2) Place urinary catheter and begin measurement of urine output. Intravenous fluids should be given to replace deficits (usually balanced electrolyte solutions) and then maintenance fluids once fluid replacement is achieved. Multiple B vitamins with pyridoxine and thiamine should be added to the maintenance fluids.

3) Administer 0.6 grams/kg body weight of 7% ethanol solution intravenously and then begin 100 mg/kg body weight/hr constant rate infusion of 7% ethanol intravenously. We now use 4-methylpyrazole (for dogs) 20 mg/kg IV, then 15 mg/kg IV 12 and 24 hours after the initial dose, then 5 mg/kg IV 36 hours after initial dose. A higher dose of 4-methylpyrazole has been recommended in cats 125 mg/kg IV initially then 31.25 mg/kg IV at 12, 24, and 36 hours. These latter doses were applied in cats experimentally intoxicated with ethylene glycol and were administered between 1 and 3 hours after ethylene glycol administration. (Often, if

animal is given 4- methylpyrazole immediately after ingestion of ethylene glycol, IV fluid diuresis and monitoring is likely all that will be necessary.)

4) Begin peritoneal dialysis with hourly continuous exchanges. During peritoneal dialysis, ethanol infusion should be doubled to 200 mg/kg/hr. Alternatively, if available, hemodialysis is more effective than peritoneal dialysis.

5) Monitor fluid therapy, urine output, PCV, TS, electrolytes, glucose, blood gas, and osmolality.

6) Administration of dopamine (3 μg/kg/min CRI) and furosemide (1 mg/kg/hr CRI) may be helpful to maintain renal vasodilation and urine output. Recently, effectiveness of dopamine in renal failure has come into question.

7) Continue peritoneal dialysis until the ethylene glycol test is negative (Generally 24–32 hours).

8) Continue 7% ethanol infusion at 100 mg/kg/hr for 10 hours after discontinuing dialysis.

10. Prognosis:

a. Prognosis is guarded to good if animal is treated immediately after ingestion of ethylene glycol.

b. Prognosis is poor if animal presents already in renal failure.

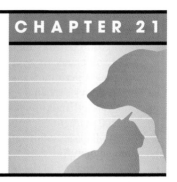

CHAPTER 21

MISCELLANEOUS EMERGENCIES

I. HEAT ILLNESS

A. Definitions

1. Heat cramps are recognized in people, characterized by muscle cramps after exercising in a warm environment, caused by salt depletion with hypotonic fluid replacement, and not clinically recognized in dogs and cats, probably because of lack of salt loss from sweating.

2. Heat exhaustion: Clinical signs in people include headache, nausea, vomiting, dizziness, weakness, irritability, cramps, and diaphoresis. Clinical signs in animals include lethargy, weakness, vomiting, diarrhea and excessive panting.

3. Heatstroke: Clinical signs are similar to those of heat exhaustion, but the hallmark of heatstroke is central nervous system (CNS) involvement, which may include depression, cortical blindness, ataxia, vestibular signs, stupor, coma, collapse with reluctance or inability to rise, and seizures. Animals may also develop bloody vomiting and diarrhea, petechiation from platelet dysfunction or disseminated intravascular coagulation (DIC), massive hypovolemic shock, and cardiac arrhythmias.

   a. Classic heatstroke occurs when an animal is left in a warm environment and cannot dissipate enough heat in relation to the environmental heat load. Examples of classic heatstroke include being locked up in a car with the windows shut or left out in the sun without water or shade on a hot day.

   b. Exertional heatstroke occurs when an animal is exercising in a warm environment.

B. Diagnosis is based on a history of exposure to a warm environment with subsequent compatible clinical signs. Body temperature may not always be increased at presentation because of cooling measures already undertaken or removal of the animal from the warm environment. Rectal temperature may range from hypothermia to >107°F.

C. Diagnostic and monitoring procedures

1. Clinical pathology: packed cell volume (PCV), total solids (TS), blood glucose, blood urea nitrogen (BUN), sodium, potassium, blood gas analysis, complete blood cell count (CBC), chemistry screen, creatinine kinase, coagulation evaluation, urinalysis, and platelet count. Common abnormalities include

   a. Increased PCV initially

   b. TS may be high initially but can become low with therapy and disease progression in more severely affected patients.

   c. Blood glucose can be profoundly low in some patients and should be observed and monitored for hypoglycemia.

   d. CBC: increased numbers of nucleated red blood cells

   e. Common abnormalities in more severely affected patients include high BUN, creatinine, ALT, and bilirubin and low cholesterol.

   f. Creatinine may be very high in some patients. Rhabdomyolysis is a major problem in people with heatstroke.

   g. Thrombocytopenia may be mild to severe. Prolonged prothrombin time (PT) and activated partial thromboplastin time (APTT) and increased fibrin split products may be noted. DIC is a common complication of heatstroke. Petechiation may occur without thrombocytopenia, suggesting platelet dysfunction or vasculitis.

h. Urinalysis: hematuria, pigmenturia (hemoglobin or myoglobin), inappropriate glucosuria, and casts. Inappropriate glucosuria and casts indicate renal damage.

2. Monitor as for any critically ill patient. Severe heatstroke patients are among the most critically ill patients and should be monitored as such. Abnormalities that can be life threatening include severe mentation changes, hypoglycemia, ventricular arrhythmias, and renal failure.

D. Therapy

1. General principles of the care of the critically ill should be applied to these patients.
2. Care is primarily supportive.
3. Cooling measures
   a. A variety of measures have been recommended including cold water/ice baths, cold water peritoneal lavage, cold water enemas, alcohol placed on the foot pads, cool fluids intravenously, and ice packs on major superficial vessels.
   b. The most effective and most easily controlled method of cooling the patient in the authors' hands is wetting it down and then cooling it with a large fan.
   c. Cold water/ice baths are not recommended because they cause peripheral vasoconstriction and shunt the hot blood to vital organs. Cold water enemas interfere with temperature monitoring, complicating patient assessment.
   d. When the rectal temperature is between 103°F (39.4°C) and 104°F (40°C), cooling measures should be discontinued to avoid rebound hypothermia.
   e. Rectal temperature should be monitored hourly until three similar rectal temperatures are obtained and then every 4 hours after that for the first 12–24 hours.
   f. If the patient becomes hypothermic, it should be warmed appropriately.
   g. A rectal temperature above normal after normalization indicates possible infection, inflammation, or inability to dissipate heat such as an upper airway obstruction and should be investigated.
4. Oxygen supplementation is warranted until proven otherwise. Most patients with heatstroke do not have respiratory oxygenation abnormalities at presentation, but supplemental oxygen may prevent organ ischemia by improving oxygen delivery to tissues.

5. Mentation abnormalities
   a. If hypoglycemic, a bolus of 0.5 g/kg of 25% dextrose should be administered, and glucose level rechecked immediately after the bolus and hourly until three consistent measurements are obtained. The intervals of glucose measurement can be extended to 4–8 hours after that. If hypoglycemia returns, a repeat bolus and constant infusion of 5% dextrose or greater may be needed.
   b. If normoglycemic or mentation abnormalities persist after correction of hypoglycemia, then cerebral edema may be present. Administer mannitol, 0.5 g/kg IV, as a slow bolus over 15 minutes.
   c. Progression of neurologic abnormalities despite therapy carries a poor prognosis.
6. Renal system: In more severely affected patients, place a urinary catheter and monitor urine output. If urine output remains subnormal (<2 mL/kg/h) despite a mean arterial pressure of at least 60 mm Hg, consider treatment for anuric or oliguric renal failure (p. 237).
7. Coagulation system: Thrombocytopenia and prolongation of PT and PTT indicate DIC, and therapy for this abnormality should be administered (p. 292).
8. Gastrointestinal
   a. Direct thermal damage and hypoperfusion can result in severe diarrhea and possible mucosal sloughing of the gastrointestinal (GI) tract.
   b. GI protectants should be administered if there is evidence of GI compromise.

9. Antibiotics are not routinely administered to heatstroke patients unless severe hypoperfusion is combined with multiorgan dysfunction or GI compromise. Then broad-spectrum antibiotics should be administered (cefoxitin, 30 mg/kg IV q6–8h, or ampicillin, 22 mg/kg IV q6–8h, combined with enrofloxacin 5 mg/kg IV BID). Aminoglycosides should be avoided in heatstroke patients because of potential renal damage from the disease.

E. Prognosis

1. Evidence of multiorgan dysfunction warrants a more serious prognosis. Serum cholesterol, albumin and total protein are lower in survivors than in nonsurvivors. Serum bilirubin and creatinine tend to be higher in nonsurvivors, and ventricular arrhythmias are more commonly detected in nonsurvivors.

2. Generally, if a patient is going to die as a result of heatstroke, it usually dies within the first 48 hours.
3. Rarely, some patients develop chronic renal dysfunction due to renal damage.

II. HYPOTHERMIA

A. General points

1. Hypothermia is any temperature below 99.5°F (37.5°C) in the dog and 100°F (37.8°C) in the cat.
2. Mild hypothermia: 90–99.5°F (32.2°C–37.5°C)
3. Moderate hypothermia: 82–90°F (27.8°C–32.2°C)
4. Severe hypothermia: <82°F (27.8°C)
5. Hypothermia can be due to
    a. Cold exposure without shelter, cold water immersion, anesthesia, systemic disease (renal disease, hypoadrenocorticism, hypothyroidism, toxin, brain dysfunction), poor or undeveloped temperature regulation (young puppies and kittens), trauma, or a combination of a predisposing environment and underlying systemic disease.
    b. Look for underlying causes that may result in hypothermia.

B. Pathophysiology

1. Most pathophysiologic changes that occur can be explained by the effect of hypothermia on sodium/potassium pump action (slows it down) and the slowing of electrical and chemical conduction. In addition, most enzymatic systems slow down with hypothermia.
2. As body temperature falls below normal, the body compensates by increasing thermogenesis through shivering and hypermetabolism. Shivering may be absent when temperature is <95°F (35°C). The animal will also curl up to minimize exposed surface area.
3. Once thermogenesis and hypermetabolism cannot compensate for heat loss, progressive hypothermia develops.
4. At approximately 95°F (35°C), peripheral vasoconstriction occurs causing blood to shunt from the peripheral sites to the core. A cold diuresis may be induced, causing loss of fluid and electrolytes.
    a. Cold-induced renal tubular enzymatic dysfunction may result in glucosuria despite normal or hypoglycemia.

    b. Fluid loss can result in decreased perfusion and activation of the renin–angiotensin system, causing even more peripheral vasoconstriction.
    c. Severely decreased renal perfusion can occur resulting in ischemia-induced acute tubular necrosis.
    d. Progressive hypovolemia, peripheral vessel vasoconstriction, cold-induced left shift of the oxygen–hemoglobin saturation curve (decreased release of oxygen to the tissues) and cold induced decrease in hepatic function all contribute to development of lactic acidosis.

5. Cardiac changes
    a. Initially tachycardia occurs, but as hypothermia progresses, bradycardia and diminished cardiac function develop.
    b. Electrocardiogram (ECG) changes
      1) Mild hypothermia: P-R, Q-T, and QRS intervals may be prolonged, and ectopic atrial beats and T-wave inversion may be noted.
      2) Moderate hypothermia: J waves (positive ECG deflection following the S wave) occur in humans but are only rarely reported in the dog.
      3) As hypothermia progresses, ventricular ectopy occurs and ventricular fibrillation is common in persons at a temperature <82°F. Take caution when handling the animal or placing central catheters because even mild mechanical irritation of the heart can result in ventricular fibrillation.

6. Respiratory system
    a. Initially is stimulated by hypothermia
    b. As metabolism decreases, less CO_2 is produced, and therefore, minute ventilation decreases.
    c. As hypothermia progresses, decreased ciliary motility and viscous bronchorrhea develop.

7. Central nervous system
    a. Neurologic dysfunction may manifest as mild depression to coma.
    b. Brain oxygen consumption decreases as hypothermia ensues and may be 16% of normal at 73°F (22.8°C). This decreased oxygen requirement may be protective as brain perfusion diminishes with progressive hypothermia.

8. Gastrointestinal: As hypovolemia develops, splanchnic vasoconstriction results in decreased GI perfusion.

a. Mucosal erosion may occur in multiple areas of the GI tract.
b. Ischemia-induced pancreatitis may occur.
c. Liver function can decrease.

9. Clinicopathologic changes
   a. Hyperkalemia may occur as hypothermia progresses, likely due to sodium/potassium cell membrane ATPase pump dysfunction.
   b. Lactic acidosis due to decreased tissue oxygen delivery to the tissues
   c. Leukopenia and thrombocytopenia secondary to perivascular tissue and splenic sequestration
   d. Both hypocoagulation and DIC might occur.
   1) Hypocoagulation might occur in vivo due to hypothermic effects on the coagulation enzymes.
   2) In vitro coagulation test results will be normal because these tests are run at normal body temperature.
   e. Hyperglycemia may develop with acute hypothermia because of decreased insulin release and increased peripheral receptor resistance to insulin. Hyperglycemia may be secondary to hypothermia-associated pancreatitis.

C. Diagnosis

1. Diagnosis is obtained by accurate measurement of a body temperature <99.5°F (37.5°C).
2. Be alert for any underlying cause.
3. Clinical pathology
   a. No clinicopathologic change is diagnostic for hypothermia.
   b. PCV and TS may be high because of dehydration. In people, hematocrit reportedly increases 2% for each 1.8°F decrease in temperature below normal.
   c. Hyperglycemia may be detected in acute hypothermia.
   d. Glucosuria may occur.
   e. Hyperkalemia may develop, possibly secondary to cell membrane sodium/potassium ATPase dysfunction.
   f. Metabolic acidosis occurs secondary to lactic acidosis.
   g. Thrombocytopenia may occur because of cold suppression of bone marrow and hepatosplanchnic sequestration.

D. Treatment

1. Assessment and approach should be as for any critically ill patient.

a. Remember that an animal with extreme hypothermia may appear dead but may not be. With extreme hypothermia, pulses may not be palpable and heartbeat may not be auscultable. An ECG should be obtained to assess for cardiac electrical activity. There is a saying that "you're not dead until you are warm and dead."
b. Hypothermic animals should be handled gently because even minor mechanical irritation of the heart can result in ventricular fibrillation.
c. Oxygen administration may reduce the risk of ventricular fibrillation.
d. If ventricular fibrillation is evident at presentation countershocks should be administered (see CPR). Repeat up to three times if ventricular fibrillation is not converted.
   1) The cold heart is relatively refractory to defibrillation. Therefore try to warm the patient to 82–86°F (27.8°–30°C) and attempt defibrillation again.
   2) The most effective way to rewarm the heart rapidly may be to perform open-chest CPR and pour warm saline into the chest. Suction the saline out before performing defibrillation.
e. The hypothermic heart may not respond to vasoactive drugs until temperature reaches approximately 86–89°F (30°–31.7°C). Repeated doses at very low temperatures because of no response may become toxic doses when the body warms.
f. The bradycardia of hypothermia does not respond to atropine. Bradycardia resolves with rewarming.
g. After immediately life-threatening problems are addressed, assess patient for the predisposing cause of hypothermia and treat on the basis of the need for immediate stabilization.
h. Hypothermic patients may have fluid deficits secondary to cold-induced diuresis. Therefore, administer an intravenous warm (about 120°F (48.9°C) if using a standard IV set), balanced electrolyte solution for fluid support.
   1) Some clinicians argue that lactated Ringer solution should be avoided because of decreased metabolism of lactate by the hypothermic liver.
   2) Fluid rate should be monitored closely because of depressed cardiac function and severe peripheral vasoconstriction.
   3) Attempt to measure blood pressure and central venous pressure (CVP) to guide fluid therapy, (with cautious placement of a

central line because of possible hypothermia-induced coagulopathy).

i. Diagnostics: Perform CBC, chemistry screen, coagulation screen, and urinalysis on moderately to severely hypothermic patients.

j. After instituting initial fluid therapy and critical patient stabilization measures, begin patient rewarming.

2. Rewarming

   a. The method or technique is based on severity, duration, and predisposing causes.

   b. There are three methods of rewarming.

   1) Passive external rewarming: Animal is covered with blankets to prevent further heat loss, and its own body is allowed to generate heat.

   a) Generally useful with mild hypothermic patients who are otherwise healthy

   b) Doesn't require special equipment

   c) Preserves peripheral vasoconstriction and allows more uniform whole body rewarming, avoiding temperature afterdrop (see 3d)

   2) Active external rewarming: Animal is covered, and external heat is applied.

   a) Active external rewarming may be provided by warm water bottles or bags, warm blankets, or warm incubators. Traditional electric heating pads should not be used because of the potential for excessive focal heat application and possible burns.

   b) The most effective way to apply this is using a forced air heating blanket (Bair Hugger, Augustine Medical Inc., Eden Prairie, MN).

   c) This method is generally used for moderately to severely hypothermic animals, debilitated animals with mild hypothermia, and animals that failed to respond to passive rewarming.

   d) Covering the animal's head so that inspired air is warm may facilitate warming.

   e) Applying warmth to the torso rather than the extremities minimizes afterdrop (see 3d below).

   f) In the absence of a commercial warming product, a hair dryer can be used to blow hot air under blankets that cover the patient.

   3) Active internal or core rewarming: Animal's core is rewarmed.

   a) Used in animals with temperatures <86°F (30°C) animals that have suffered

cardiac arrest due to hypothermia, or animals that have not responded to the other methods of rewarming.

b) Minimizes afterdrop (see 3d below) and can increase core temperature faster than the other methods

c) Methods

   i) *Peritoneal dialysis with warm 0.9% saline or peritoneal dialysis fluid at approximately 10–20 mL/kg 109°F (42.8°C). Exchanges should be performed every 30 minutes. (See peritoneal dialysis for details of technique.)*

   ii) *Warm lavage of the pleural space may also be effective. In lavage of either cavity, adequate ventilation must be ensured when administering the lavage fluid.*

   iii) *Gastric or colonic lavage 109°F (42.8°C) with 0.9% saline can be used but increases the risk of vomiting and potential aspiration and should be used only as a last resort.*

   iv) *Increase the inspired air temperature if the animal is on a ventilator or cover animal's head and allow warm air from the Bair Hugger to blow into the area of the animal's head.*

d) Afterdrop—Warming the external part of body may decrease peripheral vasoconstriction thus allowing cooler blood to circulate centrally and so decrease core temperature.

3. Pain control

   a. Persons who have experienced body temperatures <93°F (33.9°C) report substantial pain during rewarming; this has been observed in animals as well.

   b. Once temperature has reached 98°F (36.7°C), administration of narcotics for pain is recommended.

4. After initial stabilization and rewarming, monitor as for any critical patient.

5. Assess the patient for frostbite and treat accordingly (p. 406).

III. FROSTBITE

A. Actual freezing of tissues

B. Superficial frostbite involves the skin and subcutaneous tissues. No deep injuries occur, and full recovery is likely.

C. Deep frostbite involves death of skin, subcutaneous tissues, and muscle. Severe cases may include deep tendons and bone. Permanent damage may occur, with sloughing of tissues.

D. Relatively rare in small animal medicine

E. The tail, pinnae of the ears, and footpads are commonly affected in cats.

F. External genitalia and footpads are more commonly affected in dogs.

G. Three major pathways trigger the pathologic changes in frostbite:

1. Tissue freezing
2. Hypoxia
3. Release of inflammatory mediators

H. Freezing tissues form extracellular ice crystals first, then intracellular ice crystals.

1. After ice crystal formation, intracellular dehydration occurs.
2. Freezing irreversibly denatures membrane lipid–protein complexes.

I. Cold-induced vasoconstriction leads to tissue hypoxia.

1. Initially, the body responds to cooling of tissues by alternating between vasoconstriction and vasodilation of the vessels supplying the cooled area.
2. When overall body temperature becomes threatened, this alternation between constriction and dilation ceases, and persistent vasoconstriction dominates.

J. Endothelial injury, hypoxia, and local thrombosis result in release of inflammatory mediators, particularly prostaglandin F_2 (PGF_2) and thromboxane A_2 that cause further vasoconstriction, as well as platelet aggregation and continued thrombosis.

1. These are the prime mediators of progressive tissue ischemia in both cold- and heat-injured skin.
2. Levels of these mediators can be increased upon rewarming and, more importantly, during cycles of refreezing and rewarming. This is important in therapy (see below) when you want to ensure that the tissue doesn't refreeze after you rewarm it.

K. Clinical signs of frostbite

1. Four degrees of frostbite have been described in humans, but these descriptions serve no function regarding prognosis, and initial treatment of all frostbite is the same. Therefore, many clinicians have reduced the classification into superficial and deep frostbite.
2. Superficial frostbite is described in humans as numbness and a central white plaque with surrounding erythema. More severe superficial frostbite will have blisters during the first 24 hours that are filled with a clear or milky fluid and surrounded by erythema and edema.
3. Deep frostbite is characterized in humans by hemorrhagic blisters that develop to a hard, black eschar over the following 2 weeks. More severe deep frostbite is characterized by complete necrosis and loss of tissue.
4. In humans, complete demarcation between viable and nonviable tissue may not be evident for more than 3 weeks.
5. Superficial pain sensation, skin that indents when pressure is applied, and normal skin color are favorable findings on initial physical examination.
6. Hemorrhagic vesicles, nonblanching cyanotic tissue, and skin that feels "wooden" to the touch and doesn't indent with pressure are unfavorable signs.

L. Diagnosis is primarily provided by history, physical examination findings, and progression of the lesion after the fact.

M. Treatment (all based on recommendations for humans with frostbite)

1. Hypothermia may accompany frostbite and is more life threatening than frostbite itself; therefore, it should be addressed (see Hypothermia, p. 401).
2. In people, specific treatment for frostbite is focused at reversing the pathologic effects of the tissue ice crystals, vasoconstriction, and inflammatory mediator release.
3. Tissue rewarming should only be performed if refreezing will not occur. Rewarming followed by refreezing and then rewarming is more damaging than prolonged freezing.
4. The affected area should be treated gently and not rubbed aggressively, which will contribute to further tissue injury.
5. Rapid warming should be provided by soaking the affected area in a water bath within the narrow temperature range of 104–108°F (40–42.2°C) for 15–30 minutes.
  a. Water temperature outside this range may exacerbate tissue damage.
  b. Dry heat can cause uneven rewarming and possibly burn injury.
6. Inflammatory mediators are present in blisters that contain clear or milky fluid. These should be

debrided and covered with aloe vera (antiprostaglandin agent) every 6 hours. Hemorrhagic blisters should be left intact.

7. The affected area should be wrapped in a loose, protective bandage.

8. In people, immediate oral administration of ibuprofen limits the inflammatory damage that occurs with frostbite. Aspirin is not recommended because it prolongs the blockade of synthesis of prostaglandins that are beneficial for tissue healing. Definitive recommendations in animals are not available, but a single intravenous injection of Banamine (1–2 mg/kg IV) could be considered or use of other NSAIDS considered safer for dogs and cats such as ketoprofen (1–2 mg/kg SC, IM, IV).

9. Parenteral narcotic administration is required during rewarming because of the associated intense pain.

10. In people, penicillin administration is recommended during the first 72 hours to prevent infection with gram-positive organisms.

11. Long-term therapy may require staged debridement and physical therapy.

IV. NEAR DROWNING

A. Clinical signs and diagnosis

1. Near drowning is defined as survival for at least 24 hours after underwater submersion.

2. Near drowning may occur in fresh water or salt water.

3. Fresh water near drowning is characterized by
   a. Inactivation of surfactant leading to alveolar collapse/atelectasis
   b. Rapid absorption of hypotonic water from alveolus into vascular/lymphatic system
   c. Dilutional decrease in hematocrit and serum electrolyte concentrations.
   d. Possible volume overload when a large volume of water is aspirated
   e. Infection, if contaminated water is aspirated

4. Salt water near drowning is characterized by
   a. No inactivation of surfactant, therefore minimal atelectasis
   b. Alveolar flooding due to hypertonic salt water drawing fluid from intravascular space into alveolar space
   c. Hemoconcentration and increased serum electrolyte concentrations.
   d. Hypovolemia with significant aspiration due to fluid shift from intravascular to alveolar space

5. Clinical signs primarily involve respiratory and neurologic systems.

6. Acute respiratory distress results from aspiration of water into alveolus, atelectasis (fresh water), alveolar flooding (salt water), ± aspiration of gastric contents from vomiting, and possibly noncardiogenic (negative pressure) pulmonary edema caused by breathing attempts with closed glottis/laryngospasm.

7. Delayed (after 24–48 hours) respiratory distress results from infection (if contaminated water is aspirated) or development of acute respiratory distress syndrome

8. Neurologic signs result from hypoxemia, cerebral acidosis/edema, increased intracranial pressure, and electrolyte abnormalities and range from altered level of consciousness (lethargy, stupor, coma) to seizures.

9. Hypothermia may result from prolonged submersion or aspiration of a large volume of cold water.

10. Laryngospasm usually limits the volume of water aspirated to less than 22 mL/kg.

B. Emergency diagnostic and monitoring procedures

1. Chest radiographs (with minimal patient stress) are indicated and may reveal diffuse pulmonary infiltrates, caudodorsal infiltrates indicating noncardiogenic pulmonary edema, and increased vascular markings and perihilar edema suggesting volume overload or may be normal. Sand bronchograms, caused by debris in airways, indicate significant aspiration and warrant a guarded prognosis.

2. Emergency laboratory database
   a. PCV/TS may be increased or decreased if a large volume of salt or fresh water, respectively, is aspirated.
   b. Serum electrolytes may be increased or decreased if a large volume of salt or fresh water, respectively, is aspirated.
   c. In critical patients, CBC, biochemical profile, urinalysis, and coagulation assessment should be considered to determine the status of multiple organ systems.
   d. Arterial blood gas measurement is indicated in patients with respiratory distress.

3. Vital signs should be monitored with a frequency determined by severity of signs.
   a. Temperature may be normal or low; a high body temperature should prompt reconsideration of diagnosis.

b. Heart rate is usually increased but may be decreased in hypothermic patients or those with neurologic compromise.

c. Respiratory rate and effort (inspiratory *and* expiratory) are usually increased but may be depressed with hypothermia or neurologic sequelae.

d. Serial neurologic examination is indicated.

B. Treatment

1. Establish IV access for administration of fluids and drugs.

2. Type and volume of IV fluids is determined by
a. Volume and perfusion status—rapid administration of large volume (22 mL/kg IV bolus over 15 minutes, repeated up to three times if needed to resuscitate) of crystalloids and/or colloids (5 mL/kg IV repeated up to three times) in patients in shock; minimal to no fluids in patients with signs of volume overload (dilutional decrease in hematocrit, electrolyte concentration)
b. Serum electrolyte concentration
    1) Hyponatremia—Use 0.9% NaCl and/or furosemide if volume overload is present.
    2) Hypernatremia—Volume depletion is usually present; thus isotonic crystalloid (Normosol-R, lactated Ringers) is appropriate; 0.45% NaCl with 2.5% dextrose if severe or refractory hypernatremia.
    3) Overzealous correction of sodium abnormalities may cause severe neurologic sequelae and should be avoided (see pp. 85–86).
    4) Hypokalemia—Supplement fluids with KCl, 20–40 mEq/L.

3. Provide supplemental oxygen by face mask, nasal cannula, or placing the animal in an oxygen cage.
4. Ventilatory therapy, positive end-expiratory pressure (PEEP), or continuous positive airway pressure (CPAP) is indicated if respiratory distress is severe: PaO_2 <60 mm Hg, and/or $PaCO_2$ >60 mm Hg.
5. Correct hypothermia using warmed IV fluids, circulating warm water pads, and/or hot water bottles (see pp. 404–406).
6. Treatment for neurologic signs
a. Sedatives to reduce agitation—butorphanol, 0.2 mg/kg SQ, IV, q8–12h.
b. Anticonvulsants if indicated—Valium, 0.1 mg/kg IV; pentobarbital, 25–30 mg/kg IV (half rapidly, remainder to effect).

c. Refer to discussion on head trauma for complete discussion of diagnosis and treatment of elevated intracranial pressure (pp. 259–263).
7. Corticosteroids are not indicated.
8. Antibiotics are generally not indicated unless near drowning occurred in contaminated water or pulmonary infection is documented via transtracheal wash or bronchoalveolar lavage.

V. INSECT AND SPIDER BITES

A. Insect Bites

1. Most insect bites that result in reactions in small animals are caused by families of the order Hymenoptera: Apidea (bees), Vespidae (yellow jackets, wasps, hornets), Formicidae (fire ants).
2. The venom of these insects contains vasoactive amines and peptides (e.g., histamine, phospholipase, hyaluronidase, polyamines, and melittin) capable of causing allergic or toxic reactions.
3. Allergic reactions are caused by a type I (immediate) hypersensitivity response to peptides found in venom.
4. Toxic reactions are due to direct cytotoxic effects of enzymes (e.g., hyaluronidase) or vasoactive substances (e.g., kinins) found in venom.
5. Insect behavior influences the severity of the reaction.
a. Africanized bees are more aggressive and more likely to swarm (resulting in massive envenomation) than the related honeybee.
b. Yellow jacket stings may be more common in August/September when new queens and fertile males are hatching, leading to aggressive behavior known as "yellow jacket delirium."
c. Yellow jackets nest in the ground, resulting in more stings than wasps and hornets, which nest in trees, under eaves, etc.

6. Clinical signs and laboratory findings
a. Most bites/stings occur on face/head and extremities where haircoat is thin.
b. Signs may vary from mild localized toxic or allergic reactions to anaphylaxis and multisystemic effects of generalized toxic reactions associated with massive envenomation.
c. Localized toxic reactions cause swelling, redness, and pain at the site of the bite and are usually self-limiting. Treatment, if necessary, consists of removing any stinger present and disinfecting the area with dilute Nolvasan or Betadine solution.

d. Localized allergic reactions most commonly cause edema and swelling of the face/muzzle/eyelids and pinnae. A swollen foot may be present if that is where the sting occurred.

e. Generalized toxic reactions (massive envenomation) cause life-threatening and often fatal multisystem disease.

1) Presenting signs include fever, depression, weakness, and hypotension (shock).

2) Mucous membranes may be pale or hyperemic.

3) Respiratory distress may be severe because of hemorrhagic or inflammatory pulmonary infiltrates.

4) Neurologic signs include ataxia, facial paralysis, and seizures.

5) Hematemesis and bloody diarrhea are common due to toxin-induced loss of gut mucosal integrity and coagulopathy.

6) Coagulation disorders such as thrombocytopenia and DIC may occur resulting in petechial/ecchymotic hemorrhage, bleeding at venipuncture or catheter sites, ocular hemorrhage, etc.

7) Laboratory abnormalities may include anemia (nonregenerative acutely) ± spherocytosis, inflammatory leukogram, elevated liver enzymes, elevated BUN/creatinine, and possible thrombocytopenia, prolonged PT/PTT, and evidence of DIC (schistocytosis, increased fibrin/fibrinogen degradation products (FDP) and d-dimer concentrations, decreased antithrombin III (ATIII).)

f. Generalized allergic reactions range from urticaria (hives), most visible on ventrum and inguinal region where haircoat is thin, to anaphylaxis.

7. Treatment

a. Treatment of localized toxic reactions, if necessary, involves removing the stinger if present and disinfecting the wound with dilute Nolvasan or Betadine solution.

b. Treatment of localized allergic reactions

1) Diphenhydramine, 1 mg/kg SQ or IM, can be continued orally at 1 mg/kg BID prn.

2) Short-acting corticosteroid such as dexamethasone sodium phosphate. 0.1–0.2 mg/kg IV or IM; prednisolone sodium succinate, 0.5–1.0 mg/kg IV

3) Oral prednisone 0.5–1.0 mg/kg/day tapered over 5–7 days if swelling is severe

4) Most patients are treated as outpatients, though hospitalization and monitoring are indicated in animals with severe swelling.

c. Treatment of anaphylaxis (see p. 36) Anaphylaxis for treatment recommendations)

d. Treatment of generalized toxic reactions (massive envenomation)

1) For animals in severe respiratory distress, provide immediate supplemental oxygen via nasal cannula or intubation using 100% oxygen.

2) Intravenous fluids (as crystalloid) are given to restore adequate perfusion. An initial bolus of 5–10 mL/kg is administered, with subsequent volume adjusted on the basis of perfusion parameters (mucous membrane color/capillary refill time, temperature, urine production, mental state). Shock doses may be necessary in severe cases.

3) Colloids such as hetastarch, 5–10 mL/kg over 5–10 minutes, should be used in severely hypotensive patients or those with respiratory distress to speed resuscitation efforts and minimize total volume of fluids administered.

4) Diphenhydramine is given at 1 mg/kg IM.

5) Short-acting corticosteroids are given IV to potentially improve vascular integrity, stabilize lysosomal membranes, scavenge reactive oxygen species, and minimize hemolysis. Dexamethasone sodium phosphate, 1–4 mg/kg IV; prednisolone sodium succinate, 10–25 mg/kg IV

6) Blood products should be administered to correct severe anemia (using packed RBCs) or coagulopathy (using fresh frozen plasma, 6–10 mL/kg).

7) Cardiac arrhythmias are common, and ECG monitoring is needed.

B. Spider bites

1. The black widow (*Latrodectus*) and brown recluse (*Loxosceles*) are the only spiders that cause significant envenomation in dogs and cats.

2. Black widow

a. Only the female causes envenomation; the male has shorter fangs that do not penetrate the skin.

b. The female has a characteristic orange or red hourglass shape on the ventral aspect of a large, black, shiny abdomen.

c. The venom (α-latrotoxin) binds glycoproteins and gangliosides on sympathetic, parasympathetic, and neuromuscular presynaptic membranes, which causes membrane cation channels to open, allowing calcium influx that results in excessive neurotransmitter release.

d. The potency of the venom and incidence of bites is highest in late summer and early fall.

e. Clinical signs

1) Signs are severe and often fatal in cats. Dogs are less sensitive to the effects of the venom.

2) Bite causes a local reaction consisting of a central pale area surrounded by erythema (often obscured by skin pigment or haircoat).

3) Vocalization, hypersalivation, and intense abdominal pain are the most common findings in affected cats.

4) Cats may exhibit muscle spasm and rigidity of abdominal wall and rear limbs. This may progress cranially and affect the muscles of respiration.

5) Tachypnea is common because of pain and impaired respiratory muscle function.

6) Myotatic and withdrawal reflexes are normal initially but become diminished as signs progress from muscle rigidity to flaccid paresis.

7) Cats have been known to vomit the spider, either at home or on the examination room table.

f. Laboratory findings are nonspecific and include increased creatine kinase, hypocalcemia due to influx calcium into nerve terminals, hypokalemia, azotemia, and myoglobinuria.

g. Treatment goals are to provide supportive care, administer antivenom, and treat associated electrolyte disturbances.

1) An intravenous catheter is placed for administration of fluids and narcotic analgesics.

2) Antivenom—Black Widow Spider Antivenom of equine origin (Merck & Co. Inc., West Point, PA). Reconstitute one dose in 50 mL of 0.9% NaCL and give over 15 minutes.

a) *An intradermal test dose of 0.1 mL is recommended to determine potential complications (e.g., anaphylaxis).*

b) *Dramatic improvement to antivenom is usually apparent within 1–2 hours.*

3) Calcium gluconate 10%, 0.5–1.5 mL/kg IV slowly over 5–10 minutes, is given when hypocalcemia is present.

4) Glucocorticoids at antiinflammatory doses may stabilize neuronal membranes and protect against lethality of the venom.

a) *Dexamethasone sodium phosphate, 0.1–0.2 mg/kg IV*

b) *Prednisolone sodium succinate, 0.25–0.5 mg/kg IV*

5) Supplemental or assisted ventilation may be necessary in severe cases when respiratory muscles are affected.

6) Potassium supplementation, 20–40 mEq/L if IV fluids, is indicated when hypokalemia is present.

h. Prognosis is guarded unless antivenom is administered within several hours of bite. Bite may be a cause of apparent sudden death in cats living in endemic areas.

3. Brown recluse

a. The natural habitat is limited to south central Midwestern United States, with few viable reports of bites outside this range.

b. Also known as the "fiddler spider" because of the characteristic violin-shaped marking on the cephalothorax, with the neck of the violin oriented toward the abdomen.

c. Other identifying features include three pairs of eyes (most spiders have four pairs), a patternless abdomen, and fine hairs covering the legs.

d. The potent venom consists of necrotizing enzymes such as hyaluronidase, sphingomyelinase D, and other proteases that cause the characteristic dermonecrotic lesion.

e. Clinical signs

1) The bite wound causes a "bull's eye" lesion consisting of a black center within a white ischemic area surrounded by a ring of erythema.

2) The lesion may be confined to a small area, usually on an extremity or the face because of the defensive nature of most bites, or spread extensively.

3) Lesions on the side of the animal may spread downward and outward in tear-drop fashion as toxin gravitates ventrally.

4) Bites involving adipose tissue tend to be the most severe because minimal blood supply potentiates the ischemic effects of the venom.

5) Abscessation is uncommon.

6) Uncommonly, a viscerocutaneous reaction develops, resulting in systemic signs such as fever, lameness, seizures, hemolytic anemia, and/or thrombocytopenia.

   f. Treatment

    1) Smaller skin lesions may heal spontaneously, though this may take weeks to months.

    2) Severe or progressive wounds may require surgical debridement.

    3) Flap or grafting procedures may be necessary for large wounds on areas with little redundant skin (e.g., distal limbs).

    4) Broad-spectrum antibiotics are indicated with open wounds.

     a) Cephalexin, 22 mg/kg TID PO

     b) Amoxicillin/clavulanate, 12.5–25 mg/kg BID PO

     c) Clindamycin, 5.5–11 mg/kg BID PO

    5) Oxygen may inactivate sphingomyelinase and other necrotizing enzymes. Thus hyperbaric oxygen (2 atm BID for 3–4 days) or oxyhemoglobin (5–15 mL/kg IV) may be of benefit in severe or progressive cases.

    6) Dapsone, a leukocyte inhibitor, may minimize inflammation if given early, 1 mg/kg/day PO for 10 days.

    7) When systemic signs occur, administer fluids, analgesics, and glucocorticoids (if hemolysis is present).

   g. Prognosis is generally good.

VI. SNAKEBITES

A. The two main families of venomous snakes of concern are the Elapidae and the Viperidae.

1. The coral snake, cobras, mambas, kraits, and the tiger snake are members of the Elapidae family.

   a. The coral snake will not bite unless disturbed. It is generally nocturnal, reclusive, and not aggressive, making these bites less common.

   b. The elapids often hold their prey after striking. The venom of the coral snake is a powerful neurotoxin that immobilizes its prey.

   c. Minimal pain and swelling at the bite location can make diagnosis difficult. Bites often appear as a small set of round tooth marks on the lip.

   d. Clinical signs include acute flaccid quadriplegia, hyporeflexia, and respiratory paralysis. Signs can be delayed for 3–12 hours.

   e. The coral snake can be identified from the similar-looking nonpoisonous king snake and milk snake by seeing the yellow and red bands

adjacent to each other. The nonpoisonous snakes have a black band between the yellow and red bands. ("Red on yellow—kill a fellow; Red on black—venom lack").

2. The viperids (rattlesnake, cottonmouth, and copperheads) usually strike and release their prey and then search for it after it dies. Their toxins are primarily proteolytic and hemotoxic.

   a. Severity of bite depends on the amount of venom injected.

    1) Bites in the spring or from young snakes are often more toxic because they contain more venom.

    2) Bites from very large snakes are generally more toxic, especially in smaller animals.

   b. Bites on the tongue or neck may be life threatening because of progressive edema.

   c. Bites on the trunk are usually more serious than bites on the face or limb.

   d. Agonal bites often contain a large amount of venom.

   e. Approximately 20% of snakebites are "dry" and contain little or no toxic venom.

   f. Pit vipers have a triangular head, elliptical pupils, heat-seeking "pits" between the eye and nostril, and retractable front fangs.

3. Venoms

   a. The venom constituents are complex, with a mixture of enzymes, proteins, and peptides.

   b. Physiologic effects of the venoms

    1) The most common clinical effect of most venoms is an immediate decrease in systemic blood pressure because of arterial vasodilation, followed by increased peripheral vascular resistance with decreased cardiac output, hypoproteinemia, and increased PCV. The hypoproteinemia and hypovolemia may be due to increased vascular permeability and loss of fluid and protein from the vasculature.

    2) Venoms may also cause increases in bradykinins, which are potent vasodilators.

    3) Phospholipase A_2 is present in the venom of many viperids and can cause release of prostaglandins, some of which can cause vasodilation and further contribute to hypotension.

    4) Some Elapid venoms can cause hemolysis.

    5) Many rattlesnake venoms can cause platelet aggregation and thrombocytopenia.

    6) Venoms often have mixture of procoagulant and anticoagulant properties, but in general, the overall effect seems to be anti-coagulation.

7) Neurotoxicity is primarily caused by venom from elapids, although the Mojave and South American rattlesnakes also contain potent neurotoxins in their venoms. The major peripheral nervous system effects include respiratory paralysis and generalized flaccid paralysis.

8) Both elapid and rattlesnake venoms can cause muscle necrosis.

9) Renal failure can result from envenomization for a variety reasons, including myoglobinuria, hemoglobinuria, and hypovolemic shock.

10) Serious complications of snakebite envenomation include ventricular arrhythmias and cardiac failure, acute renal failure, DIC, and airway obstruction.

B. Diagnosis and clinical signs

1. The variation in the toxicity of the venom (even within an individual snake) and the sensitivity of the species being bitten causes the spectrum of clinical signs of envenomization to be wide.

2. Typically, bites of poisonous snakes tend to be much more painful than bites from nonpoisonous snakes, but this can vary quite a bit. Pit viper envenomizations tend to have local effects with immediate pain and swelling at the site. If no pain or swelling is noted within 1 hour of the bite, it is likely that no envenomization has occurred, but this is inconsistent as well.

3. Typical local signs of rattlesnake envenomization include swelling, pain, erythema, petechia, ecchymosis, bullae, cyanosis, and tissue slough.

a. The first sign is usually immediate pain and swelling at the site of the bite.

b. Usually two fang marks can be seen. Clipping hair at the site may help detection.

c. In severe cases, the tissue around the fang marks turns black within 30 minutes, and the blood oozing from the site is dark and watery.

4. Systemic signs of envenomization may include vomiting, mental confusion, hypotension, respiratory distress, weakness, rapid heart rate, shock, high body temperature, bleeding disorders, hematuria, pigmenturia, and cardiac arrhythmias.

5. Coral snake bites generally manifest with small tooth marks and minimal swelling and pain locally. Signs may be delayed for 7 hours, and then

vomiting and hypersalivation may develop. Generalized muscle and respiratory paralysis may rapidly ensue. Convulsions have been reported as well.

6. Patients that have had repeated exposures to snakebites may manifest anaphylactic-type reactions.

7. Initial evaluation should include a CBC, chemistry screen, urinalysis, platelet count, and coagulation evaluation. Aerobic and anaerobic culture of the wound is warranted, as infection may occur. No test is diagnostic for envenomation, but most dogs have echinocytosis on a blood smear.

a. Echinocytes are "burred" red blood cells that appear soon after envenomation and last 24–48 hours.

b. Echinocytosis often precedes the massive tissue necrosis and swelling that occurs with serious bites.

c. Presence of echinocytes may warrant aggressive treatment with antivenin; the lack of echinocytes and swelling may indicate a "dry" bite.

C. Treatment

1. Apply treatment as for any critically ill patient.

2. Antivenin therapy

a. No correlation exists between intradermal skin testing and anaphylactic reaction to the antivenin.

b. Antivenin may be administered in the intravenous fluids and given over 1–2 hours if no intravenous envenomation has occurred.

1) Add 1 vial of antivenin to 200 mL of crystalloid fluids and administer slowly IV.

2) Monitor the inner pinna of the ear. Hyperemia is an early indicator of an allergic reaction.

3) If hyperemia occurs, stop the infusion and give diphenhydramine (2 mg/kg IV slowly) and restart infusion at a slower rate after 5 minutes.

c. The number of vials required is related to the clinical signs, size of the patient, and location of the bite. The general recommendation for dogs is 1–3 vials given as soon as possible.

1) Smaller animals and bites on digits require more antivenin than bites on other parts of the body and larger animals, respectively.

2) There is no maximum dose, and dose is titrated to the point when pain associated with the bite is relieved. In bites that are not that painful, monitor serial physical examinations and coagulation screens until progression of the signs has subsided.

d. If signs of envenomation are present, antivenin should be given as soon as possible. Initial doses should be given within two hours of envenomization, but antivenin may still neutralize venom effectively up to 24–48 hours after the bite.

3. Corticosteroids

a. Block the action of phospholipase A_2, the primary component of most venom and the cause of most of the pathophysiology

b. Corticosteroids are not recommended if effective amounts of antivenin are used because they have no proven value and can result in unwanted side effects.

c. If antivenin is not used, corticosteroids are recommended to block phospholipase A_2 and reduce tissue inflammation and edema.

d. The recommended dose is 0.1 mg/kg dexamethasone IV or 1 mg/kg prednisone PO q12h until pain and swelling subside.

4. Antibiotics

a. Isolates from snakebites include *Staphylococcus* aureus and *S. epidermidis*, group A streptococci, and *Acinetobacter, Citrobacter,* and *Pseudomonas* spp.

b. *Clostridium tetani* has been cultured from the mouths of rattlesnakes in Arizona. Administration of tetanus toxoid has been recommended in some susceptible species.

c. Broad-spectrum antibiotics are recommended pending culture. Gram-negative, gram-positive, and anaerobic bacteria have been cultured from snakebite wounds. Therefore, combinations are recommended that may include a first- and third-generation cephalosporin, a penicillin, and enrofloxacin. Nephrotoxic antibiotics should be avoided in these patients because of the potential for renal failure in snakebite victims.

5. Antivenin provides pain relief but may not be adequate. Administration of opiates may be required.

a. Butorphanol (0.2–0.4 mg/kg SQ q4–6h)

b. Fentanyl patch (3–5 μg/kg q3 days)

c. Hydromorphone (0.1–0.2 mg/kg IV q4–6h)

d. Fentanyl CRI (3 μg/kg IV, then 3–6 μg/kg/h IV)

e. Morphine CRI (0.1–0.2 mg/kg/h IV)

6. Monitor as for any critical patients. Special attention should be paid to blood pressure, ECG, coagulation status, urine output, and swelling at the affected site. In certain areas (head, face, and neck), swelling itself can be life threatening because of airway compromise.

7. Surgical debridement may be necessary once the extent of the tissue necrosis is determined. Frequently, tissue around the bite and in dependent areas will slough after several days. The wound area should be kept clean and necrotic tissue debrided as needed until wound granulation and secondary closure occurs.

VII. ELECTROCUTION

A. General points:

1. The most common cause of electrocution of animals is biting electric cords.

2. Lightning strikes are a rare cause of electrocution in small animals.

3. Lightning strikes result in high-voltage direct current (DC).

4. Electric cord bites result in low-voltage alternating current (AC).

5. The severity of injury depends on the intensity of the electric current (voltage of source and resistance of the victim), the pathway the current flows through the body, and the duration of contact with the current. Type and extent of electrical injury also depend upon the intensity of the electric current (amperage). Voltage is related to current and resistance through Ohm's law: Voltage = Current $\times$ Resistance. During electrocution, the body's tissues provide the resistance.

6. Power lines that distribute electricity to homes, buildings, and general industry carry "low voltage" (<600V).

7. Most homes in the United States and Canada have 120V or 240V. Most regular electrical outlets are 120V; outlets for high-power appliances usually are 240V. Household voltage in other countries is usually 220V. Most household electrical injuries to dogs and cats tend to be due to 120V.

8. AC (in which electrons move through a conductor in a back-and-forth fashion) with a frequency of 60 cycles/sec is the most common type of electricity used in households. AC tends to cause tetanic muscle contractions in victims; DC does not. Therefore, AC tends to result in more serious injuries because the tetanic contractions cause the victim to clamp down on the conductor, resulting in prolonged contact with the current.

9. Lightning, batteries, defibrillators, pacemakers, and electric scalpels use DC, in which electrons flow in only one direction through the conductor.

10. Lightning voltage can exceed 1,000,000 V, but duration of conduction of current through the body is only about 1–2 msec. Thus contact is short but intense.

11. The skin is the primary layer of resistance to electrocution. Thick or dry skin provides more resistance than thin or wet skin. Moist oral mucous membranes provide minimal resistance, allowing more current to pass into the tissues.

12. Internal resistance of the body is provided by all tissues of the body other than the skin. Nerves and blood vessels provide the least resistance of the internal tissues.

13. Lightning causes injury 4 ways.
   a. Direct strike (lightning hits the victim directly)
   b. Side flash (lightning strikes an object or person near by and a secondary discharge occurs from this object or person to the victim)
   c. Stride potential (lightning hits the ground, and current enters a foot from the ground and exits through another foot)
   d. Flash over: current flows over but outside the body

B. Clinical signs

1. Cardiovascular system—asystole, ventricular fibrillation, sinus tachycardia, conduction defects and heart block, ventricular arrhythmias
   a. High-voltage DC more commonly causes asystole. Asystole can be followed by spontaneous sinus rhythm. This may account for a common owner report that the animal appeared dead but was resuscitated at home with cardiopulmonary resuscitation.
   b. Lower voltage (similar to household current) more commonly causes ventricular fibrillation.

2. Respiratory system
   a. Electric current does not injure the respiratory system directly.
   b. Immediate respiratory arrest can result from direct injury to the respiratory control center in the brain.
   c. Tetanic contraction of the thoracic muscles can occur if the thoracic respiratory muscles are in the pathway of the current. This can result in respiratory arrest due to the tetanic contractions.

   d. More commonly, neurogenic pulmonary edema occurs, manifested as respiratory distress characterized by bilaterally symmetrical harsh respiratory sounds or crackles. The edema can manifest as mild respiratory difficulty to severe distress requiring positive-pressure mechanical ventilation to maintain adequate oxygenation. Edema generally occurs within minutes of the electrocution and can progressively worsen over the next 12 hours. Most animals improve substantially within 24–48 hours or have progressed to require ventilation during this time (rare).

3. Nervous system
   a. Loss of consciousness.
   b. Autonomic dysfunction with massive release of catecholamines resulting in severe hypertension
   c. Seizures, mentation changes
   d. Respiratory center injury resulting in respiratory arrest may occur immediately during or after the electric shock.
   e. Anoxia to the brain and signs consistent with this may result from respiratory or cardiac arrest.
   f. Paresis or paralysis (usually transient) has been described in people in lightning strikes.

4. Skin and oral mucosa
   a. Conversion of electrical to thermal energy can result in burns of varying degrees.
   b. Severity of skin burns cannot be used to judge the severity of injury to underlying tissues with low-voltage electrocution.
      1) The extent and severity of skin or oral mucosa injury may not be fully evident until 1–2 days after the injury.
      2) Severity of injury to the lips, tongue, and oral mucosa may range from mild hyperemia to full-thickness burns and tissue necrosis.
   c. Oral mucosa lesions often involve the commissures of the mouth.

C. Treatment of electrical injuries

1. There are no treatments specific for electrical injuries.

2. Treatment is primarily supportive.

3. Initial treatment should be as for any critical patient.

4. Cardiac arrhythmias, if present, rarely require antiarrhythmic therapy. Antiarrhythmic therapy should be guided by severity of the arrhythmia .

5. Neurogenic pulmonary edema
   a. Furosemide, 2–4 mg/kg IV initially.
   Neurogenic pulmonary edema may range from
   a transient cardiogenic type pulmonary edema
   to a permeability edema. Furosemide may not
   be beneficial with a permeability edema, but
   the type of edema will not be evident at initial
   presentation. The major complication associated with furosemide administration is hypovolemia secondary to severe diuresis. This
   should be avoided.
   b. Positive-pressure ventilation with PEEP
   may be required in rare cases that are
   refractory to oxygen supplementation or
   cases that require prolonged periods
   of high inspired oxygen concentration
   (FiO_2 >50–60% for more than
   12–24 hours).

6. Nervous system
   a. Provide adequate oxygenation and brain
   perfusion.
   b. Treat seizures, if present, with emergency
   treatment of idiopathic epilepsy (see seizures
   pp. 267–269).

7. Oral mucosa/skin
   a. Severity and extent of injury may not be
   evident for 2–3 days.
   b. Primarily supportive care
      1) Eschar removal may be required for 2–3
      weeks.
      2) With severe lesions, nasogastric feeding
      may be required.
      3) Scarring may occur but is rare.
      4) Pain medication can be administered as
      needed.

CALIBRATION TABLES FOR THE SCHIÖTZ TONOMETER

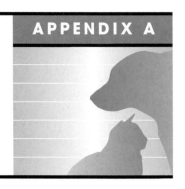

Calibration Table for Schiötz Tonometry in Dogs

Schiötz Scale Reading	IOP (mm Hg) 5.5 g wt	IOP (mm Hg) 7.5 g wt	IOP (mm Hg) 10.0 g wt
0.5	46	61	75
1.0	44	59	73
1.5	43	56	70
2.0	40	53	66
2.5	33	47	61
3.0	26	40	55
3.5	23	35	49
4.0	21	32	44
4.5	20	29	41
5.0	19	27	38
5.5	18	26	36
6.0	17	24	33
6.5	16	23	31
7.0	15	22	30
7.5	—	20	28
8.0	14	19	27
8.5	13	—	25
9.0	—	18	24
9.5	12	17	23
10.0	—	16	22
10.5	11	15	21
11.0	—	—	20
11.5	10	14	19
12.0	—	13	18
12.5	—	—	17
13.0	—	12	16
13.5	8	11	15
14.0	—	—	—
14.5	—	10	14
15.0	7	—	13
15.5	—	9	12
16.0	—	—	—
16.5	6	8	11
17.0	—	—	10
17.5	—	7	—
18.0	5	—	9
18.5	—	6	—
19.0	—	—	8
19.5	—	—	7
20.0	—	5	—

Calibration Table for Schiötz Tonometry in Cats

Schiötz Scale Reading	IOP (mm Hg) 5.5 g wt	IOP (mm Hg) 7.5 g wt	IOP (mm Hg) 10.0 g wt
0.5	44	73	—
1.0	42	71	—
1.5	40	68	—
2.0	37	65	80
2.5	33	61	76
3.0	30	56	71
3.5	27	48	66
4.0	25	42	61
4.5	24	37	56
5.0	22	34	51
5.5	21	31	47
6.0	20	29	44
6.5	18	27	40
7.0	—	25	37
7.5	17	24	35
8.0	16	22	33
8.5	15	21	31
9.0	14	20	29
9.5	13	19	27
10.0	—	18	25
10.5	—	17	23
11.0	12	16	22
11.5	11	15	20
12.0	—	14	19
12.5	10	13	18
13.0	—	12	17
13.5	9	—	15
14.0	—	11	14
14.5	8	10	13
15.0	—	—	12
15.5	—	9	11
16.0	7	8	10
16.5	—	—	9
17.0	6	7	8
17.5	—	6	7
18.0	—	—	6
18.5	5	5	5
19.0	—	—	—
20.0	—	—	—

From Pickett JP, Miller PE, Majors Ll. Calibration of the Schiötz tonometer for the canine and feline eyes. Proc Am Coll Vet Ophthalmol 1988; 19:47, with permission.

From Pickett JP, Miller PE, Majors Ll. Calibration of the Schiötz tonometer for the canine and feline eyes. Proc Am Coll Vet Ophthalmol 1988; 19:47, with permission.

NORMAL VALUES FOR THE CANINE AND FELINE ELECTROCARDIOGRAM

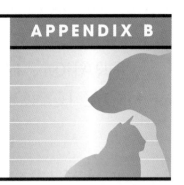

Rate

Dog — 60 to 140 beats/min for giant breeds
70 to 160 beats/min for adult dogs
Up to 180 beats/min for toy breeds
Up to 220 beats/min for puppies

Cat — Range: 120 to 240 beats/min
Mean: 197 beats/min

Rhythm

Dog — Normal sinus rhythm
Sinus arrhythmia
Wandering sinoatrial pacemaker

Cat — Normal sinus rhythm
Sinus tachycardia (physiologic reaction to excitement)

Measurements (lead II, 50 mm/sec; 1 cm = 1 mV)

Dog — P wave — Width: maximum, 0.04 sec; 0.05 sec in giant breeds
Height: maximum, 0.4 mV

P-R interval — Width: 0.06 to 0.13 sec

QRS complex — Width: maximum, 0.05 sec in small breeds
maximum, 0.06 sec in large breeds
Height of R wave[a]: maximum, 3.0 mV in large breeds
maximum, 2.5 mV in small breeds

S-T segment — No depression; not more than 0.2 mV
No elevation; not more than 0.15 mV

T wave — Can be positive, negative, or biphasic
Not greater than one-fourth amplitude of R wave
Amplitude range ±0.05–1.0 mV in any lead

Q-T interval — Width: 0.15 to 0.25 sec at normal heart rate; varies with heart rate (faster rates have shorter Q-T intervals and vice versa)

Cat — P wave — Width: maximum, 0.04 sec
Height: maximum, 0.2 mV

P-R interval — Width: 0.05 to 0.09 sec

QRS complex — Width: maximum, 0.04 sec
Height of R wave: maximum, 0.9 mV

S-T segment — No depression or elevation

T wave — Can be positive, negative, or biphasic—most often positive
Maximum amplitude: 0.3 mV

Q-T interval — Width: 0.12 to 0.18 sec at normal heart rate (range, 0.07–0.20 sec); varies with heart rate (faster rates have shorter Q-T intervals and vice versa)

Mean Electrical Axis (frontal plane)

Dog — +40 to +100°
Cat — 0 to +160° (not valid in many cats)

Precordial Chest Leads (values of special importance)

Dog — CV5RL (rV2): T wave positive, R wave not greater than 3.0 mV
CV6LL (V2): S wave not greater than 0.8 mV; R wave not greater than 3.0 mV[a]
CV6LU (V4): S wave not greater than 0.7 mV; R wave not greater than 3.0 mV[a]
V10: negative QRS complex, T wave negative except in Chihuahuas

Cat — CV6LL (V2): R wave not greater than 1.0 mV
CV6LU (V4): R wave not greater than 1.0 mV
V10: T wave negative, R/Q not greater than 1.0 mV

[a]Not valid for thin, deep-chested dogs under 2 years of age.
Modified from Tilley LP. Essentials of canine and feline electrocardiography, interpretation and treatment. 3rd ed. Baltimore: Williams & Wilkins, 1992, with permission.

CPCR Guidelines

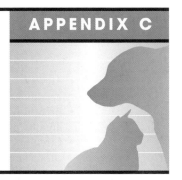

TABLE C.1
DOSAGES OF DRUGS COMMONLY USED IN CPCR

Drug	Dose	Route	Comments
Amiodarone	5–10 mg/kg	IV	May cause hypotension
Atropine	0.04 mg/kg	IV, IT, IO	Use lower dose if perfusing rhythm
Calcium gluconate	50 mg/kg	IV, IO	Not for routine use in CPCR
Epinephrine (low dose)	0.01–0.02 mg/kg	IV, IT, IO	Repeat doses in 3–5 minutes
Epinephrine (high dose)	0.1–0.2 mg/kg	IV, IT, IO	Repeat doses in 3–5 minutes
Flumazenil	0.02 mg/kg	IV, IT, IO	Benzodiazepine reversal agent
Lidocaine	2 mg/kg	IV, IT, IO	Increases defibrillation threshold
Magnesium sulfate	30 mg/kg	IV, IO	Only in hypomagnesemic patients
Mannitol	0.25–1 g/kg	IV, IO	For reduction of intracranial pressure
Naloxone	0.02–0.04 mg/kg	IV, IT, IO	Opioid reversal agent
Sodium bicarbonate	1 mEq/kg	IV, IO (not IT)	Not routinely recommended
Vasopressin	0.8 U/kg	IV, IO	Longer half-life than epinephrine

IV, intravenous; IT, intratracheal; IO, intraosseus.

TABLE C.2
QUICK REFERENCE TABLE FOR VETERINARY CPCR

Drug (conc.)	Weight (lb)	5	10	20	30	40	50	60	70	80	90	100
	Weight (kg)	2.5	5	10	15	20	25	30	35	40	45	50
	Dose	mL										
Epi low (1 : 10 000)	0.01 mg/kg	0.25	0.5	1	1.5	2	2.5	3	3.5	4	4.5	5
Epi high (1 : 1000)	0.1 mg/kg	0.25	0.5	1	1.5	2	2.5	3	3.5	4	4.5	5
Atropine (0.54 mg/mL)	0.04mg/kg	0.25	0.5	1	1.5	2	2.5	3	3.5	4	4.5	5
Lidocaine (20 mg/mL)	2 mg/kg	0.25	0.5	1	1.5	2	2.5	3	3.5	4	4.5	5
Bicarb (1 mEq/mL)	1 mEq/kg	2.5	5	10	15	20	25	30	35	40	45	50
Calcium (100 mg/mL)	50 mg/kg	1	2.5	5	7.5	10	12.5	15	17.5	20	22.5	25
Magnesium (4 mEq/mL)	0.2 mEq/kg	0.1	0.25	0.5	0.75	1	1.25	1.5	1.75	2	2.25	2.5
Vasopressin (20 units/mL)	0.8 U/kg	0.1	0.2	0.4	0.6	0.8	1	1.2	1.4	1.6	1.8	2
Amiodarone (50 mg/mL)	5 mg/kg	0.25	0.5	1	1.5	2	2.5	3	3.5	4	4.5	5
Naloxone (0.4 mg/mL)	0.04 mg/mL	0.25	0.5	1	1.5	2	2.5	3	3.5	4	4.5	5
Flumazenil (0.1 mg/mL)	0.02 mg/mL	0.5	1	2	3	4	5	6	7	8	9	10
External Defib	2–10 J/kg	20	30	50	100	200	200	200	300	300	300	360
Internal Defib	0.2–1 J/kg	2	3	5	10	20	20	20	30	30	30	50

Cardiopulmonary arrest

Begin basic life support

- **Airway**—Assess for potential airway obstruction, assess for breathing, perform intubation
- **Breathing**—Ventilate with 100% oxygen; provide **10–24 breaths/minute**
- **Circulation**—Assess for heart beat and pulses; if absent, begin external chest compressions; provide **100–120 compressions/minute**

Begin advanced life support

- **ECG and determine arrest rhythm**
- **Obtain access for drug therapy**

VF/VT

- **Defibrillate**—Deliver **2–5 J/kg (external), 0.5–1 J/kg (internal)**
   —Provide up to 3 consecutive shocks
- **Resume chest compressions**
   —Continue for 60–90 seconds
- **Drug therapy**
   Epinephrine (0.01–0.1 mg/kg IV)
   or
   Vasopressin (0.8 u/kg IV)
   Lidocaine (2 mg/kg IV)
   or
   Amiodarone (5–10 mg/kg IV)
- **Repeat defibrillation (2 x initial energy)**

Asystole/Bradycardia/PEA

- **Drug therapy**
   Atropine (0.04 mg/kg IV)
   —Lower dose, if palpable pulse or suspected vagal arrest
   Epinephrine (0.01–0.1 mg/kg IV)
   —May repeat at 3–5 minute intervals
   or
   Vasopressin (0.8 u/kg IV)
   —Given one time only
- **Consider transthoracic pacing**
   —Must be instituted early

Anesthesia-related arrest

- **Administer specific drug reversal agent**
- **Low-dose epinephrine (0.01 mg/kg) where indicated**
- **Turn off vaporizer and flush the circuit**

During CPCR

- **Consider—Interposed abdominal compressions**
- **Consider—open-chest CPCR**—Especially prolonged arrests or in large (>20 kg) patients
- **Consider sodium bicarbonate (1–2 mEq/kg IV)**—Indicated for patients with significant preexisting metabolic acidosis or in prolonged (>10 minutes) CPA
- **Consider calcium gluconate (50 mg/kg IV)**—Indicated in patients with significant hyperkalemia or ionized hypocalcemia
- **Consider magnesium sulfate (30 mg/kg IV)**—Indicated in patients with hypomagnesemia
- **Monitor ongoing resuscitation efforts**
- **Search for underlying conditions**—Run "stat" bloodwork (PCV/TS/glucose/blood gas/electrolytes)

FIGURE C-1   Algorithm for performing CPCR in veterinary patients.
(Reprinted with permission from JVECC, Blackwell Publishing.)

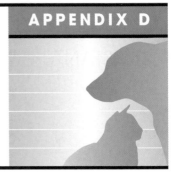

COMMON EQUATIONS

- Anion gap = (Na + K) − (HCO$_3$ + Cl); normal: 12–24 mEq/L
- Arterial–alveolar oxygen (A–a) gradient (mm Hg) = PAO$_2$ − PaO$_2$

  PAO$_2$ (room air/sea level) = 150 − (PaCO$_2$)1.2

Normal = 5–15 mm Hg (only valid when breathing room air)

PaO$_2$/FiO$_2$ ratio used when on supplemental oxygen

Normal = 500

Acute lung injury = 300

ARDS = 200

<200 = poor prognosis

- Arterial oxygen content (CaO$_2$) mL/100 mL = (1.34 × Hb × SaO$_2$) + (0.003 × PaO$_2$)
- Corrected calcium (canine) = Total Ca (mg/dL) + (3.5) − albumin (g/dL)

- Base deficit/bicarbonate requirement = (24 − HCO$_3$) × BW (kg) × 0.3 = mEq NaHCO$_3$ to correct deficit
- Fluid volume requirement (L) = % dehydration × BW (kg) + ongoing losses + maintenance requirements

Maintenance = 44 − 66 mL/kg/day or 1 mL/lb/h

- Oxygen delivery = DO$_2$ (mL/min) = Q × 1.34 × Hb × SaO$_2$ × 10

  when Q = cardiac output (normal = 29 ± 8)

If cardiac index (Q/body surface area in m^2) is used instead of Q, units for DO$_2$ are expressed as mL/min/m^2 (normal = 815 ± 234)

- Mean arterial blood pressure = systolic BP + 2(diastolic BP)/3 (normal = 70–120 mm Hg)
- Serum osmolality (mOsm/L) = 2(Na + K) + glucose (mg/dL)/20 + BUN (mg/dL)/3 (normal = 300–310 mOsm/L)

CONSTANT RATE INFUSIONS

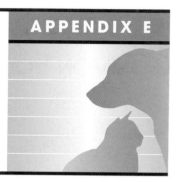

CONSTANT RATE INFUSION FORMULAS

1. $M = DWV/(R \times 16.67)$

where

M	= milligrams of drug to add to base solution
D	= dosage of drug in μg/kg/min
W	= body weight in kg
V	= volume of base solution in milliliters
R	= fluid rate in mL/h
16.67	= conversion factor

To determine the appropriate R if dosage is adjusted, the formula would be

$$R = D(adjusted)WV/(M \times 16.67)$$

2. Dosage (μg/kg/min) × BW (kg) = mg to add to 250 mL base solution at a rate of 15 mL/h

3. Dosage (μg/kg/min) × 0.36 = mg needed for 6-hour infusion.

POSTOPERATIVE ANALGESIA VIA CONSTANT RATE INFUSION

Continuous Rate Infusion of Analgesics

In small animal patients, continuous rate infusion (CRI) of opioids is an excellent way to deliver analgesia, since it eliminates peak-and-trough effects of intermittent dosing. Materials required for setting up CRI include a fluid pump, 250-mL bags of intravenous (IV) fluids (0.9 % sodium chloride or lactated Ringer's solution), fluid administration sets, and a Y-port if additional maintenance fluids are required. The basis for this system is that the 250-mL bag will last for a 25-hour period if run at 10 mL/h (*Fig. E-1*). The amount of opioid required for a 25-hour period is added to the bag. An equal volume of fluid is removed from the bag. Once the CRI is started, the rate can be increased or decreased, as the patient requires. Opioids and adjunctive agents can be administered together. Adjunctive agents amplify the analgesia and in some cases can decrease the amount of opioid required to obtain the desired effect. Common adjunctive agents include N-methyl D-aspartate (NMDA) antagonists, α_2 agonists, and local anesthetics. A loading dose of opioid and the adjunctive agent is required when the infusion is begun (*Table E-2*).

Opioids

Pure agonist opioids such as fentanyl and morphine provide excellent analgesia but can have a relatively short duration of action. Fentanyl provides approximately 30 minutes of analgesia unless it is administered as a constant infusion. The analgesic effects of morphine may last up to 4 hours, but higher doses given rapidly can induce histamine release. CRI of these opioids prevents lapses in analgesia and the induction of histamine release. Fentanyl is 100 times more potent than morphine, meaning that a higher dose of morphine is required to obtain comparable efficacy. The potency of fentanyl allows more rapid equilibration of dose changes in the CRI and may be associated with fewer adverse effects such as nausea and urine retention. Fentanyl is significantly more expensive than morphine, which may limit its use in certain cases. Butorphanol is an agonist/antagonist opioid. The duration of analgesia likely varies with the species and degree of pain, but may be less than 1 hour in dogs. A butorphanol CRI can

$$\frac{\text{Dosage (mg/kg/h)} \times \text{patient's weight (kg)} \times 25 \text{ hours}}{\text{Concentration of drug (mg/mL)}} = \text{Volume (mL) added to 250-mL bag}$$

Set rate to 10 mL/h

Example: CRI of fentanyl for a 20-kg dog

$$\frac{0.003 \text{ mg/kg/h} \times 20 \text{ kg} \times 25 \text{ hours}}{0.05 \text{ mg/mL}} = 30 \text{ mL added to 250 -mL bag}$$

$$\text{Loading dose required} = \frac{0.003 \text{ mg/kg/h} \times 20 \text{ kg}}{0.05 \text{ mg/mL}} = 1.2 \text{ mL IV}$$

FIGURE E-1 Formula for CRIs (using 250-mL base solution and dosage units in mg/mL/h).

TABLE E.1
DRUGS COMMONLY ADMINISTERED BY CONSTANT RATE INFUSION

Drug	Actions/Indication	Dosage
Atracurium besylate 10 mg/mL	Paralytic agent used for mechanical ventilation	0.3–0.5 mg/kg IV loading dose, then 4–9 μg/kg/min
Butorphanol 10 mg/mL	Analgesic for mild-to-moderate pain	Loading dose 0.2–0.4 mg/kg IV, then 0.1–0.2 mg/kg/h
Diazepam 5 mg/mL	Seizure control	4–16 μg/kg/min (0.2 mg/kg/h)
Diltiazem 5 mg/mL	Calcium channel blocker for supraventricular tachyarrhythmias	0.15–0.25 mg/kg IV over 2 min, then 1–8 μg/kg/min
Dobutamine 12.5 mg/mL	Positive inotrope, cardiogenic, or septic shock	5–20 μg/kg/min Cats: 2–5 μg/kg/min
Dopamine (low-dose) 40, 80, or 160 mg/mL	Dilates renal arteries, increases renal blood flow	1–3 μg/kg/min
Dopamine (middle dose) 40, 80, or 160 mg/mL	Positive inotrope, cardiogenic, or septic shock	4–6 μg/kg/min
Dopamine (high dose) 40, 80, or 160 mg/mL	Pressor agent, promotes peripheral vasoconstriction, increases BP	7–20 μg/kg/min
Epinephrine 1 mg/mL or 0.1 mg/mL	Anaphylaxis; cardiac and BP support	0.025–0.3 μg/kg/min
Esmolol 10 mg/mL	Short-acting β-blocker to slow HR and decrease BP (supraventricular tachycardia)	0.05–0.1 mg/kg IV, then 50–200 μg/kg/min
Fentanyl 0.05 mg/mL	Analgesic for moderate-to-severe pain	Loading dose of 0.003 mg/kg IV, then Dog: 0.002–0.005 mg/kg/h Cat: 0.001–0.0025 mg/kg/h
Furosemide 10 mg/mL	Diuretic, promotes diuresis in acute oliguric renal failure	3–8 μg/kg/min
Heparin 1000 U/mL	Prevention of thrombosis, DIC	80 IU/kg IV bolus, then 18 IU/kg/h; check PTT q6h and adjust to 1.5–2.0 × baseline PTT
Insulin (regular) 100 U/mL	Ketoacidotic diabetes	0.1 U/kg/h
Isoproterenol 0.2 mg/mL	Vasodilator, positive inotrope, bronchodilator	0.1–2.0 μg/kg/min
Ketamine 100 mg/mL	Adjunctive agent to add to opioids to increase analgesia	Loading dose 0.3–0.5 mg/kg IV, then 0.3 mg/kg/h (up to 1.2 mg/kg/h if needed).

(Continued)

TABLE E.1
(continued)

Drug	Actions/Indication	Dosage
Lidocaine 20 mg/mL	Ventricular antiarrhythmic, adjunctive agent to add to opioids for multimodal analgesia	Dog: 2–4 mg/kg IV bolus, then 25–80 μg/kg/min Cat: 0.25–0.75 mg/kg slow IV, then 10–40 μg/kg/min
Magnesium sulfate, 12.5% (1 mEq/mL)	Refractory ventricular arrhythmias in critically in patients	0.15 to 0.3 mEq/kg over 5–15 min, then 0.75–1 mEq/kg/day
Medetomidine 1.0 mg/mL	Adjunctive agent to add to opioids to increase analgesia and sedation	Loading dose 1 μg/kg IV (if immediate calming required), then 0.0015 mg/kg/h
Metoclopramide 5 mg/mL	Antiemetic	1–2 mg/kg/day (0.16–1.3 μg/kg/min)
Morphine sulfate 15 mg/mL	Analgesic for moderate-to-severe pain	Loading dose 0.2 mg/kg IM, then Dog: 0.1–0.5 mg/kg/h Cat: 0.05–0.1 mg/kg/h
Nitroprusside 10 or 25 mg/mL	Vasodilator; acute congestive heart failure	1–10 μg/kg/min (start at 2 μg/kg/min and raise q20 min by 1 μg/kg/min to desired effect)
Norepinephrine 1 mg/mL	Pressor agent, short-term BP support	0.5–2 μg/kg/min
Pancuronium 1 or 2 mg/mL	Paralytic agent used for mechanical ventilation	0.06–0.15 mg/kg, IV then 0.2–2.5 μg/kg/min
Pentobarbital 50 mg/mL	To induce coma for uncontrollable seizures, mechanical ventilation	2–15 mg/kg IV to effect, then 0.2–1.0 mg/kg/h
Phenylephrine 10 mg/mL	Vasopressor agent for refractory hypotension	5–20 μg/kg IV q10–15 min PRN, then 0.1–0.5 μg/kg/min
Procainamide 100 mg/mL	Ventricular antiarrhythmic	6–8 mg/kg IV over 5 min, then 10–40 μg/kg/min
Propofol 10 mg/mL	Short-acting nonbarbiturate anesthetic agent; CRI used for mechanical ventilation or seizure control	4–6 mg/kg slow IV, then 100–400 μg/kg/min
Vasopressin 20 U/mL	Refractory hypotension	0.001–0.004 U/kg/min
Verapamil 2.5 mg/mL	Supraventricular arrhythmias/tachycardias	0.05–0.15 mg/kg IV, then 2–10 μg/kg/min

BP, blood pressure; HR, heart rate; DIC, disseminated intravascular coagulation; PTT, partial thromboplastin time.

be effective for treating mild pain and may be more efficacious in cats than in dogs (*Table E-2*).

ADJUNCTIVE AGENTS

Adjunctive agents are frequently added to continuous opioid infusions to provide multimodal analgesia. Fentanyl, morphine, and butorphanol can be combined with ketamine. Some clinicians routinely administer morphine, lidocaine, and ketamine as a combined infusion (MLK). Low-dose

medetomidine is very useful when additional sedation and analgesia are required (*Table E-2*).

Ketamine

When used in very low doses, ketamine acts to block the NMDA receptor in the dorsal horn of the spinal cord. The NMDA receptor is an important "gatekeeper" involved in the transmission of painful (nociceptive) impulses from the peripheral to the central nervous system (CNS). The NMDA receptor is involved in long-term potentiation

TABLE E.2
DOSAGES AND SAMPLE VOLUMES FOR CONTINUOUS RATE INFUSIONS

Agent	Dosage	Drug Concentration	Loading Dose	Volume added to 250 mL bag for a 20 kg dog
Fentanyl	Dog: 2.0–5.0 μg/kg/h (0.002–0.005 mg/kg h)	0.05 mg/mL	0.003 mg/kg IV	30 mL at 0.003 mg/kg/h
	Cat: 1.0–2.5 μg/kg/h (0.001–0.0025 mg/kg/h)		0.001 mg/kg IV	
Morphine sulfate	Dog: 0.01–0.5 mg/kg/h	15 mg/mL	0.2 mg/kg IV diluted in 10 mL saline over 3 min or give IM	6.7 mL at 0.02 mg/kg/h
	Cat: 0.05–0.1 mg/kg/h		0.1 mg/kg IV diluted in 5 mL saline over 3 min or give IM	
Butorphanol	Dog and cat: 0.1–0.2 mg/kg/h	10 mg/mL	0.2 to 0.4 mg/kg IV	5.0 mL at 0.1 mg/kg/h
Ketamine	Dog and cat: 2.0–20.0 μg/kg/min (0.12–1.2 mg/kg/h) (common dosage, 0.3 mg/kg/h)	100 mg/mL	0.3–0.5 mg/kg IV	1.5 mL at 0.3 mg/kg/h
Medetomidine	Dog and cat: 1.5 μg/kg/h (0.0015 mg/kg/h)	1.0 mg/mL	1.0 μg/kg IV[a]	0.8 mL at 1.5 μg/kg/h
Lidocaine 2%	Dog: 50 μg/kg/min (3.0 mg/kg/h)	20 mg/mL	1–2 mg/kg IV	75 mL at 50 μg/kg/min

[a]Loading dose of medetomidine is only given if immediate calming is required

and central sensitization of pain. Activation of NMDA receptors by neuromodulators such as substance P and glutamate in the dorsal horn induces "wind-up" of the CNS and subsequent prolonged and exaggerated central responses to pain. Microdoses of ketamine do not cause dissociative anesthetic effects but do induce blockade of the NMDA receptor. Substantial evidence indicates that ketamine prevents the development of opioid tolerance.

Medetomidine

Medetomidine is an α_2 agonist that can be used in small doses to provide adjunctive analgesia and sedation. There are dense concentrations of α_2 receptors in the dorsal horn of the spinal cord, and the analgesic benefits of microdoses of medetomidine can be significant. Low-dose medetomidine can be administered as a CRI and is compatible with opioids and microdose ketamine. The CRI dose consists of a single full dose (40 μg/kg) administered over the entire day. This dose equates to approximately 1.5 μg/kg/h; a dosage that should not induce significant cardiovascular changes.

Lidocaine

Intravenous infusion of lidocaine can provide analgesia. There are few reports of this technique in animals. Lidocaine infusion has been shown to provide analgesia in human burn patients and cancer patients. With experimental human skin burns, intravenous lidocaine significantly inhibits the long-term inflammatory response to thermal injury. Anecdotal evidence indicates that intravenous lidocaine can provide mild visceral analgesia in the horse. Experimentally, lidocaine infusions have been shown to decrease the minimal anesthetic concentration (MAC) of halothane in ponies.

Janet Welch, MS, DVM, Dipl ACVS
Auburn University, AL

SUGGESTED READING

Cassuto J, Wallin G, Hogstrom S, et al. Inhibition of postoperative pain by continuous low-dose intravenous infusion of lidocaine. Anesth Analg 1985:64:971–974, 1985.

Doherty TJ, Frazier DL. Effect of intravenous lidocaine on halothane minimum alveolar concentration in ponies. Equine Vet J 1998;30:300–303.

Flecknell P, Waterman-Pearson A. Pain Management in Animals. Philadelphia: WB Saunders, 2000.

Gaynor JS, Muir WW III. Handbook of Veterinary Pain Management. St. Louis: Mosby, 2002.

Laulin JP, Maurette P, Corcuff JB, et al. The role of ketamine in preventing fentanyl-induced hyperalgesia and subsequent acute morphine tolerance. Anesth Analg 2002;94:1263–1269.

Massey GV, Pedigo S, Dunn NL, et al. Continuous lidocaine infusion for the relief of refractory malignant pain in a terminally ill pediatric cancer patient. J Pediatr Hematol/Oncol 2002;25:566–568.

Mattsson U, Cassuto J, Tarnow P, et al. Intravenous lidocaine infusion in the treatment of experimental human skin burns—digital colour image analysis of erythema development. Burns 2000;26:710–715.

Pypendop BH, Verstegen JP. Hemodynamic effects of medetomidine in the dog: A dose titration study. Vet Surg 1998;27:612–622.

Warncke T, Stubhaug A, Jorum E. Ketamine, an NMDA receptor antagonist, suppresses spatial and temporal properties of burn-induced secondary hyperalgesia in man: A double-blind, cross-over comparison with morphine and placebo. Pain 1997;72:99–106.

CONVERSION TABLES

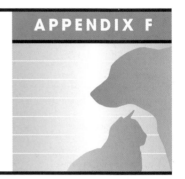

TABLE F.1
KILOGRAMS TO BODY SURFACE AREA (m²)

Common equations used to calculate body surface area:

Canine: $\dfrac{10.1 \times (\text{weight in grams})^{2/3}}{10,000}$

Canine and feline: $\dfrac{(\text{weight in kg})^{2/3}}{10}$

Feline: $\dfrac{10 \times (\text{weight in grams})^{2/3}}{10,000}$

Canine						Feline			
Kg	m²	Kg	m²	Kg	m²	Kg	m²	Kg	m²
0.5	0.06	14	0.58	28	0.92	0.5	0.063	5.5	0.311
1	0.10	15	0.60	29	0.94	1	0.1	6	0.330
2	0.15	16	0.63	30	0.96	1.5	0.131	6.5	0.348
3	0.20	17	0.66	35	1.07	2	0.159	7	0.366
4	0.25	18	0.69	40	1.17	2.5	0.184	7.5	0.383
5	0.29	19	0.71	45	1.26	3	0.208	8	0.400
6	0.33	20	0.74	50	1.36	3.5	0.231	8.5	0.416
7	0.36	21	0.76	55	1.47	4	0.252	9	0.432
8	0.40	22	0.78	60	1.55	4.5	0.273	9.5	0.449
9	0.43	23	0.81	65	1.64	5	0.292	10	0.464
10	0.46	24	0.83	70	1.72				
11	0.49	25	0.85	75	1.80				
12	0.52	26	0.88	80	1.88				
13	0.55	27	0.90	85	1.96				

TABLE F.2
CONVERSION TABLE FOR HEMATOLOGIC UNITS

	Example Values		Conversion Factors	
Analyte	Traditional	SI[a]	Traditional to SI	SI to Traditional
Hemoglobin	15.0 g/dL	150 g/L	10	0.1
HCT or PCV	45%	0.45 L/L	0.01	100
Erythrocytes	$6.0 \times 106/\text{mm}3$	$6.0 \times 10^{12}/\text{L}$	10^6	10^{-6}
MCV	$75\ \mu^3$	75 fL	No change	No change
MCH	$25\ \mu\mu\text{g}$	25 pg	No change	No change
MCHC	33 g/dL	330 g/L	10	0.1
WBC	$15.0 \times 10^3/\text{mm}^3$	$15.0 \times 10^9/\text{L}$	10^6	10^{-6}
Platelets	$250 \times 10^3/\text{mm}^3$	$250 \times 10^9/\text{L}$	10^6	10^{-6}

Modified from Bonagura JD, ed. Kirk's Current Veterinary Therapy XIII. Philadelphia: WB Saunders, 2000:1209, with permission.
[a]Système International d'Unités.

TABLE F.3
CONVERSION TABLE FOR CLINICAL BIOCHEMICAL UNITS

Analyte	Traditional Unit (with examples)	Conversion Factor	SI Unit (with examples)
Alanine aminotransferase	0–40 U/L	1.00	0–40 U/L
Albumin	2.8–4.0 g/dL	10.0	28–40 g/L
Alkaline phosphatase	30–150 U/L	1.00	30–150 U/L
Ammonia	10–80 μg/dL	0.5871	5.9–47.0 μmol/L
Amylase	200–800 U/L	1.00	200–800 U/L
Aspartate aminotransferase	0–40 U/L	1.00	0–40 U/L
Bile acids (total)	0.3–2.3 μg/mL	2.45	0.74–5.64 μmol/L
Bilirubin	0.1–0.2 mg/dL	17.10	2–4 μmol/L
Calcium	8.8–10.3 mg/dL	0.2495	2.20–2.58 mmol/L
Carbon dioxide	22–28 mEq/L	1.00	22–28 mmol/L
Chloride	95–100 mEq/L	1.00	95–100 mmol/L
Cholesterol	100–265 mg/dL	0.0258	2.58–5.85 mmol/L
Copper	70–140 μg/dL	0.1574	11.0–22.0 μmol/L
Cortisol	2–10 μg/dL	27.59	55–280 nmol/L
Creatine kinase	0–130 U/L	1.00	0–130 U/L
Creatinine	0.6–1.2 mg/dL	88.40	50–110 μmol/L
Fibrinogen	200–400 mg/dL	0.01	2.0–4.0 g/L
Folic acid	3.5–11.0 μg/L	2.265	7.93–24.92 nmol/L
Glucose	70–110 mg/dL	0.05551	3.9–6.1 mmol/L
Iron	80–180 μg/dL	0.1791	14–32 μmol/L
Lactate	5–20 mg/dL	0.1110	0.5–2.0 mmol/L
Lead	150 μg/dL	0.04826	7.2 μmol/L
Lipase, Sigma-Tietz (37°C)	≤1 ST U/dL	280	≤280 U/L
Lipase, Cherry-Crandall (30°C)	0–160 U/L	1.00	0–160 U/L
Lipids (total)	400–850 mg/dL	0.01	4.0–8.5 g/L
Magnesium	1.8–3.0 mg/dL	0.4114	0.80–1.20 mmol/L
Mercury	≤1.0 μg/dL	49.85	≤50 nmol/L
Osmolality	280–300 mOsm/kg	1.00	280–300 mmol/kg
Phosphorus	2.5–5.0 mg/dL	0.3229	0.80–1.6 mmol/L
Potassium	3.5–5.0 mEq/L	1.0	3.5–5.0 mmol/L
Protein (total)	5–8 g/dL	10.0	50–80 g/L
Sodium	135–147 mEq/L	1.00	135–147 mmol/L
Testosterone	4.0–8.0 mg/mL	3.467	14.0–28.0 nmol/L
Thyroxine	1–4 μg/dL	12.87	13–51 nmol/L
Triglyceride	10–500 mg/dL	0.0113	0.11–5.65 mmol/L
Urea nitrogen	10–20 mg/dL	0.3570	3.6–7.1 nmol/L
Uric acid	3.6–7.7 mg/dL	59.44	214–458 μmol/L
Urobilinogen	0–4.0 mg/dL	16.9	0.0–6.8 μmol/L
Vitamin A	90 μg/dL	0.03491	3.1 μmol/L
Vitamin B_{12}	300–700 ng/L	0.738	221–516 pmol/L
Vitamin E	5.0–20.0 mg/L	2.32	11.6–46.4 μmol/L
D-Xylose	30–40 mg/dL	0.06666	2.0–2.71 mmol/L
Zinc	75–120 μg/dL	0.1530	11.5–18.5 μmol/L

From Bonagura JD, ed. Kirk's Current Veterinary Therapy XIII. Philadelphia: WB Saunders, 2000: 1214, with permission.

TABLE F.4
TEMPERATURE CONVERSION

Celsius to Fahrenheit (°C × 1.8) + 32 = °F
Fahrenheit to Celsius (°F − 32) × 0.555 = °C

Celsius	Fahrenheit	Celsius	Fahrenheit
0	32.0	37.0	98.6
4.0	39.2	38.6	101.5
25.0	77.0	39.1	102.5
32.0	89.6	39.4	103

NORMAL VALUES FOR OXYGEN AND HEMODYNAMIC PARAMETERS

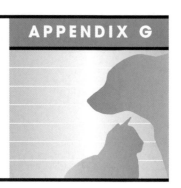

TABLE G.1
NORMAL HEMATOLOGIC VALUES

Test	Units	Dogs	Cats
WBC	$10 \times 3/mm^3$	6.0–17.0	5.5–19.5
RBC	$10 \times 6/mm^3$	5.5–8.5	6.0–10
Hemoglobin	g/dL	12.0–18.0	9.5–15
Hematocrit	%	37.0–55.0	29–45
Mean corpuscular volume	FL	60.0–77.0	41.0–54
Mean corpuscular hemoglobin	Pg	19.5–26	13.3–17.5
Mean corpuscular hemoglobin concentration	%	32.0–36.0	31–36
Platelet count (automated)	$10 \times 3/mm^3$	200–500	150–600
Platelet count (manual)	$10 \times 3/mm^3$	164–510	230–680
Neutrophils	%	60–77	35–75
	Absolute	3000–11,500	2500–12,500
Bands	%	0–3	0–3
	Absolute	0–510	0–585
Lymphocytes	%	12–30	20–55
	Absolute	1000–4800	1500–7000
Monocytes	%	3–10	1–4
	Absolute	180–1350	0–850
Eosinophils	%	2–10	2–12
	Absolute	1000–1250	0–1500
Basophils	%	0–1	0–1
	Absolute	0–100	0–100
Reticulocyte count	%	0.5–1.5	0.0–1.0
Corrected	%	0.0–1.0	0.0–1.0
Absolute	$/mm^3$	0–80,000	0–50,000

From Abbott Cell Dyne 3500; IDEXX Veterinary Services.
Caution: Normal values vary among individual laboratories.

TABLE G.2
NORMAL BIOCHEMICAL VALUES

Test	Units	Dogs	Cats
Blood urea nitrogen (BUN)	mg/dL	7–27	15–34
Creatinine	mg/dL	0.4–1.8	0.8–2.3
Cholesterol	mg/dL	112–328	82–218
Glucose	mg/dL	60–125	70–150
Alkaline phosphatase (ALP)	IU/L	10–150	0–62
Alanine aminotransferase (ALT)	IU/L	5–60	28–76
Aspartate aminotransferase (AST)	IU/L	5–55	5–55
Total protein	g/dL	5.1–7.8	5.9–8.5
Albumin	g/dL	2.6–4.3	2.4–4.1
Globulin	g/dL	2.3–4.5	3.4–5.2
Albumin/globulin ratio		0.75–1.9	0.6–1.5
Sodium	mEq/L	141–156	147–156
Potassium	mEq/L	4.0–5.6	3.9–5.3
Sodium/potassium ratio		27–40	>27.0
Chloride	mEq/L	105–115	111–125
Total CO_2	mEq/L	17–24	13–25
Anion gap	mEq/L	12–24	13–27
Calcium	mg/dL	7.5–11.3	7.5–10.8
Phosphorus	mg/dL	2.1–6.3	3.0–7.0
Total bilirubin	mg/dL	0–0.4	0.0–0.4
Direct bilirubin	mg/dL	0.0–0.1	0.0–0.1
Indirect bilirubin	mg/dL	0–0.3	0.0–0.3
Lactate dehydrogenase (LDH)	IU/L	50–380	46–350
Creatine kinase (CK or CPK)	IU/L	10–200	64–440
γGlutamyl transferase (GGT)	IU/L	0–10	1–7
Uric acid	mg/dL	0–2	0–1
Amylase	IU/L	500–1500	500–1500
Lipase	U/L	100–500	10–195
Magnesium	mEq/L	1.8–2.4	1.8–2.4
Trigiycendes	mg/dL	20–150	20–90
Bile acids:			
Fasting	μmol/L	0.0–5.0	0.0–5.0
Postprandial	μmol/L	<25	<15
Random	μmol/L	<25	<15
Total iron	μg/dL	33–147	33–134
Unsaturated iron binding capacity	μg/dL	127–340	105–205
Total iron binding capacity	μg/dL	282–386	169–325

From Hitachi Chemistry Analyzer model 747 IDEXX Veterinary Services.
Caution: Normal values vary among individual laboratories.

TABLE G.3
APPROXIMATE NORMAL RANGES FOR COMMON MEASUREMENTS IN DOGS AND CATS

	Dog	Cat
Heart rate (bpm)	60–180	140–220
Capillary refill time	<2 sec	<2 sec
Body temperature	99.5–102.5°F	100.5–102.5°F
	37.5–39.2°C	38.1–39.2°C
Systolic arterial blood pressure (mm Hg)	110–180	120–180
Mean arterial pressure (mm Hg)	90–120	100–150
Blood volume (mL/kg)	75–90	47–66
Cardiac output		
(mL/kg/min)	100–200	167 ± 39
(L/M^2/min)	4.72 ± 1.09	
Systemic resistance		
(mm Hg/mL/kg/min)	0.64 ± 0.16	
(dynes/sec/cm)	2162 ± 458	
Mean pulmonary arterial pressure (mm Hg)	14 ± 3	
Central venous pressure (cm H$_2$O)	3 ± 4	
Pulmonary artery occlusion pressure (mm Hg)	5 ± 2	
Urine output	1–2 mL/kg/h	1–2 mL/kg/h
Breathing rate (breaths/min)	10–30	24–42
Minute ventilation (mL/kg/min)	170–350	200–350
Oxygen delivery		
(mL/kg/min)	29 ± 8	
(mL/M^2/min)	815 ± 234	
Oxygen consumption		
(mL/kg/min)	4–11	3–8
(mL/M^2/min)	198 ± 53	
Arterial Po$_2$ (mm Hg)	85–105	100–115
Arterial So$_2$	>95	>95
Arterial Pco$_2$ (mm Hg)	30–44	28–35
Arterial pH	7.36–7.46	7.34–7.43
Bicarbonate (mEq/L)	20–25	17–21
Base deficit (mEq/L)	0 to −4	−1 to −8
Total plasma proteins (g/dL)	6.0–8.0	6.8–8.3
Albumin (g/dL)	2.5–3.5	1.9–3.9
Packed cell volume (%)	37–55	29–48
Hemoglobin (g/dL)	12–18	9–15.1
Sodium (mEq/L)	145–154	151–158
Potassium (mEq/L)	4.1–5.3	3.6–4.9
Chloride (mEq/L)	105–116	113–121
Total CO$_2$ (mEq/L)	16–26	15–21
Ionized calcium (mg/dL)	1.25–1.50	1.25–1.50
Lactate (mmol/L)	<2	<2
Pulse oximetry (%)	98–100	98–100
Capnography (mm Hg)	35–45	35–45

Modified from Aldrich J, Haskins SC. Monitoring the critically ill patient. In: Current Veterinary Therapy XII. Philadelphia: WB Saunders, 1995; 98–105, with permission.

TOXICOLOGY

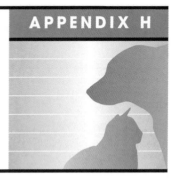

ASPCA National Animal Poison Control Center: (888) 426-4435 or (800) 548-2423

Toxic plant information: The ASPCA National Animal Poison Control web site (www.apcc.aspca.org) has a complete list of toxic and nontoxic plants listed alphabetically by common name. Information includes scientific name, toxic principle, clinical signs, and picture of plants (when available).

TABLE H.1
TOXIC AGENTS AND THEIR SYSTEMIC ANTIDOTES—DOSAGE AND METHOD OF TREATMENT

Toxic Agent	Systemic Antidote	Dosage and Method of Treatment
Acetaminophen	N-Acetylcysteine (Mucomyst, Apothecon)	150 mg/kg loading dose PO or IV, then 50 mg/kg q4h for 17–20 additional doses
Amphetamines	Chlorpromazine	1 mg/kg IM or IV; administer only half the dosage if barbiturates have been given; blocks excitation
Arsenic, mercury, and other heavy metals except cadmium, lead, silver, selenium, and thallium	Dimercaprol (BAL, Hynson, Wescott & Dunning)	10% solution in oil; give small animals 2.5–5.0 mg/kg IM q6h for 2 days then q12h for the next 10 days or until recovery. (*Note:* With severe acute poisoning, 5 mg/kg should be given only on the first day.)
	D-Penicillamine (Cuprimine, Merck)	Developed for chronic mercury poisoning; now seems most promising drug; no reports on dosage in animals; give 3–4 mg/kg q6h
Atropine, belladonna alkaloids	Physostigmine salicylate	0.1–0.6 mg/kg (do not use neostigmine)
Barbiturates	Doxapram	2% solution; give small animals 3–5 mg/kg IV only (0.14–0.25 mL/kg); repeat as necessary. (*Note:* The above is reliable only when depression is mild; in animals with deeper levels of depression, ventilatory support [and oxygen] is preferable.)
Bromides	Chlorides (sodium or ammonium salts)	0.5–1.0 g PO daily for several days; hastens excretion
Carbon monoxide	Oxygen	Pure oxygen at normal or high pressure; artificial respiration; blood transfusion
Cholecalciferol	Calcitonin (Calcimar, Rhône-Poulenc Rorer)	4 IU/kg SC or IM q8–12h
Cholinergic agents	Atropine sulfate	0.02–0.04 mg/kg, as needed
Cholinesterase inhibitors	Atropine sulfate	0.2 mg/kg, repeated as needed for atropinization; treat cyanosis (if present) first; blocks only muscarinic effects: atropine in oil may be injected for prolonged effect. Avoid atropine intoxication!

TABLE H.1
(continued)

Toxic Agent	Systemic Antidote	Dosage and Method of Treatment
Cholinergic agents and cholinesterase inhibitors (organophosphates, some carbamates; but not carbaryl, morphine, succinylcholine, or carbam piloxime)	Pralidoxime chloride (2-PAM)	5% solution; 20–50 mg/kg IM or by slow IV (0.2–1.0 mg/kg) injection (maximum dosage is 500 mg/min), repeat as needed; 2-PAM alleviates nicotinic effect and regenerates cholinesterase; phenothiazine tranquilizers are contraindicated
Copper	D-Penicillamine (Cuprimine)	See Arsenic
Coumarin-derivative anticoagulants	Vitamin K_1 (AquaMEPHYTON, 5-mg capsules or 1% emulsion, Merck)	Give 3–5 mg/kg SC or PO per day with canned food; treat 7 days for warfarin type, treat 21–30 days for second-generation anticoagulant rodenticides; oral therapy more efficacious than parenteral
	Fresh whole blood, fresh plasma, or fresh frozen plasma	Blood transfusion, 10–25 mL/kg, as required
Curare	Neostigmine methylsulfate	Solution: 1:5000 or 1:2000 (1 mL = 0.2 or 0.5 mg/mL): dosage is 0.005 mg/5 kg SC; follow with IV injection of atropine (0.04 mg/kg)
	Edrophonium chloride (Tensilon, Roche) Ventilatory support	1% solution: give 0.05–1.0 mg/kg IV
Cyanide	Methemoglobin (sodium nitrite is used to form methemoglobin)	1% solution of sodium nitrite; dosage is 16 mg/kg IV (1.6 mL/kg)
	Sodium thiosulfate	Follow with 20% solution of sodium thiosulfate at dosage of 30–40 mg/kg (0.15–0.2 mL/kg) IV; if treatment is repeated, use only sodium thiosulfate. (*Note:* Both of the above may be given simultaneously as follows: 0.5 mL/kg of combination consisting of 10 g sodium nitrite, 15 g sodium thiosulfate distilled water q.s. to 250 mL; dosage may be repeated once; if further treatment is required, give only 20% solution thiosulfate at 0.2 mL/kg.)
Digitalis glycosides, oleander, and *Bufo* toads	Potassium chloride	Dogs: 0.5–2.0 g PO in divided doses or, in serious cases, a diluted solution given IV by slow drip (ECG monitoring is essential)
	Diphenylhydantoin	25 mg/min IV until ventricular arrhythmias are controlled
	Propranolol (β-blocker)	0.5–1.0 mg/kg IV or IM as needed to control cardiac arrhythmias (ECG monitoring is essential)
	Atropine sulfate	0.02–0.04 mg/kg as needed for cholinergic and arrhythmia control
Fluoride	Calcium borogluconate	3–10 mL of 5–10% solution
Fluoroacetate (compound 1080)	Glyceryl monoacetate (monoacetin, Sigma)	0.1–0.5 mg/kg IM hourly for several hours (total 2–4 mg/kg), or diluted (0.5–1.0% solution IV; danger of hemolysis); monoacetin is available only from chemical supply houses
	Acetamide	Animal may be protected if acetamide is given before or simultaneously with compound 1080 (experimental)
	Pentobarbital	May protect against lethal dose (experimental). (*Note:* All treatments are generally unrewarding.)
Hallucinogens (LSD, phencyclidine hydrochloride [PCP])	Diazepam (Valium, Roche)	As needed—avoid respiratory depression (2–5 mg/kg)
Heparin	Protamine sulfate	1% solution; give 1.0–1.5 mg by slow IV injection to antagonize each 1 mg of heparin; reduce dose as time increases between heparin injection and start of treatment (after 30 min, give only 0.5 mg)
Iron salts	Deferoxamine mesylate (Desferal, Ciba)	Dosage for animals not yet established; dosage for humans is 5 g of 5% solution PO, then 20 mg/kg IM q4–6h; in case of shock, dosage is 40 mg/kg by IV drip over 4-hour period; may be repeated in 6 hours, then 15 mg/kg by drip q8h

TABLE H.1
(continued)

Toxic Agent	Systemic Antidote	Dosage and Method of Treatment
Lead	Calcium disodium edetate (CaEDTA)	Maximum safe dosage is 75 mg/kg per 24 hours (only for severe case); EDTA is available in 20% solution; for IV drip, dilute in 5% glucose to 0.5%; for IM, add procaine to 20% solution to give 0.5% concentration of procaine
	EDTA and BAL	BAL is given as 10% solution in oil (a) In severe cases (CNS involvement with >100 μg lead per 100 g whole blood), give 4 mg/kg BAL only as initial dose; follow after 4 hours and q4h for 3–4 days with BAL and EDTA (12.5 mg/kg) at separate IM sites; skip 2 or 3 days and then treat again for 3–4 days (b) In subacute cases with <100 μg lead per 100 g whole blood, give only 50 mg DTA/kg per 24 hours for 3–5 days
	Penicillamine (Cuprimine)	May use after either treatment (a) or (b) with 100 mg/kg per day PO for 1–4 weeks
	Thiamine hydrochloride	Experimental to treat CNS signs; 5 g/kg IV q12h for 1–2 weeks; give slowly and watch for untoward reactions
Metaldehyde	Diazepam (Valium) Triflupromazine Pentobarbital	2–5 mg/kg IV to control tremors 0.2–2.0 mg/kg IV To effect
Methanol	Ethanol	Give 1.1 g/kg (4.4 mL/kg) of 25% solution IV; then give 0.5 g/kg (2.0 mL/kg) q4h for 4 days; to prevent or correct acidosis, use sodium bicarbonate 0.4 g/kg IV; activated charcoal, 5 g/kg PO if within 4 hours of ingestion
Methemoglobinemia-producing agents (nitrites, chlorates)	Methylene blue (not recommended for cats)	1% solution (maximum concentration); give by slow IV injection, 8.8 mg/kg (0.9 mL/kg), and repeat if necessary; to prevent fall in blood pressure in cases of nitrite poisoning, use a sympathomimetic drug (ephedrine or epinephrine)
Morphine and related drugs	Naloxone hydrochloride (Narcan, Endo)	0.1 mg/kg IV; do not repeat if respiration is not satisfactory
	Levallorphan tartrate (Lorfan, Roche)	Give IV 0.1–0.5 mL of solution containing 1 mg/mL. (*Note:* Use either of the antidotes only in acute poisoning. Ventilatory support may be indicated. Activated charcoal is also indicated.)
Oxalates	Calcium	10% solution of calcium gluconate IV; give 3–20 mL (to control hypocalcemia)
Phenothiazine	Methamphetamine hydrochloride (Desoxyn, Abbott)	0.1–0.2 mg/kg; treatment for hypovolemic shock may be required
	Diphenhydramine hydrochloride	For CNS depression, 2–5 mg/kg IV to treat extrapyramidal signs

TABLE H.1
(continued)

Toxic Agent	Systemic Antidote	Dosage and Method of Treatment
Phytotoxins and botulin	Antitoxins not available commercially (attempt to obtain through Centers for Disease Control)	As indicated for specific antitoxins; examples of phytotoxins: ricin, abrin, robin, crotin
Plants		Treat signs as necessary
Red squill	Atropine sulfate, propranolol, potassium chloride	As for digitalis and oleander
Snake bite		
Rattlesnake	Antivenin (Crotalidae)	Caution: equine origin; administer 1–2 vials IV, slowly, diluted in
Copperhead	Polyvalent (Wyeth),	250–500 mL of saline or lactated Ringer's solution; also administer
Water moccasin	Trivalent Crotalidae (Fort Dodge)	antihistamines; corticosteroids are contraindicated
Coral snake	Coral Snake (Wyeth)	Caution: equine origin; may be used as with pit viper antivenin
Spider bite		
Black widow	Antivenin (Merck)	Caution: equine origin; administer IV undiluted
	Dantrolene sodium (Dantrium, Norwich-Eaton)	For neurologic signs, 1 mg/kg IV, followed by 1 mg/kg PO q4h
Brown recluse	Dapsone	1 mg/kg q12h for 10 days
Strontium	Calcium salts	Usual dose of calcium borogluconate
	Ammonium chloride	0.2–0.5 g PO 3–4 times daily
Strychnine and brucine	Pentobarbital	Give IV to effect; higher dose is usually required than that required for anesthesia; place animal in warm, quiet room
	Amobarbital	Give slow IV to effect; duration of sedation is usually 4–6 hours
	Methocarbamol (Robaxin, AH Robins)	10% solution; average first dosage is 149 mg/kg IV (range, 40–300 mg); repeat half dosage as needed
	Glyceryl guaiacolate	110 mg/kg IV, 5% solution; repeat as necessary
	Diazepam (Valium)	2–5 mg/kg; controls convulsions
Thallium	Diphenylthiocarbazone	Dogs: 70 mg/kg PO q8h for 6 days; hastens elimination but is partially toxic
	Prussian blue	0.2 mg/kg PO in 3 divided doses daily
	Potassium chloride	Give simultaneously with thiocarbazone or Prussian blue, 2–6 g PO daily in divided doses

From Bailey EM Jr, Garland T. Toxicologic emergencies. In: Murtaugh RJ, Kaplan PM, eds. Veterinary Emergency and Critical Care Medicine. St. Louis: Mosby, 1992:443–446.

IM, intramuscularly; IV, intravenously; PO, orally; SC, subcutaneously; q, every; h, hour; q.s., sufficient quantity; ECG, electrocardiogram; CNS, central nervous system.

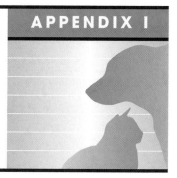

TRANSFUSION GUIDE

BLOOD COMPONENT FLOW CHART

DATE _____   Weight (kg) _____

Clinician _____   Student _____

Blood component _____   Amount _____

Primary disease _____   Reason for transfusion _____

Suggested Administration Rates for Blood and Blood Products

Normovolemic rate   3.0–6.0 mL/kg/h   (Maximum) over 6 hours

Hypovolemic rate   10–20 mL/kg/h   (Maximum) over 6 hours

Cardiac patient rate   2–4 mL/kg/h   (Maximum) over 6 hours

**Blood volume needed from the donor (mL) =

Dog: (recipient wt (kg) $\times$ 90*) $\times \left(\dfrac{\text{desired hematocrit} - \text{hematocrit of recipient}}{\text{donor hematocrit in anticoagulant}} \right)$

*use 60 in cats

Donor name or # _____

Initial Data Base	Temp	H.R.	R.R.	PCV/TS	Cross-match? Y N	Total volume transfused	30-min posttransfusion PCV/TS

Transfusion pretreatment

Drugs_____Dosage_____Route_____Time_____

Desired rate _____ mL/h

**For packed red cells, use one-half the calculated dosage for fresh whole blood.

Time in	0:0	0:10	0:20	0:30	1:0	2:0	3:0	4:0	5:0	6:0
Temp										
Pulse										
Resp rate										
Rate mL/h										

Transfusion reactions: Vomiting, increased heart rate, increased rectal temperature, diarrhea, angioedema, hypotension, collapse
If any signs occur, stop transfusion and call clinician immediately.

UNITED STATES BLOOD BANKS

Animal Blood Bank Hotline
(www.animalbloodbank.com): (800) 243-5759

"Buddies for Life" Canine Blood Bank
(www.ovrs.com): (866) 364-6877

Eastern Veterinary Blood Bank
(www.evbb.com): (800) 949-3822

Hemopet
(www.hemopet.com): (714) 891-2022
(Mon-Fri 8:30 am–5 pm PST),
(949) 378-5304 (all other times)

Midwest Animal Blood Services
(www.midwestabs.com): (877) 517-6227

Northwest Veterinary Blood Bank
(www.nwvetbloodbank.com): (306) 752-5544

Penn Animal Blood Bank: (215) 573-7222

DRUG FORMULARY

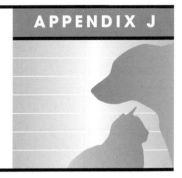

Drug (Other Names)	Pharmacology and Indications	Adverse Effects and Precautions	Dosage
Acepromazine 5-, 10-, 25-mg tablet and 10-mg/mL injection	Phenothiazine tranquilizer; used for sedation and preanesthetic purposes	May lower seizure threshold and causes α-adrenergic blockade; may cause hypotension in dehydrated animals	Restraint: 0.55–2.2 mg/kg PO or 0.055–2.2 mg/kg IV, IM Preanesthetic: 0.02–0.2 mg/kg IV, IM, SC Max (dogs) = 3 mg Max (cats) = 1 mg
Acetaminophen 120-, 160-, 325-, 500- mg tablets	Analgesic agent	Well tolerated in dogs at doses listed; high doses have caused liver toxicity. Do *not* administer to cats	Dogs: 15 mg/kg q8h PO Cats: not recommended
Acetaminophen with codeine Oral solution or tablets—many forms	Codeine is added to enhance analgesia	See Codeine and acetaminophen	Follow dosing recommendations for codeine
Acetazolamide 125-, 250-mg tablets; 500-mg vial for constitution	Carbonic anhydrase inhibitor and diuretic; used primarily to lower intraocular pressure in patients with glaucoma	Use cautiously in any animal sensitive to sulfonamides; can produce hypokalemia in some patients. Do not use in patients with acidemia.	5–10 mg/kg q8–12h PO Glaucoma: 50 mg/kg IV once
Acetylcysteine 10 or 20% solution	Decreases viscosity of secretions; used as mucolytic agent in eyes and in bronchial nebulizing solutions. As a donor of sulfhydryl group, used as antidote for intoxications (e.g., acetaminophen toxicosis in cats)	May cause bronchospasm	Antidote: 140 mg/kg (loading dose) then 70 mg/kg q4h IV or PO for 5 doses (dilute to 5% for IV use) Eye: 2% solution topically q2h. Nebulization: 4 mg in saline for 30 min q12h.
ACTH	See Corticotropin		
Activated charcoal	See Charcoal, activated.		
Albendazole 113.6-mg/mL suspension; 300-mg/mL paste; 200-mg tablets	Anthelmintic for lungworms, also *Giardia*	At approved doses there is a wide margin of safety. Adverse effects can include anorexia, lethargy, and bone marrow toxicity. At high doses has been associated with bone marrow toxicity (JAVMA 1998;213:44–46). Adverse effects are possible when administered for longer than 5 days	25–50 mg/kg q12h PO 10–21 days. For *Giardia*, use 25 mg/kg, q12h, × 5 days

Drug (Other Names)	Pharmacology and Indications	Adverse Effects and Precautions	Dosage
Albuterol 2-, 4-, 8-mg tablets; 0.083 and 0.5% solutions	β_2-Adrenergic agonist; broncho-dilator; stimulates β_2 receptors to relax bronchial smooth muscle; may also inhibit release of inflammatory mediators, especially from mast cells	Causes excessive β-adrenergic stimulation at high doses (tachycardia, tremors); arrhythmias occur at toxic doses. Avoid use in pregnant animals	Nebulization: 1.5 mL in 4 mL saline q6–12h.
Allopurinol 100-, 300-mg tablets	Prevention of urate urolithiasis	May cause skin reactions (hypersensitivity)	10 mg/kg q8h, then reduce to 10 mg/kg q24h
Aluminium 500-mg capsules	Antacid and phosphate binder for animals with hyperphos-phatemia	Generally safe; may interact with other drugs administered orally	10–30 mg/kg PO q8h (with meals)
Aluminium hydroxide gel 64-mg/mL oral liquid; 600-mg tablet	Antacid and phosphate binder for animals with hyperphos-phatemia and chronic renal failure	Generally safe; may interact with other drugs administered orally	10–30 mg/kg PO q8h (with meals)
Amikacin 50-, 250-mg/mL injection	Aminoglycoside antibacterial drug	May cause nephrotoxicosis, ototoxicity, and vestibulo-toxicity	Dog, cat: 6.5 mg/kg, q8h, IV, IM, SC, or 20 mg/kg q24h, IV, IM, SC
Aminophylline 100-, 200-mg tablets, 25-mg/mL injection	Bronchodilator; it is converted to theophylline after ingestion	Causes excitement and possible cardiac effect at high concentra-tions (see Theophylline)	Dog: 10 mg/kg q8h, PO, IM, IV Cat: 6.6 mg/kg q12h PO
Amiodarone 200 mg tablets; 50 mg/mL	Refractory arrhythmias in CPR; ventricular tachycardia; atrial fibrillation	GI, pulmonary, liver effects	5 mg/kg IV; 10–25 mg/kg PO q12h × 7days, then 7.5 mg/kg q12h × 14 days, then 7.5 mg/kg q24h
Amitriptyline (Elavil) 10-, 25-, 50-, 75-, 100-, 150-mg tablets; 10-mg/mL injection	Tricyclic antidepressant drug; inhibits serotonin uptake; used in animals to treat a variety of behavioral disorders (e.g., separation anxiety in dogs or stress-induced dysuria in cats	Antimuscarinic effects (dry mouth, rapid heart rate) and antihistamine effects (sedation)	Dog: 1–2 mg/kg, PO q12–24h, cat: 5–10 mg per cat/day, PO; (cystitis): 2 mg/kg/day (2.5–7.5 mg/cat/day)
Amlodipine besylate 2.5-, 5-, 10-mg tablets	Calcium-channel blocking drug, vasodilator; used to treat hypertension in cats and dogs	Can cause hypotension and bradycardia; use cautiously with other vasodilators	Dogs: 2.5 mg/dog, or 0.1 mg/kg, once daily PO Cats: 0.625 mg/cat initially, PO once daily, and increase if needed to 1.25 mg/cat (average is 0.18 mg/kg)
Ammonium chloride 200-mg tablets, granules	Urine acidifier used to enhance elimination of certain toxins	Do not use in patients with systemic acidemia; may be unpalatable when added to some animals' food	Dog: 100 mg/kg q12h PO Cat: 800 mg/cat (approximately ¼ to ⅓ tsp) mixed with food daily
Amoxicillin 50-, 100-, 150-, 200-, 400-mg tablets; 50-mg/mL oral liquid; 3q vial for injection	β-Lactam antibiotic	Usually well tolerated; allergic reactions are possible; diarrhea is common with oral doses	10–22 mg/kg q8–12h PO
Amoxicillin/clavulanic acid 62.5-, 125-, 250-, 375-mg tablet; 62.5-mg/mL oral liquid	β-Lactam antibiotic + β-lactamase inhibitor (clavulanate/clavulanic acid)	Same as amoxicillin	Dog: 12.5–25 mg/kg q12h PO Cat: 62.5 mg/cat q12h PO

Drug (Other Names)	Pharmacology and Indications	Adverse Effects and Precautions	Dosage
Amphotericin B (Fungizone) 50-mg vials; 100-mg/20 mL as lipid complex	Antifungal drug for blastomycosis, *Cryptococcus* infection, or histoplasmosis	Produces a dose-related nephrotoxicosis; also produces fever, phlebitis, and tremors; lipid complex formulation is less nephrotoxic	0.5 mg/kg IV (slow infusion) q48h, to a cumulative dose of 8–10 mg/kg; mix with 60 mL 5% dextrose in water and give over 15 minutes
Ampicillin 250-, 500-mg capsules, 1- and 3-g vials for injection	β-Lactam antibiotic	Hypersensitivity reactions: anorexia, vomiting, diarrhea	10–20 mg/kg q6–8h IV, IM, SC (ampicillin sodium); 20–40 mg/kg q8h PO
Ampicillin + sulbactam 1.5- and 3-g vials	Ampicillin plus a β-lactamase inhibitor (sulbactam); sulbactam has similar activity to clavulanate	Same as ampicillin	10–20 mg/kg IV, IM q8h
Ampicillin trihydrate 10- and 25-g vials	β-Lactam antibiotic	Use cautiously in animals allergic to penicillin-like drugs	Dogs: 10–50 mg/kg q12–24h IM, SC Cats: 10–20 mg/kg q12–24h IM, SC
Amprolium 9.6% oral liquid	Antiprotozoal drug; used for treatment of coccidiosis, especially in puppies	Toxicity observed only at high doses (CNS signs are due to thiamine deficiency)	1.25 g of 20% amprolium powder to daily feed, or 30 mL of 9.6% amprolium solution to 3.8 L of drinking water for 7 days
Amrinone 5 mg/mL	Positive inotrope	Limited experience in animals	1–3 mg/kg IV, followed by 30–100 μg/kg/min CRI
Antivenom (Crotalidae) Polyvalent (equine origin) 10 mL antivenom/vial when reconstituted	Neutralizes venom of all North American species of rattlesnakes, copperheads, and cottonmouth moccasins; used in the treatment of snake-bite injuries; especially acute injuries with severe tissue swelling/ecchymosis and systemic signs such as hemolysis	Hypersensitivity reaction to equine immunoglobulins that in antivenom is possible; severe reactions are uncommon	Dog: 1 vial IV; may give 2–3 or more vials if clinical signs worsen Cat: ½-1 vial IV Administer over 30–60 minutes
Apomorphine hydrochloride	Emetic drug; causes emesis via dopamine release or direct effects on CRTZ	Produces emesis before serious adverse effects occur; use cautiously in cats that may be sensitive to opiates	0.02–0.04 mg/kg IV IM, 0.1 mg/kg SC, or instill 0.25 mg in conjunctiva of eye (dissolve 6-mg tablet in 1–2 mL of saline)
Ascorbic acid (vitamin C)	Vitamin; used as acidifier	Toxicity only at very high doses	100–500 mg/animal/day (diet supplement), or 100 mg/animal q8h (urine acidification)
L-Asparaginase 10,000 U per vial	Anticancer agent; used in lymphoma protocols in combination with other drugs	Hypersensitivity, allergic reactions	400 U/kg IM weekly or 10,000 U/m² weekly × 3 weeks.
Aspirin 81-, 325-mg tablets	Nonsteroidal antiinflammatory drug; used as analgesic, antiinflammatory, and antiplatelet drug	Cats are susceptible to salicylate intoxication because of slow clearance; use cautiously in patients with coagulopathies because of platelet inhibition; GI and renal toxicity may occur	Mild analgesia: (dog) 10 mg/kg, q12h Antiinflammatory: Dog: 20–25 mg/kg q12h; cat: 10–20 mg/kg q48h Antiplatelet: dog: 5–10 mg/kg q24–48h; cat: 80 mg q48h

Drug (Other Names)	Pharmacology and Indications	Adverse Effects and Precautions	Dosage
Atenolol (Tenormin) 25-, 50-, 100-mg tablets; 25-mg/mL oral liquid; 5-mg/mL ampules for injection	β-Adrenergic blocker; Relatively selective for $β_1$-receptor; used primarily as an antiarrhythmic, or in other cardiovascular conditions to slow sinus rate	Bradycardia and heart block are possible; may produce broncho-spasm in sensitive patients	Dog: 6.25–12.5 mg/dog q12h (or 0.25–1.0 mg/kg q12–24h) Cat: 6.25–12.5 mg/cat q12h (approx. 3 mg/kg)
Atipamezole 5-mg/mL injection	$α_2$-Antagonist; used to reverse $α_2$-antagonists such as medeto-midine, xylazine, and amitraz	Safe; can cause some initial excitement in some animals shortly after reversal	Inject same volume as used for medetomidine
Atracurium 10-mg/mL injection	Neuromuscular blocking agent used to promote muscle relaxation for mechanical ventilation	Produces respiratory depression and paralysis; neuromuscular blocking drugs have no effect on analgesia	0.2 mg/kg IV initially, then 0.15 mg/kg q30 min (or IV infusion at 3–8 μg/kg/min)
Atropine 0.4-, 0.5-mg/mL for injection	Anticholinergic agent, para-sympatholytic; used primarily as adjunct to anesthesia or other procedures to increase heart rate and decrease respiratory and GI secretion; also used as antidote for organo-phosphate intoxication	Potent anticholinergic agent; do not use in patients with glaucoma, intestinal ileus, gastroparesis, or tachycardia; side effects of therapy include xerostomia, ileus, constipation, tachycardia, urine retention	0.02–0.14 mg/kg q6–8h IV, IM, SC; 0.2–0.5 mg/kg (as needed) for organophosphate and carbamate toxicosis
Azathioprine 50-mg tablets; 10-mg/mL injection	Thiopurine immunosuppressive drug; acts to inhibit T-cell lymphocyte function; used to treat various immune-mediated diseases	Bone marrow suppression is most serious concern; cats are particularly susceptible; some association with development of pancreatitis when administered with corticosteroids	Dogs: 2 mg/kg q24h PO initially then 0.5–1 mg/kg q48h Cats (use cautiously): 1 mg/kg, q48h, PO
Azithromycin 250-, 600-mg tablets; 100- or 200-mg/5 mL oral liquid; 500-mg vials for injection	Azalide antibiotic; achieves high intracellular concentrations	Has not been in common use in veterinary medicine to establish adverse effects; vomiting is likely with high doses; diarrhea may occur in some patients	Dogs: 10 mg/kg, PO, once every 5 days, or 3.3 mg/kg, once daily for 3 days. Cats: 5 mg/kg, PO every other day
Bactrim (sulfamethoxazole + trimethoprim) See Trimethoprim sulfona-mide combinations			
Benazepril (Lotensin) 5-, 10-, 20-, 40-mg tablets	ACE inhibitor; used for hypertension and heart failure	Hypotension, renal dysfunction, GI signs may occur	Dog: 0.25–0.5 mg/kg q24h, PO Cat: same
Bethanechol (Urecholine) 5-, 10-, 25-, 50-mg tablets; 5-mg/mL injection	Muscarinic, cholinergic agonist parasympathomimetic; Stimulates gastric and intestinal motility, but primarily used to increase contraction of urinary bladder	High doses of cholinergic agonists increase motility of GI tract and cause abdominal discomfort and diarrhea; can cause circulatory depression in sensitive animals	Dogs: 5–15 mg/dog q8h PO Cats: 1.25–5 mg/cat q8h PO
Bisacodyl (Dulcolax) 5-mg tablets	Laxative/cathartic; acts via local stimulation of GI motility, most likely by irritation of bowel; used primarily as laxative or for procedures in which bowel evacuation is necessary	Avoid use in patients with renal disease; avoid overuse	5 mg/animal q8–24h PO

Drug (Other Names)	Pharmacology and Indications	Adverse Effects and Precautions	Dosage
Bismuth subsalicylate (Pepto Bismol) 262 mg/15 mL; 262-mg tablets	Antidiarrhea agent and GI protectant. Antiprostaglandin action of salicylate component may be beneficial for enteritis; bismuth component is efficacious for treating infections caused by spirochete bacteria (*Helicobacter gastritis*)	Salicylate component is absorbed systemically and overuse should be avoided in animals that cannot tolerate salicylates (such as cats and animals allergic to aspirin).	1-3 mg/kg/day (in divided doses) PO.
Black widow spider antivenom (Lyovac Antivenom) 2.5 mL/vial	Equine-derived antiserum against *Latrodectus* venom; used to treat black widow spider bites	Hypersensitivity reaction to equine immunoglobulins that compose antivenom is possible; severe reactions uncommon	Dog and cat: 1 vial IV diluted in 50–100 mL D5W administered over 30–60 min
Bleomycin (Blenoxane) 15-U vials for injection	Anticancer antibiotic agent; used for treatment of various sarcomas and carcinomas	Causes local reaction at site of injection; causes pulmonary toxicity in people as well as fever and chills, but side effects are not well documented in veterinary species	Dogs; 10 U/m^2 IV or SC for 3 days, then 10 units/m^2 weekly (maximum cumulative dose 200 U/m^2)
Bupivacaine 2.5- and 5-mg/mL injection	Local anesthetic; inhibits nerve conduction via sodium channel blockade; longer-acting and more potent than lidocaine or other local anesthetics	Adverse effects rare with local infiltration; high doses absorbed systemically can cause nervous system signs (tremors and convulsions); after epidural administration respiratory paralysis is possible with high doses	1 mL of 0.5% solution per 10 cm for an epidural
Buprenorphine 0.3-mg/mL injection	Opioid analgesic; partial μ-receptor agonist, κ-receptor antagonist; 25–50 × more potent than morphine; may cause less respiratory depression than other opiates	Adverse effects are similar to those of other opiate agonists, except there may be less respiratory depression; may be less dependency from chronic use than with pure agonists	Dogs: 0.006–0.02 mg/kg IV, IM, SC, q4–8h Cats: 0.0005–0.01 mg/kg, IV, IM q4–8h
Buspirone 5-, 10-mg tablets	Antianxiety agent; acts to block release of serotonin by binding to presynaptic receptors; used for treatment of urine spraying in cats	Some cats show increased aggression; some show increased affection to owners	2.5–5 mg/cat q24h, PO (may be increased to 5–7.5 mg per cat twice daily for some cats)
Butorphanol 1-, 5-, 10-mg tablets; 0.5- or 10-mg/mL injection	Opioid analgesic; used for perioperative analgesia, chronic pain, and as an antitussive agent	Adverse effects are similar to those of other opioid analgesic drugs; sedation is common at analgesic doses; respiratory depression can occur with high doses; dysphoric effects have been observed with these agonist/antagonist drugs	Dog: (antitussive) 0.055 mg/kg q6–12h SC or 0.55 mg/kg PO; (preanesthetic) 0.2–0.4 mg/kg IV, IM, SC (with acepromazine); (analgesic) 0.2–0.4 mg/kg q2-4h Cats (analgesic): 0.2–0.8 mg/kg q2–6h, IV, SC, or 1.5 mg/kg PO q4–8h
Calcitonin salmon 200 U/mL in 2-mL vial	For vitamin D toxicity, severe hypercalcemia		4–6 U/kg SC q8–12h
Calcitriol (Rocaltrol, Calcijex) 0.25-, 0.5-μg capsules; 1- or 2-μg/mL injection	Used to treat calcium deficiency and diseases such as hypocalcemia associated with hypoparathyroidism	Overdose can result in hypercalcemia	2.5–3 ng/kg (0.0025–0.003 μg/kg) q24h PO

Drug (Other Names)	Pharmacology and Indications	Adverse Effects and Precautions	Dosage
Calcium carbonate 650-mg tablets	Used as oral calcium supplement for hypocalcemia; used as antacid to treat gastric hyperacidity; also used as intestinal phosphate binder for hyperphosphatemia	Few side effects; may decrease absorption of other drugs	5–10 mL of oral solution, q4–6h PO; for phosphate binder: 60–100 mg/kg/day in divided doses, PO
Calcium chloride 100 mg/mL	Calcium supplement; used in acute situations	Overdose with calcium is possible; do not administer solution SC, IM, because it may cause tissue necrosis	0.1–0/3 mL/kg IV (slowly)
Calcium citrate	Calcium supplement; used in treatment of hypocalcemia (e.g., in hypoparathyroidism)	Hypercalcemia possible with oversupplementation	Cats: 10–30 mg/kg q8h PO (with meals)
Calcium gluconate 100 mg/mL	Calcium supplement; used in treatment of hypocalcemia (e.g., with eclampsia)	Hypercalcemia possible with oversupplementation	0.5–1.5 mL/kg IV (slowly)
Calcium lactate	Generally same comments as for other calcium supplements		Dogs: 0.5–2.0 g/dog/day PO (in divided doses) Cats: 0.2–0.5 gm/cat/day PO (in divided doses)
Captopril 25-mg tablet	Angiotensin-converting enzyme (ACE) inhibitor; vasodilator generally used to treat hypertension and congestive heart failure	Hypotension possible with excessive doses; may cause azotemia in some patients, especially when administered with potent diuretics (furosemide); monitor electrolytes and renal function 3–7 days after starting Rx	Dogs: 0.5–2 mg/kg q8–12h PO Cats: 3.12 to 6.25 mg/cat q8–12h PO
Carbenicillin 1-, 2-, 5-, 10-, and 30-g vials for injection	β-Lactam antibiotic; active against *Pseudomonas*	Use cautiously in patients sensitive to penicillins (e.g., allergy)	40–50 mg/kg, and up to 100 mg/kg q6–8h IV, IM, SC
Carbenicillin indanyl sodium 500-mg tablets	Same as for carbenicillin; primary use is for treating infections of lower urinary tract, not for systemic infections	Same as carbenicillin	10 mg/kg q8h PO
Carboplatin 50- and 150-mg vial for injection	Anticancer agent; used for treating various carcinomas	Dose-limiting toxicosis is myelosuppression; may cause anemia, leucopenia, or thrombocytopenia; may induce renal toxicity	Dogs: 300 mg/m² q3 weeks IV Cats: 200–250 mg/m² every 4 weeks, IV
Carprofen 25-, 75-, 100-mg tablets	Analgesic agent; used primarily for treatment of musculoskeletal pain	Appears to cause lower incidence of GI ulceration and vomiting than other NSAIDs; in rare cases in dogs, carprofen has caused idiosyncratic acute hepatic toxicity (highest incidence was in Labradors); signs of toxicity appear 2–3 weeks after exposure. Do not use in cats	Dog: 2.2 mg/kg, q12h, PO Cat: doses not available Post-operative pain: 4 mg/kg IV once, then 2.2 mg/kg IV, PO, SC, IM q12h

Drug (Other Names)	Pharmacology and Indications	Adverse Effects and Precautions	Dosage
Cefaclor 250-, 500-mg capsules; 25 mg/mL oral liquid	2nd-generation cephalosporin antibiotic	All cephalosporins are generally safe; however, sensitivity can occur in individuals (allergy); rare bleeding disorders have been known to occur with some cephalosporins	4–20 mg/kg, q8h, PO
Cefadroxil 50-, 100-, 200-, 1000-mg tablets; 50-mg/mL oral liquid	Cefadroxil is a 1st-generation cephalosporin	May cause vomiting after oral administration in dogs	Dog: 22 mg/kg q12h, up to 30 mg/kg q12h PO Cat: 22 mg/kg q24h PO.
Cefazolin sodium 50- and 100-mg/50 mL for injection	Cefazolin is a 1st-generation cephalosporin	For cefazolin, use cephalothin to test susceptibility	20–35 mg/kg q8h IV, IM; for perisurgical use: 22 mg/kg every 2 hours during surgery
Cefdinir 300-mg capsules, 25-mg/mL oral liquid	Oral 3rd-generation cephalosporin; activity includes staphylococci, and many gram-negative bacilli	Similar to other oral cephalosporins	Dose not established; human dose is 7 mg/kg q12h PO
Cefixime 200- and 400-mg tablets, 20-mg/mL oral liquid	Cefixime is a 3rd-generation cephalosporin		10 mg/kg q12h PO; for cystitis: 5 mg/kg q12–24h PO
Cefotaxime 500 mg capsules, 1-, 2-, and 10-g vials for injection	Cefotaxime is a 3rd-generation cephalosporin. Cefotaxime is used when resistance is encountered to other antibiotics, or when infection is in central nervous system.		Dog: 50 mg/kg, IV, IM, SC, q12h. Cat: 20–80 mg/kg q6h IV, IM.
Cefotetan 1, 2, and 10 g vials for injection	Cefotetan is 2nd-generation cephalosporin		30 mg/kg, q8h, IV, SC
Cefoxitin sodium 1-, 2-, and 10-g vials for injection	Cefoxitin is a 2nd–generation cephalosporin; may have increased activity against anaerobic bacteria		30 mg/kg q6-8h IV
Ceftazidime 280 mg/mL	3rd-generation cephalosporin; has more activity than other cephalosporins against *Pseudomonas aeruginosa*		30 mg/kg q6h IV, IM
Ceftiofur 50-mg/mL injection	Spectrum resembles that of many of the 3rd-generation cephalosporins; used for resistant UTIs		2.2–4.4 mg/kg, SC, q24h (for urinary tract infections)
Cephalexin 250-, 500-mg tablets; 100-mg/mL oral liquid	Cephalexin is a 1st-generation cephalosporin	Use cephalothin to test susceptibility	10–30 mg/kg q6–12h PO; for pyoderma, 22–35 mg/kg, q12h, PO
Cephalothin sodium 1- and 2-g vials for injection	1st-generation cephalosporin		10–30 mg/kg q4–8h IV, IM
Cephapirin 500-mg, 1-, 2-, 4-g vials for injection	1st-generation cephalosporin		10–30 mg/kg q4–8h IV, IM

Drug (Other Names)	Pharmacology and Indications	Adverse Effects and Precautions	Dosage
Cephradine 250-, 500-mg capsules, 250-, 500-mg, 1- and 2-g vials for injection	1st-generation cephalosporin		10–25 mg/kg q6–8h PO
Charcoal, activated	Absorbent; used primarily to absorb drugs and toxins in intestine to prevent their absorption; may contain sorbitol or cathartic	Not absorbed systemically; safe for administration	1–4 g/kg PO (granules); 6–12 mL/kg (suspension)
Chlorambucil (Leukeran) 2-mg tablet	Cytotoxic agent; acts similarly to cyclophosphamide as alkylating agent; used for treatment of various tumors and immunosuppressive therapy	Myelosuppression is possible; cystitis does not occur with chlorambucil as with cyclophosphamide	2–6 mg/m^2, or 0.1–0.2 mg/kg q24h initially, then q48 h PO
Chloramphenicol and chloramphenicol palmitate 100-, 250-, 500-mg tablets, 30-mg/mL oral liquid	Antibacterial drug	Bone marrow suppression (especially in cats); avoid use in pregnant or neonatal animals; drug interactions with other drugs (e.g., barbiturates) possible because chloramphenicol inhibits hepatic microsomal enzymes	Dog: 40–50 mg/kg q8h PO Cat: 12.5–20 mg/kg q12h PO
Chloramphenicol sodium succinate 100-mg/mL injection	Injection form of chloramphenicol	Same as chloramphenicol	Dog: 40–50 mg/kg q6–8h IV, IM Cat: 12.5–20 mg/cat q12h IV, IM
Chlorothiazide (Diuril) 250- and 500-mg tablets, 50-mg/mL oral liquid and injection	Thiazide diuretic; used as diuretic and antihypertensive; since it decreases renal excretion of calcium, it also has been used to treat calcium-containing uroliths	Do not use in patient with elevated calcium levels; may cause electrolyte imbalance such as hypokalemia	20–40 mg/kg q12h PO
Chlorpheniramine maleate 4-, 8-mg tablets	Antihistamine (H-1 blocker); used for pruritus therapy in dogs and cats	Sedation is most common side effect; antimuscarinic effects (atropine-like effects) also common	Dog: 4–8 mg/dog q12h PO (up to a maximum of 0.5 mg/kg q12h) Cat: 2 mg/cat q12h PO
Chlorpromazine 25-mg/mL injection	Phenothiazine tranquilizer/ antiemetic	Causes sedation; may lower seizure threshold and causes α-adrenergic blockade; may cause hypotension; avoid use in dehydrated animals	0.5 mg/kg q6–8h IM, SC
Chlortetracycline	Tetracycline antibacterial drug; inhibits bacterial protein synthesis by interfering with peptide elongation by ribosome; bacteriostatic agent with broad-spectrum activity	Avoid use in young animals; may bind to bone and developing teeth; high doses have caused renal injury	25 mg/kg q6–8h PO
Cimetidine 100-, 150-, 200-, 300-mg tablets and 60-mg/mL injection	Histamine-2 antagonist (H-2 blocker); decreases gastric acid secretion; used to treat ulcers and gastritis	May increase concentrations of other drugs used concurrently (e.g., theophylline), because of inhibition of hepatic enzymes	10 mg/kg q6–8h IV, IM, PO (in renal failure, administer 2.5–5 mg/kg q12h IV, PO)

Drug (Other Names)	Pharmacology and Indications	Adverse Effects and Precautions	Dosage
Ciprofloxacin 250-, 500-, 750-mg tablet; 2-mg/mL injection	Fluoroquinolone antibacterial	Avoid use in dogs 4 weeks to 7 months of age; high concentrations may cause CNS toxicity, especially in animals with renal failure; use cautiously in epileptic patients; causes occasional vomiting; IV solution should be given slowly (over 30 min)	10–20 mg/kg q24h PO, IV
Cisapride 10-mg tablet	Prokinetic agent; stimulates gastric and intestinal motility; used for gastric reflux, gastroparesis, ileus, constipation	Contraindicated in patients with GI obstruction	Dog: 0.1–0.5 mg/kg q8–12h, PO (as high as 0.5–1.0 mg/kg) Cat: 2.5–5 mg/cat q8–12h, PO (as high as 1 mg/kg q8h)
Cisplatin 1-mg/mL injection	Anticancer agent; used for treating various solid tumors, including osteosarcoma	Nephrotoxicity is the most limiting factor; to avoid toxicity, perform fluid loading using sodium chloride before administration; antiemetic agents are often administered before therapy to decrease vomiting	Dogs only: 60–70 mg/m^2 q3–4 weeks IV (administer fluid for diuresis with therapy)
Clemastine 1.34- and 2.64-mg tablets; 0.134-mg/mL syrup	Antihistamine (H-1 blocker); blocks action of histamine on tissues; used primarily for treatment of allergy and pruritus	Sedation is most common side effect	Dog: 0.05–0.1 mg/kg q12h PO
Clindamycin 25-, 75-, 150-mg capsules; 25-mg/mL oral liquid; 150-mg/mL injection	Antibacterial drug with spectrum of activity primarily against gram-positive bacteria and anaerobes		Dog: 11 mg/kg q12h PO, or 22 mg/kg q24h PO Cat: 5.5 mg/kg q12h, or 11 mg/kg q24h (staphylococcal infections); 11 mg/kg q12h, or 22 mg/kg q24h, (anaerobic infections) PO Toxoplasmosis: 12.5 mg/kg PO, q12h for 4 weeks
Clomipramine 5-, 10-, 20-, 25-, 80-mg/ tablets	Tricyclic antidepressant drug (TCA); used in animals to treat variety of behavioral disorders, including obsessive-compulsive disorders and separation anxiety	Reported adverse effects include sedation, reduced appetite; other side effects associated with TCAs are antimuscarinic effects (dry mouth, rapid heart rate), and antihistamine effects (sedation); overdoses can produce life-threatening cardiotoxicity	Dog: 1–3 mg/kg/day, q12h PO Cat: 1–5 mg per cat q12–24h PO
Clonazepam (Klonopin) 0.5-, 1-, and 2-mg tablets	Benzodiazepine; used for antiseizure action, sedation, and treatment of some behavioral disorders	Side effects include sedation and polyphagia; some animals may experience paradoxical excitement	0.5 mg/kg q8–12h PO
Clorazepate 3.75-, 7.5-, 11.25-, 15-, and 22.5-mg tablets	Benzodiazepine; used for antiseizure action, sedation, and treatment of some behavioral disorders	Side effects include sedation and polyphagia; some animals may experience paradoxical excitement	2 mg/kg q12h PO
Cloxacillin 250-, 500-mg capsules; 25-mg/mL oral liquid	β-Lactam antibiotic; spectrum is limited to gram-positive bacteria, especially staphylococci	Use cautiously in animals allergic to penicillin-like drugs	20–40 mg/kg q8 h PO

Drug (Other Names)	Pharmacology and Indications	Adverse Effects and Precautions	Dosage
Colchicine 500-, 600-μg tablets; 500-μg/mL injection	Antiinflammatory agent; used primarily to treat gout and to decrease fibrosis and development of hepatic failure (possibly by inhibiting formation of collagen)	May cause vomiting, diarrhea	0.01–0.03 mg/kg q24h PO
Colony-stimulating factor	Stimulates granulocyte development in bone marrow; used primarily to regenerate blood cells to recover from cancer chemotherapy		2.5 μg/kg q12h SC
Corticotropin 800-U/mL gel	Used for diagnostic purposes to evaluate adrenal gland function; stimulates normal synthesis of cortisol from adrenal gland		Response test: collect pre-ACTH sample and inject 2.2 IU/kg IM; collect post-ACTH sample at 2 hours in dogs and at 1 and 2 hours in cats
Cosequin (glucosamine + chondroitin sulfate) (Cosequin) Capsules—regular or double strength	Cosequin is brand name for combination of glucosamine HCl and chondroitin sulfate	Adverse effects have not been reported, although hypersensitivity is possible	Dogs: 1–2 RS capsules per day (2–4 capsules of DS for large dogs) Cat: 1 RS capsule daily
Cosyntropin 250-μg/vial	Cosyntropin is a synthetic form of corticotrophin (ACTH) used for diagnostic purposes only		Response test: collect pre-ACTH sample and inject 5 μg/kg IV (dog) or 0.125 IV (cat), and collect post sample at 30, 60 min
Cyanocobalamin (vitamin B_{12})	Vitamin B analogue	Adverse effects rare except in high overdoses	Dog: 100–200 μg/day PO Cat: 50–100 μg/day PO
Cyclophosphamide (Cytoxan, Neosar) 25-, 50-mg tablets; 25-mg/mL injection	Cytotoxic agent; cytotoxic for tumor cells and other rapidly dividing cells; used primarily as adjunct for cancer chemotherapy and as immunosuppressive therapy	Bone marrow suppression is most common adverse effect; can produce severe neutropenia (usually reversible); vomiting and diarrhea may occur in some patients; dogs are susceptible to bladder toxicity (sterile hemorrhagic cystitis)	Anticancer: 50 mg/m² once daily 4 days/week PO, or 150–300 mg/m² IV, and repeat in 21 days. Immunosuppressive therapy: 50 mg/m² (approx. 2.2 mg/kg) q48h PO, or 2.2 mg/kg once daily for 4 days/week Cat: 6.25–12.5 mg/cat once daily 4 days/week
Cyclosporine 25-, 100-mg capsules/ 100 mg/mL oral liquid	Immunosuppressive drug; suppresses induction of T-cell lymphocytes	Can cause vomiting, diarrhea, anorexia; nephrotoxicity may occur. In comparison to other immunosuppressive drugs, does not cause myelosuppression	Dog: 3–7 mg/kg q12h, PO Cat: 3–5 mg/kg PO q12h
Cyproheptadine 4-mg tablet; 2-mg/5 mL oral liquid	Used as appetite stimulant (probably by altering serotonin activity in appetite center)	May cause increased appetite and weight gain	Antihistamine: 1.1 mg/kg q8–12h PO Appetite stimulant: 2 mg/cat PO
Cytarabine (cytosine arabinoside) 100-mg vial	Anticancer agent; used for lymphoma and leukemia protocols	Bone marrow suppression; causes vomiting and nausea	Dog (lymphoma): 100 mg/m² once daily, or 50 mg/m² twice daily for 4 days IV, SC Cat: 100 mg/m² once daily for 2 days

Drug (Other Names)	Pharmacology and Indications	Adverse Effects and Precautions	Dosage
Dacarbazine (DTIC) 200-mg vial	Anticancer agent; monofunctional alkylating agent; used for melanoma	Leukopenia, nausea, vomiting, diarrhea; do not use in cats	200 mg/m^2 for 5 days q3 weeks IV; or 800–1000 mg/m^2 q 3 weeks IV
Danazol (Danocrine) 50-, 100-, 200-mg capsules	May reduce destruction of platelets or RBCs in immune-mediated disease	Adverse effects have not been reported in animals	5–10 mg/kg q12h PO
Dantrolene (Dantrium) 100-mg capsule; 0.33- mg/mL injection	Muscle relaxant; also has been used for malignant hyperthermia and to relax urethral muscle in cats	Muscle relaxants can cause weakness in some animals	For prevention of malignant hyperthermia: 2–3 mg/kg IV Dog: 1–5 mg/kg q8h PO Cat: 0.5–2 mg/kg q12h PO
Dapsone (generic) 25- and 100-mg tablets	Antimicrobial drug used primarily for treatment of mycobacteria; may have some immunosuppressive properties or inhibit function of `inflammatory cells; used primarily for dermatologic diseases in dogs and cats	Hepatitis and blood dyscrasias may occur; toxic dermatologic reactions have been seen in people. *Drug interactions:* do not administer with trimethoprim (may increase blood concentrations)	1.1 mg/kg q8–12h PO
Decoquinate 6% 27.2-g/lb feed additive	Prevents development of sporozoites for intestinal coccidiosis and tissue stages of *Hepatozoon americanium*	Very safe	10–20 mg/kg (1 tsp/20 lb) missed in food q12h
Deferoxamine (Desferal) 500-mg vial	Chelating agent used to treat iron and aluminum toxicity—iron chelator to prevent reperfusion injury		10 mg/kg IV, IM q2h for two doses, then 10 mg/kg q8h for 24 hours
Desmopressin acetate (DDAVP) (DDAVP) 4- and 15-µg/mL injection; 100-µg/mL nasal spray; 0.1- and 0.2-mg tablets	Synthetic peptide similar to antidiuretic hormone (ADH); used as replacement therapy for patients with diabetes insipidus; desmopressin also has been used for treatment of patients with mild-to-moderate von Willebrand's disease prior to surgery or other procedure that may cause bleeding	No side effects reported; intranasal product is administered to dogs as eye drops; duration is 20 hours	Diabetes insipidus: 2–4 drops (2 µg) q12–24h intranasally or in eye; 0.05–0.1 mg q12h PO as needed Von Willebrand's disease treatment: 1 µg/kg (0.01 mL/kg) SC, IV, diluted in 20 mL of saline administered over 10 min
Desoxycorticosterone pivalate 25 mg/mL	Mineralocorticoid; used for adrenocorticoid insufficiency (hypoadrenocorticism); no glucocorticoid activity	Excessive mineralocorticoid effects with high doses; monitor electrolytes to determine efficacy and duration	1.5–2.2 mg/kg q 25 days IM
Dexamethasone 2- or 4-mg/mL injection; 0.25-, 0.5-, 0.75-, 1-, 1.5-, 2-, 4-, 6- mg tablets	Corticosteroid; dexamethasone has approximately 30 × potency of cortisol; Multiple antiinflammatory effects (see Betamethasone)	Multiple side effects. (See Betamethasone)	Antiinflammatory: 0.07–0.25 mg/kg q12–24h IV, IM, PO For shock, spinal injury: 2.2–4.4 mg/kg IV (of sodium phosphate form). Dexamethasone suppression test—dogs: 0.01 mg/kg IV, cats 0.1 mg/kg IV, and collect sample at 0, 4, and 8 hours

Drug (Other Names)	Pharmacology and Indications	Adverse Effects and Precautions	Dosage
Dextran (Dextran 70) 250, 500, 100 mL	Synthetic colloid used for volume expansion; high-molecular-weight fluid replacement; primarily used for acute hypovolemia and shock	Only limited use in veterinary medicine and adverse effects have not been reported; in people, coagulopathies are possible because of decreased platelet function; anaphylactic shock also has occurred	10–20 mL/kg IV to effect
Dextromethorphan	Centrally acting antitussive drug; shares similar chemical structure with opiates, but does not affect opiate receptors; appears to directly affect cough receptor	Adverse effects not reported in veterinary medicine; high overdose may cause sedation	0.5–2 mg/kg q6–8h PO
Dextrose solution 5% (D5W)	Sugar added to fluid solutions; isotonic	Do not administer for shock; large doses of hypotonic fluid cause RBC lysis	40–50 mL/kg q24h IV
Diazepam 2-, 5-mg tablet; 5- mg/mL injection	Benzodiazepine; central-acting CNS depressant; used for sedation, anesthetic adjunct, anticonvulsant, and behavioral disorders	Sedation is most common side effect; may cause paradoxical excitement; causes polyphagia; in cats, idiopathic fatal hepatic necrosis has been reported with oral diazepam	Preanesthetic: 0.5 mg/kg IV Status epilepticus: 0.5 mg/kg IV, 1 mg/kg rectal; repeat if necessary Appetite stimulant (cat): 0.2 mg/kg IV. For behavior treatment in cats: 1–4 mg per cat q12–24h PO
Dichlorphenamide 50-mg tablet	Carbonic anhydrase inhibitor; primarily used to treat glaucoma	Sulfonamide derivative; use cautiously in animals sensitive to sulfonamides; hypokalemia may occur in some patients; severe metabolic acidosis is rare	3–5 mg/kg q8–12h PO
Dicloxacillin 125-, 250-, 500-mg capsules; 12.5-mg/mL oral liquid	β-Lactam antibiotic; spectrum is limited to gram-positive bacteria, especially staphylococci	Use cautiously in animals allergic to penicillin-like drugs	11–55 mg/kg q8h PO
Diethylcarbamazine 50-, 80-, 180-, 200-, 400-mg tablet	Heartworm preventive	Safe in all species; reactions can occur in animals with microfilaria	Heartworm prophylaxis: 6.6 mg/kg q24h PO
Diethylstilbestrol (DES) 1-, 5-mg tablet; 50-mg/mL injection	Synthetic estrogen compound; used for estrogen replacement in animals; DES is most commonly used to treat estrogen-responsive incontinence in dogs; also has been used to induce abortion in dogs	Side effects may occur that are caused by excess estrogen; estrogen therapy may increase risk of pyometra and estrogen-sensitive tumors	Dog: 0.1–1.0 mg/dog q24h PO Cat: 0.05–0.1 mg/cat q24h PO
Difloxacin hydrochloride (Dicural) 11.4-, 45.4-, and 136-mg tablet	Fluoroquinolone antibacterial drug; bactericidal with broad-spectrum activity; used for variety of infections, including skin infections, wound infections, and pneumonia	Adverse effects include seizures in epileptic animals, arthropathy in young animals, vomiting at high doses	5–10 mg/kg q24h, PO (see dosing information guidelines)

Drug (Other Names)	Pharmacology and Indications	Adverse Effects and Precautions	Dosage
Digitoxin 0.05- and 0.1-mg tablet.	Cardiac inotropic agent; increases cardiac contractility and decreases heart rate; mechanism is via inactivation of cardiac muscle sodium–potassium ATPase; beneficial effects for heart failure may occur via neuroendocrine effects (alters sensitivity of baroreceptors)	Digitalis glycosides have narrow therapeutic index; may cause variety of arrhythmias in patients (e.g., heart block, ventricular tachycardia); causes vomiting, anorexia, diarrhea; adverse effects potentiated by hypokalemia, reduced by hyperkalemia	0.02–0.03 mg/kg q8h PO
Digoxin 0.0625-, 0.125-, 0.25-mg tablets; 0.05- and 0.5-mg/mL elixir	Cardiac inotropic agent; increases cardiac contractility and decreases heart rate; mechanism is via inactivation of cardiac muscle sodium–potassium ATPase; beneficial effects for heart failure may occur via neuroendocrine effects (alters sensitivity of baroreceptors); used in heart failure for inotropic effect and to decrease heart rate; used in supraventricular arrhythmias to decrease ventricular response to atrial stimulation	Digitalis glycosides have narrow therapeutic index; may cause variety of arrhythmias in patients (e.g., heart block, ventricular tachycardia); causes vomiting, anorexia, diarrhea; adverse effects potentiated by hypokalemia, reduced by hyperkalemia; some breeds of dogs (Dobermans) and cats more sensitive to adverse effects; calculate dose on basis of lean body weight	Dog: <20 kg body weight: 0.01 mg/kg q12h; >20 kg use 0.22 mg/m^2 q12h PO (subtract 10% for elixir) Dog (rapid digitalization): 0.0055–0.011 mg/kg q1h IV to effect Cat: 0.08–0.01 mg/kg q48h PO (approximately ¼ of a 0.125 mg tablet/cat)
Dihydrotachysterol 0.125-mg tablet; 0.5 mg/mL oral liquid	Vitamin D analogue; used as treatment of hypocalcemia, especially hypopara-thyroidism associated with thyroidectomy; vitamin D promotes absorption and use of calcium	Overdose may cause hypercalcemia; avoid use in pregnant animals because it may cause fetal abnormalities; use cautiously with high doses of calcium-containing preparations	0.02 mg/kg/day PO; for acute treatment, administer 0.02 mg/kg initially, then 0.01–0.02 mg/kg q24–48h PO, thereafter
Diltiazem (Cardizem, Dilacor) 30-, 60-, 90-, 120-mg tablets; 60-, 90-, 120-, 180-, 240-, 300-mg ER tablets; 5-mg/mL injection	Calcium-channel blocking drug; produces vasodilation, negative chronotropic effects; used for supraventricular arrhythmias in dogs; hypertrophic cardiomyopathy in cats	Hypotension, cardiac depression, bradycardia, AV block; may cause anorexia in some patients	Dog: 0.5–1.5 mg/kg q8h PO, 0.25 mg/kg over 2 min IV (repeat if necessary) Cat: 1.75–2.4 mg/kg q8h PO; for Dilacor XR or Cardizem, CD dose is 10 mg/kg, once daily, PO; Dilacor capsules contain 60-mg tablets for dosing cats
Dimenhydrinate (Dramamine) 50-mg tablets; 50-mg/mL injection	Antihistamine drug; converted to active diphenhydramine; used for motion sickness, vomiting		Dog: 4–8 mg/kg q8h PO, IM, IV Cat: 12.5 mg/cat q8h IV, IM, PO
Dimercaprol (BAL) (BAL in oil)	Chelating agent; used to treat lead, gold, arsenic toxicity	High doses have caused seizures, drowsiness, and vomiting; painful injection	4 mg/kg q4h IM
Dioctyl sodium sulfosuccinate	See Docusate sodium		
Diphenhydramine (Benadryl) 25-, 50-mg tablets; 2.5-mg/mL elixir; 50-mg/mL injection	Antihistamine; used for allergic disease	Sedation	2–4 mg/kg q6–8h, PO, or 1 mg/kg IM, IV (For dogs administer 25–50 mg/dog q8h IV IM PO)

Drug (Other Names)	Pharmacology and Indications	Adverse Effects and Precautions	Dosage
Diphenoxylate (Lomotil) 2.5-mg tablets	Opiate agonist; stimulates smooth muscle segmentation in intestine, as well as electrolyte absorption; used for acute treatment of nonspecific diarrhea	Excessive use can cause constipation	Dog: 0.1–0.2 mg/kg q8–12h PO Cat: 0.05–0.1 mg/kg q12h PO
Dipyridamole (Persantine) 25-, 50-, 75-mg tablets; 5-mg/mL injection	Platelet inhibitor; mechanism of action is attributed to increased levels of cAMP in platelet, which decreases platelet activation; indicated primarily to prevent thromboembolism	Adverse effects have not been reported in animals	4–10 mg/kg q24h PO
Dipyrone	No longer available commercially (previous use in animals was at 28 mg/kg q8h IV, IM, SC)		
Disopyramide (Norpace) 100-, 150-mg capsules	Antiarrhythmic agent of class 1; depresses myocardial electrophysiologic conduction rate	Not commonly used in veterinary medicine; other antiarrhythmic drugs are preferred	6–15 mg/kg q8h PO
Dobutamine (Dobutrex) 12.5 mg/mL	β-Agonist; increases heart contraction without increase in heart rate; primarily used for acute treatment of heart failure.	May cause tachycardia and ventricular arrhythmias at high doses, or in sensitive individuals; may cause seizures in cats	Dog: 5–20 μg/kg/min IV infusion Cat: 0.5–2 μg/kg/min IV infusion
Docusate calcium 60-mg tablets	Stool softener (surfactant); acts to decrease surface tension to allow more water to accumulate in the stool		Dog: 50–100 mg per dog q12–24h PO Cat: 50 mg per cat q12–24h PO
Docusate sodium 50-, 100-mg capsules; 10-mg/mL liquid	Stool softener		Dog: 50–200 mg per dog q8–12h PO Cat: 50 mg per cat q12–24h PO
Dopamine (Intropin) 40-, 80-, or 160-mg/mL	Adrenergic agonist; action is primarily to stimulate myocardium via action on cardiac β_1-receptors; there is some suggestion that lower doses of dopamine increase renal perfusion via action on renal dopaminergic receptors, however, clinical evidence for beneficial effect is lacking	May cause tachycardia and ventricular arrhythmias at high doses, or in sensitive individuals	Dog, cat: 2–10 μg/kg/min IV infusion
Doxapram (Dopram) 20-mg/mL injection	Respiratory stimulant via action on carotid chemo-receptors and subsequent stimulation of respiratory center; used to treat respiratory depression, or to stimulate respiration postanesthesia; may also increase cardiac output	No longer available from manufacturer	5–10 mg/kg IV neonate: 1–5 mg SC, sublingual, or via umbilical vein

Drug (Other Names)	Pharmacology and Indications	Adverse Effects and Precautions	Dosage
Doxorubicin (Adriamycin) 2-mg/mL injection	Anticancer agent	Most common acute effect is anorexia, vomiting, and diarrhea; dose-related toxicity also includes bone marrow suppression, hair loss (in certain breeds), and cardio-toxicity; cardiotoxicity limits the total dose administered (usually do not exceed 200 mg/m^2)	30 mg/m^2, IV q21 days. Cats, dogs <20 kg—regimen may vary with tumor type and specific protocols
Doxycycline 100-mg tablet; 10-mg/mL oral liquid; 100-mg injection vial	Tetracycline antibiotic; usually bacteriostatic; broad-spectrum activity including bacteria, some protozoa, *Rickettsia, Ehrlichia*. Drug of choice for most tick-borne infections in dogs	*Drug interactions:* Tetracyclines bind to calcium-containing compounds, which decreases oral absorption	3–5 mg/kg q12h PO IV, or 10 mg/kg q24h PO; for *Rickettsia* in dogs: 5 mg/kg q12h
Edetate calcium 20 mg/mL injection	Chelating agent. Indicated for treatment of acute and chronic lead poisoning. Sometimes used in combination with dimercaprol.	Potential nephrotoxin. Painful injection. Must remove lead from GI tract before chelation therapy.	25 mg/kg q6h SC, IM, IV for 2–5 days.
Edrophonium 10-mg/mo injection	Cholinesterase inhibitor; very short acting and ordinarily only used for diagnostic purposes (e.g., for myasthenia gravis); also has been used to reverse neuromuscular blockade of nondepolarizing agents (pancuronium)	Short acting; side effects are minimal; excessive muscarinic–cholinergic effects may occur with high doses (counteract with atropine)	Dog: 0.11–0.22 mg/kg IV Cat: 2.5 mg/cat IV
Enalapril 2.5-, 5-, 10-, 20-mg tablet	ACE inhibitor; used for vasodilation and treatment of heart failure	May cause azotemia in some patients; carefully monitor patients receiving high doses of diuretics; monitor electrolytes and renal function 3–7 days after initiating therapy and periodically thereafter	Dog: 0.5 mg/kg q12–24h PO Cat: 0.25–0.5 mg/kg q12–24h PO
Enrofloxacin 5.7-, 22.7-, and 68-mg tablets; 22.7-mg/mL injection	Fluoroquinolone antibacterial drug; bactericidal; broad-spectrum activity	Adverse effects include seizures in epileptic animals, arthropathy in dogs 4–28 weeks of age, vomiting in dogs and cats at high doses; not approved for IV use, but safe if diluted with saline and given slowly	5–20 mg/kg/day (see dosing information guidelines)
Ephedrine 25-, 50-mg capsules; 25-, 50-mg/mL injection	Adrenergic agonist; used as vasopressor, (e.g., administered during anesthesia); also has been used to treat urinary incontinence because of action on bladder sphincter muscle	Adverse effects related to excessive adrenergic activity (e.g., peripheral vasocon-, striction and tachycardia)	Urinary incontinence: 4 mg/kg, or 12.5–50 mg/dog q8–12h PO (2–4 mg/kg for cats) Vasopressor: 0.75 mg/kg, IM, SC, repeat as needed

Drug (Other Names)	Pharmacology and Indications	Adverse Effects and Precautions	Dosage
Epinephrine 1-mg/mL (1:1000) injection	Adrenergic agonist; nonselectively stimulates α- and β$_2$-adrenergic receptors; used primarily for emergency situations to treat cardiopulmonary arrest and anaphylactic shock	Overdose causes excessive vaso-constriction and hypertension; high doses can cause ventricular arrhythmias; when high doses are used for cardiopulmonary arrest, an electrical defibrillator should be available	Cardiac arrest: 10–20 μg/kg, IV (low dose); 100–200 μg/kg IV (high dose); or 200 μg/kg endotracheal (may be diluted in saline before administration) Anaphylactic shock: 2.5–5 μg/kg IV; or 50 μg/kg endo-tracheal (may be diluted in saline)
Ergocalciferol (vitamin D2) 1.25-mg tablet; 12.5- mg/mL injection	Vitamin D analogue; used for treatment of hypocalcemia	Overdose may cause hyper-calcemia; avoid use in pregnant animals because it may cause fetal abnormalities; use cautiously with high doses of calcium-containing preparations	500–2000 U/kg/day PO
Erythromycin 250-mg tablet	Macrolide antibiotic; spec-trum of activity limited primarily to gram-positive aerobic bacteria; used for skin and respiratory infections	May cause nausea, vomiting, diarrhea	10–20 mg/kg q8–12h PO Prokinetic effects at 0.5–1.0 mg/kg
Erythropoietin 2000-units/mL injection	Hematopoietic growth factor that stimulates erythropoiesis; used to treat nonregenerative anemia	Anemia may occur because of crossreacting antibodies against animal erythropoietin (reversible when drug is withdrawn)	Doses range from 35 or 50 U/kg three times/week to 400 U/kg/week SC (adjust dose to hematocrit of 0.30–0.34)
Esmolol (Brevibloc) 10-mg/mL injection	β-Blocker; selective for β1–receptor; short duration of action; indicated for short–term control of heart rate and supraventricular tachyarrhythmias	Same as other precautions for β–blockers (see Propranolol)	500 μg/kg, IV, which may be given as 0.05–0.01 mg/kg slowly every 5 min or 50–200 μg/kg/min infusion
Estradiol cypionate 2-mg/mL injection	Semisynthetic estrogen compound; used primarily to induce abortion in animals	High risk of endometrial hyperplasia and pyometra; high doses can produce leukopenia, thrombocytopenia, and fatal aplastic anemia	Dog: 22–44 μg/kg IM (total dose not to exceed 1.0 mg) Cat: 250 μg/cat IM between 40 hours and 5 days of mating
Ethanol 20%	Ethylene glycol toxicity	Sedation	Dilute to 7%, administer: 0.6 g/kg IV then 100 mg/kg/hr CRI
Etidronate disodium (Didronel) 200-, 400-mg tablets; 50-mg/mL injection	Bisphosphonate drug; used to treat osteoporosis and hypercalcemia; decreases bone turnover, inhibits osteoclast activity, retards bone resorption and decreases rate of osteoporosis	Adverse effects not reported for animals; in people, GI problems are common	
Etodolac 150–300-mg tablets	NSAID; inhibits inflammatory prostaglandins	NSAIDs may cause GI ulceration; other adverse effects caused by NSAIDs include decreased platelet function and renal injury; at high doses, etodolac caused GI ulcera-tion in dogs	Dogs: 10–15 mg/kg, once daily, PO Cats: Dose not established

Drug (Other Names)	Pharmacology and Indications	Adverse Effects and Precautions	Dosage
Famotidine (Pepcid) 10-mg tablet; 10- mg/mL injection	H-2 receptor antagonist		0.5 mg/kg q12–24h IM, SC, PO
Felbamate (Felbatol) 120-mg/mL oral liquid; 400-, 600-mg tablets	Anticonvulsant; usually used when dogs are refractory to other anticonvulsants	Not documented with use in dogs; in people, the most severe reactions have been hepatotoxicity and aplastic anemia; it may increase phenobarbital concentrations	Dog: 20 mg/kg q8h PO, max = 3000 mg/day
Fenbendazole Granules, 22.2%; 100-mg/mL oral liquid	Whipworms, *Giardia*, lungworms	Good safety margin, but vomiting and diarrhea have been reported; no known contraindications	50 mg/kg/day × 3 days, PO
Fentanyl 250-mg/5 mL injection	Synthetic opiate for analgesia	Adverse effects similar to those of morphine	Dog: 3 μg/kg IV, then CRI of 3–6 μg/kg/h Cat: 3 μg/kg IV then CRI of 1–5 μg/kg/h
Fentanyl transdermal 25-, 50-, 75-, and 100-μg/h patch	One 100 μg/h patch is equivalent to 10 mg/kg of morphine every 4 hours IM	If adverse effects are observed (e.g., respiratory depression, excess sedation, excitement in cats), remove patch and, if necessary, administer naloxone	Cats: 25 μg patch every 118 hours Dog: 10–20 kg, 50 μg/h patch every 72 hours
Ferrous sulfate	Iron supplement	High doses cause stomach ulceration	Dog: 100–300 mg/dog q24h PO Cat: 50–100 mg/cat q24h PO
Finasteride (Proscar) 5-mg tablet	Used for benign prostatic hypertrophy		0.1 mg/kg PO q24h (or 5-mg tablet q24h in 10–50 kg dogs)
Florfenicol (Nuflor) 300-mg/mL injection	Chloramphenicol derivative with same mechanism of action as chloramphenicol and broad antibacterial spectrum; it has been used in situations in which chloramphenicol is not available; only approved for use in cattle	Use in dogs and cats has been limited, therefore adverse effects have not been reported; chloramphenicol has been linked to dose-dependent bone marrow depression, and similar reactions may be possible with florfenicol; however, there does not appear to be a risk of aplastic anemia, as for chloramphenicol	Dog: 20 mg/kg q6h, PO, IM, q6h Cat: 22 mg/kg q8h IM, PO
Fluconazole (Diflucan) 50-, 100-, 150-, or 200-mg tablets; 10- or 40-mg/mL IV injection	Azole antifungal drug; efficacious against dermatophytes, and variety of systemic fungi	Adverse effects have not been reported from fluconazole administration; has less effect on endocrine function than ketoconazole; however, increased liver enzyme plasma concentrations and hepatopathy are possible; absorbed more predictably and completely than other oral azole antifungals, even on an empty stomach	Dogs: 10–20 mg/kg/day, PO Cats: 50 mg/cat q12h PO, or 50 mg/cat per day PO
Flucytosine (Ancobon) 250-mg capsule; 75-mg/mL oral suspension	Antifungal drug used primarily for cryptococcosis		25–50 mg/kg q6–8h PO (up to a maximum dose of 100 mg/kg q12h PO)

Drug (Other Names)	Pharmacology and Indications	Adverse Effects and Precautions	Dosage
Fludrocortisone (Florinef) 0.1-mg tablets	Mineralocorticoid; used as replacement therapy in animals with adrenal atrophy/ adrenocortical insufficiency	Adverse effects are primarily related to glucocorticoid effects; monitor electrolyte concentrations	Dog: 0.2–0.8 mg per dog or 0.02 mg/kg q24h PO (13–23 µg/kg) Cat: 0.1–0.2 mg per cat q24h PO
Flumazenil 0.1-mg/mL injection	Reversal agent after benzo- diazepine administration	No adverse effects reported in animals	0.2 mg (total dose) as needed IV
Flunixin meglumine (Banamine) 10-, 50-mg/mL injection	NSAID antiinflammatory drug; used primarily for short-term treatment of moderate pain and inflam- mation; not approved for small animals	Causes gastritis, GI ulceration with high doses or prolonged use; renal ischemia has also been documented; therapy in dogs should be limited to 4 consecutive days	1.1 mg/kg once IV, IM, SC, or 1.1 mg/kg/day 3 days/week PO Ophthalmic: 0.5 mg/kg once IV
5-Fluorouracil (Fluorouracil) 50-mg/mL vial	Anticancer agent	Causes mild leucopenia, thrombocytopenia. CNS toxicity; do not use in cats	Dog: 150 mg/m2 once/week IV Cat: do not use
Fluoxetine (Prozac) 10- and 20-mg capsules; 4 mg/mL oral liquid	Antidepressant drug; used to treat behavioral disorders such as obsessive-compulsive disorders and dominance aggression	Fewer adverse effects (especially antihistamine, antimuscarinic effects) than with other anti- depressant drugs; serious adverse effects have not been reported in animals, but decreased appetite may be common; in cats, nervousness or increased anxiousness have been observed	Dog: 0.5 mg/kg/day, initially PO, then increase to 1 mg/kg/day, PO (average dose is 10–20 mg/dog) Cat: 0.5–4 mg/cat q24h PO
Fomepizole	See 4-Methylpyrazole		
Furazolidone (Furoxone) 100-mg tablets	Oral antiprotozoal drug with activity against *Giardia*; may have some activity against bacteria in intestine; not used for systemic therapy	Adverse effects not reported in animals; in people, mild anemia, hypersensitivity, and disturbance of intestinal flora have been reported	4 mg/kg q12h for 7–10 days PO
Furosemide 12.5-, 20-, 50-mg tablets; 10-mg/mL oral liquid; 50-mg/mL injection	Loop diuretic; inhibits sodium and water transport in ascending loop of Henle, which produces diuresis; also may have vasodilating properties, increasing renal perfusion, and decreasing preload	Dehydration, azotemia, hypo- tension, hypokalemia	Dog: 2–6 mg/kg q8–12h (or as needed) IV, IM, SC, PO Cat: 1–4 mg/kg q8–24h IV, IM, SC, PO
Gamma globulin (human)	IMHA, ITP or other immune- mediated disease	Expensive	0.5–1.5 g/kg IV over 12 hours
Gentamicin (Gentocin) 50- and 100-mg/mL injection	Aminoglycoside antibiotic; broad-spectrum activity except streptococci and anaerobic bacteria	Nephrotoxicity is the most dose- limiting toxicity; ensure that patients have adequate fluid and electrolyte balance during therapy; ototoxicity, vestibulotoxicity also possible	Dog: 2–4 mg/kg q6–8h, or 6–10 mg/kg q24h IV, IM, SC Cat: 3 mg/kg q8h, or 9 mg/kg q24h IV, IM, SC
Glipizide (Glucotrol) 5- or 10-mg tablets	Sulfonylurea oral hypoglycemic agent; used as oral treatment in the management of diabetes mellitus, particularly in cats; this drug acts to increase secre- tion of insulin from pancreas	It may cause dose-related vomiting, anorexia, increased bilirubin, and elevated liver enzymes in some cats; causes hypoglycemia, but less so than insulin	2.5–7.5 mg/cat q12h, PO; usual dose is 2.5 mg/cat initially, then increase to 5 mg/cat, q12h

Drug (Other Names)	Pharmacology and Indications	Adverse Effects and Precautions	Dosage
Glucagon Glucagon hydro-chloride Eq. 1 mg base/vial, Glucagon recombinant 1 mg/vial	Secreted by pancreatic alpha cells; increases blood glucose concentration by inducing glycogenolysis and glyconeo-genesis; also exerts positive inotropic and chronotropic effect by increasing intra-cellular cAMP; causes ureteral relaxation; used to treat refractory hypoglycemia in patients with insulinoma or insulin overdose, to correct hypotension in β-blocker or calcium channel blocker over-dose, to increase cardiac output in refractory shock unresponsive to β-agonists, and to relieve ureteral spasm	Minimal experience in clinical practice in veterinary medicine	Dog: 0.3 mg/kg IV, IM, SC to correct hypoglycemia or 50 ng/kg once, then CRI of 10–40 ng/kg/min IV for refractory hypoglycemia; human dose for septic shock or β-blocker overdose is 70 µg/kg/min IV
Glycerin Oral solution	Used to treat acute glaucoma	No adverse effects reported	1–2 mL/kg, up to q8h PO
Glycopyrrolate 0.2-mg/mL injection	Anticholinergic drug; longer duration of action than atropine.	Adverse effects attributed to antimuscarinic (anticholinergic) effects (see Atropine)	0.005–0.001 mg/kg IV, IM, SC
Granulocyte colony-stimulating factor	Neutropenia, especially following chemotherapy		2.5–10 µg/kg/day SC × 3–5 days
Griseofulvin (microsize) (Fulvicin U/F) 125-, 250-, 500-mg tablets; 25-mg/mL oral liquid; 125-mg/mL oral syrup	Antifungal drug; activity limited to dermatophytes	Adverse effects in animals include teratogenicity in cats, anemia and leucopenia in cats, anorexia, depression, vomiting, and diarrhea; do not administer to pregnant cats	50 mg/kg q24h PO (up to a maximum dose of 110–132 mg/kg/day in divided treat-ments)
Heparin sodium 1000 and 10,000 U/mL	Anticoagulant; potentiates anticoagulant effects of anti-thrombin III; used primarily for prevention of thrombosis	Adverse effect caused by excessive inhibition of coagulation—bleeding	100–200 units/kg IV loading dose, then 100–300 units/kg q6–8h, SC Low-dose prophylaxis (dog and cat): 70 units/kg q8–12h SC Heparin CRI: 18 units/kg/h after IV loading dose
Hetastarch	Synthetic colloid used for shock, hypoproteinemia	Volume overload, increases serum amylase, possible coagulopathy	Dog: 10–20 mL/kg/day IV Cat: 10–15 mL/kg/day
Hycodan	See Hydrocodone bitartrate		
Hydralazine (Apresoline) 10-g tablets; 20-mg/mL injection	Vasodilator; antihypertensive; used to dilate arterioles and decrease afterload; primarily used for treatment of CHF and other cardiovascular disorders characterized by high peripheral vascular resistance	Hypotension, tachycardia	Dog: 0.5 mg/kg (initial dose), titrate to 0.5–2 mg/kg q12h PO Cat: 2.5 mg/cat q12–24h PO
Hydrocodone bitartrate 5-mg tablet; 1-mg/mL oral liquid	Antitussive		Dog: 0.22 mg/kg q4–8h PO Cats: no dose available Cats: no dose available

Drug (Other Names)	Pharmacology and Indications	Adverse Effects and Precautions	Dosage
Hydrochlorothiazide (Hydro–Diuril, generic) 25-, 50-, and 100-mg tablets; 10- or 100-mg/mL oral liquid	Thiazide diuretic; inhibits sodium reabsorption in distal renal tubules; used as diuretic and antihypertensive; used to treat calcium-containing uroliths	Do not use in patient with elevated calcium; may cause electrolyte imbalance such as hypokalemia	2–4 mg/kg q12h PO
Hydrocortisone 5-, 10-, 20-mg tablet	Glucocorticoid antiinflammatory drug; hydrocortisone has weaker antiinflammatory effects and greater mineralocorticoid effects than prednisolone or dexamethasone	Adverse effects are attributed to excessive glucocorticoid effects (see Betamethasone)	Replacement therapy: 1–2 mg/kg q12h PO Antiinflammatory: 2.55 mg/kg q12h PO
Hydrogen peroxide Hydrogen peroxide, 3%	Emetic agent; causes vomiting due to gastric irritation	May cause esophagitis; avoid inducing emesis if toxicant is caustic or if patient is depressed, seizuring, nonresponsive, or dehydrated	1–2 mL/kg PO (1 tsp/2–4.5 kg), repeat once if vomiting does not occur within 10 minutes
Hydromorphone	Preanesthetic, sedation, analgesia		Dog: 0.05–0.2 mg/kg IV Cat: 0.02–0.2 mg/kg IV
Hydroxyurea 500-mg capsules	Antineoplastic agent; used in combination with other anticancer modalities for treatment of certain tumors; has been used to treat polycythemia vera		Dog: 50 mg/kg PO once daily, 3 days/week Cat: 25 mg/kg PO once daily, 3 days/week
Hydroxyzine 10-, 25-, 50-mg tablet; 2-mg/mL liquid	Antihistamine, of the piperazine class; used primarily to treat pruritus in animals	Side effects of therapy are related primarily to antihistamine effects; sedation occurs in some animals	Dog: 1–2 mg/kg q6–8h PO Cat: safe dose not established
Imidocarb dipropionate	Antiprotozoal used to treat babesiosis	Painful injection; pretreatment with atropine 1.04 mg/kg SC 30 min prior to Rx may diminish cholinergic side effects	6.6 mg/kg IM, SC; repeat in 2 weeks
Imipenem 250- or 500-mg vials	β-Lactam antibiotic with broad-spectrum activity; action is similar to that of other β-lactams (see Amoxicillin); imipenem is the most active β-lactam; used primarily for serious, multiply-resistant infection	Allergic reactions may occur with β-lactam antibiotics; with rapid infusion, or in patients with renal insufficiency, neurotoxicity may occur (seizures); vomiting and nausea are possible	3–10 mg/kg, IV, IM q6–8h
Imipramine	Tricyclic antidepressant drug (TCA); used in people to treat anxiety and depression; used in animals to treat variety of behavioral disorders, including obsessive-compulsive disorders; action is via inhibition of uptake of serotonin at presynaptic nerve terminals	Multiple side effects are associated with TCAs such as antimuscarinic effects (dry mouth, rapid heart rate) and antihistamine effects (sedation); overdoses can produce life-threatening cardiotoxicity	2–4 mg/kg, q12–24h PO
Indomethacin (Indocin)	NSAID (see Flunixin meglumine)	Causes severe GI ulceration and hemorrhage in dogs do not use	Safe dose has not been established

Drug (Other Names)	Pharmacology and Indications	Adverse Effects and Precautions	Dosage
Insulin, regular crystalline 100 U/mL	Short-acting insulin used for acute management of sick diabetics; lasts 6–8 hours given SC; also used for acute hyperkalemia	Adverse effects primarily related to overdoses (hypoglycemia)	Hyperkalemia: 0.05–0.25 U/kg IV with 1–2 g glucose/unit Ketoacidosis: 0.1 U/kg/h IV CRI
Insulin, NPH isophane 100 U/mL	Intermediate insulin used to manage most chronic diabetics; last 12 hours in most	Same as above	Dog < 15 kg: 1 unit/kg q24h SC (to effect), dog > 25 kg: 0.5 units/kg q24h SC (to effect)
Insulin, ultralente 100 U/mL	Long-acting insulin; lasts 12–36 hours	Monitor glucose curve	Cat: 0.5 U/kg SC q24h
Interferon (interferon α, HuIFN–α) (Roferon) 3 million U/vial	Used to stimulate immune system in cats with FIV or FELV	Adverse effects have not been reported in animals	Cat: 15–30 U/cat PO once daily for 7 days and repeated every other week
Iodide	See Potassium iodide		
Ipecac s (Ipecac) 30-mL oral liquid	Emetic drug; for emergency treatment of poisoning	No adverse effects with acute therapy for poisoning; chronic administration can lead to myocardial toxicity	1–2 mL/kg with maximum = 15 mL/dog
Iron	See Iron sulfate		
Iron dextran	For iron deficiency anemia, especially when GI absorption is suspect		10–20 mg/kg IM
Isoproterenol (Isuprel) 0.2 mg/mL	Adrenergic agonist; stimulates both β_1- and β_2-adrenergic receptors; used to stimulate heart (inotropic and chronotropic); also used to relax bronchial smooth muscle for acute treatment of broncho-constriction	Adverse effects related to excessive adrenergic stimulation and seen primarily as tachycardia and tachyarrhythmia	0.01–0.2 μg/kg/min CRI
Isosorbide dinitrate 2.5-, 5-, 10-, 20-, 30-, 40-mg tablets	Nitrate vasodilator; causes vasodilation via generation of nitric oxide; relaxes vascular smooth muscle, especially venous; reduces preload in patients with CHF; in people, it is primarily used to treat angina	Adverse effects are primarily related to overdoses that produce excess vasodilation and hypo-tension; tolerance may develop with repeated doses	2.5–5 mg/animal q12h PO (or 0.22–1.1 mg/kg q12h PO)
Isosorbide mononitrate (Monoket) 10-, 20-mg tablets	Same comments as for isosorbide dinitrate, except that this is a biologically active form of isosorbide dinitrate; compared with isosorbide dinitrate, it does not undergo first-pass metabolism and is completely absorbed orally	Same as for isosorbide dinitrate and nitroglycerin	5 mg/dog, two doses per day, 7 hours apart PO

Drug (Other Names)	Pharmacology and Indications	Adverse Effects and Precautions	Dosage
Itraconazole (Sporanox) 100-mg capsule; 100-mg/mL oral liquid	Azole (triazole) antifungal drug; active against dermatophytes and systemic fungi, such as *Blastomyces*, *Histoplasma*, and *Coccidioides*	Vomiting and hepatotoxicosis are possible, especially at high doses; 10–15% of dogs develop high liver enzyme levels; high doses in cats caused vomiting and anorexia	Dog: 2.5 mg/kg q12h or 5 mg/kg q24h PO Cat: 5 mg/kg q12h PO For dermatophyte infection in cats: 1.5–3.0 mg/kg (up to 5 mg/kg) q24h, PO for 15 days
Ivermectin 10-mg/mL injection; 68-, 136-, 272-μg tablets; 10-mg/mL oral solution	Antiparasitic drug; neurotoxic to parasites by potentiating effects of inhibitory neurotransmitter GABA	Toxicity may occur at high doses, and in breeds in which ivermectin crosses blood–brain barrier; sensitive breeds include Collies, Australian Shepherds, Shelties, and Old English Sheepdogs; toxicity is neurotoxic and signs include depression, ataxia, difficulty with vision, coma, and death; ivermectin appears to be safe for pregnant animals; do not administer to animals under 6 weeks of age; animals with high microfilaremia may show adverse reactions to high doses	Heartworm preventative: 6 μg/kg q30days PO in dogs and 24 μg/kg q30days PO in cats Microfilaricide: 50 μg/kg PO 2 weeks after adulticide therapy Ectoparasite therapy (dogs and cats): 200–300 μg/kg IM, SC, PO Endoparasites (dogs and cats): 200–400 μg/kg weekly SC, PO
Kaopectate	Antidiarrheal compound; kaolin may act as absorbent for endotoxins and pectin may protect intestinal mucosa	Side effects are uncommon	1–2 mL/kg q2–6h PO
Ketamine 100 mg/mL	Anesthetic agent; appears to act as dissociative agent; rapidly metabolized and eliminated in most animals	Causes pain with IM injection; tremors, spasticity, and convulsive seizures have been reported; increases cardiac output more than other anesthetic agents; do not use in animals with head injury, because it may elevate CSF pressure	10 mg/kg IV following 0.5 mg/kg IV midazolam for induction or 5–10 min anesthesia, 11–33 mg/kg IM
Ketoconazole (Nizoral) 200-mg tablets; 100-mg/mL oral liquid	Azole (imidazole) antifungal drug; fungistatic; Efficacious against dermatophytes, and variety of systemic fungi, such as *Histoplasma*, *Blastomyces*, and *Coccidioides*	Adverse effects in animals include dose-related vomiting, diarrhea, and hepatic injury; enzyme elevations are common; do not administer to pregnant animals; ketoconazole causes endocrine abnormalities, most specifically, inhibition of cortisol synthesis. *Drug interactions:* Ketoconazole will inhibit metabolism of other drugs (anticonvulsants, cyclosporine, cisapride)	Dog: 10–15 mg/kg q8–12h PO For *Malassezia canis* infection: 5 mg/kg q24h PO For hyperadrenocorticism: 15 mg/kg q12h PO Cat: 5–10 mg/kg q8–12h PO
Ketoprofen 12.5-, 25-, 50-, 75-mg tablet; 10-mg/mL injection	NSAID (See Flunixin meglumine)	All NSAIDs share similar adverse effect of GI toxicity (See Flunixin); ketoprofen has been administered for 5 consecutive days in dogs, without serious adverse effects; most common side effect is vomiting; GI ulceration is possible in some animals	Dogs and cats: 1 mg/kg q24h PO for up to 5 days; initial dose can be given via injection at up to 2 mg/kg SC, IM, IV

Drug (Other Names)	Pharmacology and Indications	Adverse Effects and Precautions	Dosage
Ketorolac tromethamine (Toradol) 10-mg tablets; 15- and 30-mg/mL injection	NSAID; used for short-term relief of pain and inflammation; acts by inhibiting cyclooxygenase enzyme (COX); use of ketorolac has been evaluated clinically in dogs, but not cats	NSAIDs may cause GI ulceration; ketorolac may cause GI lesions if administered more frequently than every 8 hours. Do not administer more than 2 doses	Dogs: 0.5 mg/kg, q8–12h PO, IM, IV
L–Dopa	See Levodopa		
Lactated Ringer's solution 250-, 500-, 1000-mL bags	Crystalloid replacement fluid		Maintenance 40–50 mL/kg/day IV For shock therapy: dog: 90 mL/kg IV; cat: 60–70 mL/kg IV
Lactulose (Chronulac, generic) 10 g/15mL	Laxative; produces laxative effect by osmotic effect in colon; lactulose also has been used for treatment of hyper-ammonemia (hepatic encephalopathy)	Excessive use may cause fluid and electrolyte loss	Constipation: 1 mL/4.5 kg q8h (to effect) PO Hepatic encephalopathy Dog: 0.5 mL/kg q8h PO; cat: 2.5–5 mL/cat q8h PO
Leucovorin (Folinic acid) (Wellcovorin, and generic 5-, 10-, 15-, 25-mg tablets; 3- or 5-mg/mL injection	Leucovorin is a reduced form of folic acid, which is converted to active folic acid derivatives for purine and thymidine synthesis; it is used as antidote for folic acid antagonists; used to prevent folic acid deficiency with methotrexate or pyrimethamine		With methotrexate administration: 3 mg/m^2 IV IM PO As antidote for pyrimethamine toxicosis: 1 mg/kg q24h PO
Levamisole (Levasole, Tramisol, Ergamisol) 184-mg tablet; 50-mg tablet	Antiparasitic drug used for endoparasites in dogs and as microfilaricide; possible efficacy as an immunosuppressant	May produce cholinergic toxicity; may cause vomiting in some dogs	Dogs (hookworms): 5–8 mg/kg once PO (up to 10 mg/kg PO for 2 days) Microfilaricide: 10 mg/kg q24h PO for 6–10 days Immunostimulant: 0.5–2 mg/kg 3 times/week PO Cats: 4.4 mg/kg once PO; (for lungworms: 20–40 mg/kg q48 h for 5 treatments PO)
Levodopa (Larodopa, L-dopa)	Converted to dopamine after crossing blood–brain barrier; stimulates CNS dopamine receptors; in people, used for treating Parkinson's disease; in animals, has been used for treating hepatic encephalopathy	Adverse effects in animals have not been reported; in people, dizziness, mental changes, difficult urination, and hypotension are among the reported adverse effects	Hepatic encephalopathy: 6.8 mg/kg initially, then 1.4 mg/kg q6h
Levothyroxine sodium 0.1–0.8 tablets	Replacement therapy for treating patients with hypothyroidism		Dog: 22 μg/kg q12h PO (adjust dose via monitoring) Cat: 10–20 μg/kg/day PO (adjust dose via monitoring)

Drug (Other Names)	Pharmacology and Indications	Adverse Effects and Precautions	Dosage
Lidocaine 20-mg/mL injection	Local anesthetic. (See Bupivacaine for mechanism of action); lidocaine is also used commonly for acute treatment of cardiac arrhythmias; class 1 antiarrhythmic; decreases phase 0 depolarization without affecting conduction; not useful for supraventricular arrhythmias	High doses cause CNS effects (tremors, twitches, and seizures); lidocaine can produce cardiac arrhythmias, but has greater effect on abnormal cardiac tissue than normal tissue; cats are more susceptible to adverse effects, and lower doses should be used	Dog (antiarrhythmic): 2–4 mg/kg IV (to a maximum dose of 8 mg/kg over 10-min period); 25–75 μ/kg/min IV infusion; 6 mg/kg q1.5h IM Cat (antiarrhythmic): 0.25–0.75 mg/kg IV slowly, or 10–40 μ/kg/min infusion. For epidural (dog and cat): 4.4 mg/kg of 2% solution
Lincomycin (Lincocin) 100-, 200-, 500-mg tablets	Antibiotic, similar in mechanism to clindamycin and erythromycin; spectrum includes primarily gram-positive bacteria; used for pyoderma and other soft tissue infections	Adverse effects uncommon; lincomycin has caused vomiting and diarrhea in animals; do *not* administer orally to rodents and rabbits	15–25 mg/kg q12h PO For pyoderma, doses as low as 10 mg/kg q12h have been used
Liothyronine (Cytomel)	Thyroid supplement; liothyronine is equivalent to T3	Adverse effects have not been reported (see Levothyroxine)	4.4 μg/kg q8h PO For T_3 suppression test in cats: collect presample for T4 and T_3, administer 25 μg/q8h for 7 doses, then collect post samples for T_3 and T_4, after last dose
Lisinopril 2.5-, 5-, 10-, 20-, 40-mg tablets	ACE inhibitor; used for treatment of CHF and hypertension	Hypotension, azotemia	Dogs: 0.5 mg/kg q24h PO Cats: no dose established
Lomotil	See Diphenoxylate		
Loperamide (Imodium and generic) 2-mg tablet; 0.2-mg/mL oral liquid	Opiate agonist; stimulates smooth muscle segmentation in intestine, as well as electrolyte absorption; used for acute treatment of nonspecific diarrhea	Diphenoxylate is poorly absorbed systemically and produces few systemic side effects; however, toxicity has been observed in dogs, even at recommended doses; small dogs and Collie-type dogs may be at higher risk; in any animal, excessive use can cause constipation	Dog: 0.1 mg/kg q8–12h PO Cat: 0.08–0.16 mg/kg q12h PO
Lufenuron	Antiparasitic; used to control fleas in animals; inhibits development of hatching fleas	Adverse effects have not been reported; appears to be relatively safe during pregnancy and in young animals	Dogs: 10 mg/kg PO, q31 days Cats: 30 mg/kg PO, q30 days Cat injection: 10 mg/kg SC every 6 months
Lufenuron + milbemycinoxime (Sentinel tablets and Flavor Tabs)	Combination of two antiparasitic drugs. See Lufenuron or Milbemycin; used to protect against fleas, heartworms, roundworms, hookworms, and whipworms	See Lufenuron or Milbemycin	Administer 1 tablet, q30days; tablets are formulated for size of dog
I–Lysine	Used to treat ocular herpesvirus in cats		Cat: 250–500 mg PO q12–24h

Drug (Other Names)	Pharmacology and Indications	Adverse Effects and Precautions	Dosage
Magnesium citrate	Saline cathartic; acts to draw water into small intestine via osmotic effect; fluid accumulation produces distention, which promotes bowel evacuation; used for constipation and bowel evacuation prior to certain procedures	Adverse effects have not been reported in animals; however, fluid and electrolyte loss can occur with overuse; magnesium accumulation may occur in patients with renal impairment; *Drug interactions:* Magnesium-containing cathartics decrease oral absorption of ciprofloxacin and other fluoroquinolones	2–4 mL/kg PO
Magnesium hydroxide	Oral antacid to neutralize stomach acid and saline cathartic	Same as magnesium citrate	Antacid: 5–10 mL/kg q4–8h PO Cathartic (dog): 15–50 mL/kg PO Cathartic (cat): 2–6 mL/cat q24h PO
Magnesium sulfate	Same as magnesium citrate	See Magnesium citrate	Dog: 8–25 g/dog q24h PO Cat: 2–5 g/cat q24h PO
Mannitol 5–25% solution for injection	Hyperosmotic diuretic; increases plasma osmolality, which draws fluid from tissues to plasma; anti-glaucoma agent; used for treatment of edema and reducing intraocular pressure; mannitol also has been used to promote urinary excretion of certain toxins	Causes fluid and electrolyte imbalance; do not use in dehydrated patients; use cautiously when intracranial bleeding is suspected, because it may increase bleeding; administration that is too rapid may expand the extracellular volume excessively	Diuretic: 1 g/kg of 5–25% solution IV to maintain urine flow Glaucoma or CNS edema: 0.25–2 gm/kg of 15–25% solution over 30–60 min IV (repeat in 6 hours, if necessary)
Marbofloxacin (Zeniquin) 25-, 50-, 100-, and 200-mg tablets	Fluoroquinolone antimicrobial; same mechanism as enrofloxacin and ciprofloxacin; spectrum includes staphylococci, gram-negative bacilli, and some pseudomonads	Same precautions as enrofloxacin; may cause some nausea and vomiting at high doses; avoid use in young animals	Dog: 2.75–5.55 mg/kg PO
MCT oil	Medium-chain triglycerides; animals with poor absorption of fat (lymphangiectasia, ERI, chylothorax)	Adverse effects not reported in veterinary medicine; may cause diarrhea in some patients	1–2 mL/kg daily in food
Mebendazole (Telmintic)	Benzimidazole antiparasitic drug (See Albendazole)	Adverse effects are rare; occasional vomiting and diarrhea in dogs; some reports suggest idiosyncratic hepatic reactions in dogs	22 mg/kg (with food) q24h for 3 days
Meclizine (Antivert, generic) 12.5-, 25-, and 50-mg tablets	Used to prevent vomiting from motion sickness or vestibular disease		Dog: 25 mg q24h PO (for motion sickness, administer 1 hour prior to traveling) Cat: 12.5 mg q24h PO
Meclofenamic acid (meclofenamate sodium) (Arquel, Meclofen) 50-, 100-mg capsules	NSAID; used for treatment of arthritis and other inflammatory disorders (See Flunixin)	Adverse effects have not been reported in animals, but adverse effects common to other NSAIDs are possible (See Flunixin)	Dog: 1 mg/kg/day for up to 5 days, PO

Drug (Other Names)	Pharmacology and Indications	Adverse Effects and Precautions	Dosage
Medetomidine (Domitor) 1-mg/mL injection	α_2-Agonist (see Xylazine); used primarily as sedative, anesthetic adjunct, and analgesia	α_2-Agonists decrease sympathetic output; cardiovascular depression may occur; medetomidine causes initial bradycardia and hypertension	$750\ \mu g/m^2$ IV or $1000\ \mu g/m^2$ IM
Meglumine antimonite	Leishmaniasis		
Melarsomine (Immiticide) 25-mg/mL injection	Organic arsenical compound used for heartworm therapy; heartworm adulticide; arsenicals after glucose uptake and metabolism in heartworms	Adverse effects: Pulmonary thromboembolism (7–20 days after therapy); anorexia (13% incidence), injection site reaction (myositis) (32% incidence); lethargy or depression (15% incidence); causes elevations of hepatic enzymes;. high doses ($3\times$) can cause pulmonary inflammation and death; if high doses are administered, dimercaprol (3 mg/kg IM) may be used as antidote	Administer via deep IM injection; class 1–2 dogs: 2.5 mg/kg/day for two consecutive days; class 3 dogs: 2.5 mg/kg once, then in 1 month two additional doses 24 hours apart
Melphalan (Alkeran) 2-mg tablets	Anticancer agent; used to treat multiple myeloma and certain carcinomas	Adverse effects related to its action as an anticancer agent; causes myelosuppression	1.5 mg/m2 (or 0.1–0.2 mg/kg) q24h PO for 7–10 days (repeat every 3 weeks
Meperidine (Demerol) 50- or 100-mg tablets; 10-mg/mL oral liquid; 25-, 50-, 75-, 100-mg/mL injection	Synthetic opioid agonist	Side effects similar to those of other opiates; see Morphine	Dog: 5–10 mg/kg IV, IM as often as q2–3h (or as needed) Cat: 3–5 mg/kg IV, IM q2–4h (or as needed)
Mepivacaine (Carbocaine-V) 20-mg/mL injection	Local anesthetic of the amide class (see Bupivacaine); medium potency and duration of action, compared with bupivacaine; longer-acting than lidocaine, but equal potency	See Bupivacaine; mepivacaine may cause less irritation to tissues than lidocaine	Variable dose for local infiltration; for epidural, 0.5 mL of 2% solution q30 sec until reflexes are absent; do not exceed 8 mg/kg total dose
6-Mercaptopurine (Purinethol) 50-mg tablets	Anticancer agent; antimetabolite that inhibits synthesis of purines in cancer cells	Bone marrow suppression and anemia	$50\ mg/m^2$ q24h PO
Meropenem (Merrem)	Carbapenem β-lactam antibiotic similar to imipenem in activity	Similar risks as with other β-lactam antibiotics; meropenem does not cause seizures as much as imipenem	20 mg/kg q8h IV; for meningitis 40 mg/kg q8h IV
Mesalamine (Asacol, Mesasal, Pentasa) 400-mg tablets; 250-mg capsules	5-Aminosalicylic acid; used as treatment for colitis; is not precisely known, but suppresses inflammation in colon; component of sulfasalazine	See Sulfasalazine; mesalamine alone has not been associated with side effects in animals	Veterinary dose has not been established; the usual human dose is 400–500 mg q6–18h (also see Sulfasalazine, Olsalazine)
Metamucil	Bulk-forming laxative containing psyllium (see Psyllium for details)		

Drug (Other Names)	Pharmacology and Indications	Adverse Effects and Precautions	Dosage
Metaproterenol (Alupent, Metaprel) 10-, 20-mg, tablets; 5-mg/mL oral liquid; inhalers	β-Adrenergic agonist; β_2 specific; used primarily for bronchodilation (see Albuterol for further details)	Adverse effects related to excessive β-adrenergic stimulation (see Albuterol)	0.325–0.65 mg/kg q4–6h PO
Methazolamide 25-, 50-mg tablets	Carbonic anhydrase inhibitor; used to treat glaucoma	Use cautiously in patients sensitive to sulfonamides (see Acetazolamide, Dichlorphenamide)	2–4 mg/kg (to a maximum dose of 4–6 mg/kg) q8–12h PO
Methimazole (Tapazole) 5- and 10-mg tablets	Antithyroid drug; used for treating hyperthyroidism, primarily in cats	In cats, lupuslike reactions are possible, such as vasculitis and bone marrow changes; well tolerated by dogs	Cat: 2.5 mg/cat q12h PO × 7–14 days, then 5–10 mg/cat PO q12h, and monitor T_4 concentrations
Methocarbamol (Robaxin-V) 500-, 750-mg tablets; 100-mg/mL injection	Skeletal muscle relaxant; depresses polysynaptic reflexes; used for treatment of skeletal muscle spasms	Causes some depression and sedation of the CNS	Dog: 15–20 mg/kg PO q8h; 50–150 mg/kg IV
Methohexital (Brevital) 0.5-, 2.5-mL; 5-g vials	Barbiturate anesthetic (see Thiopental for details); methohexital is about 2–3 times more potent than pentothal, but with shorter duration	See Thiopental	3–6 mg/kg IV (give slowly to effect)
Methotrexate (MTX, Mexate, Folex, Rheumatrex, and generic) 2.5-mg tablets; 25- mg/mL injection	Anticancer agent; used for various carcinomas, leukemia, and lymphomas	Anticancer drugs cause predictable (and sometimes unavoidable) side effects that include bone marrow suppression, leukopenia, and immunosuppression; hepatotoxicity has been reported in people from methotrexate therapy. *Drug interactions:* Concurrent use with NSAIDs may cause severe methotrexate toxicity; do not administer with pyrimethamine, trimethoprim, or sulfonamides	2.5–5 mg/m² q48h PO (dose depends on specific protocol) Dogs: 0.3–0.5 mg/kg once/week IV Cats: 0.8 mg/kg IV every 2–3 weeks
Methoxamine (Vasoxyl) 20 mg/mL	Adrenergic agonist; sympathomimetic; α-adrenergic agonist; Specific for α_1-receptors; vasopressor agent for hypotension	Adverse effects related to excessive stimulation of α_1–receptor (prolonged peripheral vasoconstriction); reflex bradycardia may occur	200–250 μg/kg IM, or 40–80 μg/kg IV
Methylene blue 0.1% (generic, also called New Methylene Blue) 10-mg/mL solution	Antidote for intoxication; used to treat for methemoglobinemia; methylene blue acts as reducing agent to reduce methemoglobin to hemoglobin	Methylene blue can cause Heinz body anemia in cats, but is safe when used at therapeutic doses listed here	1.5 mg/kg IV, slowly
Methylprednisolone (Medrol) 1.2-, 4-, 8-, 18-, 32-mg tablets	Glucocorticoid antiinflammatory drug (see Betamethasone); (see also Prednisolone); methylprednisolone is 1.25× more potent than prednisolone	Same as for other glucocorticoids (see Betamethasone); manufacturer suggests that methylprednisolone causes less PU/PD than prednisolone	0.22–0.44 mg/kg, q12–24h, PO; methylprednisolone is 1.25× more potent than prednisolone

Drug (Other Names)	Pharmacology and Indications	Adverse Effects and Precautions	Dosage
Methylprednisolone acetate (Depo-Medrol) 20- or 40-mg/mL injection	Depot form of methylprednisolone; slowly absorbed from IM injection site, producing glucocorticoid effects for 3–4 weeks in some animals; used for intralesional therapy, intraarticular therapy, and inflammatory conditions	Many adverse effects possible from use of corticosteroids (see Betamethasone)	Cat: 10–20 mg/cat IM q1–3h weeks
Methylprednisolone sodium succinate (Solu-Medrol) 1-g, 2-g, 125-mg; 500-mg vials	Same as methylprednisolone, except that this is a water-soluble formulation intended for acute therapy when high IV doses are needed for rapid effect; used for treatment of shock and CNS trauma	Adverse effects are not expected from single administration; however, with repeated use, other side effects are possible (see Betamethasone)	For emergency use: 30 mg/kg IV and repeat at 15 mg/kg in 2–6 hours, IV
4-Methylpyrazole (Fomepizole) (Antizol-Vet [Fomepizole]) 5% solution in 1.5-mL vial	Antidote for ethylene glycol (antifreeze) intoxication; inhibits dehydrogenase enzyme that converts ethylene glycol to toxic metabolite; should be used early for maximum success (within 8 hours)	Methylpyrazole was safe and effective in dogs in clinical trials, but not cats	20 mg/kg initially, IV, then 15 mg/kg at 12- and 24-hour intervals, then 5 mg at 36 hours
Methyltestosterone (Android, generic) 10-, 25-mg tablets	Anabolic androgenic agent; used for anabolic actions or testosterone hormone replacement therapy (androgenic deficiency); testosterone has been used to stimulate erythropoiesis	Adverse effects caused by excessive androgenic action of testosterone; prostatic hyperplasia is possible in male dogs; masculinization can occur in female dogs; hepatopathy is more common with oral methylated testosterone formulations	Dog: 5–25 mg/dog q24–48h PO Cat: 2.5–5 mg/cat q24–48h PO
Metoclopramide (Reglan, Maxolon) 5- or 10-mg tablet; 1-mg/mL oral liquid; 5-mg/mL injection	Prokinetic drug; antiemetic; stimulates motility of upper GI tract and centrally acting antiemetic; action is to inhibit dopamine receptors and enhance action of acetylcholine in GI tract; used primarily for gastroparesis and treatment of vomiting	Adverse effects are primarily related to blockade of central dopaminergic receptors; adverse effects similar to those reported for phenothiazines (e.g., acepromazine) have been reported, in addition to behavioral changes; do not use in epileptic patients or with diseases caused by GI obstruction	0.2–0.5 mg/kg q6–8h IV, IM, PO (or 1–2 mg/kg/day via continuous IV infusion, or approximately 0.1–0.2 mg/kg/h)
Metoprolol tartrate (Lopressor) 50-, 100-mg tablets; 1-mg/mL injection	Adrenergic blocking agent; β_1-adrenergic blocker. Similar properties to propranolol, except that metoprolol is specific for β_1 receptor; used to control tachyarrhythmia and slow heart rate	Adverse effects are primarily caused by excessive cardiovascular depression (decreased inotropic effects); may cause heart block; use cautiously in animals prone to bronchoconstriction	Dog: 5–50 mg/dog (0.5–1.0 mg/kg) q8h PO Cat: 2–15 mg/cat q8h PO

Drug (Other Names)	Pharmacology and Indications	Adverse Effects and Precautions	Dosage
Metronidazole (Flagyl, and generic) 250-, 500-mg tablet; 50-mg/mL oral liquid; 5-mg/mL injection	Antibacterial and antiprotozoal drug; disrupts DNA in organism via reaction with intracellular metabolite; action is specific for anaerobic bacteria; resistance is rare; active against some protozoa, including *Giardia*	Most severe adverse effect is caused by toxicity to CNS; high doses have caused lethargy, CNS depression, ataxia, vomiting, and weakness; metronidazole may be mutagenic; fetal abnormalities have not been demonstrated in animals with recommended doses, but use cautiously during pregnancy; cats may find broken tablets unpalatable	For anaerobes: dogs: 15 mg/kg q12h or 12 mg/kg q8h, PO; cats: 10–25 mg/kg q24h, PO For *Giardia*: dogs: 12–15 mg/kg q12h for 8 days, PO; cats: 17 mg/kg (1/3 tablet/cat) q24h for 8 days
Mexiletine (Mexitil) 150-, 200-, 250- capsules	Antiarrhythmic drug; used for ventricular arrhythmias; mechanism of action is to block fast sodium channel; class IB antiarrhythmic agent	May produce arrhythmias; use cautiously in animals with liver disease	Dog: 5–8 mg/kg q8–12h PO (use cautiously)
Midazolam (Versed) 5-mg/mL injection	Benzodiazepine; action is similar to other benzodi-azepines(see Diazepam); used as anesthetic adjunct	Use very cautiously IV, especially with opiates; IV midazolam has caused serious cardiorespiratory depression	0.1–0.25 mg/kg IV IM (or 0.1–0.3 mg/kg/h IV infusion)
Milbemycin oxime (Interceptor, Interceptor Flavor Tabs, and Safe Heart)	Antiparasitic drug; action is similar to that of ivermectin; acts as GABA agonist in nervous system of parasite; used as heartworm preven-tative, miticide, and microfilaricide; used to control infections of hook-worm, roundworms, and whipworms; at high doses, it has been used to treat *Demodex* infections in dogs	In susceptible dogs (Collie breeds), milbemycin may cross the blood–brain barrier and produce CNS toxicosis (depression, lethargy, coma); at doses used for heartworm prevention, this effect is less likely	Dogs: microfilaricide: 0.5 mg/kg; *Demodex*: 2 mg/kg q24h, PO for 60–120 days; heartworm prevention and control of endoparasites: 0.5 mg/kg q30 days PO Cat: for heartworm and endoparasite control, 2.0 mg/kg q30 days PO
Mineral oil (generic)	Lubricant laxative; increases water content of stool; used to increase passage of feces for treatment of impaction and constipation	Inhalation can cause severe granulomatous pulmonary disease	Dog: 20–50 mL/dog q12h PO Cat: 10–25 mL/cat q12h PO
Minocycline (Minocin) 50-, 100-mg tablets; 10-mg/mL oral liquid	Tetracycline antibiotic; similar to doxycycline in pharmacokinetics		5–12.5 mg/kg q12h PO
Misoprostol (Cytotec) 0.1- and 0.2-mg tablets	Prostaglandin E_2 analogue; prostaglandins provide a cytoprotective role in the GI mucosa; misoprostol is used to prevent gastritis and ulcers associated with NSAID (aspirin-drugs) therapy	Adverse effects are caused by effects of prostaglandins; most common side effect is GI discomfort, vomiting and diarrhea, do *not* administer to pregnant animals; may cause abortion	Dog: 2–5 µg/kg q6–8h PO Cat: dose not established
Mitotane (o,p´-DDD) (Lysodren, op-DDD) 500-mg tablet	Adrenocortical cytotoxic agent; causes suppression of adrenal cortex; used to treat adrenal tumors and pituitary-dependent hyperadreno-corticism (PDH)	Adverse effects, especially during induction period, include lethargy, anorexia, ataxia, depression, vomiting; corticosteroid supple-mentation (e.g., hydrocortisone or prednisolone) may be admin-istered to minimize side effects	Dogs: For PDH: 50 mg/kg/day (in divided doses) PO for 5–10 days, then 50–70 mg/kg/week PO; for adrenal tumor: 50–75 mg/kg/day for 10 days, then 75–100 mg/kg/week PO

Drug (Other Names)	Pharmacology and Indications	Adverse Effects and Precautions	Dosage
Mitoxantrone (Novantrone) 2-mg/mL injection	Anticancer antibiotic; similar to doxorubicin in action (see Doxorubicin); used for leukemia, lymphoma, and carcinomas	As with all anticancer agents, certain adverse effects are predictable and unavoidable and related to drug's action; mitoxantrone produces myelo-suppression, vomiting, anorexia, and GI upset, but may be less cardiotoxic than doxorubicin	Dogs: 6 mg/m^2 IV, every 21 days Cats: 6.5 mg/m^2 IV every 21 days
Morphine (generic) 1- and 15-mg/mL injection	Opioid agonist, analgesic; prototype for other opioid agonists	Side effects from morphine administration include sedation, constipation, and bradycardia; respiratory depression occurs with high doses; cats are more sensitive to excitement than other species	Dog: 0.1–1 mg/kg IV, IM, SC (dose is escalated as needed for pain relief) q4–6h Epidural: 0.1 mg/kg; Cat: 0.1 mg/kg IM, SC, q3–6h (or as needed)
Naloxone (Narcan) 20- or 400-µg/mL injection	Opiate antagonist; naloxone may be used to reverse sedation, anesthesia, and adverse effects caused from opiates	Adverse effects are not reported; tachycardia and hypertension have been reported in people	0.01–0.04 mg/kg IV, IM, SC, as needed, to reverse opiate
Neomycin (Biosol) 200-mg/mL oral liquid	Aminoglycoside antibiotic; only administered topically or orally; systemic absorption is minimal from oral absorption; used for treatment of hepatic encephalopathy		10–20 mg/kg q6–12h PO
Neostigmine bromide, and Neostigmine methylsulfate (Prostigmin; Stiglyn) 15-mg tablets; 0.25- or 0.5-mg/mL injection	Anticholinesterase drug; used primarily for treatment of myasthenia gravis or as an antidote for neuromuscular blockade caused by nondepo-larizing neuromuscular blocking drugs	Adverse effects are related to drug's pharmacological effects: excessive cholinergic stimulation (muscarinic effects), which include diarrhea, salivation, respiratory problems, vomiting, CNS effects, muscle twitching, or weakness; atropine is used to treat overdose	2 mg/kg/day PO (in divided doses, to effect) Injection: antimyasthenic: 10 µg/kg IM, SC, as needed; antidote for neuromuscular block: 40 µg/kg IM, SC; diagnostic aid for myasthenia gravis: 40 µg/kg IM or 20 µg/kg IV
Nifedipine (Adalat, Procardia) 10-, 20-mg capsules	Calcium-channel blocking drug; more specific for vascular smooth muscle than cardiac tissue; used for smooth muscle relaxation, vasodilation	Adverse effects have not been reported in veterinary medicine; most common side effect is hypotension	Animal dose is not established; in people, the dose is 10 mg three times a day, increased in 10-mg increments to effect
Nitrofurantoin (Macrodantin, Furalan, Furatoin, Furadantin, or generic) 25-, 50-, 100-mg capsules or tablets; 5-mg/mL oral liquid	Antibacterial drug; urinary antiseptic; therapeutic concentrations are reached only in the urine; not to be used for systemic infections	Adverse effects include nausea, vomiting, and diarrhea; turns urine color rust–yellow brown; do not administer during pregnancy	10 mg/kg/day divided into four daily treatments, then, 1 mg/kg at night PO
Nitroglycerin ointment (Nitrol, Nitrobid, Nitrostat) 2% ointment, transdermal patch (0.2 mg/h)	Nitrate; nitrovasodilator; relaxes vascular smooth muscle (especially venous) via gener-ation of nitric oxide; used primarily in heart failure to reduce preload, or decrease pulmonary hypertension; in people, used to treat angina pectoris	Adverse effects from nitrates are related to their pharmacologic action; most significant adverse effect is hypotension; methemoglo-binemia can occur with accumulation of nitrates, but rare; tolerance develops with repeated use	Dog: 4–12 mg (up to 15 mg) topically q12h Cat: 2–4 mg topically q12h (or ¼ inch of ointment per cat)

Drug (Other Names)	Pharmacology and Indications	Adverse Effects and Precautions	Dosage
Nitroprusside (Nitropress) 50-mg vial	Nitrate vasodilator (see Nitroglycerin); nitroprusside is used only as a IV infusion, and patients should be monitored carefully during administration	Severe hypotension is possible during therapy; monitor patients carefully during administration; cyanide is generated via metabolism during nitroprusside treatment, especially at high infusion rates; cyanide toxicity is possible with nitroprusside therapy	Begin at 2 μg/kg/min and increase by 1 μg/kg/min q20–30 min until clinical improvement is seen; maximum dose = 10 μg/kg/min
Nystatin 100,000 units/mL oral suspension	Antifungal; oral topical for *Candida* infection	Not absorbed well; may cause GI upset	Dogs, cats: 100,000 units PO q6h
Nizatidine (Axid)	Histamine H–2 blocking drug (see Cimetidine); same as cimetidine, except up to 10× more potent	See Cimetidine and Ranitidine; side effects from nizatidine have not been reported for animals	Dog: 2.5–5 mg/kg q24h PO
Norfloxacin (Noroxin) 400-mg tablets	Fluoroquinolone antibacterial drug; narrower spectrum of activity than enrofloxacin or ciprofloxacin		22 mg/kg q12h PO
Olsalazine (Dipentum) 500-mg tablets	Antiinflammatory drug for treating colitis; two molecules of aminosalicylic acid joined by an azo bond. (see Mesalamine)	See Mesalamine	Dose not established, but 5–10 mg/kg q8h has been used (usual human dose is 500 mg twice daily)
Omeprazole (Prilosec) 20 mg capsules	Proton pump inhibitor; inhibits gastric acid secretion by inhibiting the K^+/H^+ pump; more potent and longer acting than most available antisecretory drugs; used for treatment and prevention of GI ulcers		Dog: 20 μg/dog once daily, PO (or 0.7 mg/kg, q24h) Cat: not recommended
Ondansetron (Zofran) 2-mg/mL injection; 4- or 8-mg tablets	Antiemetic drug; inhibits action of serotonin (blocks 5–HT_3 receptors); used primarily to inhibit vomiting associated with chemotherapy	Expensive	0.5 to 1.0 mg/kg, IV or oral 30 min prior to administration of cancer drugs
Orbifloxacin (Orbax) 5.7-, 22.7-, and 68-mg tablets	Fluoroquinolone antimicrobial; same mechanism as enrofloxacin and ciprofloxacin; spectrum includes staphylococci, gram-negative bacilli, and some pseudomonads	Same precautions as enrofloxacin; may cause some nausea and vomiting at high doses; avoid use in young animals	Dog and cat: 2.5 to 7.5 mg/kg once daily, PO
Ormetoprim	Trimethoprim–like drug used in combination with sulfadimethoxine. (See Primor.)		
Oxacillin (Prostaphlin, and generic) 200-, 500-mg capsules; 50-mg/mL oral liquid	β-Lactam antibiotic; inhibits bacterial cell wall synthesis; spectrum is limited to gram-positive bacteria, especially staphylococci		22–40 mg/kg q8h, PO

Drug (Other Names)	Pharmacology and Indications	Adverse Effects and Precautions	Dosage
Oxazepam (Serax) 15-mg tablet	Benzodiazepine; centrally acting CNS depressant; mechanism of action appears to be via potentiation of GABA-receptor-mediated effects in CNS; used for sedation and to stimulate appetite	Sedation is most common side effect; causes polyphagia; in cats, fatal hepatic necrosis has been reported from diazepam	Cats: appetite stimulant: 2.5 mg/cat PO
Oxtriphylline (Choledyl–SA) 400-, 600-mg tablet	Choline theophyllinate; methylxanthine broncho-dilator, similar in mechanism to theophylline	See Theophylline	Dog: 47 mg/kg (equivalent to 30 mg/kg theophylline) q12h PO
Oxyglobin (Oxyglobin)	Hemoglobin glutamer (bovine) used as oxygen-carrying fluid in dogs with anemia of varying causes	Adverse effects include skin discoloration, volume overload, and interference with blood chemistry	Dog: 10–30 mL/kg IV Cat: 5–20 mL/kg IV
Oxymorphone (Numorphan) 1.5- and 1-mg/mL injection	Opioid agonist; action is similar to that of morphine, except that oxymorphone is more lipophilic than morphine and 10–15× more potent	See Morphine	Dogs, cats: analgesia: 0.1–0.2 mg/kg IV, SC, IM (as needed), redose with 0.05–0.1 mg/kg q1–2h Preanesthetic: 0.025–0.05 mg/kg IM, SC
Oxytetracycline (Terramycin) 250-mg tablets; 100-, 200-mg/mL injection	Tetracycline antibiotic (See Tetracycline); same mechanism and spectrum as tetracycline; oxytetracycline may be more highly absorbed	Generally safe; use cautiously in young animals; see precautions for tetracycline	7.5–10 mg/kg IV, q12h; 20 mg/kg q12h PO
Oxytocin 10-, 20-U/mL injection	Stimulates uterine muscle contraction via action on specific oxytoxin receptors; used to induce or maintain normal labor and delivery in pregnant animals; does not increase milk production, but will stimulate contraction leading to milk ejection	Do not administer to pregnant bitch without pelvic radiographs and examination	Dog: 5–20 units IM, SC (repeat every 30 min up to 3 times for primary inertia) Cat: 2.5–5 units per cat, IM, IV CRI: Add 10–20 units to base solution and give to effect
2-PAM	See Pralidoxime chloride		
Pancreatic enzyme	See Pancrelipase (Viokase)		
Pancrelipase (Viokase)	Pancreatic enzyme; used to treat pancreatic exocrine insufficiency; provides lipase, amylase, and protease	Adverse effects not reported	Dog: Mix 2 tsp powder with food per 20 kg body weight, or 1–3 tsp/0.45 kg of food 20 min prior to feeding Cat: ½ tsp/cat with food
Pancuronium bromide (Pavulon) 1- or 2-mg/mL injection	Nondepolarizing neuro-muscular blocker (see Atracurium)	See Atracurium	0.1 mg/kg IV, or start with 0.01 mg/kg and additional 0.01 mg/kg doses every 30 min
Paroxetine (Paxil) 10-mg tablets	Selective serotonin reuptake inhibitor (SSRI) much like fluoxetine (Prozac) in action; used for obsessive-compulsive disorders, aggression, and other behavioral problems	Some effects similar to those of fluoxetine, but some animals tolerate paroxetine is better	Cats: ⅛ to ¼ of a 10-mg tablet daily, PO

Drug (Other Names)	Pharmacology and Indications	Adverse Effects and Precautions	Dosage
D-Penicillamine (Cuprimine, Depen) 125-, 250-mg capsules	Chelating agent for lead, copper, iron, and mercury; used primarily in animals for treatment of copper toxicity and hepatitis associated with accumulation of copper; also has been used to treat cystine calculi		10–15 mg/kg q12h PO
Penicillin G, Benzathine 150,000 U/mL	All benzathine penicillin G is combined with procaine penicillin G in commercial formulation	See Penicillin G	24,000 U/kg q48h IM
Penicillin G potassium; Penicillin G sodium 5–20 million-Unit vials	β-Lactam antibiotic; spectrum is limited to gram-positive bacteria and anaerobes	Same as for other penicillins (see Amoxicillin)	20,000–40,000 U/kg q6–8h IV, IM
Penicillin G, Procaine (generic) 300,000-U/mL injection	Same as other forms of penicillin G, except procaine penicillin is absorbed slowly, producing concentrations for 12–24 hours after injection	Avoid SC injection	20,000–40,000 U/kg q12–24h IM
Penicillin V (Pen-Vee) 250-, 500-mg tablets	Oral penicillin; otherwise same as other penicillins; not highly absorbed, and narrow spectrum compared with other penicillin derivatives	Same as other penicillin (see Amoxicillin)	10 mg/kg q8h PO
Pentazocine (Talwin-V) 30-mg/mL injection	Synthetic opiate analgesic; action as agonist–antagonist (similar to buprenorphine or butorphanol)	Adverse effects similar to those of other opiates (see butorphanol or morphine)	Dog: 1.65–3.3 mg/kg q4h IM Cat: 2.2–3.3 mg/kg IV, IM, SC
Pentobarbital (Nembutal, and generic) 50-mg/mL injection	Short-acting barbiturate anesthetic; action is via non-selective depression of CNS; pentobarbital usually is used as IV anesthetic; used to control severe seizures in animals; duration of action may be 3–4 hours	Cardiac and respiratory depression are common	25–30 mg/kg IV; inject first half of dose initially, then gradually titrate in rest of dose
Pentoxifylline (Trental) 400-mg tablets	Methylxanthine; pentoxifylline is used primarily as a rheologic agent in people (increases blood flow through narrow vessels); it may have antiinflammatory action via inhibition of cytokine synthesis; used in dogs for some dermatoses (dermatomyositis) and vasculitis	May cause similar signs as other methylxanthines (see Theophylline); nausea, vomiting have been reported in people; when broken tablet is administered to cats, the taste is unpleasant	Dog: dermatologic use: 10 mg/kg q12h PO; for other uses: 10 mg/kg q8–12 h PO, or 400 mg/dog for most animals Cats: ¼ of a 400-mg tablet (100 mg) q8–12h PO
Pepto Bismol	See Bismuth subsalicylate		

Drug (Other Names)	Pharmacology and Indications	Adverse Effects and Precautions	Dosage
Phenobarbital 15-, 30-, 60-, 100-mg tablets; 30-, 60-, 65-, 130-mg/mL injection	Long-acting barbiturate; phenobarbital's major use is as an anticonvulsant—it potentiates inhibitory actions of GABA; therapeutic range for serum concentration is 15–40 μg/mL	Adverse effects are dose related; phenobarbital causes polyphagia, sedation, ataxia, and lethargy; some tolerance develops to side effects after initial therapy; hepatotoxicity has been reported in some dogs receiving high doses	Dog: 2–8 mg/kg q12h PO Cat: 2–4 mg/kg q12h PO Status epilepticus: administer in increments of 4 mg/kg IV up to 16 mg/kg total
Phenoxybenzamine 10-mg capsules	α_1-Adrenergic antagonist; binds α_1-receptor on smooth muscle, causing relaxation; potent vasodilator; used primarily to treat peripheral vasoconstriction or to relax urethral smooth muscle	Causes prolonged hypotension in animals; use carefully in animals with cardiovascular compromise	Dog: 0.25 mg/kg q8–12h PO, or 0.5 mg/kg q24h Cat: 2.5 mg/cat q8–12h, or 0.5 mg/kg q12h PO (in cats, doses as high as 0.5 mg/kg IV have been used to relax urethral smooth muscle)
Phentolamine 5-mg vials for injection	Nonselective α_1-adrenergic blocker; vasodilator; blocks stimulation of α_1- receptors on vascular smooth muscle; primarily used to treat hypertension	May cause excess hypotension with high doses or in animals that are dehydrated; may cause tachycardia	0.02–0.1 mg/kg IV
Phenylephrine (Neo-Synephrine) 10-mg/mL injection	Specific adrenergic agonist; specific for α_1-receptor; vasopressor for severe hypotension	Same as methoxamine	0.01 mg/kg q15 min IV, 0.1 mg/kg q15 min IM, SC
Phenylpropanolamine (Dexatrim, Propagest and others) 15-, 25-, 30-, 50-mg tablets	Adrenergic agonist; used as decongestant, mild bronchodilator, and to increase tone of urinary sphincter (see Ephedrine, Pseudoephedrine)	Adverse effects are attributed to excess stimulation of adrenergic (α and β) receptors; see ephedrine; side effects: tachycardia, cardiac effects, CNS excitement, restlessness, and appetite suppression	1.5–2 mg/kg q12h PO
Phenytoin (Dilantin) 30-, 125-mg	Anticonvulsant; depresses nerve conduction via blockade of sodium channels; also classified as class 1 antiarrhythmic; commonly used as anticonvulsant in people, but not effective in dogs and not used in cats	Adverse effects: sedation, gingival hyperplasia, skin reactions, CNS toxicity; do not administer to pregnant animals	Antiepileptic: dog: 20–35 mg/kg q8h Antiarrhythmic: 30 mg/kg q8h PO or 10 mg/kg IV over 5 min
Physostigmine (Antilirium)	Cholinesterase inhibitor; antidote for anticholinergic intoxication, especially intoxication that exhibits CNS signs; major difference between physostigmine and neostigmine or pyridostigmine is that physostigmine crosses blood–brain barrier and the others do not	Adverse effects attributed to excessive cholinergic effects (treat overdoses with atropine)	0.02 mg/kg q12h IV
Phytonadione	See Vitamin K$_1$		
Phytomenadione	See Vitamin K$_1$		

Drug (Other Names)	Pharmacology and Indications	Adverse Effects and Precautions	Dosage
Piperacillin (Pipracil)	β-Lactam antibiotic of the acylureidopenicillin class; similar to other penicillins, except with high activity against *Pseudomonas aeruginosa*; also good activity against streptococci	Same precautions as for other injectable penicillins (e.g., ampicillin)	40 mg/kg IV or IM q6h
Piperazine (many)	Antiparasitic compound; produces neuromuscular blockade in parasite through inhibition of neurotransmitter, which causes paralysis of worms; used primarily for treatment of helminth (ascarid) infections	Remarkably safe in all species	44–66 mg/kg PO, administered once
Piroxicam (Feldene, and generic)	NSAID of the oxicam class; clinical effects are similar to those of other NSAIDs (see Aspirin, Flunixin); piroxicam has been used for treatment of transitional cell carcinoma in dogs	Elimination of piroxicam is slow; use cautiously in dogs; adverse effects are primarily GI toxicity (ulcers); see Flunixin	Dog: 0.3 mg/kg q48h PO Cat: dose not established
Phenytoin (Dilantin) 30-, 125-mg/mL oral suspension; 30-, 100-mg capsules; 50-mg/mL injection	Anticonvulsant; depresses nerve conduction via blockade of sodium channels; also classified as class 1 anti-arrhythmic; commonly used as anticonvulsant in people, but not effective in dogs and not used in cats	Adverse effects: sedation, gingival hyperplasia, skin reactions, CNS toxicity; do not administer to pregnant animals	Antiepileptic: dog: 20–35 mg/kg q8h Antiarrhythmic: 30 mg/kg q8h PO or 10 mg/kg IV over 5 min
Physostigmine (Antilirium) 1-mg/mL injection	Cholinesterase inhibitor; antidote for anticholinergic intoxication, especially intoxication that exhibits CNS signs; major difference between physostigmine and neostigmine or pyridostigmine is that physostigmine crosses blood–brain barrier and the others do not	Adverse effects attributed to excessive cholinergic effects (treat overdoses with atropine)	0.02 mg/kg q12h IV
Phytonadione	See Vitamin K$_1$		
Phytomenadione	See Vitamin K$_1$		
Piperacillin (Pipracil) 2-, 3-, 4-, 40-g vials for injection	β–lactam antibiotic of the acylureidopenicillin class; similar to other penicillins, except with high activity against *Pseudomonas aeruginosa*; also good activity against streptococci	Same precautions as for other injectable penicillins (e.g., ampicillin)	40 mg/kg IV or IM q6h

Drug (Other Names)	Pharmacology and Indications	Adverse Effects and Precautions	Dosage
Piperazine (many) 860-mg powder; 140- mg capsules; 170-, 340-, and 800-mg/mL oral solution	Antiparasitic compound; produces neuromuscular blockade in parasite through inhibition of neurotransmitter, which causes paralysis of worms; used primarily for treatment of helminth (ascarid) infections	Remarkably safe in all species	44–66 mg/kg PO, administered once
Piroxicam 10- or 20-mg capsules	Transitional cell carcinoma	GI ulceration	Dog: 0.3 mg/kg q24–48h
Plicamycin (old name is mithramycin) (Mithracin) 2.5-mg injection	Anticancer agent; lowers serum calcium; may have direct action on osteoclasts to decrease serum calcium; used for carcinomas and treatment of hypercalcemia	Hypocalcemia and GI toxicity have been reported; may cause bleeding problems	Dog: antineoplastic: 25–30 μg/kg/day IV (slow infusion) for 8–10 days; antihypercalcemic:25 μg/kg/day IV (slow infusion) over 4 hours
Polyethylene glycol electrolyte solution (GoLYTELY)	Saline cathartic; nonabsorbable compounds that increase water secretion into bowel via osmotic effect; used for bowel evacuation prior to surgical or diagnostic procedure	Water and electrolyte loss with high doses or prolonged use (See also Magnesium citrate)	25 mL/kg, repeat in 2–4 hours PO
Polysulfated glycosaminoglycan (PSGAG) (Adequan Canine) 1000-mg/mL injection	Large-molecular-weight compounds similar to normal constituents of healthy joints; chondroprotective; inhibits enzymes that may degrade articular cartilage; used primarily to treat or prevent degenerative joint disease	Adverse effects are rare; allergic reactions are possible; PSGAG has heparin-like effects and may potentiate bleeding problems in some animals	4.4 mg/kg IM, twice weekly for up to 4 weeks
Potassium bromide (KBr) (No commercial formulation, but can be formulated by a pharmacist)	Anticonvulsant; bromide usually is administered in combination with phenobarbital; monitor serum bromide concentrations to adjust dose; effective plasma concentrations should be 1–2 mg/mL (100–200 mg/dL), but, if used alone (without phenobarbital), higher concentrations of 2–4 mg/mL may be needed; diets high in chloride will cause shorter half-life and need for higher dose	Adverse effects are related to high levels of bromide; signs of toxicity are CNS depression, weakness, ataxia; consider using sodium bromide in patients with hypoadrenocorticism	Dog and cat: 30–40 mg/kg q24h PO; if administered without phenobarbital, higher doses of up to 40–50 mg/kg may be needed; adjust doses by monitoring plasma concentrations; loading doses of 400 mg/kg divided over 3 days have been administered
Potassium chloride (generic) 2-mEq/mL injectable solution	Potassium supplement; used for treatment of hypokalemia; usually added to fluid solutions	Toxicity from high potassium concentrations can be dangerous; hyperkalemia can lead to cardiovascular toxicity (bradycardia and arrest) and muscular weakness; oral potassium supplements can cause nausea and stomach irritation; do not exceed rate of 0.5 mEq/kg/h IV	0.5 mEq potassium/kg/day, or supplement 10–40 mEq/500 mL of fluids, depending on serum potassium

Drug (Other Names)	Pharmacology and Indications	Adverse Effects and Precautions	Dosage
Potassium citrate (generic, Urocit–K) 5-mEq tablet	Alkalinizes urine and may increase urine citric acid; used for calcium oxalate urolithiasis; also used for renal tubular acidosis	Same as potassium chloride	2.2 mEq/100 kcal of energy/day PO; or 40–75 mg/kg q12h PO
Potassium gluconate (Kaon, Tumil-K, generic) 2-mEq or 500-mg tablets; elixir	Same as potassium chloride; used for renal tubular acidosis	Same as potassium chloride	Dog: 0.5 mEq/kg q12–24h PO Cat: 2–8 mEq/day divided twice daily, PO
Potassium phosphate 3 mmol/mL phosphate and 4 mEq/mL potassium	Phosphorus supplement; used for severe hypophosphatemia associated with diabetic ketoacidosis or refeeding syndrome		0.01–0.03 mmol/kg/h IV over 6 hours; recheck phosphorus after 6 hours; repeat if necessary
Pralidoxime chloride (2–PAM) (2–PAM, Protopam chloride) 50 mg/mL	Used for treatment of organophosphate toxicosis	Adverse effects have not been reported	Cat: 20 mg/kg q8–12h (initial dose IV slowly) or IM Dog: 50 mg/kg IV slowly
Praziquantel (Droncit) 23-, 34-mg tablet; 56.8-mg/mL injection	Antiparasitic drug; used primarily to treat infections caused by tapeworms	Vomiting occurs at high doses; anorexia and transient diarrhea have been reported; safe in pregnant animals	Dog: oral dose: <6.8 kg, 7.5 mg/kg PO, once; >6.8 kg, 5 mg/kg PO, once; dog IM SC: ≤2.3 kg, 7.5 mg/kg, once; 2.7–4.5 kg, 6.3 mg/kg, once; ≤5 kg, 5 mg/kg, once Cat PO: <1.8 kg, 6.3 mg/kg PO, once; >1.8 kg, 5 mg/kg, once (for *Paragonimus*, use 25 mg/kg q8h for 2–3 days/cat IM, SC: 5 mg/kg IM SC
Prazosin (Minipress) 1-, 2-, 5-mg capsules	α_1-Adrenergic blocker; relaxes smooth muscle, especially of vasculature; prazosin is used as vasodilator and to relax smooth muscle (occasionally urethral muscle)	High doses cause vasodilation and hypotension	0.5–2 mg/animal (1 mg/15 kg) q8–13h PO
Prednisolone (Delta–Cortef, and many others) 5- and 20-mg tablets	Glucocorticoid antiinflammatory drug; potency is approximately 4× cortisol (see Betamethasone for details)	All glucocorticoids produce expected (and sometimes unavoidable) side effects; see Betamethasone for partial list of side effects	Dogs (cats often require 2× dog dose); antiinflammatory: 0.5–1 mg/kg q12–24h IV, IM, PO initially, then taper to q48h; immunosuppressive: 2.2–6.6 mg/kg/day IV, IM, PO, initially, then taper to 2–4 mg/kg q48h; replacement therapy: 0.2–0.3 mg/kg/day PO; shock, spinal trauma: see prednisolone sodium succinate
Prednisolone sodium succinate (Solu–Delta–Cortef) 10 mg/mL or 50 mg/mL	Same as prednisolone, except that this is a water-soluble formulation intended for short-term therapy when high IV doses are needed for rapid effect; used for treatment of shock and CNS trauma	Adverse effects are not expected from single administration; however, with repeated use, other side effects are possible (see Betamethasone); may cause hyperglycemia, GI ulceration, delayed wound healing	Shock: 15–30 mg/kg/IV (repeat in 4–6 hours); CNS trauma: 15–30 mg/kg IV, taper to 1–2 mg/kg q12h

Drug (Other Names)	Pharmacology and Indications	Adverse Effects and Precautions	Dosage
Prednisone 1 mg–50 mg tablets; 10- and 40-mg/mL injection; 1-mg/mL oral liquid	Same as prednisolone, except that, after administration, prednisone is converted to prednisolone	Same as prednisolone	Same as prednisolone
Primor (Ormetoprim + Sulfadimethoxine) (Primor)	Antibacterial drug; bactericidal/ bacteriostatic; broad antibacterial spectrum and active against some coccidia	Several adverse effects have been reported from sulfonamides (see Trimethoprim/Sulfonamides); no adverse effects reported from ormetoprim	27 mg/kg on first day, followed by 13.5 mg/kg q24h PO
Procainamide 250-, 375-, 500-mg capsules; 100- or 500-mg/mL injection	Antiarrhythmic drug; class I antiarrhythmic used primarily for treatment of ventricular arrhythmias; action is to inhibit sodium influx into cardiac cell via sodium channel blockade	Adverse effects include cardiac arrhythmias, cardiac depression, tachycardia, and hypotension; in people, procainamide produces hypersensitivity effects (lupus-like reactions), but these have not been reported in animals; drug interactions: cimetidine may increase plasma concentrations	Dog: 10–30 mg/kg q6h PO (q8h for CR–continuous release), (to a maximum dose of 40 mg/kg), 8–20 mg/kg IV, IM; 25–50 μg/kg/min IV infusion Cat: 3–8 mg/kg IM PO q6–8h
Prochlorperazine (Compazine) 5-mg/mL injection	Phenothiazine; centrally acting dopamine (D_2) antagonist; used for sedation, tranquilization, and as antiemetic	Causes sedation and other side effects attributed to other phenothiazines (see Acepromazine)	0.1–0.5 mg/kg q6–8h IM, SC
Propantheline bromide (Pro-Banthine) 7.5- or 15-mg tablet	Anticholinergic (antimuscarinic) drug; blocks acetylcholine receptor to produce parasympatholytic effects (atropine-like effects); used to decrease smooth muscle contraction and secretion of GI tract; used to treat vagus-mediated cardiovascular effects	Side effects are attributed to excess anticholinergic (antimuscarinic) effects	0.25–0.5 mg/kg q8–12h PO
Propionibacterium acnes injection 0.4 mg/mL	Immunostimulant for recurrent pyoderma, FeLV, FIV		Dogs: 0.03–6.07 mL/kg 2×/week for 10 weeks Cats: 0.5 mL 2×/week for 2 weeks, then 1×/week for 20 weeks or until cat is seronegative
Propofol (Rapinovet [veterinary]; Diprivan [human]) 10 mg/mL	Anesthetic; used for induction or producing short-term general anesthesia; propofol may be used as induction agent, followed by inhalation with halothane or isoflurane	Apnea and respiratory depression is most common adverse effect; adverse effects attributed to general anesthetic properties	6.6 mg/kg IV slowly over 60 sec; constant-rate IV infusions have been used at 2 mg/kg/h
Propranolol (Inderal) 10-, 20-, 40-, 60-, 80- and 90-mg tablets; 1-mg/mL injection	β-Adrenergic blocker; nonselective for $β_1$- and $β_2$-adrenergic receptors; class II antiarrhythmic; used primarily to decrease heart rate, decrease cardiac conduction, tachyarrhythmia, and decrease blood pressure	Adverse effects related to $β_1$-blocking effects on heart; causes cardiac depression, decreases cardiac output; $β_2$-blocking effects can cause bronchoconstriction; decreases insulin secretion	Dog: 20–60 μg/kg over 5–10 min IV, 0.2–1 mg/kg PO q8h (titrate dose to effect) Cat: 0.4–1.2 mg/kg (2.5–5 mg/cat) PO q8h

Drug (Other Names)	Pharmacology and Indications	Adverse Effects and Precautions	Dosage
Prostaglandin F$_{2\alpha}$ (Dinoprost) (Lutalyse) 5-mg/mL injection	Prostaglandin induces luteolysis; has been used to treat pyometra in animals or to induce abortion	Side effects include vomiting, diarrhea, and abdominal discomfort	Pyometra (dog): 0.1–0.2 mg/kg, once daily for 5 days SC; (cat): 0.1–0.25 mg/kg, once daily for 5 days SC Abortion (dog): 0.025–0.05 mg (25–50 mcg)/kg q12h IM; (cat): 0.5–1 mg/kg IM for 2 injections
Protamine sulfate 10 mg/mL	Low-molecular-weight, strongly basic, cationic protein; binds to heparin to form inactive complex; used in all species to treat hemorrhage caused by heparin overdosage	Rapid infusion causes hypotension, bradycardia, pulmonary hypertension, and respiratory distress; a "rebound" anticoagulant effect may occur several hours after administration due to release of heparin from protamine–heparin complexes or extravascular stores (weak intrinsic anticoagulant properties of protamine not thought to cause clinical bleeding)	1 mg for every 100 U heparin to be inactivated; decrease dose by 50% for every 30 minutes that have lapsed since heparin dose; administer over 1–3 min; do not exceed 50 mg per 10 min
Pseudoephedrine (Sudafed, and many others [some formulations have other ingredients]) 30-, 60-mg tablets; 120-mg capsules; 6-mg/mL oral liquid	Adrenergic agonist; similar to ephedrine, phenylpropanolamine in action; used to increase peripheral resistance, as a decongestant, and in animals to treat urinary incontinence	Side effects attributed to adrenergic effects (excitement, rapid heart rate, arrhythmias) (see Ephedrine, Phenylpropanolamine)	0.2–0.4 mg/kg (or 15–60 mg/dog) q8–12h PO
Psyllium (Metamucil, and others)	Bulk-forming laxative; use for treatment of constipation and bowel evacuation; action is to absorb water and expand to provide increased bulk and moisture content to the stool, which encourages normal peristalsis and bowel motility	Adverse effects have not been reported in animals; intestinal impaction can occur with overuse or in patients with inadequate fluid intake	1 tsp/5–10 kg (added to each meal)
Pyrantel pamoate (Nemex, Strongid) 180-mg/mL paste, 50-mg/mL oral suspension	Antiparasitic drug	No adverse effects reported	Dog: 5 mg/kg once PO and repeat in 7–10 days Cat: 20 mg/kg once PO
Pyridostigmine bromide (Mestinon, Regonol) 60-mg tablets; 12-mg/mL oral liquid; 5-mg/mL injection	Anticholinesterase; same as for neostigmine, except that pyridostigmine has longer duration of action	Same as for neostigmine, except that adverse effects may persist longer; drug interactions: since this product contains bromide, use cautiously in patients already receiving bromide (e.g., potassium bromide for epilepsy)	Antimyasthenic: 0.02–0.04 mg/kg q2h IV, or 0.5–3 mg/kg q8–12h PO Antidote for muscle blockade: 0.15–0.3 mg/kg IM, IV
Pyrimethamine (Daraprim) 25-mg tablets	Antibacterial, antiprotozoal drug; activity of pyrimethamine is more specific against protozoa than bacteria; used for toxoplasmosis, hepatozoonosis, neosporosis	When administered with trimethoprim/sulfonamide combinations, anemia has been observed; folic or folinic acid has been supplemented to prevent anemia, but benefit of this treatment is unclear	Dog: 0.5–1 mg/kg q24h PO for 2 days, then 0.25 mg/kg q24h for 2 weeks Cats: 0.5–1 mg/kg q24h PO for 14–28 days

Drug (Other Names)	Pharmacology and Indications	Adverse Effects and Precautions	Dosage
Quinidine gluconate (Quinaglute, Duraquin) 324-mg tablets; 80-mg/mL injection	Antiarrhythmic drug; class I antiarrhythmic; acts to inhibit sodium influx via blockade of sodium channels; used to treat ventricular arrhythmia and occasionally atrial fibrillation	Side effects more common with quinidine than with procainamide and include nausea and vomiting; adverse effects: hypotension, tachycardia (due to antivagal effect) *Drug interactions:* coadministration with digoxin may increase digoxin concentrations	Dog: 20 mg/kg q6h IM; 6–20 mg/kg q6–8h PO (of base)
Quinidine polygalacturonate (Cardioquin) 275-mg tablets (contain 167 mg of quinidine)	Same as quinidine gluconate	Same as quinidine gluconate	Dog: 6–20 mg/kg q6h PO (of base) (275 mg quinidine polygalacturonate = 167 mg quinidine base)
Quinidine sulfate (Cin-Quin, Quinora) 100-, 200-, 300-mg tablets; 200-, 300-mg capsules; 200-mg/mL injection	Same as quinidine gluconate	Same as quinidine gluconate	Dog: 6–20 mg/kg q6–8h PO (of base); 5–10 g/cat PO (added to food each day)
Ranitidine (Zantac) 75-, 100-, 300-mg tablets; 150- or 300-mg capsules; 25-mg/mL injection	H-2 antagonist (see Cimetidine for details); same as cimetidine except 4–10× more potent and longer-acting; promotility agent that stimulates gastric motility	Ranitidine may have fewer effects than cimetidine on endocrine function and drug interactions	Dog: 2 mg/kg q8h IV, PO Cat: 2.5 mg/kg q12h IV, 3.5 mg/kg q12h PO
Retinoids	See Isotretinoin (Accutane), Retinol (Aquasol–A), or Etretinate (Tegison)		
Retinol	See Vitamin A (Aquasol–A).		
Riboflavin (vitamin B_2)	See Vitamin B_2		
Rifampin (Rifadin) 150-, 300-mg capsules	Antibacterial. Spectrum of action includes staphylococci and mycobacteria; streptococci also susceptible bacteria; used in people primarily for treatment of tuberculosis	*Drug interactions:* multiple drug interactions are possible; induces P-450 enzymes; drugs affected include barbiturates, chloramphenicol, and corticosteroids	10–20 mg/kg q24h PO
Ringer's solution (generic)	IV solution for replacement	Monitor pulmonary pressure when infusing high doses	40–50 mg/kg day IV, SC, IP
Salicylate	See Acetylsalicylic acid (aspirin)		
Selegiline (Deprenyl) (Anipryl) 2-, 5-, 10-, 15-, and 30-mg tablets	Acts to inhibit specific monoamine oxidase (MAO type B); specifically, it appears to inhibit degradation of dopamine in CNS; in people, it is primarily used to treat Parkinson's disease and other neurodegenerative diseases (in combination with levodopa); in dogs, it is approved to control clinical signs of pituitary-dependent hyperadrenocorticism (Cushing's disease) and to treat cognitive dysfunction in geriatric dogs	At high doses in dogs, hyperactivity has been observed (doses >3 mg/kg)	Dogs: begin with 1 mg/kg q24h PO; if no response within 2 months, increase dose to maximum of 2 mg/kg q24h PO Cats: dose not established

Drug (Other Names)	Pharmacology and Indications	Adverse Effects and Precautions	Dosage
Sodium bicarbonate 1 mEq/mL	Alkalizing agent; antacid; used to treat systemic acidosis or to alkalize urine, increase plasma and urinary concentrations of bicarbonate	Adverse effects attributed to alkalizing activity; *Drug interactions:* when administered orally, interaction may occur to decrease absorption of other drugs (partial list includes anticholinergic drugs, ketoconazole, fluoroquinolones, tetracyclines)	Acidosis: 0.5–1 mEq/kg IV; renal failure: 10 mg/kg q8–12h PO Alkalization of urine: 50 mg/kg q8–12h PO (1 tsp is approximately 2 g)
Sodium chloride 500, 1000 mL	Sodium chloride is used for IV infusion as replacement fluid	Not a balanced electrolyte solution; long-term infusion may cause electrolyte imbalance	40–50 mL/kg/day IV, SC, IP
Sodium chloride 7%	Concentrated sodium chloride used for short-term treatment of hypovolemia		2–8 mL/kg IV
Sotalol (Betapace) 80, 160, 240 mg	Nonspecific β (β_1 and β_2) adrenergic blocker (class II antiarrhythmic), action is similar to propranolol (1/3 potency); however, its beneficial effect may be caused more by the other antiarrhythmic effects; in addition to being a class II antiarrhythmic drug, sotalol may have some class III (potassium-channel blocking) activity	Like many antiarrhythmics, it may have some proarrhythmic activity; negative inotropic effects may cause concern in some animals with poor contractility	Dogs: 1–2 mg/kg q12h PO (begin with 40 mg/dog q12h and increase to 80 mg if no response) Cats: 1–2 mg/kg q12h, PO
Spironolactone (Aldactone) 25-, 50-, 100-mg tablets	Potassium-sparing diuretic; acts to interfere with sodium reabsorption in distal renal tubule; spironolactone competitively inhibits the action of aldosterone; used for treating high blood pressure, and congestion caused by heart failure	Can produce hyperkalemia in some patients; do not use in dehydrated patients; *Drug interactions:* NSAIDs may interfere with action; avoid supplements high in potassium	2–4 mg/kg/day (or 1–2 mg/kg q12h) PO
Succimer (Chemet) 100-mg capsule	Used in treatment of lead toxicosis; chelates lead and other heavy metals, such as mercury and arsenic	No known adverse effects	10 mg/kg q8h, PO for 5 days, then 10 mg/kg q12h PO for 2 more weeks
Sucralfate (Carafate) 1 gm tablets; 200 mg/mL suspension	Gastric mucosa protectant; antiulcer agent; binds to ulcerated tissue in GI tract to aid healing of ulcers; some evidence suggests that sucralfate may act as a cytoprotectant (via prostaglandin synthesis); used to treat or prevent ulcers	*Drug interactions:* may decrease absorption of other orally administered drugs via chelation with aluminum (such as fluoroquinolones and tetracyclines)	Dog 0.5–1 g q8–12h PO Cat: 0.25 g q8–12h PO
Sufentanil citrate (Sufenta) 50-μg/mL injection	Opioid agonist; action of fentanyl derivatives is via μ-receptor (see Fentanyl, Morphine); sufentanil is 5–7× more potent than fentanyl; 13 to 20 μg of sufentanil produces analgesia equal to 10 mg of morphine	Adverse effects similar to those of other opiates (see Morphine)	2 μg/kg IV, up to a maximum dose of 5 μg/kg

Drug (Other Names)	Pharmacology and Indications	Adverse Effects and Precautions	Dosage
Sulfadiazine (combined with trimethoprim in Tribrissen) 500-mg tablets	Synergistic with trimethoprim; broad spectrum of activity, including some protozoa (toxoplasmosis, hepatozoonosis); bacteriostatic	Adverse effects associated with sulfonamides include allergic reactions, type II and III hypersensitivity, hypothyroidism (with prolonged therapy), keratoconjunctivitis sicca, and skin reactions	15–30 mg/kg PO, IV q12h (with trimethoprim)
Sulfadimethoxine (Albon, Bactrovet, and generic) 125-, 250-, 500-mg tablets; 50-mg/mL oral liquid	See Sulfadiazine	See Sulfadiazine	55 mg/kg PO (loading dose), followed by 27.5 mg/kg q12h PO
Sulfamethazine (many brands [e.g., Sulmet])	See Sulfadiazine	See Sulfadiazine	100 mg/kg PO (loading dose), followed by 50 mg/kg q12h PO
Sulfamethoxazole (Gantanol)	See Sulfadiazine	See Sulfadiazine	100 mg/kg PO (loading dose) followed by 50 mg/kg q12h PO
Sulfasalazine (Sulfapyridine + Mesalamine) (Azulfidine) 500-mg tablet	Sulfonamide + antiinflammatory drug; used for treatment of colitis along with dietary therapy; sulfonamide has little effect, salicylic acid (mesalamine) has antiinflammatory effects (see Mesalamine)	Adverse effects are all attributed to sulfonamide component (see Sulfadiazine); keratoconjunctivitis sicca has been reported	10–30 mg/kg q12h PO (see also Mesalamine, Olsalazine)
Sulfisoxazole (Gantrisin) 500-mg tablets; 100-mg/mL oral liquid	See Sulfadiazine; sulfisoxazole is primarily used only for treating urinary tract infections	See Sulfadiazine	50 mg/kg q8h PO (urinary tract infections)
Taurine	Nutritional supplement for cats; used in prevention and treatment of ocular and cardiac diseases (cardiomyopathy) caused by taurine deficiency	Adverse effects have not been reported	Dog: 500 mg q12h PO Cat: 250 mg/cat q12h PO
Telesol	See Tiletamine		
Terbutaline (Brethine, Bricanyl) 2.5-, 5-mg tablets; 1-mg/mL injection	β-Adrenergic agonist; β$_2$-specific; used primarily for bronchodilation	Adverse effects related to excessive β-adrenergic stimulation; see Albuterol for list of adverse effects	Dog: 1.25–5 mg/dog q8h PO or 3–5 μg/kg SC Cat: 0.1–0.2 mg/kg q12h SC (or 0.625 mg/cat, 1/4 of 2.5 mg tablet) q12h PO
Tetracycline (Panmycin) 200-, 500-mg capsule; 100-mg/mL oral liquid	Tetracycline antibiotic; usually bacteriostatic; broad-spectrum activity including bacteria, some protozoa, rickettsia, *Ehrlichia*	Tetracyclines in general may cause renal tubular necrosis at high doses; tetracyclines can affect bone and teeth formation in young animals; tetracyclines have been implicated in drug fever in cats; hepatotoxicity may occur at high doses in susceptible individuals; *Drug interactions:* tetracyclines bind to calcium-containing compounds, which decreases oral absorption	15–20 mg/kg q8h PO; or 4.4–11 mg/kg q8h IV, IM

Drug (Other Names)	Pharmacology and Indications	Adverse Effects and Precautions	Dosage
Theophylline 100-, 125-, 200-, 250-, 300-mg tablets; oral solution and injection	Methylxanthine broncho-dilator	Adverse effects: nausea, vomiting, diarrhea; with high doses, tachycardia, excitement, tremors, and seizures are possible; cardio-vascular and CNS adverse effects appear to be less frequent in dogs than in people; plasma concentra-tions should be 10–20 μg/mL	Dog: 9 mg/kg q6–8h PO Cat: 4 mg/kg q8–12h PO (see also Aminophylline)
Theophylline sustained-release 100-, 200-, 300-, and 450-mg tablets (Theo-Dur); 50–200 mg capsules (Slo-Bid)	Same as theophylline; sustained-release preparations are used to decrease frequency of administration	Same as theophylline	Dog: 20 mg/kg q12h (Theo-Dur); 30 mg/kg q12h (Slo-Bid) PO Cat: 25 mg/kg q24h (at night) for Theo-Dur and Slo-Bid, PO
Thiabendazole (Omnizole, Equizole) 2- or 4-g/oz oral liquid	Benzimidazole anthelmintic (see Fenbendazole, Albendazole)	Adverse effects uncommon	Dog: 50 mg/kg q24h for 3 days, repeat in 1 month; respiratory parasites: 30–70 mg/kg q12h PO Cat (Strongyloides): 125 mg/kg q24h for 3 days
Thiacetarsamide sodium (Caparsolate) 10 mg/mL	Organic arsenical used for treatment of heartworm infections; adulticide	Adverse effects are common, especially anorexia, vomiting, hepatic injury; pulmonary thromboembolism may occur as consequence of heartworm kill; if adverse effects occur, treatment should be discontinued	Dog: 2.2 mg/kg IV twice daily for 2 days Cat: Not recommended
Thiamine (vitamin B₁) 100- and 500-mg/mL injection	Vitamin B₁ used for treatment of thiamine deficiency	Adverse effects are rare because water-soluble vitamins are easily excreted; riboflavin may discolor the urine	Dog: 10–100 mg/dog/day PO Cat: 100–250 mg SC or IM q12h until signs resolve, then 10 mg/kg PO q24h × 21 days
Thiopental sodium (Pentothal)	Ultrashort–acting barbiturate; used primarily for induction of anesthesia or for short duration of anesthesia (10–15 min procedures); anesthesia is produced by CNS depression, without analgesia; anesthesia is terminated by redistribution in the body	Severe adverse effects are caused by respiratory and cardiovascular depression; overdoses are caused by rapid or repeated injections; avoid extravasation outside of vein	Dog: 10–25 mg/kg IV (to effect) Cat: 5–10 mg/kg IV (to effect)
Ticarcillin (Ticar, Ticillin) 1-, 3-, 6-, 20-, and 30-g vials	β-Lactam antibiotic; action similar to that of ampicillin/amoxicillin; spectrum similar to carbenicillin; ticarcillin is primarily used for gram-negative infections, especially those caused by *Pseudomonas*	Adverse effects are uncommon; however, allergic reactions are possible; high doses can produce seizures and decrease platelet function; *Drug interactions:* do not combine in same syringe or in vial with aminoglycosides	33–50 mg/kg q4–6h IV, IM
Ticarcillin + clavulanate (Timentin) 3-g vials	Same as ticarcillin, except clavulanic acid has been added to inhibit bacterial β-lactamase and increase spectrum	Same as ticarcillin	Dose according to rate for ticarcillin

Drug (Other Names)	Pharmacology and Indications	Adverse Effects and Precautions	Dosage
Tiletamine + zolazepam (Telesol, Zoletil)	Anesthetic; combination of tiletamine (dissociative anesthetic agent similar in action to ketamine) and zolazepam (benzodiazepine similar in action to diazepam); produces short-duration (30 min) anesthesia	Wide margin of safety; side effects include excessive salivation (may be antagonized with atropine), erratic recovery, and muscle twitching; deep IM injection	5–7 mg/kg IM
Tobramycin (Nebcin) 40-mg/mL injection	Aminoglycoside antibacterial drug; mechanism of action and spectrum similar to amikacin, gentamicin	Adverse effects similar to amikacin, gentamicin	2–4 mg/kg q8h IV, IM, SC
Tocainide (Tonocard) 400-, 600-mg tablets	Antiarrhythmic drug; considered an oral analogue of lidocaine; class I antiarrhythmic	In dogs, anorexia and GI toxicity have been reported; arrhythmia, vomiting, ataxia also are possible (in one study, 35% of dogs showed GI effects)	Dog: 15–20 mg/kg q8h PO Cat: no dose established
Triamcinolone (Vetalog, Trimtabs, Aristocort, generic) 0.5- and 1.5-mg tablets; 10 mg/mL injection	Glucocorticoid antiinflammatory drug (see Betamethasone for details); potency is approximately equal to that of methylprednisolone (about 5× cortisol and 1.25× prednisolone), although some dermatologists suggest that potency is higher	Adverse effects are similar to those of other corticosteroids (see β-Methasone)	Antiinflammatory: 0.5–1 mg/kg q12–24h PO, then taper dose to 0.5–1 mg/kg q48h PO (manufacturer recommends doses of 0.11–0.22 mg/kg/day)
Triamcinolone acetonide (Vetalog) 2- or 6-mg/mL injection	Same as for triamcinolone, except that injectable suspension is slowly absorbed from IM or intralesional injection site; used for intralesional therapy of tumors and purposes similar to those of methylprednisolone acetate	See Methylprednisolone acetate; when used for ocular injections, there is some concern that granulomas may occur at injection site	0.1–0.2 mg/kg IM, SC, repeat in 7–10 days;. intralesional: 1.2–1.8 mg, or 1 mg for every cm diameter of tumor every 2 weeks
Triamterene (Dyrenium) 50-, 100-mg capsules	Potassium-sparing diuretic; similar in action to spironolactone, except that spironolactone has competitive inhibiting effect of aldosterone, triamterene does not	See Spironolactone	1–2 mg/kg q12h PO
Trientine hydrochloride (Syprine) 250-mg capsules	Chelating agent; used to chelate copper when a patient cannot tolerate penicillamine; generally less effective than penicillamine	Adverse effects have not been reported in animals	10–15 mg/kg q12h PO
Triflupromazine (Vesprin) 10-, 20-mg/mL injection	Phenothiazine; similar in action to other phenothiazines, except triflupromazine may have stronger antimuscarinic activity than the others; used for antiemetic action		0.1–0.3 mg/kg IM PO q8–12h

Drug (Other Names)	Pharmacology and Indications	Adverse Effects and Precautions	Dosage
Trimeprazine tartrate (Temaril) 2.5-mg/5 mL oral liquid; 2.5-mg tablets	Phenothiazine with anti-histamine activity (similar to promethazine); used for treating allergies and motion sickness; combination product containing prednisone (Temaril-P) is used for pruritus	Adverse effects similar to those of promethazine	0.5 mg/kg q12h PO
Trimethobenzamide (Tigan) 100-mg/mL injection; 100-, 250-mg capsules	Antiemetic; mechanism of action is not understood	Adverse effects not reported in animals	Dog: 3 mg/kg q8h IM, PO Cat: not recommended
Trimethoprim + sulfadiazine (Tribrissen) 30-, 120-, 240-, 480-, 960-mg tablets	Combines the antibacterial drug actions of trimethoprim and a sulfonamide; together, the combination is synergistic, with a broad spectrum of activity	Adverse effects primarily caused by sulfonamide component (see Sulfadiazine)	15 mg/kg q12h PO, or 30 mg/kg q12–24h PO (for *Toxoplasma*: 30 mg/kg q12h PO)
Trimethoprim + sulfamethoxazole (Bactrim, Septra, and generic forms) 480-, 960-mg tablet; 240-mg/5 mL oral liquid	Combines the antibacterial drug actions of trimethoprim and a sulfonamide; together, the combination is synergistic, with a broad spectrum of activity	Adverse effects primarily caused by sulfonamide component (see Sulfadiazine)	15 mg/kg q12h PO, or 30 mg/kg q12h–24h PO
Tylosin (Tylocine, Tylan, Tylosin tartrate) 2.2-g/teaspoon powder	Macrolide antibiotic (see Erythromycin for mechanisms of action and spectrum of activity); used for colitis and inflammatory bowel disease	May cause diarrhea in some animals; do not administer orally to rodents or rabbits	Dogs and cats: 7–15 mg/kg q12–24h PO Dogs (for colitis): 1 mg/kg q8h with food
Ursodiol (Ursodeoxycholate) (Actigall) 300-mg capsules	Hydrophilic bile acid; anti-cholelithic; used for treatment of liver diseases; increases bile flow; in dogs, may alter pool of circulating bile acids, dis-placing the more hydrophobic bile acids; in people, used to prevent or treat gallstones	Adverse effects not reported in animals; may cause diarrhea	10–15 mg/kg q24h PO
Valproic acid 125-, 250-, 500-mg tablets; 250-mg capsules; 50-mg/mL oral liquid	Anticonvulsant; used usually in combination with phenobarbital to treat refractory epilepsy in animals; action is not known, but may increase GABA concentrations in the CNS	Adverse effects have not been reported in animals, but hepatic failure has been reported in people; sedation may be seen in some animals; do not use in pregnant animals; *Drug interactions:* may cause bleeding if used with drugs that inhibit platelets	Dog: 60–200 mg/kg q8h PO; or 25–105 mg/kg/day PO, when administered with phenobarbital
Vancomycin (Vancocin, Vancoled) 0.5–10-g vials for injection	Antibacterial drug; mechanism of action is to inhibit cell wall and cause bacterial cell lysis (via different mechanism than β-lactams); spectrum includes staphylococci, streptococci, and enterococci (but not gram-negative bacteria); used primarily for treatment of resistant staphylococci and enterococci	Adverse effects have not been reported in animals; administer IV; causes severe pain and tissue injury if administered IM or SC; do not administer rapidly; use slow infusion, if possible (e.g., over 30 min)	Dog: 15 mg/kg q6–8h IV infusion Cat: 12–15 mg/kg, q8h, IV infusion

Drug (Other Names)	Pharmacology and Indications	Adverse Effects and Precautions	Dosage
Vasopressin (ADH) (Pitressin) 20 U/mL	Used to diagnose diabetes insipidus in water deprivation test; also used as a vasopressor agent during CPR and in patients with severe hypotension	Doses are adjusted on the basis of water intake and urine output monitoring (see also Desmopressin)	10 U IV, IM for water deprivation test; 0.8 U/kg IV for cardiac arrest; 0.001–0.004 U/kg/min constant rate infusion
Verapamil (Calan, Isoptin) 2.5-mg/mL injection	Calcium channel-blocking drug; produces vasodilation, negative chronotropic effects; used to treat supraventricular tachyarrhythmias	Hypotension, cardiac depression, bradycardia, AV block; may cause anorexia in some patients	Dog: 0.05 mg/kg q 10–30 min IV (maximum cumulative dose is 0.15 mg/kg); oral dose is not established
Vinblastine (Calan, Isoptin) 1-mg/mL injection	Similar to vincristine; some-times used as an alternative to vincristine; do not use to increase platelet numbers (may actually cause thrombocytopenia)	Does not produce neuropathy, as vincristine does, but there may be a higher incidence of myelo-suppression; causes tissue necrosis if injected outside vein	1 mg/m^2 IV (slow infusion) once/week
Vincristine (Oncovin, Vincasar, generic)	Anticancer agent; used in combination chemotherapy protocols; vincristine also increases numbers of functional circulating platelets and is used for thrombocytopenia	Generally well tolerated; less myelosuppressive than other anticancer drugs; neuropathy has been reported, but is rare; constipation can occur; very irritating to tissues; avoid extra-vasation outside of vein during administration	Antitumor: 0.5–0.7 mg/m^2 IV (or 0.025–0.05 mg/kg) once/week; for thrombocytopenia: 0.02 mg/kg IV once/week
Viokase	See Pancrelipase		
Vitamin C (Ascorbic acid) (see Ascorbic acid)	Used to treat vitamin C deficiency and occasionally used as urine acidifier	Adverse effects have not been reported in animals; high doses may increase risk of oxalate stones in bladder	100–500 mg/day
Vitamin E (Alpha Tocopherol) (Aquasol E, and generic)	Vitamin considered an anti-oxidant; used as supplement and in treatment of some immune-mediated dermatoses	Side effects have not been reported	100–400 U q12h PO (or 400–600 U q12h PO for immune-mediated skin disease)
Vitamin K$_1$ (Phytonadione, Phytomenadione) (Aqua MEPHYTON [injection], Mephyton [tablets]; Veta-K1 [capsules]) 2- or 10-mg/mL injection; 5- or 25-mg tablet	Vitamin K$_1$ used to treat coagulopathies caused by anticoagulant toxicosis (warfarin or other rodenticides)	Anaphylactoid reactions possible with IV administration	Short-acting rodenticides: 1 mg/kg/day, IM, SC, PO for 10–14 days Long-acting rodenticides: 2.5–5 mg/kg/day, IM, SC, PO for 3–4 weeks; test PT in 24 hours; if high, continue treatment for a total of 6 weeks (IM injections may cause hematoma formation in coagulopathic animals)
Warfarin (Coumadin, generic) 1–10-mg tablets	Anticoagulant; depletes vitamin K$_1$, which is responsible for generation of clotting factors; used to treat hypercoagulable disease, prevent thromboembolism	Adverse effects are attributable to decreased clotting; monitor PT and maintain at 1.5–2× baseline; *Drug interactions:* Other drugs may potentiate warfarin's action including aspirin, chloramphenicol, phenylbutazone, ketoconazole, cimetidine)	Dogs: 0.1–0.2 mg/kg q24h PO Cats (thromboembolism): start with 0.5 mg/cat/day and adjust dose based on clotting time assessment

Drug (Other Names)	Pharmacology and Indications	Adverse Effects and Precautions	Dosage
Xylaxine (Rompun, and generic) 20- or 100-mg/mL injection	α_2-Adrenergic agonist; used primarily for anesthesia and analgesia; often used in combination with other drugs (e.g., ketamine)	Produces sedation and ataxia; cardiac depression, heart block, and hypotension are possible with high doses; produces emesis after IV injection, especially in cats	Dog: 1.1 mg/kg IV, 2.2 mg/kg IM Cat: 1.1 mg/kg IM (emetic dose is 0.4–0.5 mg/kg IV)
Yohimbine (Yobine) 1-mg/mL injection	α_2-Adrenergic antagonist; used primarily to reverse actions of xylazine or detomidine	High doses can cause tremors and seizures	0.11 mg/kg IV, or 0.25–0.5 mg/kg SC, IM
Zidovudine (AZT) (Retrovir) 10-mg/mL oral liquid; 10-mg/mL injection	Antiviral drug; in people, used to treat AIDS; in animals, has been used experimentally for treatment of FeLV and FIV viral infection in cats; AZT acts to inhibit the viral enzyme reverse transcriptase, which prevents conversion of viral RNA into DNA	Anemia and leukopenia are adverse effects; monitor the PCV in treated cats and perform a CBC periodically	Cats: 15 mg/kg q12h, PO, to 20 mg/kg q8h PO (doses as high as 30 mg/kg/day also have been used)

Modified from Papich MG. Drug Formulary. In: Tilley LP, Smith FWK Jr. The 5–Minute Veterinary Consult: Canine and Feline. 2nd ed. Baltimore: Lippincott Williams & Wilkins, 2000.

Abbreviations: IM, intramuscular; IV, intravenous; OTC, over the counter (without prescription); Rx (prescription only); PO, per os (oral); SC, subcutaneous; U, units; mL, milliliters; μg, micrograms.

Disclaimer for Dose Tables: Doses listed are for dogs and cats, unless otherwise noted. Many of the doses listed are extra-label or are human drugs not approved for animals administered in an extra-label manner. Doses listed are based on best available information at the time of table editing. The authors cannot ensure efficacy or absolute safety of drugs used according to recommendations in this table. Adverse effects may be possible from drugs listed in this table of which authors were not aware at the time of table preparation. Veterinarians using this table are encouraged to consult current literature, product labels and inserts, and the manufacturer's disclosure information for additional information on adverse effects, interactions, and efficacy not identified at the time these tables were prepared.

GUIDELINES FOR ANESTHESIA IN ANIMALS WITH CRITICAL PROBLEMS

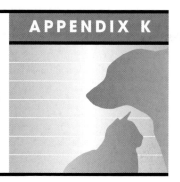

Problem	Major Concerns	Conditions to Avoid	Procedures to Assure	Anesthetic Guidelines
Respiratory	All anesthetic agents are potent respiratory depressants			
Upper airway obstruction	Complete obstruction—hypoxemia, hypercapnia	Slow induction	Calm smooth induction; Preoxygenation; Rapid access to airway	*Avoid:* Inhalational induction Opioid induction *Consider:* Propofol, thiobarbiturate, or ketamine-valium induction
Bronchospasm	Worse obstruction—hypoxemia, hypercapnia	Slow induction	Calm smooth induction; Preoxygenation; Rapid access to airway	*Avoid:* Inhalation induction Barbiturates *Consider:* ketamine-valium induction, anticholinergic premed
Pneumothorax	Worsening pneumo-thorax—hypoxemia, hypercapnia	Exaggerated breathing efforts; positive pressure ventilation	Calm smooth induction; Preoxygenation; Rapid thoracentesis	*Avoid:* Inhalation induction; High pressure ventilation *Consider:* Ket/val or propo-fol induction with immedi-ate thoracocentesies +/− chest drain
Diaphragmatic hernia	Destabilized ventilation/perfusion relationships—hypoxemia	Slow induction; watch for cyanosis with change in positioning	Calm smooth induction; Preoxygenation; Rapid access to airway; Positive pressure ventilation; Monitor oxygenation	*Avoid:* Inhalational induction *Consider:* Ket/val, thio-barbituate propofol induction
Pneumonia; Pulmonary edema	Additional small airway/alveolar collapse—hypoxemia which may not resolve after recovery	Apnea	Calm smooth induction; Preoxygenation; Rapid access to airway; Positive pressure ventilation	*Avoid:* Inhalational induction; Protracted recovery *Consider:* Opioid/diazepam or ket/val induction in debilitated patients; propofol for bronchoalveo-lar lavage
Cardiovascular	All anesthetic agents are potent cardiovascular depressants	Excitement, struggling; overdose; fluid overload	Pre-oxygenate; titrate drugs to effect	*Avoid:* (Propofol), (Barbiturates) *Consider:* Preanesthetics and inhalation induction

Problem	Major Concerns	Conditions to Avoid	Procedures to Assure	Anesthetic Guidelines
Hypotension-prone*	Myocardial depression/vasodilation—excessive hypotension	Excessive myocardial depression; excessive vasodilation	Optimize circulating volume; monitor arterial blood pressure (ABP)	*Avoid:* (Inhalational induction)#; (propofol); (barbiturates); phenothiazines; alpha$_2$-agonists *Consider:* Ket/val or narcotic/valium induction
Dilative cardiomyopathy	Additional myocardial depression	Excessive myocardial depression; excessive fluid infusion; hypertension	Monitor and support central venous pressure (CVP) and forward blood flow parameters	*Avoid:* (Inhalational induction); Propofol; (barbiturates) acepromazine, alpha$_2$-agonists *Consider:* Ket/val or narcotic/benzodiazepine combination
Hypertrophic cardiomyopathy	Inability to relax in diastole	Fluid overload; bradycardia; tachycardia	Keep preload high	*Avoid:* (Opioids); anticholinergics; ketamine; β$_1$-agonists *Consider:* etomidate, propofol
Ventricular arrhythmias	Worsening arrhythmia—poor cardiac output; ventricular fibrillation	All common anesthetic problems, acid-base and electrolyte imbalances	Monitor ECG; lidocaine as necessary	*Avoid:* Barbiturates; halothane; alpha$_2$-agonists; anticholinergics *Consider:* Narcotic/Acepromazine combination
Atrial fibrillation	Excessive heart rate interferes with diastolic filling and cardiac output	Excessive tachycardia	Monitor ECG, ABP	*Avoid:* Anticholinergics; ketamine *Consider:* Etomidate Narcotic/Benzodiazepine
Atrioventricular valve insufficiency	Decreased stroke volume effectiveness	High end-diastolic volumes (aggressive fluid infusion; bradycardia)—worsens regurgitant volume	Monitor forward blood flow parameters; CVP; Preoxygenate	*Avoid:* Propofol, alpha$_2$-agonists *Consider:* Narcotic/benzodiazepine combination, telazole, etomodate
Aortic stenosis	Poor ability to increase cardiac output	High preload; bradycardia; hypotension	Monitor ABP	*Avoid:* Acepromazine; (propofol) *Consider:* Etomodate, Telazole, ket/val
Patent ductus arteriosus	Hypotension prior to ligation; hypertension after ligation	Aggressive fluid infusion	Monitor ABP, ECG, CVP	*Consider:* Ket/val or narcotic/benzodiazepine induction, inhalation
Abdomen				
Gastric torsion	Impaired: 1) ventilation, 2) venous return to heart, 3) perfusion of stomach 4) perfusion of other abdominal organs; ventricular arrhythmias; metabolic acidosis	All common anesthetic problems	Treat shock; decompress stomach; monitor ventilation and oxygenation ABP, CVP, ECG; electrolyte status. Low dose of acepromazine (0.01 mg/kg IV) may prevent catecholemine induced arrhythmias after volume loading	*Avoid:* Propofol, barbiturates, alpha$_2$-agonists *Consider:* Narcotic/benzodiazepine + inhalation

Problem	Major Concerns	Conditions to Avoid	Procedures to Assure	Anesthetic Guidelines
Cesarean section	Exhausted patients are more prone to anesthetic effects; ventilation impairment; fetal depression	All common anesthetic problems; anesthetic over-dosage (base dose on non-pregnant lean body weight)	Monitor ABP; newborn "thriftiness" (naloxone to reverse opioids; doxapram to reverse other anesthetics) Consider caudal epidural	*Avoid:* Methoxyflurane; enflurane; alpha$_2$-agonists; (opioids increase ADH release); (phenothiazines block dopamine receptors); high dose ketamine or telazole
Anuric renal failure	Fluid, urea nitrogen (etc), potassium and hydrogen ion retention	Fluid under- or overload	CVP and skin turgor; ABP; ECG; electrolytes—potassium and acid–base	As for the hypotension-prone
Peritonitis; pancreatitis	Hypovolemia; hypo-proteinemia; toxemia	Fluid under-loading	CVP, ABP, ECG	As for the hypotension-prone
Severe liver disease	Inability of liver to produce important blood constituents: albumin, coagulation factors, glucose; Inability of liver to metabolize anesthetic drugs.	Hypotension; vasoconstriction	CVP; ABP	As for the hypotension-prone *Avoid:* methoxyflurane; enflurane; (halothane); alpha$_2$-agonists; (phenothiazines); long-acting barbiturates (or repeated doses) Consider low dose midazolam and narcotic, isoflurane
GI obstruction	Hypovolemia; hypo-proteinemia; toxemia; vomiting and aspiration	Hypovolemia	CVP, ABP, ECG	As for the hypotension-prone
CNS				
Seizure prone patients or procedures	Precipitating or worsening of the seizures			*Avoid:* Ketamine; phenothiazines, telazole *Consider:* Barbiturates, propofol
Intracranial disease	Increased intracranial pressure; decreased cerebral perfusion; worsening the cerebral dysfunction; herniation	Hypotension; hyper-tension; hypoxemia; hypercapnia; hyper-thermia; venous outflow impairment; induction/recovery excitement; seizures	ABP, CVP; normoventilation	*Avoid:* Ketamine; (inhalationals); alpha$_2$-agonists; phenothiazines *Consider:* Barbiturates, propofol
Ophthalmic				
Glaucoma	Increases in intraocular pressure may worsen the retinal damage	Induction and recovery excitement; increased muscle tone		*Avoid:* Ketamine; anticholinergics; sympathomimetics, Telazol *Consider:* Narcotic/ace combination
Near-perforated corneal ulcer	Increases in intraocular pressure may rupture the globe	Induction and recovery excitement/ trauma; increased muscle tone		*Avoid:* Ketamine, Telazol *Consider:* Narcotic/ acepromazine combination

*Hypotension-prone patients include any severe illness, trauma, shock, old age
#Agents to avoid in parentheses are precautions, not contraindications

INDEX

In this index, page numbers in *italics* designate figures; page numbers followed by the letter "t" designate tables; page numbers followed by the letter "b" designate boxes; (*see also*) cross-references refer to related topics or more detailed subtopic listings.

ABCs of life support, 3, 4t, 5b, 7b, 16–19
Abdominal auscultation, 189
Abdominal conditions, anesthesia guidelines, 486–487t
Abdominal counterpressure, 17–18
Abdominal drainage, in penetrating wounds, 218
Abdominal effusion, 192
Abdominal evaluation, 10, 189
Abdominal radiography, 189–190, *190, 197*
   in hepatitis, 211
   in hyperadrenocorticism, 311–312
   in reproductive disorders, 334
Abdominal trauma, 10
Abdominal ultrasound
   in hepatitis, 211
   in hyperadrenocorticism, 311–312
   in reproductive disorders, 334–335
Abdominocentesis, 10, 190–191
   in acute pancreatitis, 203
   in peritonitis, 220
   in protein-losing enteropathy, 217
Abnormal ongoing fluid losses, 67–68, 69t
Abortion, spontaneous, 339
ABP (arterial blood pressure), 73–74
Abscess
   bite wound, 375–376
   prostatic, 247, 335
Absent pulses, 7
Acaricidal dips, in sarcoptic mange, 379
AC/DC current, 414–415
ACE inhibitors, in renal disease, 245
Acepromazine, 43, 44t, 54t, 438t
   in epistaxis, 294
   in feline thromboembolism, 180
   in tracheal collapse, 126
Acepromazine/atropine, 48
Acepromazine/oxymorphone, 48
Acetaminophen, 52, 52t, 438t
   toxicity, 52, 211, 288, 432t
Acetaminophen/codeine, 438t
Acetazolamide, 438t
   in glaucoma, 359
   in urinary incontinence, 278
Acetylcholine, in organophosphate poisoning, 393
Acetylcysteine, 438t
   in acetaminophin poisoning, 387
Acid(s)
   ascorbic (vitamin C), 387, 440t, 483t
   bile, 192
   boric, toxicity, 398
   folic, 428t

   folinic (leucovarin), 460t
   lactic, 75–76
   meclofenamic, 462t
   uric, biochemical units, 428t
   valproic, 482t
Acidosis
   addition, 66
   intracellular/CSF, sodium bicarbonate and, 21t
   lactic, 76
      in hypothermia, 405
   metabolic, 66, 320 (*see also* Metabolic acidosis)
   mineral, 317
A CRASH PLAN mnemonic, 7, 7b
ACTH stimulation test, 297, 310, 312
Activated charcoal, 386, 438t, 445t
Acute bacterial prostatitis, 339–340
Acute blindness, 362–363, *363*
Acute fulminant myasthenia gravis, 254
Acute metritis, 338
Acute moist (pyotraumatic) dermatitis, 376
Acute on chronic renal failure, 243–244
Acute renal failure, 83, 226, 235–237
   causes, 235, 236t
   treatment, 236–237
   vs. chronic, 235–236
Acute respiratory distress syndrome (ARDS), 36
   in near drowning, 408
Acute stomatitis/oral ulcers, 207–208
Acute vestibular disease, 272
Addison's disease (primary hypoadrenocorticism), 309–311
   pseudo-, 310
Addition (organic) acidoses, 66
Admixture, venous, 81
Advanced cardiac life support, 19–23, 20t, 21t, 26b (*see also* Cardiac life support; Cardiopulmonary resuscitation)
Agglutination test, microscopic, 243
Agonist-antagonist opioids, 51, 51t
Agonist opioids, 49–51, 50t, 51t
Agonists, for cardiopulmonary resuscitation (CPR), 20t
Airway
   emergency establishment of, 16
   treatment priorities, 5b
Airway disease, lower, 144–155 (*see also under* Respiratory emergencies)
Airway obstruction, upper airway, 118–127 (*see also under* Respiratory emergencies)
Alanine aminotransferase, 428t
Albendazole, 438t
Albumin, 59t, 60, 85, 428t
   molecular size, 59t
Albumin/globulin concentration assay, 192
Albuterol, 439t
   in COPD, 150
   in feline bronchial asthma syndrome, 144, 147, 148
   in smoke inhalation, 149
Alkali exposure, 361